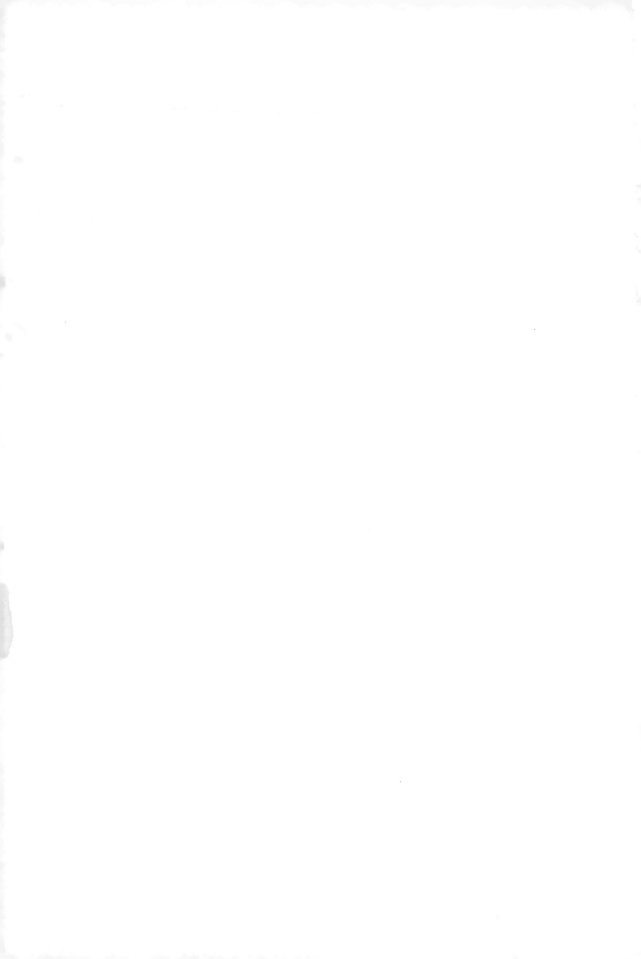

# A History of Medicine

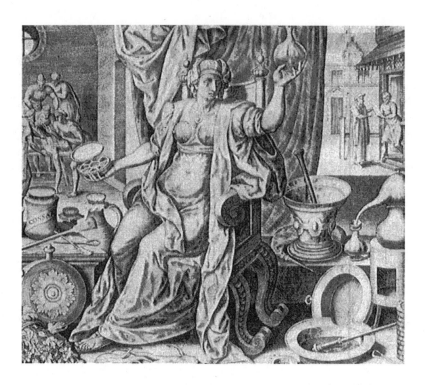

Panacea

# A
# $\mathscr{H}$istory
# of
# $\mathscr{M}$edicine

## SECOND EDITION

**Lois N. Magner**

**informa**

healthcare

New York   London

First published in 2005 by Taylor & Francis Group.

This edition published in 2011 by Informa Healthcare, Telephone House, 69-77 Paul Street, London EC2A 4LQ, UK.

Simultaneously published in the USA by Informa Healthcare, 52 Vanderbilt Avenue, 7th Floor, New York, NY 10017, USA.

Informa Healthcare is a trading division of Informa UK Ltd. Registered Office: 37–41 Mortimer Street, London W1T 3JH, UK. Registered in England and Wales number 1072954.

A CIP record for this book is available from the British Library.

Library of Congress Cataloging-in-Publication Data available on application

ISBN-13: 9780824740740

Orders may be sent to: Informa Healthcare, Sheepen Place, Colchester, Essex CO3 3LP, UK
Telephone: +44 (0)20 7017 5540
Email: CSDhealthcarebooks@informa.com
Website: http://informahealthcarebooks.com/

For corporate sales please contact: CorporateBooksIHC@informa.com
For foreign rights please contact: RightsIHC@informa.com
For reprint permissions please contact: PermissionsIHC@informa.com

Printed in the United States of America

To Ki-Han and Oliver, as always

# Preface

"Health is a state of complete physical, mental and social well-being, and not merely the absence of disease or infirmity." (The World Health Organization)

My primary purpose in writing and revising this book has been to provide an updated introduction to the history of medicine. Although the text began as a "teaching assistant" for my own one-semester survey course, I hope that this new edition will also be of interest to a general audience, and to teachers who are trying to add historical materials to their science courses or science to their history courses. As in the previous edition of this book, I have tried to call attention to major themes in the history of medicine, the evolution of theories and methodologies, and the diverse attitudes and assumptions with which physicians and patients have understood health, disease, and healing.

Many changes have taken place in the history of medicine since the 1940s, when Henry E. Sigerist (1891–1957) called for a new direction in the field, a move away from the study of the great physicians and their texts towards a new concept of medical history as social and cultural history. From an almost exclusive focus on the evolution of modern medical theories, scholars turned to new questions about the social, cultural, economical, and political context in which healers and patients are embedded. Profoundly influenced by concepts and techniques borrowed from sociology, psychology, anthropology, and demography, the new social and cultural historians of medicine emphasized factors such as race, class, and gender, as well as institutional and professional affiliations. Some arguments about the nature of the field remain, but there is general agreement that medical history is not simply an account of the path from past darkness to modern scientific enlightenment.

Given the vitality and diversity of the field today, finding a satisfactory way to present an introductory survey of the history of medicine has become increasingly difficult. Thus, a selective approach, based on a consideration of the needs and interests of readers who are first approaching the field, seems appropriate. I have, therefore, selected particular examples of theories, diseases, professions, healers, and scientists, and attempted to allow them to illuminate themes that raise fundamental questions about health, disease, and history. The book is arranged in a roughly chronological, but largely thematic manner.

Medical concepts and practices can provide a sensitive probe of the intimate network of interactions in a society, as well as traces of the introduction, diffusion, and transformation of novel or foreign ideas and techniques. Medical problems concern the most fundamental and revealing aspects of any society—health and disease, wealth and poverty, birth, aging, disability, suffering, and death. All people, in every period of history, have dealt with childbirth, disease, traumatic injuries, and pain. Thus, the measures developed to heal mind and body provide a valuable focus for examining different cultures and contexts. Perhaps immersion in the history of medicine can provide a feeling of kinship with patients and practitioners past and present, a sense of humility with respect to disease and nature, and a critical approach to our present medical problems.

The history of medicine can throw light on changing patterns of health and disease, as well as questions of medical practice, professionalization, institutions, educations, medical costs, diagnostics, and therapeutics. Since the end of the nineteenth century, the biomedical sciences have flourished by following what might be called the "gospel of specific etiology"—that is, the concept that if we understand the causative agent of a disease, or the specific molecular events of the pathological process, we can totally understand and control the disease. This view fails to take into account the complex social, ethical, economical, and geopolitical aspects of disease in a world drawn closer together by modern communications and transportation, while simultaneously being torn apart by vast and growing differences between wealth and poverty.

Public debates about medicine today rarely seem to address fundamental issues of the art and science of medicine; instead, the questions most insistently examined concern health care costs, availability, access, equity, and liability. Comparisons among the medical systems of many different nations suggest that despite differences in form, philosophy, organization, and goals, all have experienced tensions caused by rising costs and expectations and pressure on limited or scarce resources. Government officials, policy analysts, and health care professionals have increasingly focused their energy and attention on the management of cost containment measures. Rarely is an attempt made to question the entire enterprise in terms of the issues raised by demographers, epidemiologists, and historians as to the relative value of modern medicine and more broadly based environmental and behavioral reforms that might significantly affect patterns of morbidity and mortality.

Skeptics have said that we seem to exchange the pestilences of one generation for the plagues of another. At least in the wealthier, industrialized parts of the world, the prevailing disease pattern has shifted from one in which the major killers were infectious diseases to one in which chronic and degenerative diseases predominate, associated with a demographic shift from an era of high infant mortality to one with increased life expectancy at birth and an aging population. Since the end of the nineteenth century, we have seen a remarkable transition from a period where prevention was expensive (e.g., installation of sewer systems) and therapy was basically inexpensive (e.g., bleeding and purging) to one where therapy is expensive (e.g., coronary by-pass operations) and prevention is inexpensive (e.g., exercise and low-cholesterol diets). The demand for high cost diagnostic and therapeutic technologies seems insatiable, but it may well be that improvements in health and the overall quality of life are better served by a new commitment to social services and community health rather than more sophisticated scanners and specialized surgeons. After years of celebrating the obvious achievements of biomedical science, as exemplified by such contributions as vaccines, anesthesia, insulin, organ transplantation, and the hope that infectious epidemic diseases would follow smallpox into oblivion, deep and disturbing questions are being raised about the discrepancy between the costs of modern medicine and the role that medicine has played in terms of historical and global patterns of morbidity and mortality. Careful analysis of the role of medicine and that of social and environmental factors in determining the health of the people indicates that medical technology is not a panacea for either epidemic and acute disease, or endemic and chronic disease.

A general survey of the history of medicine reinforces the fundamental principle that medicine alone has never been the answer to the ills of the individual or the ills of society, but human beings have never stopped looking to the healing arts to provide a focus for cures, consolation, amelioration, relief, and rehabilitation. Perhaps a better understanding of previous concepts of health, healing, and disease will make it possible to recognize the sources of contemporary problems and the inherent limitations and liabilities of current paradigms.

Once again I would like to express my deep appreciation to John Parascandola and Ann Carmichael for their invaluable advice, criticism, and encouragement during the preparation of the first edition of this book. Of course, all remaining errors of omission and commission remain my own. Many thanks also to the students who took my courses, read my books, and let me know what was clear and what was obscure. I would also like to thank the History of Medicine Division, National Library of Medicine, for providing the illustrations used in this book and the World Health Organization for the photograph of the last case of smallpox in the Indian subcontinent. I would like to thank Marcel Dekker, Inc. for inviting me to prepare a second edition of *A History of Medicine*.

*Lois N. Magner*

# Contents

# 1

# Paleopathology and Paleomedicine

## INTRODUCTION

One of our most appealing and persistent myths is that of the Golden Age, a time before the discovery of good and evil, when death and disease were unknown. But, scientific evidence—meager, fragmentary, and tantalizing though it often is—proves that disease is older than the human race and was not uncommon among other species. Indeed, studies of ancient fossil remains, skeletons in museum collections, animals in zoos, and animals in the wild demonstrate that arthritis is widespread among a variety of medium and large-sized mammals, including aardvarks, anteaters, bears, and gazelles. Evidence of infection has been found in the bones of prehistoric animals, and in the soft tissues of mummies. Modern diagnostic imaging techniques have revealed evidence of tumors in fossilized remains. For example, researchers performing CT-scans of the brain case of a 72-million-year-old gorgosaurus discovered a brain tumor that probably impaired its balance and mobility. Other abnormalities in the specimen suggested that it had suffered fractures of a thigh, lower leg, and shoulder.

Thus, understanding the pattern of disease and injury that afflicted our earliest ancestors requires the perspective of the paleopathologist. Sir Marc Armand Ruffer (1859–1917), one of the founders of paleopathology, defined it as the science of the diseases that can be demonstrated in human and animal remains of ancient times. Paleopathology provides information about health, disease, death, environment, and culture in ancient populations.

In order to explore the problem of disease among the earliest humans, we will need to survey some aspects of human evolution, both biological and cultural. In *Descent of Man and Selection in Relation to Sex* (1871) Charles Darwin argued that human beings, like every other species, evolved from previous forms of life by means of natural selection. According to Darwin, all the available evidence indicated that "man is descended from a hairy, tailed, quadruped, probably arboreal

1

in its habits." Despite the paucity of the evidence available to him, Darwin suggested that the ancient ancestor of modern human beings was related to that of the gorilla and the chimpanzee. Moreover, he predicted that the first humans probably evolved in Africa. Evidence from the study of fossils, stratigraphy, and molecular biology suggests that the separation of the human line from that of the apes took place in Africa about five million to eight million years ago.

The fossilized remains of human ancestors provide valuable clues to the past, but such fossils are very rare and usually incomplete. South African anatomist Raymond Dart made the first substantive discovery of human ancestors in Africa in the 1920s when he identified the famous fossils known as *Australopithecus africanus* (South African Ape-man). The most exciting subsequent twentieth-century discoveries of ancient human ancestors are associated with the work of Louis and Mary Leakey and that of Donald Johanson. Working primarily at sites in Olduvai Gorge and Laetoli in Tanzania, Mary and Louis Leakey identified many hominid fossils, including *Australopithecus boisei* and *Homo habilis*. Johanson's most important discovery was the unusually complete skeleton of a primitive australopithecine (*Australopithecus afarensis*), commonly referred to as Lucy. New hominid remains discovered at the beginning of the twenty-first century stimulated further controversy about the earliest hominid ancestors, as well as those of the chimpanzee.

Paleoanthropology is a field in which new discoveries inevitably result in the re-examination of previous findings and great debates rage over the identification and classification of tiny bits of bones and teeth. Further discoveries will no doubt add new insights into the history of human evolution and create new disputes among paleoanthropologists. Scientists also acknowledge that pseudopaleopathologic conditions can lead to misunderstanding and misinterpretation because they closely resemble disease lesions, but are primarily the result of postmortem processes. For example, because the primary chemical salts in bones are quite soluble in water, soil conditions that are conducive to leaching out calcium can cause changes in bones like those associated with osteoporosis. Despite all the ambiguities associated with ancient remains, many traumatic events and diseases can be revealed by the methods of paleopathology.

Insights from many different disciplines, including archeology, historical geography, morphology, comparative anatomy, taxonomy, genetics, and molecular biology have enriched our understanding of human evolution. Changes in DNA, the archive of human genealogy, have been used to construct tentative family trees, lineages, and possible patterns of early migrations. Some genes may reveal critical distinctions between humans and other primates, such as the capacity for spoken language.

Anatomically modern humans first emerged some 130,000 years ago, but fully modern humans, capable of sophisticated activities, such as the production of complex tools, works of art, and long distance trade, seem to appear in the archaeological record about 50,000 years ago. However, the relationship between modern humans and extinct hominid lines remains controversial.

The Paleolithic Era, or Old Stone Age, when the most important steps in cultural evolution occurred, coincides with the geological epoch known as the Pleistocene or Great Ice Age, which ended about 10,000 years ago with the last retreat of the glaciers. Early humans were hunter-gatherers, that is, opportunistic omnivores who learned to make tools, build shelters, carry and share food, and create uniquely human social structures. Although Paleolithic technology is characterized by the manufacture of crude tools made of bone and chipped stones and the absence of pottery and metal objects, the people of this era produced the dramatic cave paintings at Lascaux, France, and Altamira, Spain. Presumably, they also produced useful inventions that were fully bio-degradable and, therefore, left no traces in the fossil record. Indeed, during the 1960s feminist scientists challenged prevailing assumptions about the importance of hunting as a source of food among hunter-gatherers. The wild grains, fruits, nuts, vegetables, and small animals gathered by women probably constituted the more reliable components of the Paleolithic diet. Moreover, because women were often encumbered by helpless infants, they probably invented disposable digging sticks and bags in which to carry and store food.

The transition to a new pattern of food production through farming and animal husbandry is known as the Neolithic Revolution. Neolithic or New Stone Age peoples developed crafts, such as basket-making, pottery, spinning, and weaving. Although no art work of this period seems as spectacular as the Paleolithic cave paintings in France and Spain, Neolithic people produced interesting sculptures, figurines, and pottery.

While archeologists and anthropologists were once obsessed with the *when* and *where* of the emergence of an agricultural way of life, they are now more concerned with the *how* and *why*. Nineteenth-century anthropologists tended to classify human cultures into a series of ascending, progressive stages marked by the types of tools manufactured and the means of food production. Since the 1960s new analytical techniques have made it possible to test hypotheses about environmental and climatic change and their probable effect on the availability of food sources. When the idea of progress is subjected to critical analysis rather than accepted as inevitable, the causes of the Neolithic transformation are not as clear as previously assumed. Given the fact that hunter-gatherers may enjoy a better diet and more leisure than agriculturalists, prehistoric or modern, the advantages of a settled way of life are obvious only to those who are already happily settled and well fed. The food supply available to hunter-gatherers, while more varied than the monotonous staples of the agriculturalist, might well be precarious and uncertain.

Recent studies of the origins of agriculture suggest that it was almost universally adopted between ten thousand and two thousand years ago, primarily in response to pressures generated by the growth of the human population. When comparing the health of foragers and settled farmers, paleopathologists generally find that dependence on a specific crop resulted in populations that were less well nourished than hunter-gatherers, as indicated by height, robustness, dental conditions, and so forth. In agricultural societies, the food base became narrower with dependence on a few or even a single crop. Thus, the food supply might have been adequate and consistent in terms of calories, but deficient in vitamins and minerals. Domestication of animals, however, seemed to improve the nutritional status of ancient populations. Although the total human population apparently grew very slowly prior to the adoption of farming, it increased quite rapidly thereafter. Prolonged breast feeding along with postpartum sexual prohibitions found among many nomadic societies may have maintained long intervals between births. Village life led to early weaning and shorter birth intervals.

The revolutionary changes in physical and social environment associated with the transition from the way of life experienced by small mobile bands of hunter-gatherers to that of sedentary, relatively dense populations also allowed major shifts in patterns of disease. Permanent dwellings, gardens, and fields provide convenient niches for parasites, insects, and rodents. Stored foods are likely to spoil, attract pests, and become contaminated with rodent excrement, insects, bacteria, molds, and toxins. Agricultural practices increase the number of calories that can be produced per unit of land, but a diet that overemphasizes grains and cereals may be deficient in proteins, vitamins, and minerals.

Lacking the mobility and diversity of resources enjoyed by hunters and gatherers, sedentary populations may be devastated by crop failures, starvation, and malnutrition. Migrations and invasions of neighboring or distant settlements triggered by local famines may carry parasites and pathogens to new territories and populations. Ironically, worrying about our allegedly unnatural and artificial modern diet has become so fashionable that people in the wealthiest nations have toyed with the quixotic idea of adopting the dietary patterns of ancient humans or even wild primates. In reality, the food supply available to prehistoric peoples was more likely to be inadequate, monotonous, coarse, and unclean.

## PALEOPATHOLOGY: METHODS AND PROBLEMS

Because direct evidence of disease among ancient human beings is very limited, we will have to seek out a variety of indirect approaches in order to reach at least a tentative understanding of the prehistoric world. For example, studies of our closest relatives, the great apes and monkeys, have shown that living in a state of nature does not mean freedom from disease. Wild primates suffer from many disorders, including arthritis, malaria, hernias, parasitic worms, and impacted teeth. Our ancestors, the first "naked apes," presumably experienced disorders and diseases similar to those found among modern primates during a lifespan that was truly "nasty, brutish, and short." Nevertheless, prehistoric peoples gradually learned to adapt to harsh environments, quite unlike the mythical Garden of Eden. Eventually, through cultural evolution, human beings changed their environment in unprecedented ways, even as they adapted to its demands. By the domestication of animals, the mastery of agricultural practices, and the creation of densely populated settlements, human beings also generated new patterns of disease.

Paleopathologists must use a combination of primary and secondary evidence in order to draw inferences about prehistoric patterns of disease. Primary evidence includes bodies, bones, teeth, ashes, and charred or dried remains of bodies found at sites of accidental or intentional human burials. Secondary sources include the art, artifacts, and burial goods of preliterate peoples, and ancient documents that describe or suggest the existence of pathological conditions. The materials for such studies are very fragmentary, and the over-representation of the hard parts of bodies—bones and teeth—undoubtedly distorts our portrait of the past.

Indeed the possibility of arriving at an unequivocal diagnosis through the study of ancient remains is so small that some scholars insist that the names of modern diseases should *never* be conferred on ancient materials. Other experts have systematically cataloged paleolithic ailments in terms of congenital abnormalities, injury, infection, degenerative conditions, cancers, deficiency diseases, and that all-too-large category, diseases of unknown etiology.

Nevertheless, by combining a variety of classical and newly emerging techniques, scientists can use these fragmentary materials to gain new insights into the patterns of ancient lives. The study of human remains from archaeological contexts may also be referred to as bio-archaeology, a field that encompasses physical anthropology and archaeology.

Funerary customs, burial procedures, and environmental conditions, such as heat, humidity, soil composition, can determine the state of preservation of human remains. Cremation, in particular, could create severe warping and fragmentation of the remains. Bodies might be buried in the ground shortly after death, covered with a mound of rocks (cairn burial), or placed on a scaffold and exposed to the elements. Both nomadic and settled people might place a body in some type of scaffold as a temporary measure if the death occurred when the ground was frozen. Later, the skeletal remains could be interred with appropriate ceremonies. In some cemeteries the dead might be added to old graves, causing the commingling of bones. Added confusion arises from ritual mutilation of the body, the admixture of grave goods and gifts, which may include body parts of animals or grieving relatives, and distortions due to natural or artificial mummification. Burrowing animals and looters might also disturb burial sites and change the distribution of bones. Catastrophes, such as floods, earthquakes, landslides, and massacres, may provide information about a large group of individuals during one moment in time.

Despite the increasing sophistication and power of the new analytical techniques employed in the service of paleopathology, many uncertainties remain, and all results must still be interpreted with caution. Since the last decades of the twentieth century, scientists have exploited new methods, such as DNA amplification and sequencing, the analysis of stable isotopes of carbon and nitrogen, and scanning electron microscopy in order to ask questions about the health, lifestyle, and culture of ancient peoples. Scanning electron microscopy has been used to examine patterns of tooth wear and enamel defects caused by stress and growth disruption, and the effect of workload on the structure of limb bones. Where possible, chemical investigations of trace elements extracted from ancient bones and hair can provide insights into ancient dietary patterns and quality of life. Lead, arsenic, mercury, cadmium, copper, and strontium are among the elements that can be identified in hair.

The analysis of stable isotopes of carbon and nitrogen provides insights into bone chemistry and diet, because the ratios of the stable isotopes of carbon and nitrogen found in human and animal remains reflect their ratios in the foods consumed. Thus, the relative importance of plant and animal foods in the diet of prehistoric populations can be estimated. Differences in ratios found in human bones for different time periods may reveal changes in diet. For example, scientists determined the relative amounts of carbon 13 and nitrogen 15 in the bones of human beings living in various parts of Europe more than twenty thousand years ago. These studies suggested a diet that was high in fish, shellfish, and waterfowl. Analyses of the isotopes in the bones of Neanderthals, in contrast, suggested that their dietary proteins came largely from the flesh of larger prey animals.

Today, and presumably in the past, most infections involved soft tissue rather than bones, but bones and teeth are the primary source of paleopathological information. Scientists can subject skeletal remains to X-rays, CT (computer tomographic) imaging, chemical analysis, and so forth. The bones may reveal evidence about an individual's history of health and disease, age and cause of death.

Specific injuries identifiable in ancient remains included fractures, dislocations, sprains, torn ligaments, degenerative joint disease, amputations, penetrating wounds, bone spurs, calcified blood clots, nasal septal deformities, and so forth. Projectile weapons, such as spears and arrows, have been found in fossilized vertebrae, sternum, scapula, humerus, and skulls. But projectile tips embedded in bone are rare, either because healers extracted them, or, most likely, the projectile point that caused a fatal injury lodged in soft tissues. In some cases long-term survival occurred after penetrating wounds, as indicated by projectile parts that were incorporated into the injured bone and retained as inert foreign objects.

In favorable cases, the type of injury and the length of time that elapsed between the traumatic event and death can be estimated. Bones usually heal at relatively predictable rates. Survival and healing suggest some form of treatment, support, and care during convalescence. Some skeletons exhibit fractures that resulted in deformities that must have caused difficulty in walking, chronic pain, and degenerative joint disease. The fact of survival suggests the availability of effective assistance during convalescence and after recovery. During healing, bone is usually replaced by bone. Sometimes, however, healing is faulty; complications include osteomyelitis, delayed or nonunion, angular deformities, bone spurs in adjacent soft tissues, calcified blood clots, growth retardation, aseptic necrosis, pseudoarthrosis (fibrous tissue is substituted for bone), and degenerative joint disease (traumatic arthritis).

Bone is a dynamic living tissue constantly being modified in response to the stimulus of growth, and to physiological and pathological stresses. Many factors, such as age, sex, nutrition, hormones, heredity, and illness, affect the bones. Heavy labor or vigorous exercise can result in increases in bone mass. Degenerative processes change the size, shape, and configuration of the skeleton and its individual bones. The skeleton can be modified by inflammation of the joints (arthritis) and by decreases in bone density (osteoporosis).

Bones respond to changes in their environment, especially the mechanical environment created by body weight and muscle forces. The morphology of a bone, therefore, records the mechanical forces exerted on it during life. Usually, paleopathologists are interested in bones that display obvious pathology, but normal bones can provide evidence of body size, behavior, degree of sexual dimorphism, activities, workloads, and posture. Bones may, therefore, testify that an individual habitually performed heavy lifting, pushing, pulling, carrying, standing, stooping, walking, running, or squatting. For example, a peculiarity of the ankle joint, known as a squatting facet, is found in people who spend much of their times in a squatting position. Thus, the absence of squatting facets distinguishes those who sat in chairs from those who did not.

Most diseases do not leave specific signs in the skeleton, but tuberculosis, yaws, syphilis, and some fungal infections may leave diagnostic clues. Twentieth century studies suggest that the skeleton is affected in about one to two percent of tuberculosis patients. The kinds of bone lesions caused by syphilis are generally different from those caused by tuberculosis. Congenital syphilis may produce the so-called Hutchinson's incisor defect. Leprosy often results in damage to the bones of the face, fingers, and toes. Because hormones regulate the growth and development of all parts of the body, a malfunction of the endocrine glands may leave signs in the bones. Some peculiarities in ancient skeletal remains have been attributed to abnormalities of the pituitary and thyroid glands. However, because of recent changes in patterns of disease, physicians, unlike paleopathologists, rarely see the results of historically significant severe, untreated infectious diseases. Various cancers may be identifiable in skeletal remains. Although primary bone cancers are probably rare, many other cancers may spread to the bone. Some relatively uncommon conditions, such as osteomyelitis and various benign tumors of the bone and cartilage, have been of particular interest to paleopathologists because they are easily recognized.

Various forms of malnutrition, such as rickets, scurvy, and anemia, may cause abnormalities in the structure of the bone (porotic hyperostosis). Rickets was rare during Neolithic times, but became increasingly common as towns and cities grew. Osteomalacia, an adult form of rickets, can cause collapse of the bones of the pelvis, making childbirth a death sentence for mother and fetus. The presence of calcified blood clots in many skeletons might reflect the prevalence of scurvy in a particular population. Given heavy or chronic exposure, some soil elements, such as arsenic, bismuth, lead, mercury, and selenium, can cause toxic effects that leave their mark on the bones. Porotic hyperostosis is a pathological condition characterized by porous, sieve-like lesions that are found in ancient human skulls. These lesions may be caused by malnutrition and infectious diseases—iron deficiency anemia or inflammatory processes, bleeding associated with scurvy, or certain diseases (rickets, tumors). Generally, it is difficult to determine the specific cause of such defects. Moreover, postmortem damage can simulate these conditions.

Although tooth decay and cavities are often thought of as the results of a modern diet, studies of contemporary primitives and research on ancient skeletons disprove this assumption. Dental problems and diseases found in human remains include dental attrition due to diet, temporomandibular joint derangement, plaque, caries, abscesses, tooth crown fractures, tooth loss, and so forth. Analysis of dental microwear patterns by scanning electron microscopy and microwear measurements began in the 1980s. Microscopic pits, scratches on tooth surfaces, and surface attrition reveal patterns of wear caused by abrasive particles in food. Abrasive wear could lead to infection and tooth loss. Dental disorders were often worse in women, because of the effects of pregnancy and lactation, and the use of teeth and jaws as tools.

In general, the condition of bones and teeth provides a history of health and disease, diet and nutritional deficiencies, a record of severe stresses or workload during life, and an approximate age at death. Bone fractures provide a record of trauma, which might be followed by infection or by healing. Before the final closure of the epiphyses, the growing bones are vulnerable to trauma, infections, and growth disorders. Stresses severe enough to disrupt growth during childhood result in transverse lines, usually called Harris lines or growth arrest lines, which are visible in radiographs of the long bones of the body. Because Harris lines suggest severe but temporary disturbance of growth, a population suffering from chronic malnutrition has fewer transverse lines than one exposed to periodic or seasonal starvation. Starvation, severe malnutrition, and severe infection may also leave characteristic signs in the teeth, microdefects in dental enamel known as pathological striae of Retzius, enamel hypoplasias, or Wilson bands. Severe episodes of infant diarrheas, for example, can disrupt the development of teeth and bones. Scanning electron micrography makes it possible to observe disruptions in the pattern of these lines, but there is still considerable uncertainty about the meaning of pathological striae of Retzius.

Archaeological chemistry, the analysis of inorganic and organic materials, has been used in the discovery, dating, interpretation, and authentication of ancient remains. This approach provides many ways of reconstructing ancient human cultures from bits of stone tools, ceramics, textiles, paints, and so forth. By combining microscopy with chemical analysis, scientists can recover information about the manufacture and use of ancient artifacts because such objects carry with them a "memory" of how they were manipulated in the past. Perhaps the most familiar aspect of archaeological chemistry is the carbon-14 method for dating ancient remains. Carbon-14 dating is especially valuable for studying materials from the last ten thousand years, the period during which the most profound changes in cultural evolution occurred.

Multidisciplinary groups of scientists have combined their expertise in archaeology, chemistry, geophysics, imaging technology, and remote sensing as a means of guiding nondestructive investigations of sensitive archeological sites. As the techniques of molecular biology are adapted to the questions posed by paleopathologists, new kinds of information can be teased out of the surviving traces of proteins and nucleic acids found in some ancient materials. Improvements in instrumentation allow archaeologists to analyze even smaller quantities of biological materials. For example, by using mass spectrometry and lipid bio-markers chemists can distinguish between human and other animal remains.

## MUMMIES AND SIGNS OF DISEASE

In rare instances, the soft parts of prehistoric bodies have been preserved because of favorable burial and climatic conditions or through human ingenuity. Whether sophisticated or primitive, mummification techniques have much in common with the preservation of foods and animal hides. Especially well-preserved bodies have been recovered from the peat bogs of northwestern Europe. Peat has been used as a fuel for millennia, giving clumsy peat-gatherers a chance to sacrifice themselves for the future enlightenment of paleopathologists. Some of the "bog bodies" were apparently victims of strange forms of punishment or religious rituals. Sacrificial victims were fed a ceremonial meal, stabbed in the heart, clobbered over the head, strangled with ropes that were deliberately left around their necks, and then pushed into the bog.

Mummified bodies have also been found in the southwestern United States, Mexico, Alaska, and the Aleutian Islands. In the Western hemisphere natural mummification was more common than artificial methods, but the prehistoric people called the Basket-Makers deliberately dried cadavers in cists or caves, disarticulated the hips, wrapped the bodies in furs, and stuffed them into large baskets. Peruvian mummification techniques allowed the "living corpses" of chiefs, clan ancestors, and Incan rulers to be worshipped as gods. Such mummies provide suggestive evidence for the existence of tuberculosis, hookworm, and other diseases in pre-Columbian America.

Where conditions favor the preservation of organic matter, coprolites (fossilized human feces) may be found in or near prehistoric campsites and dwellings. Indeed, for the dedicated paleopathologist, the contents of cesspools, latrine pits, and refuse piles are more precious than golden ornaments from a palace. Because certain parts of plants and animals are undigestible, information about diet, disease, seasonal activities, and cooking techniques can be inferred from the analysis of pollen grains, charcoal, seeds, hair, bits of bones or shells, feathers, insect parts, and the eggs or cysts of parasitic worms in coprolites. Moreover, the distribution of coprolites in and about ancient dwellings may reflect prevailing standards of sanitation.

Patterns of injury may provide clues to environment and occupation. For example, fractures of the leg bones were more common in Anglo-Saxon skeletons than fractures of the forearm. These leg injuries are typically caused by tripping in rough terrain, especially if wearing clumsy footwear. In ancient Egypt, broken arms were more common than fractures of the leg bones.

The bones may also bear witness to acts of violence, mutilation, or cannibalism. Evidence concerning cannibalism remains highly controversial, but the ritualistic consumption of the ashes, brains, or other parts of departed relatives was practiced until recently by members of certain tribes as a sign of respect for the dead. A disease known as *kuru*, a degenerative brain disease found among the Fore people of Papua New Guinea, has been linked to ritual cannibalism. In 1976 Daniel Carleton Gajdusek (1923–), American virologist and pediatrician, won the Nobel Prize in Physiology or Medicine for his work on kuru. While conducting epidemiological field work in New Guinea, Gajdusek was introduced to a strange neurological disorder found among Fore women and children. Gajdusek concluded that the disease was transmitted by ritual cannibalism, in which women and children ate the brains of those who had died of kuru. After the ritual was abandoned, the disease eventually disappeared. Having demonstrated that the disease could be transmitted to chimpanzees, Gajdusek suggested that kuru was caused by a "slow virus." Scientists later determined that kuru was caused by prions, the "proteinaceous infectious particles" associated with Creutzfeldt–Jakob disease, mad-cow disease, and other spongiform encephalopathies.

Evidence of infectious diseases and parasitic infestations has been found in the tissues of mummies. Eggs of various parasitic worms have been found in mummies, coprolites, and latrine pits. These parasites cause a variety of disorders, including schistosomiasis (snail fever) and the gross enlargement of the legs and genitals called elephantiasis or pachydermia. Depictions of deformities suggesting elephantiasis are found in prehistoric artifacts. Schistosomiasis is of special interest because stagnant water, especially in irrigated fields, serves as a home for the snail that serves as the intermediate host for this disease. The incidence of schistosomiasis in a population may, therefore, reflect ancient agricultural and sanitary practices.

Ancient artifacts provide a uniquely human source of pseudodiagnoses, because of the vagaries of fashion in the art world. Without knowledge of the conventions peculiar to specific art forms, it is impossible to tell whether a strange and unnatural image represents pathology or deliberate distortion. Masks and pottery may depict abnormalities, artistic exaggeration, or the structural needs of the artifact, as in flat-footed and three-legged pots. Striking abnormalities may be matters of convention or caricature. For example, the Paleolithic statues known as "Stone Venuses" or "fat female figurines" may be fertility symbols, or examples of idiosyncratic ideas of beauty, rather than actual portrayals of obesity.

## ICEMAN

Perhaps the most remarkable of all naturally mummified bodies was discovered in 1991, emerging from a melting glacier in the Tyrolean Alps near the current border between Italy and Austria. Thought to be the oldest mummy in the world, this Neolithic hunter was dubbed the Iceman. Radiocarbon dating indicated that the body was about 5,100 to 5,300 years old. The Iceman was about 159 cm (5 feet, 2.5 inches) tall, between 45 and 50 years old, tattooed, arthritic, and infested with parasitic worms. Analysis of pollen associated with the body, indicated that he died in the spring or early summer. The tools and weapons found with the Iceman included an axe, a dagger, a bow, a quiver made of animal skins, arrows, and articles for fire-making. Because the axe and dagger were made of copper rather than bronze and his hair contained high levels of copper and arsenic, he might have been a coppersmith. His clothing included skins from eight different animal species, including goat and deerskins, a cape made of woven grasses, shoes made of calf skin, and a bearskin hat. Analysis of the contents of his intestines indicated that his last meal included meat (probably ibex and venison), along with various grains and other plant foods.

At first investigators thought that the Iceman had died of a fall, or the cold, but closer examination of the body revealed that a flint arrow-head had lodged in his shoulder. In addition to shattering the scapula the arrow must have torn through nerves and major blood vessels and paralyzed the left arm. Because of the presence of defensive wounds on his hands and traces of blood from several individuals on the Iceman's weapons, researchers suggest that he died in a violent fight with several men.

## PALEOMEDICINE AND SURGERY

Evidence of disease and injuries among ancient humans and other animals is incomplete for epidemiological purposes, but more than sufficient to establish the general notion of their abundance. Therefore, we would like to be able to determine when uniquely human responses to the suffering caused by disease and injury began. For example, a CT scan of a 36,000-year-old Neanderthal skull which had obviously suffered a blow with a sharp stone implement revealed a degree of healing around the wound. To have survived the injury for at least several months would have required care and perhaps wound treatment by other members of the group. Such cases lead to the question: at what stage did human beings begin to administer care that would be recognized as a form of medicine or surgery?

Clues to the existence of paleomedicine must be evaluated even more cautiously than evidence of disease. For example, the "negative imprints" that appear to be tracings of mutilated hands found in Paleolithic cave paintings may record deliberate amputations, loss of fingers to frostbite, magical symbols of unknown significance, or even some kind of game. Early humans may have learned to splint fractured arms or legs to alleviate the pain caused by the movement of injured limbs, but there is little evidence that they learned to reduce fractures. Moreover, well-healed fractures can be found among wild apes. Thus, the discovery of healed fractures, splints, and crutches, does not necessarily prove the existence of prehistoric bonesetters.

Ancient bones and skulls may try to tell us many things, but the enemies of preservation often mute their testimony and generate false clues leading to pseudodiagnoses. Except for violent deaths in which a weapon remains in the body, ancient bones rarely disclose the cause of death. A hole in the skull, for example, might have been caused by a weapon, the bite of a large carnivore, postmortem damage caused by burrowing beetles, a ritual performed after death, or even a surgical operation known as trepanation. A discussion of a Peruvian trepanned skull at the 1867 meeting of the Anthropological Society of Paris stimulated the search for more examples of prehistoric surgery. Eventually, trepanned skulls were discovered at Neolithic sites in Peru, Europe, Russia, and India. The origin and dissemination of this prehistoric operation remain controversial, but the procedure certainly appeared in both the Americas and the Old World before the voyages of Columbus. Whether the operation developed in one culture and spread to others or evolved independently in different regions is still the subject of heated debate. It is impossible to determine just how frequently such operations were performed, but some scholars believe that the operation was performed more frequently during the Neolithic period than in later prehistoric times.

Although trepanation is sometimes mistakenly referred to as "prehistoric brain surgery," a successful trepanation involves the removal of a disk of bone from the cranium, without damage to the brain itself. When scientists first encountered such skulls, they assumed that the operation must have been performed after death for magical purposes. However, anthropologists have discovered that contemporary tribal healers perform trepanations for both magical and practical reasons. Prehistoric surgeons may also have had various reasons for carrying out this difficult and dangerous operation. The operation might have been an attempt to relieve headaches, epilepsy, or other disorders. In some cases, the operation might have been a rational treatment for traumatic injuries of the skull. Perhaps it was also performed as a desperate measure for intractable conditions, rather like lobotomy, or as a form of shock therapy or punishment. Despite the lack of reliable anesthesia or antiseptic technique, evidence of well-healed trepanations indicates that many patients survived, and some even underwent additional trepanations.

Three major forms of trepanation were used by prehistoric surgeons. One technique involved creating a curved groove around the selected area by scraping away bone with a sharp stone or metal instrument. When the groove became deep enough, a more-or-less circular disk, called a button or roundel, could be removed from the skull. Boring a series of small holes in a roughly circular pattern and then cutting out the button of bone with a sharp flint or obsidian knife was the method most commonly used in Peru. The patient could wear the disk as an amulet to ward off further misfortunes. In some regions, surgeons performed partial or perhaps symbolic trepanations. That is, the potential disk was outlined with a shallow crater, but left in place. Some skulls bear thin canoe-shaped cuts that form a rectangular shape, but square or rectangular excisions may have been reserved for postmortem rituals.

Another prehistoric operation that left its mark on the skull is called "sincipital mutilation." In this operation, the mark is the scarring caused by cauterization (burning). Neolithic skulls with this peculiar lesion have been found in Europe, Peru, and India. In preparation for the application of the cauterizing agent, the surgeon made a T- or L-shaped cut in the scalp. Cauterization was accomplished by applying boiling oil, or ropes of plant fibers soaked in boiling oil, to the exposed bone. In either case, permanent damage was done to the thick fibrous membrane covering the bone.

Most of the prehistoric victims of this operation were female, which might mean that the procedure had a ritualistic or punitive function rather than a therapeutic purpose. During the Middle Ages, this operation was prescribed to exorcise demons or relieve melancholy. Doubtless, the operation would dispel the apathy of even the most melancholic patient, or would give the hypochondriac a real focus for further complaints.

In looking at the decorative motifs for which the human frame serves as substrate, objectivity is impossible. What is generally thought of as cosmetic surgery in our society—face-lifts, nose jobs, and liposuction—would be considered mutilations in societies that treasured double chins, majestic noses, thunder thighs, and love handles. While most of the cosmetic surgery of prehistoric times has disappeared along with the soft parts of the body, some decorative processes affected the bones and teeth. Such customs include deforming, or molding the skulls of infants, and decorating or selectively removing teeth. Unusually shaped heads might also reflect traditional methods of caring for or transporting infants. For example, cradle-board pressure during infancy can alter the contours of the skull. Considerable evidence remains to suggest that tattooing and circumcision were not uncommon in ancient times. Direct evidence can only be found in well-preserved mummies, but studies of similar customs in contemporary traditional societies can expand our understanding of the myriad possibilities for prehistoric cosmetic surgery.

Since the 1990s, women's health reformers have been attempting to end the traditional practice of female circumcision, also known as female genital mutilation, which is still practiced in more than 25 countries in Africa and the Middle East. Generally, the painful ritual is performed with crude instruments, without anesthesia or antiseptics. Although the ritual is prohibited by many African nations, it is often performed secretly. The World Health Organization estimates that 130 million girls and women have undergone some form of cutting of the clitoris. In the most extreme form of female circumcision, still practiced widely in Somalia and Ethiopia, the outer labia are sliced off and the remaining tissue is sewn shut. Female circumcision is seen as a way of ensuring chastity and was often practiced as a coming of age ritual and a prerequisite to marriage.

## HEALING RITUALS, TRADITIONS, AND MAGIC

Paleopathologists must make their deductions about the antiquity of infectious diseases with limited and ambiguous data; however, their conclusions must be consistent with modern biomedical knowledge. Infectious diseases have affected human evolution and history in complex and subtle ways. Endemic and epidemic diseases may determine the density of populations, the dispersion of peoples, and the diffusion of genes, as well as the success or failure of battles, invasions, and colonization. Thus, one way to test hypotheses about disease in ancient times is to examine the pattern of disease among contemporary peoples whose culture entails features similar to those characteristic of prehistoric societies.

Even if transistor radios, communication satellites, and television have turned the world into a global village, it is still possible to find people who live in relative isolation, maintaining a way of life that seems little changed from the Old Stone Age. Until recently, anthropologists and historians generally referred to such people as "contemporary primitives." Of course, in terms of biological evolution, contemporary primitives are as far removed from Paleolithic peoples as any professor of anthropology, but the patterns of their lives may be similar to those of early hunter-gatherers, nomadic followers of semidomesticated animals, or proto-agriculturalists. Because cultural patterns are a product of history, not biology, the term "traditional society" is now generally substituted for the term "primitive," which carries a rather pejorative connotation. The newer terminology is, however, somewhat confusing because of the various shades of meaning associated with the term "traditional." Where possible, we shall use the term "traditional society"; where necessary for clarity, we shall refer to "tribal societies" or "so-called primitives."

Many pathogens are species specific, but diseases like bubonic plague, malaria, yellow fever, and tuberculosis are formidable exceptions to this rule. Wild or domesticated animals can serve as reservoirs for many diseases transmitted to humans directly or via insect vectors. The survival of pathogens that are species specific depends on the pathogen's virulence, the size and population density of the host group, the immune response mounted by the host, and the pathogen's ability to find new victims. Certain pathogens can only be transmitted during the acute phase of the disease, because the pathogen disappears upon recovery or death. When such an organism is introduced into a small population, virtually all individuals become infected and recover or die. Such diseases could not establish permanent residence among small bands of Stone Age peoples. New disease patterns became part of the price paid for living in large, densely populated, permanent towns and cities which, as Thomas Jefferson warned, were "pestilential to the morals, the health, and the liberties of man."

Pathogens that remain in the host during convalescence, persist in chronic lesions, or establish permanent residence in healthy carriers are likely to find new victims even among small bands of people. Some diseases are caused by commensal organisms—those that live harmlessly in or on their host until some disturbance triggers the onset of illness. Commensalism indicates a long period of mutual adaptation; thus, such diseases may be the most ancient. Variant forms of proteins, such as sickle cell hemoglobin, may reflect evolutionary adaptations in the host population to ancient scourges like malaria.

It is often assumed that modern and so-called primitive people differ in their susceptibility and resistance to disease. Comparisons of crude mortality rates for "moderns" and "primitives" are, however, likely to be very misleading. Mortality rates during an epidemic may reflect the kind of care given to the sick rather than some mysterious quality called "resistance." During an explosive epidemic in a small, isolated population, there may be no healthy adults left to feed infants and care for the sick. Those who might have survived the epidemic may, therefore, die because of the lack of food, water, and simple nursing care.

In general, the trait shared by all forms of ancient medicine is a supernatural orientation, a belief in magic. In this context, magic is not a trivial concept; the belief in magic has influenced and shaped human behavior more deeply and extensively than scientific or rationalist modes of thought, as we are pleased to call our own way of explaining the world. In societies where magical and scientific beliefs coexist, one cannot predict which will be stronger or more influential. Even today, people may vacillate between alternative systems of medicine, depending on particular circumstances, perhaps relying on modern medicine for a broken arm and magical medicine for "spirit possession."

Magic plays an important role in many cultures; it provides answers to questions that cannot be answered by existing logical or rational knowledge. Magic may be so closely related to religion that it is difficult to define the borderline between them. The primary difference between a prayer and a spell is the assumption that magical practices, correctly performed, *must* bring about the desired reaction. A prayer, in contrast, is an appeal for aid from a supernatural being who has the power to grant or deny the request.

In primitive medicine, the supernatural is involved in all aspects of disease and healing. Because disease and misfortune are attributed to supernatural agents, magic is essential to the prevention, diagnosis, and treatment of disease. All events must have a cause, visible or invisible. Thus, diseases for which there are no obvious immediate causes must be caused by ghosts, spirits, gods, sorcery, witchcraft, or the loss of one of the victim's special souls. Illness calls for consultation with those who have the power to control the supernatural agents of disease: the shaman, medicine man, wise woman, diviner, priest, soul-catcher, or sorcerer. A close examination of the roles and powers assigned to such figures reveals many specific differences, but for our purposes the general term "healer" will generally suffice. Most societies, however, differentiate between the healers and herbalists who dispense ordinary remedies and the shamans or priest-like healers who can intercede with the spirits that affect weather, harvests, hunting, warfare, conception, childbirth, disease, and misfortune.

Although the shaman or medicine man performs magical acts, including deliberate deceptions, he or she is neither a fake nor a neurotic. The shaman is likely to be as sincere as any modern physician or psychiatrist in the performance of healing rituals. When sick, the medicine man will undergo therapy with another medicine man, despite knowledge of all the tricks of the trade.

For the shaman, the cause of the disorder is more significant than the symptoms because the cause determines the manner of treatment, be it herbs or exorcisms. Diagnostic aids may include a spirit medium, crystal gazing, and divination. Having performed the preliminary diagnostic tests, the healer might conduct a complex ritual involving magic spells, incantations, the extraction of visible or invisible objects, or the capture and return of the patient's lost soul. To drive out or confuse evil spirits, the shaman may give the patient a special disguise or a new name, offer attractive substitute targets, or prescribe noxious medicines to transform the patient into an undesirable host.

The shaman may dispense powerful drugs and closely observe the patient, use knowledge of animal behavior for diagnostic tests, and dispense powerful drugs, but it is the ritual, with its attempts to compel the cooperation of supernatural powers, that is of prime importance to healer, patient, and community. For example, certain traditional healers had their patients urinate on the ground near an ant hill. The behavior of the ants would provide a low-cost diagnostic test for diabetes. Outsiders may see the healing ritual in terms of magical and practical elements, but for healer and patient there is no separation between the magical and empirical aspects of therapy. In a society without writing or precise means of measuring drug concentrations and time intervals, strict attention to ritual may provide a means of standardizing treatment, as well as a reassuring atmosphere. The shaman cannot isolate and secularize pharmacologically active drugs, because of the holistic nature of the healing ritual. But the problem of evaluating remedies and procedures is more difficult than generally assumed. Thus, a modern physician is no more likely to conduct a double-blind trial of generally accepted remedies than the traditional medicine man.

Practitioners of "modern medicine" find it difficult to believe that the obvious superiority of scientific medicine has not caused the disappearance of all other systems of healing. Yet traditional and alternative systems of medicine continue to flourish in America, Europe, Africa, China, India, and the Middle East. On the other hand, traditional medicine has been influenced by modern theory and practice. Today's shaman may dispense both penicillin and incantations in order to combat both germs and evil spirits.

Ultimately, the success of any healing act depends on a combination of social, psychological, pharmacological, and biochemical factors. Where infant mortality is high and life expectancy low, the healer is unlikely to confront many cases of metabolic diseases among the young, or the chronic degenerative diseases of the elderly. Many perceptive practitioners of the healing arts have acknowledged that, left to themselves, many diseases disappear without any treatment at all. Thus, if a healing ritual extends over a long enough period, the healer will be credited with curing a self-limited disease. Given the dubious value of many remedies, recovery is often a tribute to the patient's triumph over both the disease and the doctor.

Because of the uncertainties involved in evaluating the treatment of disease, historians of medicine have often turned to the analysis of surgical operations as a more objective measure of therapeutic interventions. But even here there are difficulties in comparing practices carried out under greatly differing circumstances, by different kinds of practitioners, with different goals and objectives. One surprising aspect of so-called primitive surgery is the fact that surgical operations for purely medical reasons may be rare or nonexistent in a particular tribe, although the shaman may wield the knife with great skill and enthusiasm for ceremonial, decorative, or judicial purposes. Ritual scarification, for example, may signify caste, adulthood, or the "medicine marks" thought to provide immunization against disease, poisons, snakebites, and other dangers. Just how effective such protection might be is open to question, but there have been reports of African healers who impregnated "medicine cuts" with a mixture of snake heads and ant eggs. When twentieth century scientists discovered how to detoxify toxins with formalin, which is present in ant eggs, the African ritual suddenly seemed less bizarre.

Although amputation for ritual purposes or punishment is not uncommon in tribal and ancient societies, interest in medically indicated amputation is rare. Some native American surgeons, however, amputated frozen fingers and, in Africa, the Masai are noted for successfully amputating fractured limbs. Some prehistoric peoples performed amputations as a form of punishment or as part of mourning rituals. Mutilations of the genital organs are often components of puberty rites. Circumcision and clitorectomy are the most common operations, but some tribes practiced more exotic mutilations.

Traditional surgeons developed many ingenious methods of closing wounds. Sewing is, of course, an ancient skill, but in the absence of antiseptic techniques, applying needle and thread to a wound is likely to lead to serious infection. There is a better chance of success when the skewer and thread method, which is commonly used to close a stuffed turkey, is applied to wounds. A remarkable technique devised by surgeons in Africa, India, and the Americas depended on the use of particular species of termites or ants. The appropriate insect was brought into contact with the wound and stimulated to bite. When the insect's body was broken off, the jaws remained as natural suture clamps.

To combat bleeding, traditional surgeons used tourniquets or cauterization or simply packed the wound with absorbent materials and covered it with bandages. Masai surgeons, however, repaired torn blood vessels with suture thread made from tendons. Wound dressings often contained noxious materials, such as cow dung and powdered insects, as well as ingredients that might function as astringents and antiseptics. Traditional wound dressings might contain pharmacologically valuable ingredients, such as ergot, which is present in rye smut, but symbolic values are likely to predominate. The odds of finding penicillin, or other effective antibiotics in earth taken from a recent grave are actually vanishingly small.

Traditional surgeons were often quite skillful in the treatment of fractures and dislocations, although the treatment might be considered incomplete until the appropriate incantations were recited over the splints or a lizard's head was tied to the wound. The shaman could also encourage the patient by symbolic acts such as breaking the leg of a chicken and applying remedies to the unfortunate fowl.

One of the major duties of the Western surgeon, or barber-surgeon, until quite recent times was the practice of therapeutic and prophylactic bleeding. Selecting the proper vein for bleeding was an important aspect of treatment. Rather than opening a vein, traditional healers usually carried out bleeding by means of scarification or cupping. Unlike their Europeans counterparts, traditional healers generally thought that extracting large amounts of blood from the body was very dangerous.

Despite certain special exceptions, traditional surgery was generally limited in scope and quality. Part of the problem was undoubtedly lack of systematic knowledge of anatomy, asepsis, anesthesia, and the failure of a small tribal unit to provide enough "clinical material" for the healer to develop surgical skills through repetition. However, ideas, rather than materials, were often the limiting factors. The influence of the supernatural view of nature fosters a fear of bodily mutilation, other than those considered fashionable. Moreover, the use of surgical mutilation as punishment for the most shameful crimes produced negative associations with surgery.

Although rituals and spells may be the most dramatic aspects of primitive medicine, the medicine man may also use pharmacologically active and effective drugs. Natural product chemists are just beginning to exploit the ethnobotany of so-called primitive peoples. Plant and animal sources provided the traditional healer with analgesics, anesthetics, emetics, purgatives, diuretics, narcotics, hallucinogens, cathartics, febrifuges, and perhaps even oral contraceptives. From the primitive pharmacopoeia, modern medicine has adopted salicylic acid, quinine, ipecac, cocaine, ephedrine, colchicine, digitalis, ergot, and many other drugs.

Probably more than half of the prescriptions written by modern physicians involve drugs extracted from plants or their synthetic equivalents. Nature provides such a formidable array of natural products that the great problem has always been knowing where to begin the search for medicinal substances. Although many folk remedies may be nothing more than placebos, if only 10 to 25 percent of the drugs in so-called primitive pharmacopoeias are pharmacologically active, the potential for the discovery of new drugs is prodigious. The limiting factor in evaluating such remedies may well be the disappearance of traditional societies, with their rich, but fragile oral traditions and their intimate knowledge of their endangered environment. In Africa, it is said that a library vanishes every time an old person dies. It is also true that a potential drugstore vanishes every time a unique bit of the natural environment is destroyed.

Primitive medicine has often been dismissed as mere superstition, but it has much in common with the medical practices of ancient civilizations and with the folk beliefs that persist and even flourish alongside modern medicine. Accounts of the medicine of primitive or traditional societies often overemphasize exotic and magical aspects, leaving the impression that an unbridgeable chasm exists between such medical systems and those of modern societies. The customs that seem bizarre in other cultures are, however, sometimes similar to our own quaint and charming folk practices.

When we analyze traditional and folk medicine, the apparent chaos of specific details can generally be reduced to a few almost universal themes. Indeed, as we survey the history of medicine, the same themes will often reappear in only slightly different forms. Folk medicine, like primitive medicine, generally views disease as a malevolent invader and the body as a battlefield. Our vocabulary for illness still reflects this idea: we are "attacked" by disease, and we "fight off" infection until the disease is "expelled" from our system. Thus, it would not be unreasonable to expect to cure a patient by luring the invader out of the body and transferring it to a suitable receiver. For example, a desperate parent might force a dog to eat a sandwich containing hair from a child with whooping cough. If the dog coughed, the child would recover. A related approach, generally known as *dreckapothecary*, uses remedies designed to drive out the invader by dosing the patient with vile, nauseating, and disgusting concoctions. Presumably, saturating the patient with remedies containing excrements, noxious insects, rancid fat, foul smelling plants, and so forth, will make the body an unattractive abode for a fastidious invader.

The *doctrine of signatures* is another guiding principle of folk medicine. According to this concept, God has furnished the world with diseases and remedies and has taught us that nothing exists without a purpose. Therefore, we may assume that God has marked potential remedies with some sign hinting at their medicinal virtues. For example, a plant remedy for jaundice might sport yellow flowers and remedies for heart disease might be found in plants with heart-shaped leaves.

Many folk remedies require the parts and products of animals. Selection of the appropriate remedy may be guided by either the principle of *opposites* or the principle of *similars*. For example, if roasted rabbit brains failed to cure excessive timidity, courage might be found in the blood of a ferocious beast. Lowly animals such as mice and moles were used in remedies for warts, coughs, fevers, fits, and bedwetting, but no creature has served the healing art as diligently as the leech. According to folk beliefs, this natural medical device can selectively remove the "bad blood" from arthritic joints and reduce the swelling of a black eye. Insects and insect products remain important components of folk remedies. Those who might ridicule the use of spider webs to stop bleeding may laud the virtues of honey in the treatment of bee stings, coughs, colds, rheumatism, and tuberculosis.

In addition to herbs, animal parts and products, and minerals, folk remedies include charms, spells, prayers, relics, amulets, and images of gods or saints. Rings containing quicksilver were probably just as effective in warding off headaches as copper bracelets are in curing arthritis. Tar-water tea, an American folk remedy prepared by soaking ropes from old ships in cold water, was popularized in Europe by Bishop George Berkeley (1685–1753), who praised it as a panacea cheap enough to be used by the poorest people and safe enough for infants. According to the good bishop, the violent opposition of physicians and apothecaries to such inexpensive folk remedies proved that doctors feared only an outbreak of good health.

On the other hand, we should remind ourselves that the ingredients in many traditional remedies are so exotic, nauseating, or toxic that the prescriptions were more likely to scare people out of their illness than to cure them. When faced with the choice of consuming "boiled black bugs and onions," or pleading guilty to good health, many marginally ill and malingering patients must have chosen the latter course. In modern societies, the spells and rituals that once surrounded the taking of remedies have virtually disappeared. But vestiges of these actions remain in the "old wives' tales" told by people entirely too sophisticated to believe such stories any more than they would worry about a broken mirror or Friday the thirteenth.

## SUGGESTED READINGS

Ammerman, A. J., and Cavalli-Sforza, L. L. (1984). *The Neolithic Transition and the Genetics of Populations in Europe.* Princeton, NJ: Princeton University Press.

Aufderheide, A. C., and Rodriguez-Martín, C. (1998). *The Cambridge Encyclopedia of Human Paleopathology.* New York: Cambridge University Press.

Brothwell, D. R., and and Brothwell, P. (1998). *Food in Antiquity: A Survey of the Diet of Early Peoples.* Baltimore, MD: Johns Hopkins University Press.

Cockburn, A., Cockburn, E., and Reyman, T. A., eds. (1980). *Mummies, Disease, and Ancient Cultures,* 2nd ed. New York: Cambridge University Press.

Cohen, M. N., and Armelagos, G. J., eds. (1983). *Paleopathology and the Origins of Agriculture.* New York: Academic Press.

Conrad, L. I., and Dominik, W., eds. (2000). *Contagion: Perspectives from Pre-Modern Societies.* Burlington, VT: Ashgate.

Fowler, B. (2002). *Iceman: Uncovering the Life and Times of a Prehistoric Man Found in an Alpine Glacier.* Chicago, IL: University of Chicago Press.

Gilbert, R. I., and Mielke, J. H., eds. (1985). *The Analysis of Prehistoric Diets.* New York: Academic Press.

Herrmann, B., and Hummel, S., eds. (1994). *Ancient DNA: Recovery and Analysis of Genetic Material from Paleontological, Archaeological, Museum, Medical, and Forensic Specimens.* New York: Springer-Verlag.

Larsen, C. S. (1999). *Bioarchaeology: Interpreting Behavior from the Human Skeleton.* New York: Cambridge University Press.

Ortner, D. J., and Aufderheide, A. C., eds. (1991). *Human Paleopathology: Current Syntheses and Future Options.* Washington, DC: Smithsonian Institution Press.

Roberts, C. A., and and Manchester, K. (1995). *The Archaeology of Disease.* Ithaca, NY: Cornell University Press.

Rothschild, B. M., and and Martin, L. D. (1993). *Paleopathology: Disease in the Fossil Record.* Boca Raton, FL: CRC Press.

Sandford, M. K., ed. (1993). *Investigations of Ancient Human Tissue: Chemical Analyses in Anthropology.* Langhorne, PA: Gordon and Breach.

Stead, I. M., Bourke, J. B., and and Brothwell, D. (1986). *Lindow Man. The Body in the Bog.* Ithaca, NY: Cornell University Press.

Steinbock, R. T. (1976). *Paleopathological Diagnosis and Interpretation: Bone Diseases in Ancient Human Populations.* Springfield, IL: Thomas.

Ubelaker, D. H. (1999). *Human Skeletal Remains: Excavation, Analysis, Interpretation,* 3rd ed. Washington, DC: Taraxacum.

Waldron, T. (1994). *Counting the Dead: The Epidemiology of Skeletal Populations.* New York: John Wiley and Sons.

# 2

# Medicine in Ancient Civilizations: Mesopotamia and Egypt

## INTRODUCTION

The Greeks thought it easy to define "civilization": it referred to the qualities of citizens—free men living in cities. Today the concept is regarded as more complex, subtle, and problematic. The term "culture" is used to encompass all the ways of life and customary behaviors invented by human beings. Civilization is, therefore, a particular kind of culture, characterized by increasing complexity in social, economic, and political organization, a settled life, a food supply in excess of subsistence levels, occupational specialization, writing and reckoning, and innovations in the arts and sciences—all maintained by a large number of people over a significant period of time.

The first civilizations developed in the period between about 3500 and 1500 B.C.E. in a few delimited areas of the world. Historians continue to pose questions about the nature of the factors that cause the development of civilizations and those that nurture their growth. No simple, definitive answer seems possible, but a variety of causes involving some complex balance between the bounties and challenges of geographic, climatic, and economic factors have been suggested. Presumably, it is significant that four of the earliest civilizations developed in river valleys: the Nile River of Egypt, the Tigris-Euphrates in the Middle East, the Indus River in India, and the Yellow River in China.

Because the evidence from the earliest periods is ambiguous and fragmentary, the question of which civilization was the first to appear has been the subject of endless debate. We will, therefore, ignore these controversies and look instead at some of the major centers of civilization to see what they can tell us about health, disease, and ancient medicine.

25

## MESOPOTAMIA

Mesopotamia, the land between the Tigris and Euphrates Rivers, was the arena of the growth and decay of many civilizations, including those known as Sumerian, Chaldean, Assyrian, and Babylonian. Although Egyptian civilization is better known, we will begin our survey of ancient civilizations with Sumer to emphasize the point that other, less familiar areas also became urban and literate at a very remote date.

Sumer flourished some four thousand to five thousand years ago, but by the first century, its language had vanished and its writings, in the form of cuneiform characters inscribed on clay tablets, were indecipherable. Scholars believe that the wedge-shaped symbols evolved from pictures used in an early accounting system into abstract signs that represented sounds of speech. Most Sumerian tablets dealt with mundane economic and administrative transactions, but thousands of others record myths, fables, and ideas about science, mathematics, and medicine. Scholars have even discovered cuneiform tablets containing recipes, which provide intriguing clues to eating, drinking, and the role of cults and feasting in the ancient world. Other traces of the extent and complexity of ancient Mesopotamian civilization have recently been revealed by surveillance satellites. These photographs reveal traces of previously unknown settlements and networks of roads long buried under the sands of the Middle East. Some of the roads were probably constructed four thousand to five thousand years ago to link the cities of Mesopotamia to neighboring settlements and distant farmlands.

In Sumer, the mastery of agricultural techniques led to dramatic changes in population density and the establishment of the bureaucratic apparatus needed for planning, storage, and redistribution of crops. The great mass of people lived as peasants, but their productivity supported a small urban elite of priests, warriors, and noblemen. Because law and medicine were ascribed to divine origins, the priests also assumed the roles of judges, lawyers, and physicians.

The cuneiform texts pertaining to medicine can be divided into three categories: therapeutic or "medical texts," omen collections or "symptom texts," and miscellaneous texts that incidentally provide information on diseases and medical practices. After analyzing numerous texts, scholars divided the medical traditions of Sumer into two categories, which have been called the "scientific" and the "practical" schools. According to this scheme, the "scientific practitioners" were the authors and users of the symptom texts. In contrast, members of the practical school concentrated on empirical medical practices and were the authors and users of the medical texts.

The medical texts of the practical school followed a formal arrangement typical of Mesopotamian scribal practice. Each text contained a series of units or cases following the same general format: "If a man is sick (and has the following symptoms) . . ." or "If a man suffers from (such and such) pain in (wherever it was) . . ." The description of the list of symptoms was followed by instructions for the medicines needed, their preparation, the timing and means of administration. The healer "discovered" the significant symptoms by listening to the patient's account of the illness, not by performing a direct physical examination of the patient's body. Although most units conclude with the comforting promise that the patient would get well, certain symptoms presaged a fatal outcome.

In contrast, the "conjurer," "diviner," or "priest-healer" looked at the patient's symptoms and circumstances as omens that identified the disorder and predicted the outcome of the disease. Unlike his "practical" counterpart, the diviner performed a direct physical examination in order to discover signs and omens. Clearly the gods were at work if a snake fell onto the sick man's bed, because this omen indicated that the prognosis was favorable. But wine-colored urine was a portent of progressive, debilitating illness and pain. If the priest could not wrest sufficient information from his direct examination of the patient, he could find signs in the viscera of sacrificial animals. Omens provided by animal livers were applied to the patient, whose liver was inaccessible.

Although there are many uncertainties in interpreting ancient texts, tentative diagnoses of some of the disorders discussed in the cuneiform tablets are sometimes possible. Mesopotamian physicians were probably familiar with a wide range of diseases, including schistosomiasis, dysentery, pneumonia, and epilepsy. Malnutrition would obviously correlate with the periodic famines alluded to in various texts, but even when food supplies were adequate in quantity, the daily diet was probably monotonous and unbalanced. Descriptions of eye disorders, paralysis, swollen bellies, and the "stinking disease" are consistent with various vitamin deficiency diseases. A combination of poor quality foods and chronic infestation with various parasites would amplify the problem of malnutrition and retard the growth of children.

Because illness was regarded as a divine punishment for sins committed by the patient, healing required the spiritual and physical catharsis obtained by combining confession and exorcism with purgative drugs. Sumerian prescriptions include about 250 vegetable and 120 mineral drugs, as well as alcoholic beverages, fats and oils, parts and products of animals, honey, wax, and various kinds of milk thought to have medical virtues. Medical texts, like almost all Mesopotamian tablets, were anonymous. But some medical tablets provide enthusiastic personal endorsements and testimonials for particular remedies. Medications are said to have been tested or discovered by unimpeachable authorities, such as sages and experts. Some remedies were praised for their antiquity or exclusivity. Of special interest is a small cuneiform tablet containing about a dozen recipes recorded by a Sumerian physician about four thousand years ago. This tablet appears to be the oldest written collection of prescriptions.

The separation of magical and empirical aspects of medicine is a very recent development. Thus, it should not be surprising that Mesopotamian patients considered it prudent to attack disease with a combination of magic and medicine. A healer who was both priest and physician could increase the efficacy of drugs by reciting appropriate incantations. Although the healer needed some knowledge of anatomy and drug lore, precise knowledge of magical rituals was more important because errors in this department could alienate the gods.

Hordes of demons and devils were thought to cause diseases and misfortune; each evil spirit tended to cause particular disorders. As in the case of folk medicine and so-called-primitive medicine, Mesopotamian healers also attempted to rid their patients of disease-causing demons by the administration of noxious remedies. Enveloped in the aroma of burning feathers, and liberally dosed with dog dung and pig's gall, the patient hardly seemed an inviting abode for demons and devils. The magician might also try to transfer the demon into a surrogate victim, such as an animal or a magical figure. Sometimes healers engaged disease-causing demons in a formal dialogue, as in a conversation between the priest and the "tooth worm" recorded about 2250 B.C.E. While an incantation entitled "The Worm and the Toothache" hardly sounds like a major epic, this dialogue is a rich source of cosmological concepts and creation myths.

Mesopotamian pharmaceutical texts reflect familiarity with fairly elaborate chemical operations for the purification of crude plant, animal, and mineral components. Plants and herbs were so important to ancient medicine that the terms for "medicine" and "herbs" were essentially equivalent. Drugs made from seeds, bark, and other parts of plants were dissolved in beer or milk and administered by mouth, or mixed with wine, honey, and fats and applied externally. In retrospect, it is logical to assume that the wine used in wound dressings provided some benefit as an antiseptic. Whether red or white, wine is a better antiseptic than 10 percent alcohol, but red wine seems to be the beverage of choice for fighting infection.

According to the Mesopotamian legend known as the Gilgamesh Epic, human beings lost possession of the most powerful, life-giving herb in creation through the carelessness of Gilgamesh, a powerful hero-king who was two-thirds god and one-third human (by what genetic mechanism these ratios were generated is not clear). The hero of the ancient epic was apparently based on the exploits of a real king who ruled Babylonia about 2700 B.C.E. Some six hundred years after his death, legends about the life of Gilgamesh were collected in the form of an epic poem. Thus, *The Epic of Gilgamesh* provides insights into the lives and beliefs of the people who lived in the land between the Tigris and Euphrates rivers in the second and third millenniums B.C.E.

Despite his god-like qualities, Gilgamesh learns that he, like all human beings, must inevitably succumb to illness and death. When his friend Enkidu was stricken with a serious illness, Gilgamesh swore that he would never give up hope of saving him "until a worm fell out of his nose" (a striking omen of impending death). After many trials and tribulations, and an awesome journey through the realm of darkness, Gilgamesh learned the secret of the herb of life and swam to the bottom of the waters where the marvelous plant grew. Before he could take the herb of health and healing back to Uruk, the exhausted hero stopped to rest. While Gilgamesh slept, a mysterious serpent slithered out of his hiding place and ate the herb of life. As a result, the snake shed its old skin and was instantly rejuvenated while Gilgamesh wept for himself and all of suffering mankind. According to the epic, when Gilgamesh returned from his journey, he engraved the story of all his adventures and the wonders of the city of Uruk on a clay tablet for the instruction of posterity. Thus, ever since the time of Gilgamesh, each time a snake sheds its old skin its rebirth reminds human beings that they must grow old and die. Nevertheless, the epic tells us, even though great heroes may die they become immortalized in the written record of their great deeds.

## HAMMURABI'S CODE OF LAWS

When the Greek historian Herodotus visited Babylonia in the fifth century B.C.E., he reached the remarkable conclusion that the Babylonians had no doctors. The sick, he said, were taken to the marketplace to seek advice from those who had experienced similar illnesses. This story proves only that we should not take the tales told by tourists too seriously. As we have seen, Mesopotamia had a complex medical tradition. Both the empirical and the magical approach to healing were well established, but eventually the balance of power apparently tilted in favor of the magician. Evidence about the various kinds of healers who practiced the art in the region can be extracted from the most complete account of Babylonian law, the Code of Hammurabi. Today, Hammurabi (fl. 1792–1750 B.C.E.), Babylonia's most famous king, is of more interest for the code of laws bearing his name than for his military and political triumphs.

Hammurabi founded the Babylonian empire that unified and ruled southern Mesopotamia (Sumer and Akkad) for almost two centuries. The Babylonian empire was eventually destroyed and, in 538 B.C.E., the last of the Babylonian kings surrendered to the Persian ruler Cyrus the Great and Babylonia became part of the Persian Empire. Toward the end of his reign, Hammurabi commissioned the creation of a great stele portraying the king receiving the insignia of kingship and justice from the gods. Below this portrait were inscribed the 282 clauses or case laws now referred to as the Code of Hammurabi. According to the inscription, the gods who had made Babylon a great and everlasting kingdom called upon Hammurabi to "bring about the rule of righteousness in the land, to destroy the wicked and the evil-doers; so that the strong should not harm the weak." In an epilogue to the Code, Hammurabi called himself the "wise king," who had taught his people righteous laws and pious statutes, and established order in his kingdom.

The code governs criminal and civil matters such as the administration of justice, ownership of property, trade and commerce, family relations, labor, personal injuries, and professional conduct. Replete with harsh punishments, the Code of Hammurabi reveals the relationships that governed Babylonia's priests, landowners, merchants, peasants, artisans, and slaves. The penalty for many infractions, such as theft or harboring a runaway slave, was death, but many other crimes were punished by amputations. Various clauses refer to illness, adoption, prostitution, wet nursing, pregnancy, miscarriages, and malpractice by doctors and veterinarians. Some laws actually did promote Hammurabi's promise that the laws would protect the weak. For example, a man could take a second wife if his first wife became ill, but he had to support his sick wife and allow her to remain in his house.

Criminal penalties were based on the principle of *lex talionis*, literally, the "law of the claw," that is, an eye for an eye, a tooth for a tooth. Retribution or punishment was designed to fit the crime: amputation of the hand that struck the father, or blinding the eye used to pry into secrets. Such punishments are generally referred to as "judicial mutilation." Given the number of clauses that specify amputations as punishment for various offenses, one could imagine a fairly lively business for specialists in judicial mutilation. The penalties specified by the laws fell with different degrees of severity on the three classes that made up Babylonian society: gentlemen, or seigniors; commoners, or plebeians; and slaves, whose lowly status was indicated by a physical mark. Slaves apparently carried a 30-day warranty against certain disorders. For example, if a slave was attacked by epilepsy within one month of purchase, the seller had to reclaim that slave and return the purchase price.

The laws of special interest to the history of medicine—those pertaining to surgeons, veterinarians, midwives, and wet nurses—follow the laws dealing with assault. Nine paragraphs are devoted to the regulation of medical fees and specifications concerning the relationship between the status of the patient and the appropriate fees and penalties. The severe penalties set forth for failures suggest that practitioners would be very cautious in accepting clients and would shun those that looked hopeless or litigious. The laws also reflect a profound distinction between medicine and surgery. The physicians, who dealt with problems that would today be called "internal medicine," were of the priestly class and their professional conduct was not governed by the criminal laws pertaining to assault and malpractice.

Because internal disorders were caused by supernatural agents, those who wrestled with such diseases were accountable to the gods. Wounds were due to direct human error or aggression. Therefore, those who wielded the "bronze knife" were accountable to earthly authorities. Fees and penalties for surgical operations were substantial. If a doctor performed a major operation and saved the life or the eyesight of a seignior, his fee was 10 shekels of silver. The fee was reduced by half for operating on a commoner, and was only two shekels when the patient was a slave. However, if the surgeon performed such an operation and caused the death of a seignior, or destroyed his eye, the doctor's hand should be cut off. If the physician caused the death of a slave, he had to provide a replacement. If he destroyed the eye of a slave, he had to pay the owner one-half his value in silver.

Just what operation was involved in "opening the eye-socket" or "curing" the eye is a matter of some dispute. The operation could have been the couching of a cataract (destruction of a lens that had become opaque) or merely lancing an abscess of the tear duct. While such an abscess causes intense pain, it does not affect vision, whereas cataracts lead to blindness. Probing or lancing might help in the case of an abscess, but if poorly done such interventions could cause blindness. Presumably eye surgery was only twice as difficult as setting a broken bone, or healing a sprain, because the fee for such services was five shekels of silver for a seignior, three for a commoner, and two for a slave. The veterinarian, also called the "doctor of an ox or an ass," carried out various surgical operations, including castration of domesticated animals.

Women served as midwives, surgeons, and even palace physicians in Mesopotamia, but the Code of Hammurabi does not specifically mention female doctors. The laws did, however, refer to women who served as wet nurses (women who provided breast milk for the infants of other women). If a seignior gave his son to a wet nurse and the child died, her breasts could be cut off if she had taken in other infants without informing the parents. Obviously, such a woman would never commit that offense again.

In excavating the remains of ancient Mesopotamian cities, archaeologists continue to unearth thousands of cuneiform tablets. Most refer to mundane business transactions and political matters, but as new texts are painstakingly deciphered our picture of Mesopotamian civilizations may well undergo profound changes.

## EGYPT

Egyptian civilization has fascinated travelers and scholars since Herodotus initiated the tradition of Nile travelogues. To Greeks and Romans, Egypt was an ancient and exotic land, with peculiar customs, especially in terms of gender roles. Shops and markets in Egypt were run by women and men did the weaving. Collecting Egyptian antiquities was already fashionable in Roman times, but modern Egyptology begins with the discovery of the Rosetta Stone, a slab of black basalt inscribed with a message in three forms of writing: hieroglyphic Egyptian, demotic Egyptian, and the Greek alphabet. Formal hieroglyphs, "the words of the gods," were not only a way of writing, but also a form of artistic expression. Egyptian scribes developed a simplified script known as demotic, but by the fifth century, other forms of writing were adopted and the ancient writings became indecipherable.

The development of the first true writing system has generally been credited to ancient Sumer, but in the 1990s, archaeologists discovered pictures and symbols inscribed on a limestone cliff in Egypt that might challenge that chronology. The carvings, including a tableau measuring 18 by 20 inches, appear to depict the exploits of a legendary king who played a critical role in the foundation of Egyptian civilization. Although these inscriptions were apparently created about 5,250 years ago, they seem to resemble later hieroglyphs. Some scholars believe the inscription represents an early stage of writing, or proto-hieroglyphs. Similar symbols—inscribed on ivory, bone, and pottery—were found by archaeologists excavating a royal tomb at Abydos, which supports the conclusion that they represent the beginning of Egyptian script. These findings suggest that phonetic elements were present in Egyptian inscriptions before the Mesopotamian symbols reached their mature format.

Popular ideas about ancient Egypt have been shaped by romantic images of the elaborate tombs of the Pharaohs, such as Howard Carter's 1922 discovery of the tomb of Tut-ankh-Amen, who had ruled for a brief period during the Eighteenth Dynasty. Egyptologists had previously explored many tombs in the Valley of the Kings near Luxor, but most had been thoroughly plundered by grave robbers over the centuries. Interest in Egyptian antiquities, as well as legends of a "Pharaoh's Curse," were revived by the remarkable findings in the tomb and the deaths of 12 of the archaeologists present at the opening of the tomb during the next seven years.

The tomb contained hundreds of precious objects, including the Pharaoh's mummy, in a gold coffin, nested within two outer coffins. Tut-ankh-Amen, was only nine when he assumed the throne in 1333 B.C.E. Studies of his mummy confirmed the tradition that he was only about 18 when he died and proved that he was significantly less handsome than his beautiful golden death mask would suggest. Studies of the king's mummy and his clothing indicate that he had abnormally wide hips, an abnormal curvature of the spine, and fusion of the upper vertebrae. Researchers note that these findings are consistent with a disorder called Klippel-Feil syndrome, a rare spinal disorder that involves anomalies of the musculoskeletal system, kidneys, heart, and nervous system. If Tut-ankh-Amen had Klippel-Feil syndrome he would have had difficulty walking. The discovery of more than a hundred walking sticks among his grave goods seems to support this theory.

Ancient Greek writers from Homer to Herodotus praised the physicians of Egypt for their wisdom and skill, but the Greeks also knew Egypt as the "mother country of diseases." Certainly, ancient Egyptian skeletons, portraits, writings, and, above all, mummies provide ample evidence of the crushing burden of disease in the ancient world. Although mummified bodies have been found in many parts of the world, for most people the term "mummy" conjures up the Egyptian mummy, as seen in museums and late-night horror shows. The term comes from a Persian word for bitumen (natural asphalt), reflecting the mistaken notion that ancient Egyptian bodies had been preserved and blackened by soaking in pitch.

For the ancient Egyptians, life after death was of paramount importance, but success in the afterlife depended on preservation of the body so that the soul would have a suitable place to dwell. Within their tombs, wealthy Egyptians were surrounded by grave goods meant to provide for their comforts in the next world. In addition to the treasures that lured grave robbers (and archaeologists) to even the most well-protected tombs, mummies were accompanied by "texts" painted on the walls of their tombs and coffins and written texts known as the Book of the Dead. These "books" contained collections of spells and maps to guide the recently departed along the path taken by the dead. The tombs of some of Egypt's earliest known pharaohs provide evidence of human sacrifices. Scholars concluded that the kings of the first dynasty were already so powerful and so obsessed with the afterlife that court officials, servants, and artisans were killed so that they could serve their ruler in the afterlife. Some of the grave goods included the names and titles of those dispatched to serve their pharaoh.

In predynastic Egypt (before 3100 B.C.E.), bodies were wrapped in skins or linen and interred in shallow graves in the desert. If the body was not discovered by jackals or otherwise disturbed, the hot dry sand would draw out moisture from the soft tissues, leaving the body looking rather like tanned leather, but still recognizable several thousand years later. Simple sand burials continued to be the norm for peasants, but during the Dynastic Period, the burial chambers of pharaohs and other

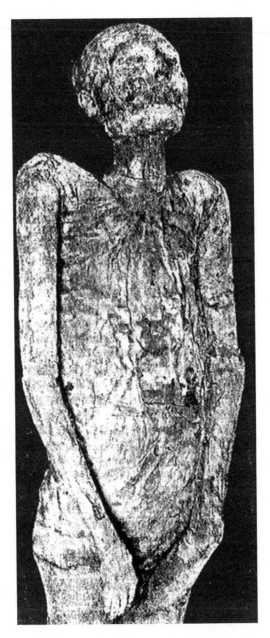

**An Egyptian mummy.**

notable individuals became increasingly elaborate. Unfortunately, putting bodies in relatively cool, damp, underground tombs allowed the forces of putrefaction to prevail. If the pharaoh were to enjoy both an elegant resting place and a well-preserved body, new methods of preparing the corpse for eternal life were essential.

Much has been made of the "mysteries" of Egyptian mummification, but the basic steps were simple: removing the viscera, thoroughly drying the cadaver, and wrapping the desiccated corpse. Over the course of almost three thousand years, the methods and quality of workmanship of the embalmers varied, but the basic methodology remained essentially the same.

Desiccation could have been achieved by techniques used to preserve food and hides, such as salting fish or pickling vegetables. Perhaps there was some aesthetic obstacle to preserving a pharaoh like a pickle. A secret and mysterious procedure would surely provide a better passage to eternity. In place of hot, dry sand, or a vinegar brine, embalmers used natron, a naturally occurring mixture of salts, as a drying agent and removed the organs most susceptible to rapid decay. The heart, which was regarded as the "seat of the mind," was left inside the body.

Herodotus left the best known account of embalming, but his discussion contains much doubtful material and represents a late, possibly degenerate, state of the art. According to Herodotus, there were three methods of mummification, which varied in thoroughness and price. For the "first class" procedure, the embalmers drew out the brain through the nose with an iron hook. The intestines were removed through a cut made along the flank, the abdominal cavity was washed with palm wine and aromatics, the belly was filled with exotic spices, and the eviscerated body was kept in natron for 70 days. When embalming was completed, the corpse was washed, wrapped in bandages of fine linen, smeared with gum, and enclosed in a wooden case shaped like a person.

If the embalmers were asked to follow a more economical course, they would omit the removal of the brain and the incision into the abdominal cavity. Instead, they injected "cedar oil" into the belly through the anus and embalmed the body in natron. Seventy days later, they removed the plug from the anus and allowed the oil and dissolved bowels to escape. The cadaver, now reduced to skin and bones, was returned to the relatives. Poorer people could only expect a simple purge to cleanse the belly and 70 days of embalming.

Herodotus was apparently mistaken about certain details of the embalming process. Other sources indicate that the embalmers used juniper oil rather than cedar oil and that the entire mummification process took 70 days, of which 40 were devoted to dehydrating the body by packing it, inside and out, with bags of natron pellets. Sometimes, the embalmers resorted to simplified procedures, neglecting evisceration and employing onions and garlic in place of the proper aromatic preservatives. Poor workmanship and outright fraud are manifest in mummy packs where the viscera were badly mutilated, bones broken or lost, and animal remains or pieces of wood were used to fill out the form. Chemists have attempted to recreate and analyze the components of ancient preservatives. Some scientists believe that an extract of cedar wood was used because cedar contains a chemical called guaiacol that is not present in juniper oil. Chemists were able to compare their cedar wood preparation with surviving samples of unused embalming material. The cedar wood preparation prevented the growth of bacteria and was quite effective in preserving animal tissues.

One of the most peculiar uses of Egyptian mummies was the medieval practice of grinding mummies into a powder used as a remedy for wounds and bruises. By the end of the sixteenth century, "mummy powder" could be found in every apothecary shop in Europe. The irony of making medicines by destroying remains meant to secure eternal life was noted by English physician Sir Thomas Browne (1605–1682), author of *Religio Medici* (1642), who observed that mummies spared by time and previous conquerors "avarice now consumeth. Mummy is become merchandise . . . and Pharaoh is sold for balsams."

Long after the vogue of "mummy powder" had passed, William Konrad Roentgen's (1845–1923) discovery of X-rays revived Western interest in Egyptian antiquities. During the initial wave of excitement, some eight thousand mummies were studied in a rather crude and hurried manner. At the School of Medicine in Cairo, the formidable trio composed of Sir Grafton Elliot Smith (1871–1937), anatomist, Sir Marc Armand Ruffer (1859–1917), bacteriologist, and Alfred Lucas (1867–1945), chemist, pioneered methods of analyzing mummified tissues and experimented with mummification methods.

More recently, paleopathologists have subjected mummies to X-ray examination, CT scanning, electron microscopy, chemical analyses, immunological evaluations, and other analytic techniques that provide significant data with minimal damage. Biochemical techniques have been used to detect malaria, various forms of anemia, and the eggs of parasitic worms. Well-preserved mummies offer information about parasitic diseases, trauma, infections, metabolic and genetic defects. For example, biochemical studies of the mummy of a man who died about 1500 B.C.E. provided evidence for what is probably the earliest known case of alkaptonuria, a metabolic disease due to the absence of an enzyme needed to break down the amino acids phenylalanine and tyrosine.

The first lessons learned from modern autopsies and X-ray studies of mummies concerned the health hazards associated with the life-giving Nile. The fertile soil and irrigation ditches fed by the Nile River harbored hordes of parasitic worms. Calcified eggs found in mummies reflect the prevalence of schistosomiasis (bilharzia or snail fever) in ancient Egypt. At least five species of schistosomes are known to infect humans: *Schistosoma mansoni, S. japonicum, S. mekongi, S. intercalatum,* and *S. haematobium.* The snail in which the parasitic worm (schistosome) completes an essential stage of its life cycle flourishes in stagnant irrigation canals. Human infections begin when the free-swimming larval form of the parasite penetrates the skin of the new host. Changing form, the parasites enter the capillaries and lymphatic vessels and begin their migration to various organs. Severe infestations can result in damage to the lungs, liver, intestines, and urinary tract. Although schistosomiasis does not kill outright, the chronic irritation caused by the worm and its eggs leads to increasing mental and physical deterioration throughout the victim's life. Mature worms produce eggs throughout their three to five year lifespan. When eggs are excreted in fresh water, they produce a new form that infects certain freshwater snails. After a reproductive stage in the snail, new parasites are produced that attack mammalian hosts and continue the cycle.

Epidemiologists estimate that schistosomiasis now affects about two hundred million people in sub-Saharan Africa, Brazil, Venezuela, the Caribbean, China, Indonesia, the Philippines, Cambodia, and Laos. Despite major advances in control, schistosomiasis continues to spread to new geographic areas. Environmental changes that result from the development of water resources and the growth and migration of populations can facilitate the spread of schistosomiasis. For example, the construction of the Aswan High Dam in Egypt virtually eliminated *S. haematobium* from the Nile Delta, but it allowed the establishment of *S. mansoni* in upper Egypt.

Winds as well as waters were the source of debilitating conditions. Winds blowing in from the desert carried fine particles of sand that lodged in the lungs and caused sand pneumoconiosis, a disorder similar to the black lung disease found among coal miners. Sand pneumoconiosis can be detected by electron microscopy of mummified lung tissue, but because only the elite were mummified, it is not possible to tell how common this disorder was among the masses of peasants. Another disorder of the lungs known as anthrocosis was the result of the inhalation of carbon particles coming from burning wood.

Sand particles found in bread and other foods consumed by both the rich and the poor caused a severe form of dental attrition. Frequent sandstorms contaminated most foodstuffs, adding grit to everything, while the soft stones used for milling grain added their share of residue. Very few mummies had healthy teeth. Sometimes the teeth were so worn down at the crown that the pulp or even the root was exposed. On the other hand, cavities were fairly rare and standards of cleanliness were very high. Obsessive about cleanliness and personal hygiene, the ancient Egyptians used natron as a cleansing agent for the mouth. They also chewed on reeds to cleanse and massage the teeth and gums.

Other disorders found in mummies include tuberculosis, hardening of the arteries, and arthritis. Worn down by these ever present hazards, helpless in the face of disease and traumatic accidents, even the most privileged were unlikely to attain a life span greater than 40 years. Probably few of these ancient Egyptians actually resembled the life-like, idealized portraits that adorned their coffins and tombs. Evidence of atherosclerosis, a condition associated with various disorders of the heart and blood vessels, including stroke, heart attacks, and peripheral vascular disease, has been found in Egyptian mummies. During mummification the aorta was often left in the mummy. Ruffer reported that atheromas, just like those found in the arteries of his contemporaries, could be found in almost all of the arteries he had been able to salvage from Egyptian mummies. Nevertheless, some examples of remarkable longevity did occur. For example, studies of the mummy of Rameses II indicated that he had suffered from arthritis, atherosclerosis, calcification of the temporal arteries, and dental lesions with infectious complications. Although he was presumably physically and mentally feeble during the last years of his life, Rameses II was 90 years of age when he died.

Before the introduction of modern techniques for determining the age of ancient materials, Egyptologists depended on indirect methods, such as evaluating the decorations on the coffin and the name and grave goods of the deceased person. But identifications were generally tentative and sometimes incorrect because many tombs and mummies had been vandalized by grave robbers. Egyptian priests rescued and rewrapped many royal mummies, but the bodies often ended up in mismatched coffins with new identities. Researchers are now able to convert data from CT scans into realistic three-dimensional (3D) images of mummies without removing the outer wrappings. Using this method, scientists can explore previously unknown aspects of Egyptian burial rituals and find artifacts placed inside mummies, such a ceramic bowl that appeared in images of the head of a three thousand-year-old mummy.

Carbon-14 dating can be used to estimate the age of mummies, if uncontaminated samples of flesh or bone collagen are used. But it is difficult to remove impurities from the mummification materials in tissue samples and rather large parts of the body must be sacrificed in order to study bone collagen. X-ray analysis can provide valuable data about medical and dental diseases, estimates of age at death, and morphological variations. It can also spare modern scholars from the embarrassing mistakes that sometimes occurred when nineteenth century archaeologists, trying to enliven their lectures, unwrapped the mummy of some great Egyptian prince only to find the body of a princess or, worse yet, a baboon. In addition to diagnosing the ills of ancient pharaohs, modern medical techniques have been used to "cure" mummies suffering from "museum ailments" caused by improper storage, display, and the ravages of insects, fungi, and bacteria.

The abundance of diseases that flourished in Egypt provides a rationale for Herodotus' observation that the whole country swarmed with highly specialized physicians dedicated to care of the eyes, head, teeth, stomach, and obscure ailments. Not all ancient physicians were specialists, but there is evidence that specialists, lay physicians, priests, and magicians worked in harmony and referred patients to each other as appropriate. One specialist called Iri, Shepherd of the Anus (or Keeper of the Bottom), held a place of honor among court physicians. Often referred to as the first proctologist, the Keeper of the Royal Rectum might have served primarily as the pharaoh's enema-maker. According to Egyptian mythology, the enema itself had a noble origin: it was invented by the god Thot.

High standards of professional behavior were expected of the physician, who was told: "Do not mock at the blind; do not scoff at dwarfs; do not injure the lame, do not sneer at a man who is in the hand of God (of unsound mind)." Medical specialization in ancient Egypt was primarily the result of the religious doctrine that no part of the body was without its own god. Like the gods they served, priest–physicians tended to specialize in a particular organ or disease. Pharmacists traced the origin of their art to Isis, who had imparted the secrets of remedies to her son Horus. All who participated in the work of the Houses of Life attached to the temples, as well as the embalming establishments, claimed the god Anepu as their patron. However, responsibility for the "necessary art" as a whole was eventually ascribed to Imhotep, the first physician known to us by name.

A prodigy and master of all fields of learning, Imhotep designed and built the famous Step Pyramid of Sakkara, served the Pharaoh Zoser (or Djoser, r. 2630–2611 B.C.E.) as vizier, minister of state, architect, chief priest, sage, scribe, magician–physician, and astronomer. Imhotep, no less than Asclepius, the Greek god of medicine, is a powerful symbol and true ancestral god of the healing profession. Imhotep's career as a healer can be divided into three phases: first, as a physician in the court of Zoser; second, as a medical demigod (ca. 2600–525 B.C.E.); and third, as a major deity (ca. 525 B.C.E.–550).

When Imhotep died, the sick flocked to the temple that had been built over his grave. The cult of Imhotep eventually spread from Memphis throughout Egypt and Nubia. Excavations of the temples of Imhotep suggest that "temple sleep," or therapeutic incubation, so closely associated with the Greeks, was really of Egyptian origin. Priests carefully tended to the sick and encouraged their expectation that the god would appear and effect miraculous cures. The priests used "holy water," baths, isolation, silence, suggestion, and therapeutic dreams in their healing rituals. As a god who healed the sick, granted fertility to barren women, protected against misfortune, and gave life to all, Imhotep understandably became one of the most popular gods. Although worship of Imhotep sharply declined by the end of the second century, he remained a major deity in Memphis into the fourth century.

Some scholars have argued that magic was the motive force behind almost all the achievements of the Egyptians, but others have defended

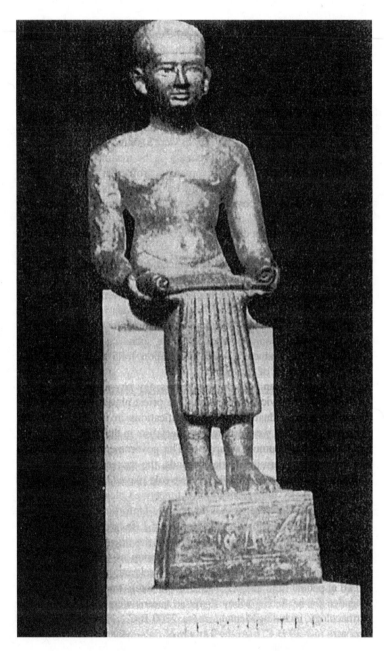

**Imhotep, the Egyptian god of medicine.**

the ancients against the charge that their medicine was little more than superstition and magic. Operating within the context of ancient society, physician and patient expected incantations and charms to increase the efficacy of treatment; certainly they would do no harm. Spells and stories about the healing acts of the gods were a source of comfort and hope that enhanced the effect of remedies and surgical procedures. For example, before changing a bandage, the healer could offer a prayer, such as: "The one whom the god loves, him he shall keep alive." This prayer could be turned into a spell by adding: "It is I whom the god loves, and he shall keep me alive."

Many aspects of the evolution of the medical profession in ancient Egypt remain obscure; even the etymology of the word for physician is unclear. Some scholars interpret the hieroglyph for physician—an arrow, a pot, and a seated man—as "the man of the drugs and lancet," or "opener of the body," while others suggest "man of pain," or "the one who deals with disease." Worse yet, the same term was also used for the "tax valuer."

Priest–physicians were expected to conduct a detailed examination of the patient to observe symptoms and elicit signs. The physician noted general appearance, expression, color, swellings, stiffness, movements, odors, respiration, perspiration, excretions, and listened to the patient's account of the history of the illness. The physician was allowed to touch the patient to study the quality of the pulse, abdomen, tumors, and wounds. Functional tests, such as having the patient move in particular ways, were conducted to elicit information, follow the course of the disease, and evaluate the success of treatment.

Not all of the Egyptian healers were priests; lay physicians and magicians also offered their special services to the sick. The priest–physician enjoyed the highest status, but some individuals acquired qualifications in two or three categories. Physicians and surgeons were assisted by specialists in the art of bandaging, a skill that had its origin in mummy wrapping. The government paid lay physicians to oversee public works, armies, burial grounds, the sacred domains, and the royal palace. Despite uncertainty about the precise role played by the institutions known as the Houses of Life in the religious, medical and intellectual life of ancient Egypt, they seem to have functioned along the lines of an "open college" or "think tank," rather than a formal school or temple. Unfortunately, the collections of papyrus scrolls that were stored at the Houses of Life have not survived.

A woman physician known as Peseshet held the title "Lady Director of Lady Physicians," indicating that Peseshet supervised a group of women practitioners. An interesting group of women surgeons used flint chisels and stick drills with which they worked at a patient until blood was drawn. Such treatments were especially recommended for headache. Many Egyptian queens were well versed in medicine and pharmacology, including Mentuhetep (ca. 2300 B.C.E.), Hatsheput (ca. 1500 B.C.E.), and Cleopatra (60–30 B.C.E.). At the Temple of Sais, near the Rosetta Mouth of the Nile, there was a medical school where

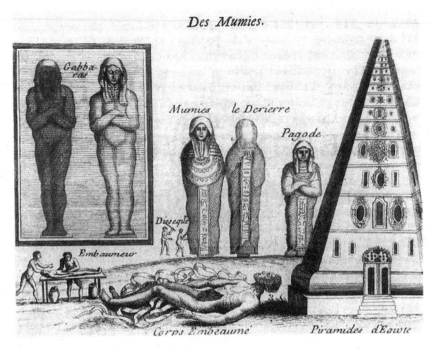

*Des Mumies.*

**Egyptian mummies, pyramids, and the embalming process as depicted in a seventeenth century French engraving.**

women professors taught obstetrics and gynecology to female students. Women may have studied at the medical school at Heliopolis.

According to Egyptian medical theory, human beings were born healthy, but were innately susceptible to disorders caused by intestinal putrefaction, visible or occult external entities, and strong emotions, such as sorrow, unrequited love, and homesickness. The body was constantly threatened by noxious winds caused by changes in the weather, or by spirits and ghosts. Worms and insects represented exogenous causes of disease, but the term *worms* included both real and imaginary agents, or a misperception of bits of tissue, mucus, or blood clots that appeared in feces and wounds. Whether disease was due to visible or occult causes, cure required forcing the morbid agents from the body by purging or exorcism. Healer and patient would expect to see signs of the departing invader in the excretions and secretions of the patient.

Many threats to health were avoidable, intermittent, or random, but intestinal decay was a constant and inescapable danger. Obviously, food was needed to sustain life, but as it passed through the intestinal tract it was subject to the same putrid processes that could be observed in rotting foods, wounds, and unembalmed corpses. If the products of decay were strictly confined to the intestines, eating would not be so dangerous, but putrid intestinal materials often contaminated the system of channels that carried blood, mucus, urine, semen, water, tears, and air throughout the body, causing localized lesions and systemic diseases. Health could only be maintained by frequent use of emetics and laxatives to purge the body of intestinal putrefaction. Convinced that the rectum was a particularly dangerous center of decay, the Egyptians relied on remedies designed to soothe and refresh the orifice and keep it from twisting or slipping. Thus, the Keeper of the Royal Rectum truly deserved the honors due to a specialist with primary responsibility for the health of the pharaoh.

Herodotus noted the Egyptian concern with internal sources of decay and reported that three days each month were set aside for purging the body with emetics and enemas. These prophylactic purges were not the only preventive measures taken by the Egyptians in their pursuit of health. Cleanliness of body was even more valued by the Egyptians than by the Greeks. Rules for the disinfection of dwellings and proper burial of the dead sprang from a combination of hygienic and religious motives. Fear of exacerbating intestinal putrefaction by the ingestion of impure foods and drink encouraged protective food inspection and dietary restrictions. Despite the preoccupation with diet and health, overeating, drunkenness, disorders due to unwholesome foods, famine, and starvation were not uncommon.

Popular accounts of Egyptian medicine have presented it as either "mere superstition" or as a mysteriously advanced science, but neither extreme is correct. The ancient Egyptians could distinguish magic and medicine as separate activities, but they expected the effects of the combination to be synergistic. The efficacy of magic rested upon the spell, the rite, and character of the practitioner. Words used in the spell were so powerful in both their written and spoken forms that objects over which an incantation had been spoken became protective amulets. Spells were recited over a mixture of drugs before giving them to the patient. Many remedies were noxious substances meant to make the patient too repulsive an abode for disease-causing demons. Patients suffering from conditions that might be ascribed to "suggestion," might be challenged or even cured with noxious remedies such as charred beetles mixed with fat. Ritual acts or gestures added power to words. Rituals varied from simple symbolic acts, such as tying knots in a thread in order to bind up the agents of disease, to elaborate ceremonies combining music, dance, drugs, and divination. Other magical methods were based on the principle of transfer. For example, a migraine headache might be transferred to a fish applied to the affected side of the head.

## THE MEDICAL PAPYRI

Unfortunately, except for a few fragmentary medical papyri, the texts used for teaching the art of medicine in the Houses of Life have been lost. The eight surviving medical papyri were composed between about 1900 and 1100 B.C.E., but they are probably compilations and copies of older medical texts. In modern translations, the surviving medical papyri constitute only about two hundred printed pages.

Remedies and case histories taken from the Ebers, Smith, and Kahun papyri provide the most significant insights into ancient Egyptian ideas about health and disease, anatomy and physiology, and magic and medicine. The other medical texts include collections of remedies, aphrodisiacs, incantations against disease, descriptions of fertility tests, and spells for the safety of pregnant women and infants.

The Ebers papyrus, which was probably written about 1500 B.C.E., is the longest, most complete, and most famous of the medical papyri. Named after Georg Ebers, who obtained the papyrus in 1873 and published a facsimile and partial translation two years later, it is an encyclopedic collection of prescriptions, incantations and extracts of medical texts on diseases and surgery taken from at least forty older sources. The Ebers papyrus was apparently planned as a guide for the three kinds of healers: those who dealt with internal and external remedies, surgeons who treated wounds and fractures, and sorcerers or exorcists who wrestled with the demons of disease.

Although the ancients did not see any reason for a strict separation between natural and supernatural diseases, there was a tendency for what might be called "realistic" prescriptions to be grouped together with diseases that could be treated with a reasonable chance of success. Incurable disorders are generally clustered together with more magically oriented practices. Healers were warned against causing additional suffering by undertaking useless treatments. In hopeless cases, ointments and incantations were preferable to the knife.

Many recipes, at least in translation, call for incomprehensible, exotic, or seemingly impossible ingredients, like Thot's Feather and Heaven's Eye, which may have been cryptic or picturesque names for ordinary medicinal herbs. No doubt Egyptian pharmacists would have ridiculed prescriptions calling for "fox's gloves" (digitalis), "pretty lady" (belladonna), or "male duck" (mandrake).

About seven hundred drugs, combined in a variety of ways to create more than eight hundred formulas, are found in the Ebers papyrus. Drugs were administered as pills, ointments, poultices, fumigations, inhalations, snuffs, gargles, suppositories, enemas, and so forth. Physicians apparently relied on specialized assistants and drug collectors, but sometimes they prepared their own remedies. In contrast to Mesopotamian custom, Egyptian prescriptions were precise about quantities.

Although components were usually measured by volume rather than by weight, the instruments used in the preparation of drugs included balances, as well as mortars, mills, and sieves.

Remedies fortified by spells were said to open and close the bowels, induce vomiting, expel worms and demons, cure fevers, rheumatism, cough, bloody urine, dysentery, and a plethora of other diseases. Hemorrhages, wounds, and crocodile bites could be dressed with a mixture of oil, honey, and roasted barley, and covered with fresh meat. Other prescriptions called for crocodile dung, human urine, myrrh, beans, dates, and ostrich eggs. Gold, silver, and precious stones were identified with the flesh and limbs of gods; thus, they were used in amulets and talismans to ward off disease. Less exotic minerals, such as sulfur, natron, and heavy metal salts, were commonly associated with skin diseases, but one interesting ointment called for burnt frog in oil. Minerals were used either in their native form or as powders recycled from broken pottery, bricks, or millstones.

Diseases of the eye were apparently as much a problem in ancient Egypt as they are today in many parts of the Middle East, India, and Africa. Blindness was not uncommon, as indicated by various documents and paintings. For a disorder that was probably night blindness (a common sign of vitamin A deficiency), roasted ox liver was enthusiastically recommended. Another remedy for impaired eyesight consisted of honey, red ochre, and the humor of a pig's eye, which the healer poured into the patient's ear.

Rheumatism is the diagnosis suggested by descriptions of chronic aches and pains in the neck, limbs, and joints. Treatment for this painful condition included massages with clay or mud and ointments containing herbs, animal fat, ox spleen, honey, wine dregs, natron, and various obscure materials. The recommendation that certain remedies be applied to the big toe suggests that gout was one of these painful disorders.

Not all prescriptions in the medical papyri were for life-threatening conditions. The medical texts also contain recipes for cosmetics and hair restoratives, such as a mixture of burnt hedgehog quills mixed with oil. Another ingenious recipe could be applied to the head of a woman one hated in order to make her hair fall out. Cosmetics generally reflect only vanity and the tyranny of fashion, but cleansing unguents, perfumes, and pigments probably had valuable astringent and antiseptic properties.

Another example of the lighter side of ancient medicine comes from the study of masticatories or quids, materials that are chewed but not swallowed. The masticatory favored by the Egyptians was the stem of the papyrus plant. The Greeks thought the Egyptian habit of chewing papyrus stems and spitting out the residue was ludicrous and squalid, until they too took up the custom. Resin-based pellets and balls of natron and frankincense were chewed to purify and sweeten the breath. Other masticatories were said to prevent disorders of the teeth and gums.

The Kahun papyrus, which was probably composed about 1900 B.C.E., consists of fragments dealing with gynecology and veterinary medicine, including methods for detecting pregnancy, predicting the sex of the fetus, and preventing conception. One of the contraceptives was basically a pessary (vaginal suppository) containing crocodile dung. Other prescriptions call for a plug (rather like a contraceptive sponge) made with honey and natron, an extract of the acacia plant, and a gum-like material. Later contraceptive prescriptions kept the spirit of the Egyptian recipe, but substituted elephant dung for that of the crocodile. Greek observers noted that the Egyptians seemed to regulate the size of their families without infanticide. This suggests that even the most noxious and bizarre pessaries might work if they functioned as mechanical barriers, or spermicides, or caused a total lack of interest in sexual intercourse. Prolonged lactation, which tends to suppress ovulation, and a three-year interval between births were considered essential for the health of mother and child.

Although midwives were probably the main childbirth attendants, physicians were acquainted with various gynecological conditions, including prolapse of the uterus, cancer, leucorrhoea, dysmenorrhea, amenorrhea, and menopause. Because the uterus was thought to be a mobile organ that could cause mischief by wandering about the body, doctors prescribed special fumigants to lure it back to its proper position. Complex and noxious mixtures were recommended for wandering uterus, abnormal delivery, and miscarriage. Such remedies were said to warm the breasts, cool the womb, regulate menstruation, and increase milk production. Generally, these medicines were taken as fumigants, douches, or suppositories, but in some cases, the woman simply sat on the remedy. Fertility tests were based on the assumption that in fertile women free passages existed between the genital tract and the rest of the body. Therefore, when the woman sat on a test substance, such as date flour mixed with beer, vomiting proved that conception could occur and the number of vomits corresponded to the number of future children. Once pregnancy was established, the physician studied the effect of the patient's urine on the germination and growth of wheat and barley seedlings in order to predict the sex of the child. Of course, such tests had at least a fifty–fifty chance of being correct.

Ancient texts indicate that women gave birth while squatting on so-called magical bricks decorated with religious symbols and images of the gods that protected the health of mothers and infants. A remarkable example of these birth bricks was discovered by archaeologists excavating the ruins of Abydos, an ancient city in southern Egypt. A painted brick found among the artifacts in a 3,700-year-old house depicted a mother with her newborn baby, female assistants, and Hathor, the cow goddess associated with birth and motherhood. An image of the sun god and his guardians presumably invoked magical protection for the fragile life of the newborn babe.

Egyptian physicians were remarkably specialized, but there is no mention of pediatrics, a field based on the age of the patient rather than specific parts of the body, as a separate area of specialization. There were, however, remedies and spells for the health of infants and prescriptions for obscure childhood diseases, bed-wetting, retention of urine, cough, and teething. For example, chewing on a fried mouse was recommended to ease the pain of cutting teeth and an old letter boiled in oil was said to cure retention of urine. Since the child was commonly breast-fed for three years, remedies could be given to the mother or wet nurse.

Since the Egyptians made mummies of humans and other animals, they had the opportunity to study comparative anatomy. Archaeologists have discovered the skeletons or mummies of lions, baboons, ibis, fish, cats, dogs, and crocodiles in tombs and special cemeteries. Nevertheless, despite centuries of experience with mummification, Egyptian anatomical concepts remained rudimentary. The embalmers, who belonged to a special guild of craftsmen, were not practicing physicians or disinterested scientists. Even the embalmers seem to have been ambivalent about the task of opening the body. As part of the ritual that preceded this act, a man called the scribe drew a mark along the flank. The man who actually made the incision was symbolically abused and driven away with stones and curses.

Haruspicy, divination through the study of animal organs, offered another source of anatomical information. Since the structure, size, and shape of organs used for divination were important omens, haruspicy probably provided a greater impetus to anatomical study than mummification. Support for this hypothesis is found in the animal-like hieroglyphic signs used for human organs. Egyptologists have catalogued names for over a hundred anatomical signs; many names apply to parts of the all-important alimentary canal. The nerves, arteries, and veins, in contrast, were poorly understood and essentially undifferentiated.

Physiological and pathological phenomena were explained in terms of the movement of fluids in a system of channels that brought nourishment to the body just as the flooding of the Nile brought nourishment to the land. A complicated system of vessels carried blood, mucus, water, air, semen, urine, and tears. The heart, the "seat of the mind," was clearly regarded as a major gathering place for the vessels, but there was another confluence of channels in the vicinity of the anus. Because the rectum and anus were associated with dangerous decaying matter, the arrangement of the vessels exposed the entire system to contamination with the products of internal decay.

As a sign of its special significance, the heart was left in the body during mummification. "Weighing the heart" was an important step in the judgment of the dead by the gods. Afraid that their hearts might not measure up, the Egyptians carefully fortified their tombs with magical amulets designed to secure successful judgments. By weighing the heart of the dead, the gods could measure their moral worth. In the living, the physician measured health by placing his fingers on the pulses of the head, neck, stomach, and limbs, because the heart spoke out through the vessels of the body. Indeed, knowledge of the heart and its movements was called the "physician's secret." The physician knew that fainting occurred when the heart could no longer speak. If the heart and its vessels became contaminated with decaying matter or heat from the rectum, the patient would experience illness, debility, and ultimately loss of consciousness.

In 1862, Edwin Smith (1822–1906), a pioneer Egyptologist, purchased a papyrus scroll that had been found in a grave near Luxor. Smith's attempts to decipher the document were not very successful. But when James Henry Breasted (1865–1935) completed his translation of the scroll in 1930, he revolutionized ideas about the relative weight of magic, empiricism, and surgery in Egyptian medicine. Breasted envisioned the Smith papyrus as a document in a class by itself, because it was a systematic collection of case histories that offered the physician important anatomical and physiological information. Sections of the Smith papyrus were copied from texts so ancient that the idioms and concepts in the originals had already become virtually incomprehensible. Therefore, the scribe who compiled the document had to include explanations that would make the text useful to his contemporaries, thus providing valuable information for modern Egyptologists.

The 48 cases preserved in the Smith papyrus were arranged systematically from head to foot in order of severity. Each case consists of a title, instructions to the physician, the probable prognosis, and the proper treatment. Ailments were divided into three categories: those that were almost definitely curable, those that were treatable, but uncertain, and incurable disorders for which no treatment should be attempted.

The section called the "Book of Wounds" describes treatments for fractures, dislocations, bites, tumors, ulcers, and abscesses. Broken bones were set in splints made from ox bones, supported by bandages soaked in quick-setting resin. Recognizing the poor prognosis for compound or open fractures (fractures in which the broken ends of the bone have pierced the skin), the doctor who was prepared to "contend with" simple or closed fractures considered an open fracture an ailment beyond treatment. Plasters or adhesive bandages were generally used to close wounds, but some injuries called for sutures. The Egyptian surgeon used a variety of bandages, adhesive plasters, splints, braces, drains, plugs, cleansers, and cauteries, as well as bronze implements, including scalpels and needles. Excavations at the tomb of a Fifth Dynasty physician revealed many bronze surgical implements, as well as statues of gods and goddesses.

Although the Egyptians were familiar with the sedative effects of opium and henbane, there is no direct evidence of their use as surgical anesthetics. A scene depicting male circumcision accompanied by a text that states: "This is to render it agreeable," has been interpreted as evidence of anesthesia. However, the inscription that accompanies a similar depiction of this operation says: "Hold him so that he does not fall." Since circumcision was a religious ritual, it fell within the province of the priest and would not be discussed in a medical treatise. The surgical tools used in circumcision are shown in some Egyptian temples. One illustration seems to represent an initiation ritual, but there is debate about whether a priest is being circumcised or doing a circumcision.

Although Amenhotep II and III were circumcised, the mummies presumed to be those of their predecessors, Amenhotep I and Ahmose I, were uncircumcised. Studies of early male mummies indicate that male circumcision was not uncommon in the Old Kingdom, but the practice was probably more common among priests and royalty in later periods. Although there are panels depicting the male operation, no such pictures of female circumcision, now generally known as female genital mutilation, are known. Even today there is a similar pattern; the circumcision of a boy is a public celebration, but that of a girl is conducted privately, without celebration.

Female circumcision, which consists of excising the clitoris and other external female genitalia, persists in the region today. Infibulation, the most extreme form of female genital mutilation involves removing the entire clitoris, the labia minora, and parts of the labia majora. The Greek geographer Strabo, who visited Egypt about 25 B.C.E., reported that it was customary among the Egyptians to circumcise male children and excise females. The operation was generally done when children were about 14 and almost ready for adult roles.

Unfortunately, the "Books of Wounds" is incomplete. The scribe apparently stopped writing in the middle of an interesting account of afflictions of the spine and left the rest of that "page" blank. When he resumed work, he apparently turned to another source and copied out recipes to "transform an old man into a youth of twenty" and incantations against "the wind of the pest of the year." This abrupt transition may be symptomatic of the gradual transformation of priorities in Egyptian culture over the millennia, during which engineering, astronomy, science, and medicine stagnated, while superstition and magic flourished.

In 322 B.C.E. Alexander the Great (356–323 B.C.E.) conquered Egypt and brought it into the sphere of Hellenistic culture. How much the

Greeks learned from the Egyptians and how much they taught them is difficult to determine. By this late stage, much of the esoteric knowledge of ancient Egypt had been forgotten, although medicine, mathematics, and technology would flourish once again, at least for a brief time, in the great city of Alexandria in Egypt. Under the Roman Empire, Egypt played an important role in the network of maritime and overland trade routes that linked Rome to Arabia and India, as well as Egypt. Trade items included ivory, tortoise shells, drugs, slaves, peppercorns, frankincense, and myrrh. Port cities along the Egyptian shore of the Red Sea supported maritime trade routes that rivaled the Silk Road, but they were eventually abandoned, buried by desert sands, and forgotten.

## SUGGESTED READINGS

Andrews, C. (1978). *Egyptian Mummies.* Cambridge, MA: Harvard University Press.

Avalos, H. (1995). *Illness and Health Care in the Ancient Near East: The Role of the Temple in Greece, Mesopotamia, and Israel.* Atlanta, GA: Scholars Press.

Bottéro, J. (2001). *Everyday Life in Ancient Mesopotamia.* Baltimore, MD: Johns Hopkins University Press.

Breasted, J. H., ed. (2001). *Ancient Records of Egypt.* Urbana, IL: University of Illinois Press.

Brothwell, D. R., and Chiarelli, B. A., eds. (1973). *Population Biology of the Ancient Egyptians.* New York: Academic Press.

Brothwell, D. R., and Sandison, A. T., eds. (1967). *Diseases in Antiquity. A Survey of the Diseases, Injuries, and Surgery of Early Populations.* Springfield, IL: C. C. Thomas.

Bryan, C. P. (1974). *Ancient Egyptian Medicine: The Papyrus Ebers.* Chicago, IL: Ares Publishers.

Bucaille, M. (1991). *Mummies of the Pharaohs. Modern Medical Investigation* (Trans. by A. D. Pannell and M. Bucaille). New York: St. Martin's Press.

Cockburn, A., and Cockburn, E., eds. (1980). *Mummies, Disease, and Ancient Cultures.* Cambridge: Cambridge University Press.

Ehrich, R. W., ed. (1992). *Chronologies in Old World Archaeology*, 3rd ed. Chicago, IL: University of Chicago Press.

Estes, J. W. (1990). *The Medical Skills of Ancient Egypt.* Massachusetts: Science History Publications/Neal Watson.

Foster, B. R., Frayne, D., and Beckman, G. M., eds. (2001). *The Epic of Gilgamesh: A New Translation, Analogues, Criticism.* New York: Norton.

Ghalioungui, P. (1973). *The House of Life: Magic and Medical Science in Ancient Egypt.* Amsterdam: B. M. Israel.

Ghalioungui, P. (1987). *The Ebers Papyrus: A New English Translation, Commentaries and Glossaries.* Cairo: Academy of Scientific Research and Technology.

Harris, J. E., and Wente, E. F. (1980). *An X-Ray Atlas of the Royal Mummies.* Chicago, IL: University of Chicago Press.

Hurry, J. B. (1978). *Imhotep, the Vizier and Physician of King Zoser, and Afterwards the Egyptian God of Medicine.* New York: AMS Press.

Johns, C. H. W., trans. (2000). *The Oldest Code of Laws in the World: The Code of Laws Promulgated by Hammurabi, King of Babylon, B.C. 2285–2242.* Union, NJ: Lawbook Exchange, Ltd.

Majno, G. (1975). *The Healing Hand. Man and Wound in the Ancient World.* Cambridge, MA: Harvard University Press.

Nunn, J. F. (1996). *Ancient Egyptian Medicine.* Norman, OK: University of Oklahoma Press.

Oppenheim, A. L. (1976). *Ancient Mesopotamia: Portrait of a Dead Civilization.* Chicago, IL: University of Chicago Press.

Romm, J. S. (1998). *Herodotus.* New Haven, CT: Yale University Press.

Ruffer, M. A. (1921). *Studies in the Paleopathology of Egypt.* Edited by R. L. Moodie. Chicago, IL: University of Chicago Press.

Schrnandt-Besserat, D. (1996). *How Writing Came About.* Austin, TX: University of Texas Press.

# 3

# The Medical Traditions
# of India and China

In surveys of the history of medicine, the invention of science and rational medicine was generally credited to the Greek natural philosophers who lived during the sixth century B.C.E. Accustomed to tracing the roots of Western culture back to Greece, with some slight concessions to those civilizations mentioned in the Bible, European scholars generally ignored the evolution of medicine, science, and philosophy in India and China. This peculiarly narrow focus is especially unfortunate in the history of medicine because, unlike the ancient medical traditions of Mesopotamia and Egypt, those of India and China are still very much alive. Recent scholarship, however, has made it clear that the very different paths taken in pursuit of health, healing, and systematic inquiry in China and India are well worth exploring. Historians have come to realize that the scientific and medical traditions that developed in China and India were complex, productive, and different from European traditions in fundamental respects. Many questions remain, but there is little doubt that the most interesting questions about the evolution of science and medicine in different civilizations are related to what thinkers, investigators, and healers in ancient cultures thought they were doing, rather than the trivial question of who did what first.

## INDIA

Densely populated, with a mixture of races, languages, cultures, and religions, the Indian subcontinent is a world of bewildering complexity. In the 1920s, the study of Indian history was revolutionized by the discovery of the wonders of Mohenjo-daro and Harappa, two major cities that were part of the forgotten Indus River Civilization that had flourished from about 2700 to 1500 B.C.E. Recent excavations are now yielding evidence of the extensive trade relations that existed between Egypt and India some two thousand years ago. Scholars previously assumed that the ancient maritime trade between India and Rome was the product of Roman enterprise, but studies of once thriving Egyptian port cities suggest that the ships involved in these long and dangerous voyages might have been built in India and operated by Indian crews. The Silk Road, an Asian network of camel caravan routes, served as the primary cultural and commercial link between China and Europe between about 100 B.C.E. and the fifteenth century. However, the maritime trade route between Egypt and India might have served as another link with the Far East.

Memories of the growth, turmoil, and decay that characterized early Indian civilization have survived in the form of four texts known as the *Vedas*, which are revered by the Hindus as sacred books of divinely inspired wisdom. The *Vedas* are accompanied by later commentaries known as the *Brahmanas* and the *Upanishads*, which explain the older texts and speculate about the nature of the universe and the human condition. The traditional Indian healing art is known as *Ayurvedic* medicine.

Many aspects of Indian history are vague until the fourth and third centuries B.C.E., when the Indus Valley region was conquered, first by the Persians and then by the forces of Alexander the Great (356–323 B.C.E.). Although Alexander spent less than two years in India, the invasion led to cultural exchanges between the Greek-speaking world and the peoples of India. During the turmoil that followed the death of Alexander, Chandragupta Maurya was able to drive out the remaining Macedonian officials and establish his own empire. His grandson, Asoka, who reigned from about 272 to 232 B.C.E., was able to bring most of India under the domination of the Maurya Dynasty. The *Artha Sastra*, on the science of politics and administration, is said to have been written for Chandragupta. It contains many laws that are of interest to the history of medicine, such as those regulating medical practitioners, midwives, nurses, drugs and poisons, prostitution, sanitation, and public health. The judicial mutilations prescribed for improper behaviors would have provided employment for legions of surgeons. For example, the penalty for a person who had insulted his parents or teachers was amputation of the tongue.

Initially regarded as a cruel despot, King Asoka became so overwhelmed with remorse over the bloodshed and misery he had caused that he renounced warfare and became a Buddhist. Buddhism originated in India in the sixth century B.C.E. in the teachings of Buddha, "The Enlightened One," and developed as a protest against the strict stratification of Hindu society and the religious rituals controlled by the Brahmanic priests.

Buddha's teachings emphasized universal love, service, and the peace of mind brought about by the abandonment of desire. According to the great stone edicts posted throughout his empire, Asoka devoted himself to peace and righteousness through good deeds, compassion, religious tolerance, and purity. Giving up the sport of hunting and the eating of flesh, Asoka offered animals as well as humans his protection and established rest houses, facilities for the care of the sick, and other charitable institutions.

Although the edicts of Asoka suggest that free hospitals and dispensaries were widely distributed throughout ancient India, other lines of evidence are ambiguous. One fifth-century Chinese traveler described Indian hospitals that cared for the poor and the sick, but noted that these institutions were privately endowed rather than state supported. Other observers commented on rest houses sponsored by the king where travelers and the poor could find physicians and medicines, as well as food and drink. Medical aid was apparently available at some temples and schools. Charitable hospitals seem to have been more characteristic of neighboring countries that imported Buddhism and Indian medical philosophy. Later visitors to India were amazed to find hospitals for animals and asserted that charity and mercy were more likely to be given to cows and dogs than to human beings.

During the reign of Asoka, Buddhist monks held the great "Council of Patna" (250 B.C.E.) to determine which texts should be regarded as authentic tenets of their religion and how its members should be organized. Buddhist missionaries traveled to Syria, Egypt, Greece, Tibet, and China. Although Buddhism became well established in other parts of the world, in India the ancient Vedic traditions eventually reasserted themselves. After the reign of Asoka, the history of India became a series of assassinations, betrayals, and invasions by Greeks, Scythians, Muslims, Mongols, and Europeans. Independence from Great Britain in 1947 led to riots, mass migrations, massacres, and ultimately partition into Hindu and Muslim regions. In 1950, India became a sovereign democratic republic; Pakistan became a separate Islamic republic in 1956.

Thus, although Buddhism exerted a profound impact in many of the countries that imported both Buddhism and Indian medicine, Ayurvedic medicine remained intimately linked to Hindu religious traditions. The universe portrayed by Indian religions was of immense size and antiquity, undergoing endless cycles of development and decay. Human beings were enmeshed in this universal cycle by reincarnation into positions higher or lower in the complex caste system. As interpreted by Brahmanic priests, India's caste system was a reflection of the order of nature found in the hymn of creation in the *Rigveda*. From the sacrifice that created the world, the *brahmans* (priests) arose from the head, the *kshatriyas* (warriors and nobles) from the arms, the *vaisyas* (farmers, merchants, and craftsmen) from the thighs, and the *sudras* (laborers, servants, and slaves) from the feet. The four major castes gave rise to more than three thousand subcastes and the "untouchables."

Growing within and beyond the boundaries of the mythic lore and epic battles of gods, conquerors, and castes, Indian medicine developed in a series of distinct phases: prehistoric, Vedic, and Ayurvedic. According to Hindu mythology, Brahma, the First Teacher of the Universe, was the author of *Ayurveda,* or *The Science of Life,* an epic consisting of a hundred thousand hymns and the source of all knowledge pertaining to drugs and medicine. The divine sage Dhanvantari, who arose from the cosmic ocean bearing the miraculous potion that conferred immortality on the gods, taught Ayurvedic lore to a long line of sages before it was finally committed to writing. The texts that have survived are said to be only shadows of the lost *Ayurveda* composed by Brahma.

While the authorship and time of composition of the *Vedas* cannot be determined with any precision, the *Rigveda* is said to represent materials from the period 4500 to 2000 B.C.E. and the *Atharvaveda* is probably a compilation of materials created during the period from 1500 to 1000 B.C.E. In Vedic hymns and legends, gods and healers wrestled with demonic forces and performed rites that consecrated mysterious remedies against disease and pestilence. All medicines, including more than a thousand healing herbs, were said to be derived from heaven, earth, and water. Although the origin of Ayurvedic theory is uncertain, its materia medica may have evolved from Vedic or even prehistoric drug lore.

The *Vedas* contain many references to medical lore, anatomy, wounds, diseases, healers, demons, drugs, charms, and spells. Along with a complex pantheon of gods, the ancient Hindus believed in a vast array of disease-causing demons. Because disease was the result of sin or the work of demons, cure required confession, spells, incantations, and exorcism. Vedic healers prepared herbal remedies and charms against the demons that caused fevers, fractures, wounds, and venomous bites. Specific remedies and surgical techniques could only be therapeutic when combined with the appropriate ritual, but the roles of magicians, physicians, and surgeons were differentiated to some extent. Surgeons treated wounds and snakebites, removed injured eyes, extracted arrows, amputated limbs, and fitted patients with artificial legs. If the skulls discovered at two Harappan sites are representative of a lost tradition, Indian surgeons also practiced trepanation.

Additional insights into the practice of Indian medicine and surgery can be gleaned from ancient laws, monuments, inscriptions, surgical instruments, artwork, and the stories told by travelers, pilgrims, and foreign invaders. A study of contemporary folklore and the work of traditional healers may also throw light on ancient practices. However, the most direct guide to ancient Indian medicine is found in the classics of Ayurvedic medicine. These texts are fundamental sources

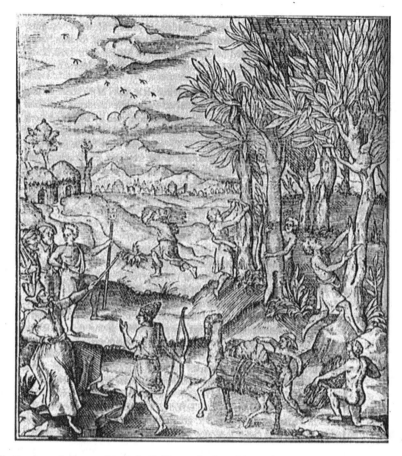

**Gathering cinnamon bark in India as depicted in a sixteenth century woodcut.**

for a civilization in which the oral tradition remained a dominant force, but given the complexity of Indian history and the diversity of its cultures, they must be regarded as portraits of the ideal physician rather than the typical practitioner.

## AYURVEDIC MEDICINE, THE SCIENCE OF LIFE

Ayurveda, the learned system that forms the basis of the traditional medicine widely practiced in India today, is called "the science of life." The practitioner who has come to understand the science of life is known as the *vaidya*. The physician, the medicine, the attendant, and the patient constitute the four pillars of Ayurvedic medicine. The task of the physician was to exercise good judgment about his duties, the attendant was expected to prepare medicines and perform nursing duties, and the patient's role was to provide an accurate history of the disease and follow the physician's instructions. It was important for the physician to assess his patient and his assistant carefully, because when therapy was unsuccessful only the physician's competence would be questioned.

Properly speaking, Ayurveda is composed of eight branches: internal medicine, diseases of the head, surgery, toxicology, demonic diseases, pediatrics, rejuvenation, and aphrodisiacs. The primary objective of the science of life was the maintenance of health, rather than the treatment of disease. Health was not simply the absence of disease, but a state attained and enjoyed only by vigorous pursuit of an elaborate, individualized program of prophylactic measures prescribed by the Ayurvedic doctor.

Caraka, Susruta, and Vagbhata, the semilegendary authors of the classic texts that illuminate the eight branches of Ayurvedic medicine, are honored as the "Triad of Ancients." Although many colorful stories have become associated with these sages, there is little definitive biographical information about any of them. Traditionally, Caraka is said to have lived sometime between 1000 and 800 B.C.E., but Western scholars have placed him as late as the first century. In any case, the *Caraka Samhita* (the collected writings attributed to Caraka) probably reached its present form in the first century. Honored as the first great treatise of Indian medicine, the text describes hundreds of drugs and classifies them in terms of the diseases for which they are useful.

Susruta is said to have practiced medicine and surgery about 600 B.C.E. While the *Susruta Samhita* (the collected writings attributed to Susruta) might be considered more systematic than the *Caraka Samhita* in its treatment of pharmacology, its emphasis on the art of surgery is of particular interest. Because Vagbhata's text mentions both Caraka and Susruta, he is obviously the most recent author, but his biography is similarly obscure. Other classics of Ayurveda dealt with obstetrics, gynecology, and pediatrics. A fourteenth century text still popular with practicing vaidyas includes a description of pulse diagnosis, which reflects the absorption and adaptation of foreign techniques into Ayurvedic theory and practice.

According to Caraka, the attainment and maintenance of health and happiness was a necessary and noble pursuit. Diseases obstructed the attainment of humanity's highest goals, but Ayurveda, the most sacred of the sciences, benefited human beings in their present and future lives. The *Caraka Samhita* provides a guide to the three forms of medicine: mantras and religious acts; diet and drugs; and psychic therapy, or subjection of the mind.

Both Caraka and Susruta devoted considerable attention to the characteristics that distinguished the true physician from pretenders to the art. Understanding the anatomy, physiology, and development of the human body, as well as the origin and evolution of the universe, a wise physician was never in doubt about the etiology of disease, recognized the earliest and most subtle signs and symptoms, and knew which diseases were easily cured and which were incurable.

Because physicians were members of a professional group rather than a specific caste, a practitioner could accept students from all of the three upper castes. Students were expected to live with and serve their teacher until the master was satisfied that their training was complete. Access to the classics could only be obtained by listening to a master physician read and explain the texts. It was the student's duty to memorize the sacred texts and demonstrate competence in medicine and surgery. Using fruits, vegetables, meats, and manikins, the apprentice developed his surgical skills before operating on patients. For example, he learned to make incisions by operating on cucumbers and practiced venesection on the veins of dead animals or lotus stems.

The good physician exhibited four primary qualifications: theoretical knowledge, clarity of reasoning, wide practical experience, and personal skill. Sympathetic and kind to all patients, the physician devoted himself to those who could be cured while maintaining a sense of detachment toward those who would die. The surgeon must have courage, steady hands, sharp instruments, a calm demeanor, unshakable self-confidence, and the services of strong-nerved assistants. Although the physician must never desert or injure a patient, he was not obligated to accept patients who were known criminals, or those suffering from incurable diseases. Yet, the ideal doctor would strive with all his might to cure his patient even if he placed his own life at risk.

Ayurvedic physiology explained bodily functions in terms of the three *dosas*, the primary fluids, humors, or principles—*vata*, *pitta*, and *kapha*—which are usually translated as wind, bile, and phlegm. Although the basic principles of Indian humoral pathology are similar to those of Greek medicine, the Ayurvedic system provides additional complications. The three Ayurvedic humors, in combination with blood, determined all vital functions. The body was composed of a combination of the five elements—earth, water, fire, wind, and empty space—and the seven basic tissues. Bodily functions were also dependent on five separate winds, the vital soul, and the inmost soul. Some Ayurvedic healers were interested in the art of pulse diagnosis, life breath (*prana*), and channels (*nadis*), concepts that are reminiscent of classical Chinese medical theory.

Health was the result of a delicate and harmonious balance among the primary humors that was easily disturbed by accidents, wounds, stress, and demonic possession. Thus, illness could be thought of as the result of an imbalance among wind, bile, and phlegm, or, in a more philosophical exposition, as the physiological result of abuse of the body, errors in judgment, and the passage of time. The degree of derangement determined whether the disease would be minor, major, or incurable. Except for a few perfectly balanced individuals, all human beings were born with some degree of discord among the three humors that created a predisposition to particular diseases. Discord among the three humors produced a disturbance in the blood. Therefore, the physician had to remove "bad blood" by venesection or leeching, and restore humoral balance by prescribing an appropriate diet.

Choosing a proper dietary regimen was a formidable task that had religious as well as medical and physiological aspects. Although there is no doubt among historians that the early Hindus ate meat, modern Hindu fundamentalists consider vegetarianism and the prohibition on beef-eating hallmarks of Hindu identity. In several Indian states, it is against the law to kill a cow. Yet, evidence from the Vedas, epic poems, and archaeological sites indicates that the "holiness" of the cow is a relatively recent myth. Early Indian traditions included the sacrifice of oxen and other animals to Vedic gods, and the consumption of such animals as part of the ordinary diet. Some historians believe that the taboo on meat-eating was the result of the evolution of the Hindu, Buddhist, and Jain doctrines of reincarnation and nonviolence. Themes woven throughout the Indian medical classics suggest a fundamental relationship between foods and the cosmological order. Vegetarianism, nonviolence, and compassion for all beings were fundamental to health, healing, and the social order. Nevertheless, Ayurvedic prescriptions sometimes contradicted the ideal Hindu concept of nonviolence and vegetarianism. For particular patients, the physician might even prescribe broths made from lion or tiger meat.

Diagnosis was a daunting mission; more than a thousand diseases were alluded to in the ancient texts. Fever was given pride of place as the "king of all bodily diseases." When the fever was intermittent, the intervals between the peak periods provided the key to prognosis. Interest in the intervals between episodes of fever, which is also found in Greek medicine, probably reflects experience with the patterns of malarial fevers.

Accurate diagnosis was the key to selecting the proper treatment for curable disease. After listening closely to the patient's narrative concerning the illness, the physician studied the patient's general appearance, abnormalities, internal noises, blood, body fluids, and excretions. The physician employed palpation (touch) and auscultation (listening), elicited latent symptoms by using drugs as therapeutic tests, and assessed the odor and taste of secretions and discharges. If a physician did not want to taste the secretions himself, he could assign this task to his students, or feed them to insects and observe their reactions. The most famous diagnostic taste test provided information about the "honey urine disease," which presumably was the disease now known as diabetes. Contemporary Ayurvedic practitioners assert that recognition of the microbial origin and infective nature of certain diseases is implicit in the classics texts. Perhaps the ancients suspected a parasitic origin for leprosy and smallpox, but the "parasitic agents" that transmitted epidemic diseases were more likely to be disease-causing demons than micro-organisms. Nevertheless, methods of coping with an invisible demonic agent may be quite effective against microbes. For example, rituals performed while worshiping the goddess Sitala might have included inoculation for smallpox.

The art of therapeutics incorporated the five canonical therapies. Various kinds of massage, anointment with oils, and yoga were regarded as therapeutic. For example, yoga, a complex system of postures, meditation, and breath control, was used to calm the mind and establish harmony between mind and body. Contemporary advocates of yoga claim that it promotes good health and has therapeutic value in the treatment of physical, psychosomatic, and psychiatric disorders. Originally, however, yoga developed as a means of self-realization, rather than a therapeutic approach. Some forms of yoga, such as Kundalini Yoga, which is part of Tantra Yoga, are said to specifically promote mental health and the functioning of the nervous system. Tantra Yoga teaches that the body contains six nerve centers, or *chakras*. This form of yoga was popularized by Sir John Woodroff (Arthur Avalon), author of *The Serpent Power* (1919). Practitioners of this form of yoga expected to experience a remarkable sense of awakening or even the release of supernatural powers by stimulating the Kundalini power and directing it toward the brain.

A wealth of remedies, all part of Ayurvedic pharmacology, allowed Caraka to assert that with proper treatment even aged and infirm patients might regain youthful powers. Almost one thousand drugs derived from plant sources are referred to in the major Ayurvedic classics, but many are unidentifiable materials or "divine drugs" such as soma. Vedic myths say that Brahma created soma to prevent old age and death, but the identity of this "king of plants" was a mystery to later sages. Healers also prepared remedies based on minerals, gems, metals, and animal products, such as honey, milk, snakeskin, and excrements. For diseases involving corruption of the bodily humors, the proper remedies included internal cleansing, external cleansing, and surgery. Diseases caused by improper diet called for remedies that accomplished internal cleansing, but physicians often began treatment with a seven-day fast. Some patients recovered during this period and needed no other remedies; presumably, some died and also needed no further remedies.

Mundane drugs typically came from well-known plants. Some were assigned multiple uses. For example, senna, which was prepared from cassia, was probably used by Ayurvedic healers for at least two thousand years. Recipes including senna were recommended as laxatives, and for skin diseases, eye problems, coughing, and fevers. Another traditional Indian medicine made from the resin of a tree that grows in India, Pakistan, and Afghanistan has been used to treat various illnesses for two thousand years. Scientists who have been searching for pharmacological agents in traditional remedies discovered that sap from the guggul tree (*Commiphora mukul*) contains a compound that helps regulate cholesterol levels.

## SURGERY, ANATOMY, AND DISSECTION

Perhaps the most striking aspect of ancient Indian medicine was the range of surgical interventions and the level of success claimed by the disciples of Susruta and Caraka. Vedic myths speak of remarkable operations on men and gods, such as a cure for impotence achieved by transplanting the testes of a ram to the afflicted god Indra. Ayurvedic texts describe more prosaic but still formidable operations such as cesarean section, lithotomy (removal of bladder stones), couching the cataract, tonsillectomy, amputations, and plastic surgery. Thus, the Ayurvedic surgical tradition offers an interesting challenge to Western assumptions that systematic human dissection, animal vivisection, and the rejection of humoral pathology are essential for progress in surgery. In ancient India, surgeons mastered many major operations without these supposed prerequisites.

While the therapeutic use of the knife was accepted in India, for the upper castes contact with cadavers and use of the knife on the dead were prohibited by custom and religion. Nevertheless, Susruta taught that physicians and surgeons must study the human body by direct observation in order to gain essential knowledge of the structure and function of its parts. While acknowledging religious prohibitions against contact with dead bodies, Susruta justified the study of anatomy—the science of being—as a form of knowledge linked to higher phenomena, including the relationship between humans and gods.

Ingeniously working his way around religious prohibitions against the use of the knife on dead bodies, Susruta proposed an unusual form of anatomical investigation. If a body was complete in all its parts, neither too old nor too young, and if death had not been caused by protracted illness or poison, it was suitable for dissection. After removing the excrements from the intestines, the anatomist should cover the body with grasses, place it in a cage made of fine mesh, and leave it to steep in a quiet pond. Seven days later the anatomist could gradually remove successive layers of skin and muscle by gently rubbing the body with soft brushes. According to Susruta, this process rendered the most minute parts of the body distinct and palpable. There is, however, little evidence that teachers of Ayurvedic medicine followed Susruta's prescription for human dissection.

One aspect of human anatomy that all students were expected to have mastered was the complex system of "vital points," or *marmas*, distributed throughout the body. The *marmas* appear to be sites where major veins, arteries, ligaments, joints, and muscles unite and where injuries are likely to be incapacitating or fatal. The classical system included 107 points, each of which had a specific name and special properties. When examining an injured patient, the physician's first task was to determine whether a wound corresponded to one of the *marmas*. If injury to a *marma* would lead to death, the surgeon might amputate the limb at an auspicious site above the *marma*. In venesection, or any form of surgical intervention, the surgeon had to avoid damage to the *marmas*.

Bleeding and cauterization were among the most routine surgical operations. Cauterization, Susruta taught, was the method of choice for treating hemorrhages and diseases that resisted medicinal remedies. Moreover, he believed that the healing properties of the actual cautery (red-hot irons) were vastly superior to those of the potential cautery (chemically induced burns). Bloodletting was considered an excellent remedy, but it had to be done cautiously because blood was the source of strength, vitality, and longevity. Leeching was recommended as the most propitious form of bleeding, because leeches were thought to have a preference for vitiated blood rather than healthy blood.

According to Susruta, all surgical operations could be described in terms of their most basic techniques. That is, all operations were variations on excising, incising, probing, scarifying, suturing, puncturing, extracting solid bodies, and evacuating fluids. Preparations for any surgical operation were exacting, involving special attention to the patient, the operating room, and the "one hundred and one" surgical instruments. One reason for the large number of surgical tools was the preference for instruments resembling various animals. If the lion-mouth forceps did not fit the task, the surgeon could try the hawk, heron, or crocodile-mouth version. Surgeons also needed tables of different shapes and sizes for particular operations and a "fracture-bed" for stretching fractured or dislocated limbs. Above all, the surgeon must see to it that the room used for surgery was carefully prepared to insure cleanliness and comfort.

Medical care of pregnant women encompassed efforts to ensure male offspring, management of diet, easing the pains of labor, safe delivery, and the postnatal care of mother and child. Normally, childbirth was managed by midwives, but in difficult deliveries, a surgeon might be needed to perform operations in which the fetus was turned, flexed, mutilated, or destroyed. If natural delivery was impossible, or if the mother died in childbirth, Susruta recommended cesarean section. Certain signs foretold the outcome of pregnancy. If, for example, the mother was violent and bad-tempered, the child might be epileptic, while the child of an alcoholic woman would suffer from weak memory and constant thirst. Failure to gratify the wishes of a pregnant woman might cause the child to be mute, lame, or hunchbacked. A malformed child might also be the result of misdeeds in a prior life, physical or emotional injury to the mother, or an aggravated condition of the three humors.

Indian surgeons apparently developed techniques for dealing with the major problems of surgery, that is, pain and infection. Fumigation of the sickroom and the wound before surgery in the pursuit of cleanliness might have reduced the dangers of infection, but the effectiveness of such techniques is an open question. Claims that the ancients had discovered potent and reliable anesthetic agents are likely to be somewhat exaggerated, since both Caraka and Susruta recommended wine before surgery to prevent fainting and afterwards to deaden pain. In some cases, patients had to be bound hand and foot in preparation for surgery. Burning Indian hemp (marijuana) may have released narcotic fumes, but references to drugs called "producer of unconsciousness" and "restorer of life" remain obscure.

The *Susruta Samhita* describes many difficult operations, such as couching the cataract, lithotomy, opening the chest to drain pus, and the repair of torn bellies and intestines. Various kinds of threads and needles were used for closing wounds, but when the intestines were torn, large black ants were recommended as wound clips. Plastic surgery, especially the art of reconstructing noses, lips, and ears, was probably the most remarkable aspect of the Indian doctor's achievements. Noses and ears were at risk among Indian warriors, who worked without protective masks or helmets, and among the general run of sinners and criminals. In India, as in Mesopotamia, justice was meted out by mutilation and amputation. Even those who led peaceful, blameless lives might need a plastic surgeon. For example, earlobes were sometimes stretched beyond endurance by the large, heavy earrings worn to ward off misfortune.

Repairs of noses, lips, and ears were made with the "sensible skin-flap" technique. Using a leaf as his template, the surgeon would tease out a patch of "living flesh" (now called a pedicle flap) from the patient's cheek or forehead in order to create a new nose. After scarifying the patch, the physician quickly attached it to the site of the severed nose and covered the wound with an aesthetically pleasing bandage. Because a pedicle flap used as a graft must remain attached to its original site, the free end can only be sewn to an area within easy reach. After the graft had grown attached to the new site, the base of the flap was cut free. If the surgeon had superb skill, steady hands, and sharp razors, the operation could be completed in less than two hours.

During the nineteenth century, British colonialism gave Western doctors the opportunity to investigate traditional Indian medical and surgical practices. While working at the Madras Ophthalmic Hospital in the 1910s, Dr. Robert Henry Elliot assembled a collection of 54 eyeballs in a study of the Indian operation for cataracts. Elliot found evidence of many serious complications, but, since all the eyes were collected from blind patients, these cases represented only the failures of traditional surgeons. Unfortunately, Elliot never observed a traditional practitioner at work, but his informants claimed that practitioners often told the patient that surgery was unnecessary. Then, while pretending to examine the eye, the operator suddenly pushed a needle through the cornea and detached the lens. Immediately after the operation, the surgeon tested the patient's vision, bandaged the eyes, collected his fees, and advised the patient to rest for at least 24 hours. Scornfully, Elliot noted that this would allow the operator to disappear before the outcome of the case could be ascertained.

Although cleanliness was a major precept for Susruta and Caraka, Elliot claimed that it was of no concern to contemporary traditional practitioners. Moreover, unscrupulous practitioners recklessly operated on patients suffering from optic atrophy or glaucoma rather than cataract. Reports by colonial observers might provide some valuable insights into traditional Indian surgical practices, but these accounts cannot be directly related to the ancient Indian science of life. The wandering empiric, crudely performing illegal operations in the shadow of colonial power, had only the most tenuous links to the scholarly practitioners envisioned by Susruta and Caraka.

Unfortunately, although in theory India has a vast primary health care system, with public clinics for every three thousand to five thousand people, the clinics are often closed because of the lack of doctors, nurses, medicines, safe water, and electricity. Villagers are forced to rely on traditional healers and private "doctors" who have no formal medical training. Such healers give injections of antibiotics and intravenous glucose drips, despite the lack of sterile equipment.

Western science and medicine have won a place in India, but Ayurvedic medicine and religious healing traditions still bring comfort to millions of people suffering from physical and mental illnesses. In much of rural India today, treatment for mental illness is more likely to take place in a traditional "healing temple" than in a clinic or hospital. When Western-trained psychiatrists evaluated patients treated at such temples, they found some cases of paranoid schizophrenia, delusional disorders, and manic episodes. After an average stay of five weeks, many patients had improved significantly, as measured on a standard psychiatric ranking. Psychiatrists attributed the improvement in symptoms to cultural factors, expectations, and the temple's supportive, nonthreatening, and reassuring setting.

As demonstrated by the popularity of health spas and resorts featuring traditional Ayurvedic principles of health, healing, and nutrition, Ayurvedic concepts have now reached a global audience. Instead of dismissing Ayurveda as "mere superstition," scholars in India are finding valuable medical insights and inspiration in the ancient texts. Like students of traditional Chinese medicine, followers of Ayurveda see their ancient traditions as a treasure-house of remedies and healing practices. Indeed, at the end of the twentieth century, there were more than 6,000 licensed Ayurvedic pharmacies in India, about 1,500 Ayurvedic hospitals, and over 100 Ayurvedic colleges registered in the New Delhi Central Council of Indian Medicine. The Council continues to issue regulations that govern Ayurvedic education for undergraduate and postgraduate students.

## CHINESE MEDICINE: CLASSICAL, TRADITIONAL, AND MODERN

Until recently, Western historians of science and medicine generally ignored China, except for a few exotic items and inventions that could be rationalized as crude precursors of technologies brought to fruition in the West, such as gunpowder and printing. Fortunately, the work of Joseph Needham, Nathan Sivin, Paul Unschuld, and other scholars has helped redefine the place of Asian studies in the global history of science and medicine. Scholars have suggested that a fundamental difference between Greek and Chinese thought was the competitiveness of early Greek political and intellectual life. In contrast, the power of autocratic rulers in China forced scholars toward consensus positions. Consequently, while Greek thinkers were free to criticize their mentors and rivals, Chinese scholars accepted aspects of change that Greek philosophers rejected. Thus, Chinese astronomers and Chinese physicians made very different assumptions about the movement of the heavenly bodies and the movement of the blood.

Most elements of the ancient learned systems have essentially disappeared, or survive only in folklore as quaint vestiges of the past, but supporters of Chinese medicine maintain that it is and always has been a viable scientific enterprise. Traditional Chinese medicines and healing techniques have gained a significant place in the alternative or integrative medicine practiced in the Western world today. Certainly, classical Chinese medicine is remarkable for its persistence and adaptability. In practice, the system exhibits an exceptional level of flexibility. A patient of Chinese medicine might receive 10 different prescriptions. Rather than conclude that most of these prescriptions must be useless, the patient might find many of them satisfactory and effective.

More than any other culture, China has maintained its traditional medicine not only in folk remedies, but also in mature and respected forms. In part, this unique stability can be attributed to a profound reverence for the past and a system of writing perhaps six thousand years old. Although many scholars have discounted the earliest chapters in China's historical narratives, recent archaeological and archival discoveries will doubtlessly transform much mythology into history and much history into mythology. Since the 1970s, Chinese archaeologists have experienced a golden age of discovery. Ancient tombs have yielded treasures ranging from panels of magnificent wall paintings and manuscripts written on bamboo or silk to well-preserved bodies, skeletons, and hordes of life-sized terra-cotta figures of warriors complete with weapons and horses from the Ch'in Dynasty (221–206 B.C.E.) and the Han Dynasty (206 B.C.E.–220 A.D.). Archaeologists and art scholars think that these remarkable terra-cotta warriors, horses, chariots, musicians, and farm animals once served as symbolic escorts into the afterlife for members of the nobility.

Much of China's history is obscured by warfare and chaos until the Ch'in unification in 221 B.C.E. To enforce his goal of total reorganization, the Emperor Shih Huang-ti ordered the destruction of all surviving manuscripts in order to erase unacceptable historical traditions. Exceptions were made only for texts dealing with medicine, drugs, divination, agriculture, and forestry. During the centuries of conflict, scholars as well as peasants assimilated the concepts that formed the framework of classical Chinese medicine: belief in the unity of nature, yin–yang dualism, the theory of the five phases, and a medical practice based on the theory of systematic correspondences.

Some elements of this system can be traced back to China's Bronze Age, the period of the Shang Dynasty, which was already flourishing by the fifteenth century B.C.E. Scholars once consigned the Shang Dynasty to the realm of legend, but excavations begun in the 1930s have provided evidence that the Shang era served as the formative period of Chinese culture. So-called oracle bones, inscribed with an archaic but essentially mature form of written Chinese, have provided valuable insights into this semilegendary era.

Oracle bones used in divination ceremonies were made of various materials, including the shoulder blades of oxen, goats, and sheep, turtle shells, antlers, and even human skulls. According to Shang beliefs, the well-being of the living was dependent on the will of the ancestral spirits that rule the world. If the ancestors were displeased, their hostility could cause disease, crop failures, and military defeats. In order to address questions about battles, harvests, illness, and epidemics to the ancestral spirits, appropriate bones or shells were carefully prepared for the king and his diviners. During the divination ritual, pairs of antithetical questions were addressed to the spirits; for example, "Will the king recover from his illness" and "Will the king not recover from his illness?" Heat was applied to the oracle bone with a heated bronze rod, a burning stick, or a glowing piece of charcoal. If the bones had been properly prepared, heat would result in the appearance of a pair of cracks resembling the written character "pu," a vertical line joined about midpoint from the right by a perpendicular line (⊢). If the angle between the lines was close to the perpendicular, the answer was yes; if not, the answer was no.

Shang writings and divination were essentially forgotten until the end of the nineteenth century even though oracle bones could be found in almost every traditional Chinese apothecary shop. When physicians included "dragon bones" in their prescriptions for disorders ranging from lung diseases to anxiety and nocturnal emissions, apothecaries used bits of ancient bones and shells, including many that had served as ancient oracles. Since nineteenth century fossil hunters discovered that collections of dragon bones often contained valuable fossils, hundreds of thousands of oracle bones have been collected. How many were pounded into medicines over the centuries can only be imagined.

## THE THREE CELESTIAL EMPERORS: FU HSI, SHEN NUNG, AND HUANG TI

History yields to mythology in accounts of the Three Celestial Emperors, who are revered as the founders of Chinese civilization. Fu Hsi, who is said to have reigned about 2000 B.C.E., is the legendary founder of China's first dynasty. His most important inventions included writing, painting, music, the original eight mystic trigrams, and the yin–yang concept. The *I Ching* or *Canon of Changes*, honored as the most ancient of Chinese books, is ascribed to Fu Hsi.

The invention of the fundamental techniques of agriculture and animal husbandry are attributed to Shen Nung, the second Celestial Emperor. When the Emperor, who was also known as the Divine Peasant, saw his people suffering from illness and poisoning, he taught them to sow the five kinds of grain and he personally investigated a thousand herbs so that the people would know which were therapeutic and which were toxic. In his experiments with poisons and antidotes, Shen Nung is said to have taken as many as seventy different poisons in one day. Having collected many remedies in the first great treatise on herbal medicine while setting a magnificent example of unselfish devotion to medical research, Shen Nung died after an unsuccessful experiment.

During his hundred-year reign, Huang Ti, the last of the legendary Celestial Emperors, gave his people the wheel, the magnet, an astronomical observatory, the calendar, the art of pulse measurement, and the *Huang-ti Nei Ching (The Inner Canon of the Yellow Emperor)*, a text that has inspired and guided Chinese medical thought for over 2,500 years. Like many ancient texts, the *Nei Ching* has been corrupted over the centuries by additions, excisions, and misprints. Scholars agree that the existing text is very ancient, perhaps dating back to the first century B.C.E., but the time of its composition is controversial. Most historians believe that the text in existence today was compiled at the beginning of the T'ang Dynasty (618–907). Other medical texts have sometimes overshadowed it, but most of the classics of Chinese medicine may be considered interpretations, commentaries, and supplements to the Yellow Emperor's *Canon*.

Although *The Inner Canon* is revered as one of the oldest and most influential of the classical Chinese medical texts, studies of medical manuscripts that were buried with their owner, probably during the second century B.C.E., and recovered in Mawangdui, Hunan, in the 1970s, have provided new insights into early Chinese medical thought. As newly recovered texts are analyzed, scholars are beginning to illuminate the philosophical foundations of Chinese medicine and the ways in which the learned physicians of the fourth to first centuries B.C.E. were able to separate themselves from shamans and other popular healers. Physicians apparently were still exploring approaches to physiology, pathology, and therapy that differed from those found in the *Inner Canon*. Therapeutics in the older texts included medicinal drugs, exorcism, magical and religious techniques, and surgical operations, but acupuncture, the major therapeutic technique in the *Inner Canon*, was not discussed in the Mawangdui manuscripts.

As it exists today, the *Nei Ching* is a collection of sometimes contradictory ideas and interpretations forced into a supposedly integrated conceptual system. The *Inner Canon* is cast in the form of a dialogue between Huang Ti and Ch'i Po, his Minister of Health and Healing. Together, Emperor and Minister explore a medical philosophy based on the balance of yang and yin, the five phases (also called the five elements), and the correlations found among them and almost every conceivable entity impinging on human life, from family and food to climate and geography. The terms yin and yang are generally taken to represent all the pairs of opposites that express the dualism of the cosmos. Thus, whereas yin is characterized as female, dark, cold, soft, earth, night, and empty, yang represents male, light, warm, firm, heaven, day, full, and so forth. Yang and yin, however, should be understood as "relational concepts," that is, not firm or soft per se, but only in comparison to other states or entities.

The original meanings of the characters for yin and yang are obscure, but light and shade appear to be fundamental aspects. The original characters might have represented the banks of a river, one in the shade and the other in the sun, or the shady side and the sunny side of a hill. Applying these concepts to the human body, the outside is relatively yang, the inside is relatively yin, and specific internal organs are associated with yang or yin.

Huang Ti taught that the principle of yin–yang is the basis of everything in creation, the cause of all transformations, and the origin

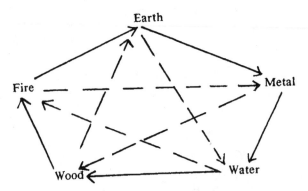

The five phases. As individual names or labels for the finer ramifications of yin
and yang, the five phases represent aspects in the cycle of changes. The five phases
are linked by relationships of generation and destruction. Patterns of destruction
may be summarized as follows: water puts out fire; fire melts metal; a metal ax
cuts wood; a wooden plow turns up the earth; an earthen dam stops the flow of
water. The cycle of generation proceeds as water produces the wood of trees;
wood produces fire; fire creates ash, or earth; earth is the source of metals; when
metals are heated, they flow like water.

of life and death. Yin and yang generate the five phases: wood, fire,
earth, metal, and water. Because the terms yang and yin are essentially
untranslatable, they have been directly adopted into many languages.
But the same lack of meaningful correspondence applies to the *wu-hsing*,
a term that was usually translated as "five elements," because of a false
analogy with the four elements of the ancient Greeks. The Chinese term
actually implies passage, transition, or phase, rather than stable, homo-
geneous chemical constituents. In recent years, scholars have invented
new terms such as "five conventional values" and "five evolutive
phases" to convey a more precise meaning. For the sake of simplicity,
we shall use the term "five phases."

Chinese philosophers and scientists created an elaborate system to
rationalize the relationships of the five phases to almost everything else.
Thus, the sequences of creation and destruction among the five phases provided a foundation for classical concepts of human physiology.

## CLASSICAL CHINESE CONCEPTS OF ANATOMY

One aspect of Chinese medicine that is likely to seem especially strange to
the modern reader is the classical approach to human anatomy. However,
if classical Chinese anatomy is properly thought of in terms of function
rather than structure, distinctions between anatomy and physiology
become irrelevant. Anatomy, in the Western sense, did not form the basis

of classical Chinese medical theory or practice. Western anatomists study the body as if dealing with an assemblage of bits and pieces belonging to a machine. In contrast, classical Chinese anatomy is concerned with the dynamic interplay of functional systems rather than specific organs. Within classical Chinese medical concepts, the term "liver" does not mean the material substance used to create pâté, but the functional sphere within the body that corresponds to wood, spring, morning, quickening, and germination. Because of its emphasis on *function* rather than *structure*, Chinese anatomy can incorporate organs that have no physical substrate, such as the remarkable triple-warmer. Rather like *id, ego*, and *superego* in psychology, the triple-warmer has functions, but no specific location.

Other intriguing entities that have no direct counterpart in Western anatomy and physiology have been called the "life gate" and the "potential fire." Some scholars believe that classical Chinese theories about the "life gate" and the "potential fire" might be related to modern endocrinology. Joseph Needham called such classical theories "physiological alchemy." Classic Chinese medical texts refer to the "life gate" as the repository of the primary life energy (*ch'i* or *qi*), which originated from the kidneys. In the male, this repository stores the essence and in the female it sustains the uterus. The theory of "potential fire" was ascribed to a physician who lived during the Yüan Dynasty (1271–1368), which indicates that new entities and forces continued to appear in Chinese medical thought. The "potential fire", which originated in the abdomen, was controlled by body fluids, like the blood. Another form of "fire" was associated with the heart and was related to mental activities. Normally, these two kinds of "fires" kept each other in balance, but an excess of "potential fire" could lead to loss of control over the emotions. Followers of this school of thought tried to maintain health by focusing on physical and spiritual harmony, and the management of food and environment. They also claimed that they could cure diseases that could not be healed by ordinary means.

In the *Inner Canon*, the yin and yang, and the five phases, are closely related to the five "firm organs" (heart, spleen, lungs, liver, kidneys) and the five "hollow organs" (gall bladder, bladder, stomach, large intestines, small intestines). Residing deep within the body, the five firm organs, or viscera, are classified as yin and function as storage facilities, reservoirs, or depots. Located relatively close to the exterior of the body, the five hollow organs, or bowels, are classified as yang, and assumed the functions of elimination. Interactions among the various organs were made possible by linking them through a system of conduits rather like irrigation channels.

Because of the vital importance of irrigation to agriculture in China, the functions of the conduits in the body were often compared to the hydraulic works maintained by the government. For example, the triple-warmer was analogous to officials who were charged with planning the construction of ditches and sluices. For the body to work properly, the organs, like the officials of the state, must dutifully assist one another. Thus, when the system functioned harmoniously, the heart acted with insight and understanding like the king's minister, while the liver acted like the military leader responsible for strategic planning.

The system of fivefold correspondences could have created an embarrassing discrepancy between medical philosophy and medical practice, because acupuncture and moxibustion techniques had become standardized around a system of six pairs of conduits or acupuncture tracts. The problem was resolved by adding the pericardium or heart-enclosing network and the triple-warmer to the list of firm and hollow organs, respectively.

Despite considerable debate about various details, there is little argument about the fact that Chinese scholars accepted the relationship between the heart and the circulation of the blood long before these concepts were incorporated into Western science and medicine by William Harvey (1578–1657) in the seventeenth century. Westerners generally coped with the challenge to Harveian originality by dismissing Chinese concepts of the circulation as obscure mysticism "improved" by loose translations. Philosophical arguments, rather than dissection, presumably led Chinese physicians to the concept of the ceaseless circulation of some vital substance—which might be translated as blood, or breath, or energy—within the body's network of channels.

Although the *Nei Ching* assumes that the movement of blood is controlled by the heart and the movement of energy by the lungs, scholars disagree as to the meaning and the implications of the terms that are variously translated as blood, breath, or energy. Chinese physicians believed that because blood was a vital substance that nourished the body, the loss of blood was debilitating. In contrast to Western doctors, Chinese physicians rejected the practice of bloodletting, which was an important therapeutic component of Western medicine up to the twentieth century.

According to Chinese medical philosophy, disease was basically caused by an imbalance of yin and yang, resulting in a disorder of one of the five phases, expressed as a dysfunction of the corresponding organ and the organs controlled by the injured organ. Therefore, all therapies were directed toward restoration of a state of harmony. In accordance with the fivefold system, the *Nei Ching* described five methods of treatment: curing the spirit by living in harmony with the universe, dietary management, acupuncture, drugs, and treatment of the bowels and viscera, blood, and breath. In prescribing any preventive or therapeutic regimen, the physician had to carefully consider the influence of geography, climate, and local customs.

With a sense of sorrow and disappointment, the Yellow Emperor and his Minister recalled that, in a previous golden age, human beings practiced temperance and lived in harmony with nature for over one hundred vigorous years. Later, people disregarded the ways of nature and became feeble, short-lived, and subject to many diseases. For example, the people of the East ate fish and craved salt; this diet injured the blood and caused ulcers. Winds, or "noxious airs," caused much illness because they penetrated the body, disturbed the harmony of yin and yang, and diminished vital energy. Generally, winds caused chills and fevers, but specific winds associated with the changing seasons were linked to particular dangers. Disturbances of the harmonious relationship between mind and body could also cause illness.

For diagnosis and prognosis, the Chinese physician relied on *sphygmology*, a very complicated examination of the pulse. Because of the intimate connection between the tracts and vessels through which yang and yin flowed, the study of yin in the blood could reveal problems of yang in the tracts. Thus, by listening to the waves of blood generated by the heartbeat, the physician could detect disease in various parts of the body. The physician was expected to study fifty pulses, recognize more than two hundred variations, and know those that indicated the imminence of death. Pulses could be weak, strong, rough, smooth, sharp as a hook, fine as a hair, dead as a rock, deep as a well, or soft as a feather. The volume, strength, weakness, regularity, or irregularity of the pulse revealed the nature of the disease, whether it was chronic or acute, its cause and duration, and the prospects for death or recovery.

Sphygmology revealed incipient illness and allowed the physician to prescribe preventive measures or manage the course of therapy. Other kinds of diagnostic clues might be necessary, especially when dealing with children. Through close inspection, the physician could find diagnostic clues in the sounds made by the patient when talking, moaning, laughing, or weeping, and in the colors of various parts of the body. For example, inspection of the tongue could reveal 30 different shades of color that provided evidence of disease or the possibility of death. Physicians also had to recognize various types of difficult and skeptical patients, such as those who were arrogant, miserly, or addicted to overeating and dissipations, and those who had more faith in magicians and quacks than physicians.

## SAGES, PHYSICIANS, HEALERS, AND QUACKS

According to Huang Ti, the great sages of ancient times did not treat those who were already ill. Instead, they gave the benefit of their instruction to those who were healthy, because seeking remedies after diseases had already developed was as foolish as waiting until a war broke out to cast weapons. In theory, superior physicians guided the healthy patient; inferior physicians treated the sick. While the scholar practiced preventive medicine and took no fee for his work, hordes of healers without scholarly pretensions—surgeons, apothecaries, magicians, fortune-tellers, peddlers, and assorted quacks—were eager to collect fees and quite willing to serve sick and stupid patients. The typical practitioner was accused of being more interested in fees and favors than theories and philosophy.

Although the education and activities of physicians in the Imperial Service are hardly typical of the general practice of medicine in China, many interesting innovations are associated with the evolution of this institution. For example, the institutions of the Chou indicate that during the Chou Dynasty (ca. 1122–221 B.C.E.,) the government conducted yearly examinations of those who wished to practice medicine. Schools of medicine were established in almost every province, but most practitioners were trained by apprenticeship, and lower-class healers were largely self-taught. For the Imperial Service, the salaries of successful applicants were determined by how well they had placed in the examinations. Rank and salary for physicians serving the government were determined by an analysis of their success rate. Physicians who cured all of their patients were ranked first class; the lowest grade contained those who could not cure more than sixty percent of their patients. This took into account the belief that half of the patients would probably have recovered without any treatment at all. Veterinarians were also ranked according to their rate of successful treatment.

The Chou Imperial Service included Food Physicians, Physicians for Simple Diseases, Ulcer Physicians (surgeons), Physicians for Animals, and the Chief-of-Physicians, who supervised the others. Physicians for Simple Diseases were assigned the task of testing the five kinds of breaths, the five kinds of sounds, and the five colors to determine whether the patient was dead or alive. The Imperial College of Medicine consisted of about 30 physicians attached to the Imperial palaces. Physician-scholars of the highest rank gave lectures on the classics to junior colleagues. These physicians had access to the Imperial Library's collection of 12,000 works on medicine and the natural sciences. Obviously, very few people were served by the sages. Lowly practitioners of public medicine and street medicine far outnumbered those involved in court medicine. A rather diffuse system of public assistance may have existed in theory, but it was never sufficiently funded to have a significant impact on the medical needs of the populace.

Patients who were more worried about demons and spirits than the five phases found their medical practitioners on street corners, along with astrologers, geomancers, and fortune-tellers, or made their way to monasteries where healers dispensed medical advice and amulets with equal enthusiasm. Protective measures for dealing with magical forces included charms, prayers, exorcisms, incantations, amulets, and talismans. A talisman might resemble an official imperial document, except that the named official was a high-ranking demon who ordered demons lower in the hierarchy to cease and desist from causing illness and misfortune.

Driving out demons might require drugs compounded from powerful poisons or highly odoriferous materials. To prevent the poison from killing the patient, the prescription or drug could be worn as a charm or burned as a fumigant. A worm spirit, known as the *ku*, figured prominently among the demon diseases described in both scholarly literature and folklore. Elaborate beliefs developed about the *ku* spirit, including the belief that the only way for the original victim to rid himself of the *ku* was to provide another host. *Ku* antidotes included prayers, charms, drugs, and centipedes (because centipedes consume worms). Law codes show that belief in *ku* magic survived into the nineteenth century. The penalties for *ku* magic were quite severe, including bizarre methods of executing the criminal and his whole family.

Physicians with scholarly training or aspirations tried to separate their profession from magic and sorcery, and disparaged the remedies prescribed by folk practitioners and quacks, but sometimes they too offered prescriptions that combined medicine with magic. One example of a mixed prescription used in the treatment of digestive complaints consisted of magic characters written on thick, yellow paper with medicinal pigments. The prescription was burnt to a powdery ash, which was added to hot water and taken as a medicinal tea.

Written sources generally reflect scholarly interest in medical theory, but occasional glimpses of actual interactions between physicians and their patients appear in collections of cases histories, biographies, diaries, and advice literature. According to case histories from the Ming Dynasty (1368–1644), physicians used the "four examinations" in order to make a diagnosis. That is, they followed appropriate steps in looking, listening and smelling, asking, and touching (pulse measurement), depending on the condition and sex of the patient. Although pulse measurement was usually considered the most reliable part of the examination, physicians also claimed the ability to diagnose and advise patients they had not seen in person. If the physician thought that death was inevitable, or the disease was inappropriate for medical intervention, he could refuse to treat that patient. As in other ancient medical systems, it was important for the physician to predict death and avoid responsibility for such failures of treatment. Frequent references to the deficiencies of other practitioners seem to reflect fierce competition between physicians. Case histories and autobiographies suggest that even elite physicians were often forced to travel in search of patients. Some physicians visited patients at fairly predictable intervals, only to discover that some of their patients sought out other healers or foolishly medicated themselves when dissatisfied with the intervals between visits or the nature of their prescriptions.

Texts from late imperial China suggest an ancient and complex body of theories and practices related to gender-based concepts of the body and its functions. Generally, however, classical texts focused on the distribution of energy in the male body. Discussions of "women's medicine" usually dealt with female fertility, the diseases specific to women, and remedies appropriate for women at different stages of life. Physicians apparently used similar methods of diagnosis for women and men, but during the Ming Dynasty male physicians were generally not allowed to examine women directly. Little is known about female practitioners, other than midwives, but a Ming Dynasty writer noted that women usually sought out female healers for themselves and their children.

## ACUPUNCTURE AND MOXIBUSTION

Drug lore, herbal medicine, and magical practices are essentially universal aspects of traditional and ancient medical systems. Chinese medicine is unique, however, in the development of the techniques known as *acupuncture* and *moxibustion* and the sophisticated rationalizations that justified these very ancient practices. Both acupuncture and moxibustion could be used to restore the free flow of yin and yang that was essential to health.

For at least 2,500 years, acupuncture, the art of inserting needles at specific points on the surface of the body, has been a part of Chinese medicine. Moxa or moxibustion, a related technique in which burning tinder made from the powdered leaves of *Artemisia vulgaris* (mugwort or wormwood) is applied to specific points on the skin, may be even more ancient than the art of needling. Acupuncture has attained considerable notoriety and a degree of acceptance in the West, but moxibustion has been largely ignored. Although moxibustion may produce burns and scars, practitioners claim that the pain is not unpleasant. Skeptics, however, find it difficult to imagine a burn associated with a "pleasant pain."

The goddesses Scarlet and White are said to have given the secret of acupuncture to the Yellow Emperor, who then devised nine kinds of needles from flint and bone. According to obscure and fragmentary references to the use of pointed stones to open abscesses and cure disease in China's semi-legendary past, marvelous needle-like stone implements were found at the foot of a jade-crowned mountain. Unfortunately, the series of steps leading from opening abscesses with sharp stones to the sophisticated system described in the *Nei Ching* remains obscure.

In the *Nei Ching*, the total number of acupuncture points is said to be 365. However, Huang Ti seems to name only about 160. The number 365 may represent a theoretically perfect system symbolically correlating the number of degrees in the celestial circle, the days in the year, and the number of parts in the human body. The points are said to be distributed along a complex system of tracts, channels, or meridians that make their way through the body. In its mature form, the acupuncture system consists of twelve main tracts, each of which carries the name of the solid or hollow organ with which it is primarily associated. The system also accommodates various auxiliary tracts and organs. For outside observers, the most disconcerting aspect of this system is probably the lack of any apparent relationship between the organ or disorder being treated and the site of the therapeutic acupuncture point.

Theoretically, acupuncture practitioners gain access to the system of tracts that are said to distribute energy throughout the body by inserting needles into specific points where the tracts are close to the surface. The idea that the acupuncturist can extract, purge, or drain energy by needling points on the tracts may reflect the evolution of the system from its empirical foundation as a means of draining pus or blood from an abscess. In the course of treating localized lesions, practitioners may have discovered that needling particular points elicited generalized effects. Certain sensations are supposed to show that the points were properly selected. These include warmth, numbness, and the feeling that these sensations are traveling slowly up or down the limbs or trunk. If the points are the primeval basis of the system, it is possible that the subjective sensation of a response traveling through the body when points are needled gave rise to maps of the tracts.

Much ink has been spilled in Western writings over whether the tracts enjoy a true physical existence. While the functional aspects of the tracts remain a fundamental principle of classical Chinese medicine, it is possible that the system of vessels is essentially a mnemonic device that allows practitioners to learn how to associate diverse physiological phenomena with empirically determined points. Aspiring physicians could learn the art of acupuncture from illustrated manuals and by practicing on specially prepared bronze models or wooden dolls. Ultimately, the physician had to leave behind idealized models and work with patients who were large or small, fat or thin, male or female, old or young. According to scholar-physicians, the most dangerous aspect of the acupuncture system is the possibility of misuse by ignorant or evil practitioners, because the system included a number of "forbidden points." Inserting needles at forbidden points could cause serious damage or even death.

Acupuncture was especially recommended for all disorders involving an excess of yang. Moxibustion was thought to be preferable when yin was in excess. However, the relationships among yin and yang, the five phases, and the organs are so complex that the use of either method could be justified. Moxa was generally recommended for chronic conditions, such as tuberculosis, bronchitis, and general weakness, but it was also used for toothache, headache, gout, diarrhea, and some psychological disorders. Pao Ku, wife of the alchemist Ko Hung (254–334), was famous for treating skin diseases with moxibustion. Officials of seventh century China would not undertake a journey unless protected against foreign diseases and snakebites by fresh moxibustion scars. In modern China, physicians have been experimenting with moxa in the treatment of influenza, chronic bronchitis, and infections of the respiratory tract.

Today, there are professional acupuncturists in Russia, Europe, North America, and South America, as well in Asia. Nevertheless, the legal status of practitioners in some countries remains ambiguous. Until the 1970s, the legal status of acupuncture was of no interest to the American medical community. Traditional Chinese medicine was dismissed as pure quackery. What could be more bizarre than killing pain by sticking needles into people (unless, of course, the needles were hypodermics full of narcotics)? Practitioners of alternative and unorthodox medicine, however, were often eager to explore the potential of acupuncture, acupressure, and moxibustion. As acupuncturists increasingly gained both notoriety and clients, the medical profession began to pay attention. The American Medical Association took the position that acupuncture was folklore, not science, but that it could only be performed by licensed physicians because needling was an invasive procedure. In 1975, Nevada became the first state to establish a state Board of Chinese Medicine and require that physicians and nonphysicians pass an examination to qualify as licensed acupuncturists. Although other states have established licensing procedures, the status of acupuncturists and other practitioners of Chinese medicine is often ambiguous.

## DRUG LORE AND DIETETICS

According to the *Nei Ching*, a diet balanced in accordance with the five-fold system of correspondences will promote health and longevity, strengthen the body, and drive out disease. The first remedies were to be found among the herbs, trees, plants, and animals that served as foods. But medical theory and folklore taught that normally harmless foods could be dangerous under special circumstances, such as pregnancy. For example, if a pregnant woman consumed the meat of a hare, the child would be mute and lack an upper lip; eating mule meat would cause a difficult birth. Dietary physicians also warned against eating foods that were spoiled, meat that moved by itself, and apricots with two pits.

The use of tea illustrates the overlap between foods and drugs. For about six thousand years, the Chinese have been making a beverage from the leaves of the tea shrub. Tea contains small amounts of nutrients, but it is rich in physiologically active alkaloids, including caffeine, theobromine, and theophylline. Perhaps the most important health aspect of tea drinking in the ancient world, and in many regions of the world even today, was the use of vigorously boiling water. In general, the boundary between medical prescriptions and dietary prescriptions was not as sharply defined in many ancient traditional systems as it is in modern Western medicine. Yet, modern medicine is once again focusing on the role of diet as an aid to good health, disease prevention, and longevity.

The importance of dietary management is illustrated in a classic text presented to the Mongol Emperor at the Yüan court in 1330 by Hu Szu-hui, who served as court dietary physician for more than 10 years. Hu's *Proper and Essential Things for the Emperor's Food and Drink* explains early Chinese and Mongolian ideas about the importance of dietetics. For historians, the book is of special interest for the medical and hygienic ideas it contains rather than the recipes. Still, it is interesting to consider both the medical and culinary values of entries such as Roast Wolf Soup and Boiled Sheep's Heart. Most such recipes were said to increase *ch'i*, but some were more specifically valued for conditions like backache and agitation of the heart. The text suggests foods that promote longevity, warns against certain foods or combinations of foods, and gives special attention to proper diets for pregnant women. Edible plants and animals were carefully classified in terms of medical theories of systematic correspondence.

When dietary measures were insufficient, physicians could search for remedies among the many known drugs. Because the nature of drugs was often violent, scholars warned against recklessly prescribing or consuming them. Nevertheless, when brought together in the proper proportions, drugs could accomplish wonderful effects. Some five thousand native plants are in common use as medicinal herbs, and modern scientists are attempting to isolate specific active ingredients from traditional remedies. For guidance in this quest, they often turn to the *Pen-ts'ao Kang Mu*, an encyclopedic study of medicine, pharmacology, botany, and zoology, complied by Li Shih-Chen (1518–1593), China's "prince of pharmacists." Published in 1596 by his sons, Li's great work included close to two thousand drugs from the animal, vegetable, and mineral kingdoms, more than eight thousand prescriptions, references to over nine hundred other texts, and more than a thousand illustrations. Today, experts in Asian medicine hope that high-volume screening and rigorous clinical trials will demonstrate the value of traditional Chinese herbal remedies. For example, in 2003, the U.S. Food and Drug Administration approved a phase II trial to test the efficacy of one such remedy in treating non-small-cell lung cancer.

The three classes of drugs—vegetable, animal, and mineral—were said to correspond to heaven, man, and earth. Animal organs were highly regarded as sources of remarkable "vital principles," such as tiger liver for courage and snake flesh for endurance. Among the more prosaic and presumably effective remedies were sea horse powder and seaweed, which are good sources of iodine and iron, for goiter and chronic fatigue, and ephedra for lung diseases and asthma. Generally, the Chinese exhibited admirable skepticism about foreign "wonder drugs," but expeditions were launched in response to rumors that Indian physicians had discovered the herb of immortality. Many Chinese healers, however, considered ginseng, the "queen of medicinal herbs," as the equal of India's wonder drug.

Medical therapy can take two general forms: healers can attempt to strengthen the body so that it can heal and defend itself, or they can attack the agents of disease directly. The primary goal of Chinese medicine is to enhance the body's ability to regulate itself and to restore the normal balance of energy. The reverence inspired by ginseng illustrates the classical Chinese approach to healing. Ginseng has been used as a tonic, rejuvenator, and aphrodisiac. Modern researchers have called it an "adaptogen," a substance that increases resistance to all forms of stress, from disease to misfortune. Li Shih-Chen described an ingenious experiment to demonstrate the effect of ginseng: select two men of about the same size and have both run a certain distance after giving ginseng to one of the runners. At the end of the test, the man given ginseng would not be fatigued, whereas the other man would suffer shortness of breath. The same test could be used to determine whether a given specimen was genuine ginseng.

The gathering and preparation of ginseng were surrounded by a rich body of folklore, ritual, and myth. Because metal implements would destroy the virtues of a ginseng root, only wooden knives and earthenware pots could be used in its preparation. Wild ginseng was said to assume a luminous glow and walk about at night disguised as a bird or a child who lured ginseng hunters to their death. China's emperors established ginseng monopolies, appointed their own gatherers, and kept the best roots for themselves.

Classical sources describe ginseng as a tonic for the five viscera: it opens the heart, quiets fears, expels evil effluvia, improves understanding, invigorates the body, and prolongs life. Ginseng is prescribed for fatigue, anemia, insomnia, arthritis, disorders of the nerves, lungs, and stomach, impotence, tuberculosis, and so forth. Ginseng is sometimes marketed as an aphrodisiac. Herbalists claim that it increases stamina and allows even very elderly men to become fathers, in addition to preventing baldness, gray hair, wrinkles, and age spots.

The Chinese materia medica also included typical examples of *dreckapothecary*—remedies made of noxious and repulsive ingredients, such as dried salamander, donkey skin, medicinal urines, and human parts and products. Human bones were among the ingredients in remedies used to treat syphilis. According to a text by Ming Dynasty physician Wang Ji (1463–1539), a magician claimed that he could cure syphilis with a preparation made from the bones of a dead infant. After the bones were roasted, the resulting ashes were ground into a powder and mixed with alcohol. The patient was advised to take the remedy on an empty stomach. Wang Ji objected that a preparation made by roasting bones in a fire would be fierce and violent. Other physicians, however, objected to the use of human bones in medicines on the ground that it was incompatible with the role of medicine as the "art of benevolence." Smallpox inoculation can also be thought of as a "medicine derived from man." To provide protection against 40 forms of the "heavenly blossom disease," doctors collected the crusts from pustules of a mild case of smallpox. The powdered material was blown into the nostrils; males snorted the powder through the left nostril and females via the right side.

Chinese alchemists developed a very different approach to human health and longevity. Alchemy generally conjures up the image of mystics and quacks vainly attempting to turn lead into gold. Alchemists were, however, also associated with the search for the mysterious elixir of life. To an unusual extent, Chinese alchemists were obsessed with both the theoretical aspects of gold-making (and gold-faking) and "macrobiotics," that is, the search for the great drugs of well-being and immortality. Ko Hung (ca. 300), an eminent alchemist, Taoist adept, and physician, taught that minor elixirs could provide protection from ghosts, wild animals, and digestive disorders. More powerful elixirs could restore those who had just died, while superior elixirs would confer immortality.

## SURGERY

In contrast to India, surgery generally remained outside the domain of China's scholarly, elite medicine. Presumably, reluctance to mutilate the body and the lack of dissection-based anatomy inhibited the development of surgery in China, but such obstacles are not necessarily insurmountable. Indeed, forensic medicine reached a high level of sophistication in China, as indicated by a text known as *The Washing*

*Away of Wrongs* (1247), which is considered the world's first treatise on forensic medicine.

When confronted with their apparent failure to establish a respected surgical tradition, Chinese scholars contended that the efficacy of their preventive and therapeutic medicine obviated the need for surgical interventions. Nevertheless, Chinese history provides accounts of physicians who performed miraculous operations. Interactions between China and India during the transmission of Buddhism may have inspired such stories, although they did not lead to the integration of surgery into classical Chinese medical traditions.

The most famous Chinese surgeon, Hua T'o (ca. 145–208), was credited with the invention of anesthetic drugs, medicinal baths, hydrotherapy, and medical gymnastics. Master of acupuncture and a brilliant diagnostician, Hua T'o could reputedly cure migraine headaches with one acupuncture needle. One of his most unusual cases involved a patient suffering from a painful tumor between the eyes. When Hua T'o skillfully opened the tumor, a canary flew out and the patient was completely cured. Although canary-filled tumors may be a rarity in medical practice, headaches and chronic pains are not, and Hua T'o usually cured such disorders with acupuncture. Unfortunately, when consulted by the Emperor Ts'ao Ts'ao, the surgeon recommended trepanation as a treatment for his intractable headaches. Suspecting that such drastic surgery might be part of an assassination plot, Ts'ao Ts'ao ordered Hua T'o's execution. Unable to smuggle his writings out of prison, Hua T'o took the secrets of his great discoveries with him. The lost secrets of Hua T'o supposedly included ointments that prevented and cured infection as well as miraculous anesthetics.

According to tradition, of all the operations invented by Hua T'o, the only one to survive and enjoy considerable usage was his technique for castration. This operation provided the eunuchs employed as civil servants and palace attendants. Descriptions of castration as practiced in 1929 note that despite the crudeness of the operation most patients healed in about a hundred days, although about two percent died as the result of hemorrhage or infection.

## THE CHINESE CULTURAL SPHERE

Although the nations surrounding China were heavily influenced by Chinese medical philosophy, the direction of exchange is sometimes obscure. Shared medical traditions have different creation myths in each state within the Chinese cultural sphere. For example, in Korea, the invention of moxa and stone acupuncture needles was attributed to Tan Gun, the legendary founder of that nation. Many medicinal substances were exported from Korea to China, before Korea exported

Chinese medicine to Japan. Due to Korea's geographical situation, the history of medicine in the peninsula was intimately linked to developments in China, Japan, and other Asian countries. During the Three Kingdoms period (37 B.C.E.–935 A.D.), scholars adapted the Chinese writing system to the Korean language. The date for the introduction of Buddhism into Korea is usually given as 372, when a Chinese monk brought Buddhist scriptures and images. Having adopted Buddhism from China, Korean monks and scholars traveled to China and India in search of further enlightenment. Buddhism also figures prominently in early interactions between Korea and Japan. Surviving historical records suggest that disease germs as well as religious artifacts were involved in these transactions.

Korean physicians were very much influenced by Chinese medical philosophy, and used Chinese medical terms in describing disease, but they also reinterpreted Chinese texts in terms of local conditions and added information obtained from Indian sources. Scholarly discussions of disease generally followed the principles set forth in the Chinese medical literature, but the study of Korea's traditional folk remedies stimulated the development of an independent line of medical scholarship that recognized the importance of local conditions. Such texts include the *Emergency Remedies of Folk Medicine* (1236), a medical encyclopedia entitled the *Compilation of Native Korean Prescriptions* (1433), and the *Exemplar of Korean Medicine* (1610).

*Emergency Remedies of Folk Medicine* mainly deals with the use of local drugs, but it also describes symptoms of various diseases and methods of cure in terms of classical Chinese medicine. Medical emergencies described in the text include food poisoning, the bites of poisonous insects and wild animals, stroke, nightmares, drowning, falls, alcoholism, epilepsy, fainting, hemorrhages, internal bleeding, and so forth. The text also described the symptoms of malaria, the "three-day fever" that was much feared throughout the region, and its treatment with various local medicines.

Chinese records suggest very early opportunities for the spread of smallpox and other diseases through direct and indirect trade with India, Rome, and Arabia. The *Exemplar of Korean Medicine* states that smallpox was introduced into northern China from Central Asia by the Huns about the time that the Han Dynasty replaced the Chou Dynasty. Smallpox was probably brought to Korea from China by the end of the sixth century and then transmitted from Korea to Japan.

Another kind of argument about China's relationship with the Western world is exemplified by Gavin Menzies's controversial claim that Ming Dynasty explorers, led by Admiral Zheng He, discovered the Americas in 1421. In 1405, Zheng launched a great fleet of ships on the first of seven expeditions. Between 1405 and 1433, Zheng allegedly led the fleet to places as distant as Sumatra, India, Sri Lanka, Somalia,

Kenya, and the Americas. Most scholars believe that Chinese explorers and travelers did bring back stories of an exotic world outside the sphere of Chinese influence, but China's rulers apparently concluded that what the outside world had to offer was insignificant. Menzies, author of *1421: The Year China Discovered America*, gained considerable notoriety for his theory that Admiral Zheng discovered America before Columbus. He has also argued that DNA evidence confirms his thesis. According to Menzies, some Chinese sailors and concubines who accompanied the Ming Dynasty admiral remained in the Americas, established settlements, and interbred with indigenous peoples.

## MEDICAL PRACTICE IN MODERN CHINA

When the People's Republic of China was founded in 1949, Chairman Mao Zedong (1893–1976) declared that traditional Chinese medicine and pharmacology constituted a great treasure-house that must be explored and improved. Mao's call for the use of both traditional and Western-trained doctors was a pragmatic response to China's desperate need to expand the pool of health care workers to serve 540 million people, typically living in impoverished, rural areas without public health, sanitary, or medical facilities. Circumstances impelled China into a unique experiment in the integration of past and present, East and West. The revival of traditional medicine was launched with the Great Leap Forward (1958–1960), gained momentum during the Cultural Revolution (1966–1969), and peaked in the aftermath of this ideological frenzy.

China's health care system was dedicated to dealing with common and recurrent diseases, public health work, and the eradication of major endemic disorders. The motto adopted by the Chinese medical system was: "Eradicate the four pests!" The official four pests were rats, flies, mosquitoes, and sparrows. Cockroaches, fleas, lice, bedbugs, snails, and mice were also targeted for eradication, but listing all of them would have ruined a good motto.

By the 1980s, China had established a health care system that is generally conceded to be a model for other developing countries. Sensitive measures of health in Shanghai in 1980, such as infant mortality and life expectancy at birth, compared favorably with New York City. Western visitors were impressed by Chinese experiments in medical education and the restructuring of medical practice, which obligated the physician to share diagnostic and therapeutic responsibilities with a newly empowered array of lay and paramedical personnel. Preventive medicine and basic primary health care were provided by legions of "barefoot doctors," midwives, and nurses. The use of herbal remedies, acupuncture, and moxibustion remains the core of medical practice, but traditional doctors also study microbiology and pharmacology. China's colleges of Western medicine include training in traditional medicine.

The development of acupuncture anesthesia has been hailed in China as another great leap forward. Inspired by the thoughts of Chairman Mao, hospital workers began to wonder whether the pain-relieving effects of needling that had been exploited in the treatment of post-surgical distress might be used in place of chemical anesthetics during surgery. Even in China, the prospect of acupuncture anesthesia was greeted with some skepticism, but in the 1960s acupuncture anesthesia was being used in about sixty percent of all surgical operations. Modern acupuncturists argue that, in contrast to chemical anesthesia, needling allows the body to mobilize all its defense mechanisms, while maintaining normal physiological functions.

The revival of interest in acupuncture and herbalism has not been accompanied by commensurate attention to the theoretical basis of traditional medicine. Separated from its theoretical framework, Chinese medicine could become merely a hodge-podge of empirical remedies, rather than a sophisticated philosophical system capable of providing guidance and inspiration for both patients and practitioners. Chinese philosophy and medicine have, however, always demonstrated a remarkable capacity for syncretism and adaptation. China is a living civilization, in which the traditional arts are intimately linked to their modern counterparts. Perhaps the thoughts of both Huang Ti and Chairman Mao will be subsumed and integrated into a new synthesis, still reflecting the goals of the Three Celestial Emperors for the perfection of Chinese medicine as a source of peace of mind, health, strength, and long life.

## SUGGESTED READINGS

Arnold, D. (2000). *The New Cambridge History of India*. Vol. 3, Part 5: Science, Technology and Medicine in Colonial India. New York: Cambridge University Press.

Bowers, J. Z., Hess, J. W., Sivin, N., and eds. (1989). *Science and Medicine in Twentieth-Century China: Research and Education.* Ann Arbor, MI: University of Michigan Press.

Buell, P., and Andersen, E. N. (2000). *A Soup for the "Qan": Chinese Dietary Medicine of the Mongol Era as seen in Hu Szu-Hui's, "Yin-Shan Cheng-yao."* New York: Kegan Paul International.

Furth, C. (1998). *A Flourishing Yin: Gender in China's Medical History, 960–1665.* Berkeley, CA: University of California Press.

Harper, D. (1997). *Early Chinese Medical Literature.* New York: Columbia University Press.

Hsu, E., ed. (2001). *Innovation in Chinese Medicine.* New York: Cambridge University Press.

Huff, T. E. (2003). *The Rise of Early Modern Science: Islam, China, and the West,* 2nd ed. New York: Cambridge University Press.

Jaggi, O. P. (2000). *Medicine in India: Modern Period.* New York: Oxford University Press.

Keightley, D. N. (1985). *Sources of Shang History: The Oracle-Bone Inscriptions of Bronze Age China.* Berkeley, CA: University of California Press.

Kuriyama, S. (1999). *The Expressiveness of the Body and the Divergence of Greek and Chinese Medicine.* Cambridge, MA: MIT Press.

Leslie, C., and Young, A., eds. (1992). *Paths to Asian Medical Knowledge.* Berkeley, CA: University of California Press.

Li Shih-Chen. (1973). *Chinese Medical Herbs.* Trans. by F. Porter Smith and G. A. Stuart. San Francisco, CA: Georgetown Press.

Liu, Y. (1988). *The Essential Book of Traditional Chinese Medicine.* 2 Vols. New York: Columbia University Press.

Lloyd, G. E. R., and Sivin, N. (2002). *The Way and the Word: Science and Medicine in Early China and Greece.* New Haven, CT: Yale University Press.

Lu, G.-D., and Needham, J. (1980). *Celestial Lancets. A History and Rationale of Acupuncture and Moxa.* New York: Cambridge University Press.

Majno, G. (1975). *The Healing Hand. Man and Wound in the Ancient World.* Cambridge, MA: Harvard University Press.

Majumdar, A. (1998). *Ayurveda: The Ancient Indian Science of Healing.* New Delhi: Wheeler Publishing.

McKnight, B. E. (1981). *The Washing Away of Wrongs: Forensic Medicine in Thirteenth-Century China.* Ann Arbor, MI: University of Michigan.

Needham, J. (1954–2000). *Science and Civilisation in China.* Vols. 1–7. New York: Cambridge University Press.

Porkert, M., with Ullmann, C. (1990). *Chinese Medicine.* New York: H. Holt.

Ray, P., and Gupta, H. N. (1965). *Charaka Samhita. A Scientific Synopsis.* New Delhi: National Institute of Sciences of India.

Scheid, V. (2002). *Chinese Medicine in Contemporary China: Plurality and Synthesis.* Durham, NC: Duke University Press.

Selin, H., ed. (2003). *Medicine Across Cultures: History and Practice of Medicine in Non-Western Cultures.* Dordrecht: Kluwer Academic.

Singhal, G. D., and Patterson, T. J. S. (1993). *Synopsis of Ayurveda: Based on a Translation of the Susruta Samhita.* New York: Oxford University Press.

Sivin, N. (1995). *Medicine, Philosophy and Religion in Ancient China: Researches and Reflections.* Brookfield, VT: Variorum.

Strickmann, M. (2002). *Chinese Magical Medicine.* Palo Alto, CA: Stanford University Press.

Unschuld, P. U. (1985). *Medicine in China. A History of Pharmaceutics.* Berkeley, CA: University of California Press.

Unschuld, P. U. (1998). *Chinese Medicine.* Brookline, MA: Paradigm Publications.

Unschuld, P. U. (2003). *Huang Di Nei Jing Su Wen: Nature, Knowledge, Imagery in an Ancient Chinese Medical Text.* Berkeley, CA: University of California Press.

Veith, I. (2002). *The Yellow Emperor's Classic of Internal Medicine.* Berkeley, CA: University of California Press.

Wujastyk, D., ed. and trans. (1998). *The Roots of Ayurveda. Selections from Sanskrit Medical Writings.* New Delhi: Penguin Books India Ltd.

Zimmermann, F. (1999). *The Jungle and the Aroma of Meats. An Ecological Theme in Hindu Medicine.* Delhi: Motilal Banarsidass.

Zysk, K. G. (1993). *Religious Medicine: The History and Evolution of Indian Medicine.* New Brunswick, NJ: Transaction Publishers.

# 4

# Greco-Roman Medicine

In contrast to the gradual evolution found in Egyptian, Indian, and Chinese history, Greek civilization seems to have emerged suddenly, much like Athena from the head of Zeus. Although this impression is certainly false, it is difficult to correct because of the paucity of material from the earliest stages of Greek history. Whatever their origins, the intellectual traditions established in ancient Greece provided the foundations of Western philosophy, science, and medicine. The early history of Greece can be divided into two periods: the Mycenaean, from about 1500 B.C.E. to the catastrophic fall of Mycenaean civilization about 1100 B.C.E., and the so-called Dark Ages from about 1100 to 800 B.C.E.. Very little information from the latter period has survived, nor is it clear what forces led to the collapse of the early phase of Greek civilization. As in India, distant memories of warfare, chaos, misfortune, and victory were transmitted in the form of myths and legends. Much of this material was gathered into the great epic poems known as the *Iliad* and the *Odyssey*, which are traditionally attributed to the ninth-century poet known as Homer. Deep within these stories of life and death, gods and heroes, exotic lands, home and family, are encoded ancient concepts of epidemic disease, the vital functions of the body, the treatment of wounds, and the roles played by physicians, surgeons, priests, and gods.

Greek medicine, as portrayed by Homer, was already an ancient and noble art. Apollo appears as the most powerful of the god-physicians, as well as the god of prophecy. Apollo could cause epidemic disease as a form of punishment or restore and heal the wounded. In search of the god's advice and guidance, the ancients flocked to his famous oracle at the Temple of Apollo at Delphi. Originally a shrine to Gaea, the earth goddess, the site was said to be the center of the world. Before transmitting the words of the god, the oracle, who was always a woman known as the Pythia, would enter a small chamber, inhale the sweet-smelling vapors coming from a fissure in the earth, and succumb to a trace-like state. Sometimes, after inhaling the intoxicating fumes, the oracle would go from trance to delirium to death. When nineteenth-century archaeologists excavating the temple failed to find the legendary chamber, they rejected Plutarch's theory of intoxicating fumes coming from deep within the earth. But in 2001, scientists discovered a previously unknown conjunction of geological faults beneath the temple grounds. They suggested that the ground waters below the Pythia's chamber could have carried various chemicals, including ethylene, a gas that has been used as an anesthetic. Inhaling ethylene produces euphoria, but an overdose can be fatal.

In the Homeric epics, priests, seers, and dream readers dealt with the mysterious plagues and pestilences attributed to the gods. When angered, the gods could cause physical and mental disorders, but they might also provide sedatives and antidotes to save those they favored. In the *Iliad*, the skillful physician is praised as a man more valuable than many others.

Given the large number of war injuries so poignantly described by Homer, skillful doctors were desperately needed. In some instances, however, warriors treated their comrades or bravely extracted arrows from their own limbs. Wound infection, traumatic fever, and deaths due to secondary hemorrhages were probably uncommon, because the wounded rarely lingered long enough to develop such complications. The mortality rate among the wounded was close to 80 percent.

Medical treatment in the *Iliad* was generally free of magical practices, but when medicine failed, healers might resort to incantations and prayers. Sometimes, the surgeon would suck the site of a wound, perhaps as an attempt to draw out poisons or some "evil influence" in the blood. After washing the wound with warm water, physicians applied soothing drugs and consoled or distracted the patient with wine, pleasant stories, or songs. Unlike the complex Egyptian and Indian wound poultices, Greek wound remedies were "simples" derived from plants. Unfortunately for the Greek warriors, their physicians did not know the secret of Helen's famous Egyptian potion, *nepenthe*, which could dispel pain and strife and erase the memory of disease and sorrow. Indeed, the specific identities of most of the drugs referred to by Homer are obscure, although various sources suggest that the soothing agents, secret potions, and fumigants used by healers and priests of this time period probably included warm water, wine, oil, honey, sulfur, saffron, and opium.

Modern Western medicine traces its origins to the rational, scientific tradition associated with Hippocrates, but even the secular physicians of classical Greece traced their art back to Asclepius, the god of medicine. Asclepius, who was said to be the son of Apollo, appears in the *Iliad* as heroic warrior and "blameless physician." According to Homer, Chiron, the wise and noble centaur, taught Asclepius the secrets of the drugs that relieve pain and stop bleeding. The sons of Asclepius were also warriors and healers; their special talents presage the future division of the healing art into medicine and surgery. The cunning hands of Machaon could heal all kinds of wounds, but it was Podalirius who understood hidden diseases and their cure. When Machaon was injured, his wound was simply washed and sprinkled with grated goat cheese and barley meal. The methods Machaon used to cure the hero Menelaus were only slightly more complicated. After extracting the arrow that had pierced the hero's belt, Machaon sucked out the blood and sprinkled the wound with soothing remedies that Chiron had given to Asclepius.

The magical and shamanistic practices that once flourished in Greece left their traces in myths, poems, and rituals, such as the annual festival held in honor of Melampus, founder of a long line of seers, who had acquired knowledge of divination from Egypt. Combining elements of purification and "psychotherapy" with strong purgative drugs, Melampus was able to cure disorders ranging from impotence to insanity. Melampus is also said to have taught Orpheus how to use healing drugs.

The story of Orpheus incorporates the shamanistic elements of the healer who enters the underworld in pursuit of a departed soul, and the dismemberment and reconstitution of the shaman. As the son of the muse Calliope, Orpheus possessed skill in healing and supernatural musical gifts. When his beloved wife Eurydice died, Orpheus descended into Hades where he charmed the gods of the underworld into allowing him to bring back her soul. His failure to comply with all the conditions surrounding her release led to the failure of his mission. Contrary to the explicit instructions he had received from the gods, Orpheus turned to look at Eurydice before she had completed the journey from Hades back to the world of the living. A distraught Orpheus realized he had lost Eurydice once again. Finally, the unfortunate Orpheus was torn to pieces by wine-crazed followers of Dionysus, the god of wine. Preternaturally musical to the end, the spirit of Orpheus continued to sing as his head floated to Lesbos.

## PHILOSOPHY AND MEDICINE

Shamanistic, religious, and empirical approaches to healing seem to be universal aspects of the history of medicine. Where Greek medicine appears to be unique is in the development of a body of medical theory associated with natural philosophy, that is, a strong secular tradition of free enquiry, or what would now be called science. Scholars have suggested that the fundamental difference between Greek and Chinese thought was the competitiveness of early Greek political and intellectual life. Whereas Chinese thinkers sought consensus, Greek thinkers openly criticized their teachers, rivals, and peers. Unlike previous civilizations, the Greeks were not primarily organized around agriculture and a strong central government or priesthood. The city-state became their unit of organization and, because Greece was relatively overpopulated in relation to cultivatable land, trade, colonization, and industry were encouraged.

The earliest Greek natural philosophers were profoundly interested in the natural world and the search for explanations of how and why the world and human beings came to be formed and organized as they were. Natural philosophy developed first, not in the Athens of Socrates, Plato, and Aristotle, but on the Aegean fringes of the mainland of Asia Minor. By the sixth-century B.C.E., Greek philosophers were attempting to explain the workings of the universe in terms of everyday experience and by analogies with craft processes rather than divine interventions and supernatural agents. Many of the earliest Greek philosophers are known only through a few fragments of their work, but enough has survived to reveal their ingenious theories as the seed crystals that were to stimulate the subsequent evolution of Western physics, astronomy, biology, and medicine.

Pythagoras of Samos (ca. 530 B.C.E.) is said to have been the first Greek philosopher with a special interest in medical subjects. Although the Pythagorean concept of a universe composed of opposite qualities is reminiscent of Chinese yin-yang philosophy, the Pythagorean approach was apparently inspired by mathematical inquiries. Just as numbers formed the two categories, "odd" and "even," so could all things be divided into pairs of opposites. The harmony, or proper balance of pairs of qualities, such as hot and cold, moist and dry, was especially important in matters of health and disease.

Although the medical theories of Alcmaeon of Croton (ca. 500 B.C.E.) have much in common with those of Pythagoras, the exact relationship between them is uncertain. Both Alcmaeon and Pythagoras believed that pairs of opposites were the first principles of existence. Health, according to Alcmaeon, was a harmonious blending of each of the qualities with its appropriate opposite, such as moist and dry, cold and hot, bitter and sweet. Disease occurs when one member of a pair appears in excess; an excess of heat causes fever, an excess of cold causes chills. The idea that the systematic dissection of animals would provide a means of understanding the nature of human beings was attributed to Alcmaeon. Despite the loss of most of his writings, Alcmaeon was one of the first physician-philosophers to exert a significant influence on the course of Greek medical and scientific thought.

A paradoxical blend of philosophy and mysticism is part of the legacy of Empedocles (ca. 500–430 B.C.E.). Echoing themes common to shamanism, Empedocles boasted that he could heal the sick, rejuvenate the aged, raise the dead, and control wind and weather. Numerous references to him in later medical writings suggest great fame and success as a healer, but it was his theory of the four elements that became a major theme in the history of medicine. According to Empedocles, all things were composed of mixtures of four primary and eternal elements: air, earth, water, and fire. Changes and transformations in the cosmos and the human body were simply reflections of the mixing and unmixing of the eternal elements.

## HIPPOCRATES AND THE HIPPOCRATIC TRADITION

Many of the early Greek philosophers and medical writers have been largely forgotten, but the name Hippocrates (ca. 460–360 B.C.E.) has become synonymous with the phrase "Father of Medicine." The establishment of medicine as an art, a science, and a profession of great value and dignity has been associated with the life and work of Hippocrates. Yet surprisingly little is known about his life. Indeed, some historians insist that Hippocrates was neither the author of the Hippocratic collection nor even a real person. For the sake of simplicity and tradition, we shall use the name Hippocrates as the exemplar of the ideal physician of antiquity and for any of the authors of the medical texts attributed to Hippocrates. Presumably, these texts were written by physicians who practiced medicine in accordance with the principles known to us as Hippocratic medicine.

Although Hippocrates was widely praised and respected in antiquity, many of the most fascinating biographical details were supplied several centuries after his death. Historians note that, in response to changing cultural and social circumstances, the idea of Hippocrates and Hippocratic medicine have been subjected to cycles of construction, reconstruction, and transformation ever since antiquity. It was probably during the Renaissance that the modern picture of Hippocrates emerged. Today, the image of Hippocrates is invoked as a model for the ideal physician and the philosophy of humanistic holism.

According to ancient biographers, Hippocrates was born on the island of Cos, lived a long, exemplary life, and died in Larissa when 95 or perhaps 110 years old. In genealogical tables constructed by his later admirers, Hippocrates traced his ancestry back to Asclepius on his father's side and to Hercules on the maternal side. Plato and Aristotle spoke of Hippocrates with respect, despite the fact that he taught medicine for a fee. Not all ancient writers praised Hippocrates. The Father of Medicine was accused of burning down the medical library at Cos in order to eliminate competing medical traditions. An even more unflattering story accused Hippocrates of plagiarizing the prescriptions of Asclepius before destroying the god's temple and claiming clinical medicine as his own invention. Another legend says that the great doctor

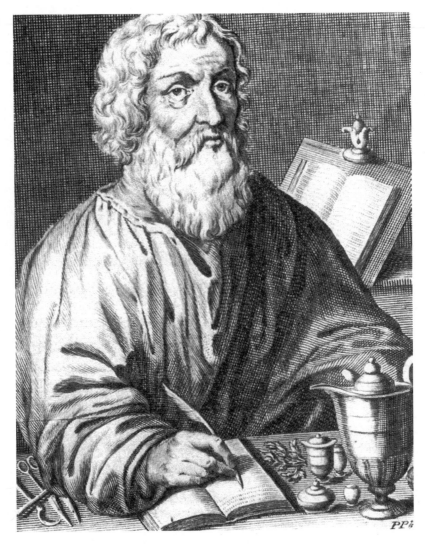

**Hippocrates.**

never thought about collecting fees and was always ready to admit his errors.

Whatever uncertainty there may be about Hippocrates himself, the collection of some fifty to seventy essays and texts attributed to him is undoubtedly the foundation of Western medicine. Ironically, as scholars gained more information about the writings of the ancients, they had to admit to less and less certainty about distinctions between the "genuine" and the "spurious" works of Hippocrates. Nevertheless, throughout Greek, Roman, and medieval times, the texts that had made their way into the Hippocratic collection remained authoritative and worthy of study, interpretation, and commentary. In Western history, Hippocratic medicine is revered for its emphasis on the patient instead of the disease, observation rather than theory, respect for facts and experience rather than philosophical systems, "expectative therapy" (rather like "watchful waiting") as opposed to "active intervention," and the Hippocratic motto: "At least do no harm."

One of the most important and characteristic expressions of Hippocratic medicine is found in the text known as *On Ancient Medicine*. A major thesis of this work is that nature itself has strong healing forces. The purpose of the physician, therefore, was to cultivate techniques that would work in harmony with natural healing forces to restore the body to a harmonious balance. Other characteristics of the Hippocratic texts are perceptive descriptions of the symptoms of various diseases, insights into medical geography and anthropology, and explorations of the idea that climate, social institutions, religion, and government can affect health and disease.

By assigning explanations for the phenomena of health and disease to nature and reason, the Hippocratic physician rejected superstition, divination, and magic. In other words, if the world was uniform and natural, all phenomena were equally part of nature. If the gods were responsible for any particular phenomenon, they were equally responsible for all phenomena. Thus, nature was everywhere both natural and divine. While Hippocrates ridiculed the deceptions practiced in the name of religious healing, he was not opposed to prayer and piety. "Prayer indeed is good," Hippocrates conceded, "but while calling on the gods one must oneself lend a hand." Skepticism was also appropriate with respect to the claims of philosophers, because, according to Hippocrates, one could learn more about nature through the proper study of medicine than from philosophy alone.

The true physician understood that disease was a natural process, not the result of possession, supernatural agents, or punishment sent by the gods. Disease could be interpreted as punishment only in the sense that one could be punished for transgressing against nature by improper behaviors. Thus, to care for his patient, the physician must understand the constitution of the individual and determine how health was related to food, drink, and mode of life.

In a fundamental sense, *dietetics* was the basis of the art of healing. According to Hippocrates, human beings could not consume the rough food suitable for other animals; thus, the first cook was the first physician. From such crude beginnings, the art of medicine developed as people empirically discovered which diets and regimens were appropriate in sickness and in health. As medicine became more sophisticated, physicians became skilled and knowledgeable craftsmen. As knowledge about human beings and nature accumulated, philosophers propounded theories about the nature of human life and derived therapeutic systems from their theories. Medicine and philosophy interacted to their mutual benefit, but Hippocrates refused to be bound by any rigid medical dogma, or therapeutic system, such as treatment by "similars" or "opposites." The experienced physician knew that some diseases were cured by the use of opposites and others by the use of similars. That is, in practice, the physician discovered that some "hot" diseases in some patients could be cured by cooling medicines, while others might require warming remedies.

While the physician must not be bound by philosophical systems, neither should a practitioner of the healing art ever act as an unthinking technician. The true physician understood the principles guiding his course of action in each case, as related to the nature of man, disease, diagnosis, remedies, and treatment. Moreover, this display of medical knowledge and proper behavior helped win the trust of the patient.

In the absence of legally recognized professional qualifications and standards, virtually anyone could claim to be a physician. Thus, to secure his reputation and compete with quacks and magicians, the physician had to prove that medicine was an art and a science that could promote health and cure disease. Complaints about ignorant physicians and outright quacks appear in many Hippocratic texts, suggesting that the profession was already plagued by impostors who were bringing disrepute to the art.

The related problems of professional recognition, standards of practice, and ethical obligations are addressed in several Hippocratic texts. However, the well-known formula known as the "Hippocratic Oath" may have been composed and popularized long after the death of Hippocrates. There is little doubt that the Oath was originally Greek, as indicated by various ancient manuscripts and inscriptions on Greek temples. There are many uncertainties about the origins, usage, purpose, and meaning of the Oath, but there is considerable evidence to suggest that the text honored as the nucleus of Western medical ethics was actually a "neo-Pythagorean manifesto." During the Roman era, Greek physicians like Scribonious Largus, personal physician to the Emperor Claudius, cited the Hippocratic Oath as proof of their good intentions and reliability. However, the Oath apparently had limited influence until it was essentially adopted as a useful bridge between antiquity and Christianity.

Although the Oath includes the promise to practice medicine for the benefit of the patient, a prohibition against giving anyone a lethal drug, or using medical knowledge to cause the sick any danger or injury, it was primarily a private contract between a new physician and his teacher, not, as commonly assumed, a promise from practitioner to patient. Indeed, the Greeks had no official medical practice act to enforce such contracts. Presumably, it was love of the art, joined with love of man and fear of dishonor, more than the swearing of oaths that made the Hippocratic physician conform to the highest standards of medical ethics.

The fact that the Hippocratic Oath prohibits prescribing a "destructive pessary" may be the most compelling evidence that the Oath represents the precepts of the Pythagoreans rather than Greek physicians in general, because this prohibition was essentially unique to that sect. The ancients generally accepted abortion and infanticide as means of population control. Surgical abortions were condemned because they were more dangerous than childbirth, not because they were necessarily immoral. Moreover, unwanted infants could be "exposed." Generally, midwives dealt with normal childbirth, abortion, and assorted "female complaints," but the physician could prescribe appropriate fumigations, fomentation, washes, and pessaries. Although the Hippocratic texts discuss the diseases of women in some detail, Hippocrates acknowledged that women were often so reluctant to discuss their problems with physicians that simple illnesses became incurable. According to some calculations, gynecological texts make up about a quarter of the Hippocratic collection.

Within the ethical framework of antiquity, very different patterns of medical treatment were considered appropriate to the rich and the poor. For the rich, the aesthetic pursuit of health was far more significant than the mere absence of disease. Striving for optimum health required a complex, time-consuming regimen and presupposed that the patient could assign complete control over food, drink, exercise, rest, and other aspects of life to the most skillful physician. Patients who were free but poor could expect an intermediate kind of pragmatically designed medical care, without the benefits of individualized regimens. Remedies that acted swiftly were appropriate for patients lacking time and money, because the poor must either recover quickly and resume their work or die and so be relieved of all further troubles. The Hippocratic texts indicate that the physician did not necessarily refuse to treat slaves, or to adapt dietetic therapy to the needs of the poor. But various sources suggest that, for the most part, the treatment of slaves was rather like veterinary medicine and was carried out by the doctor's servants.

Ideally, the Hippocratic physician did not practice medicine merely for the sake of money, but like other craftsmen who had perfected their skills, the physician was entitled to a fee for his services. The ethical physician was expected to consider the status of the patient in determining the size of the fee. He was not to argue about fees before treating a patient, especially in acute illnesses, because extra worries might interfere with the patient's recovery. Patients without money who hoped to acquire the services of the ideal physician described in the Hippocratic texts were well advised to remember the Greek proverb "There is no skill where there is no reward."

Many noble sentiments about the practice of medicine and the relief of suffering are found in the Hippocratic texts, but the limits of the art were sharply defined. Knowing that it was impossible to cure all patients, the physician had to determine which patients would die in order to avoid blame. Thus, the injunction against treatment in diseases that were necessarily fatal was a fundamental principle of Hippocratic medicine. Unlike the temple priest, who had the authority of the gods to protect and excuse him, the secular physician was in a peculiar, highly vulnerable position. Only skill, success, and a rigorous commitment to the ethical standards of the profession protected the physician. Ultimately, the physician was a craftsman, who was judged by his patients—not by a peer review committee—according to the results of his art.

## THE NATURE OF DISEASE AND THE DOCTRINE OF THE FOUR HUMORS

The modern physician and patient are especially eager for a precise *diagnosis*—the ceremonial naming of the disease—but this was of little importance to the Hippocratic physician. His main preoccupation was *prognosis*, which meant not only predicting the future course of the disease, but also providing a history of the illness. This recital of past and future was a factor in impressing the patient and family with the knowledge and skill of the physician. It also was essential in predicting crises and deaths so that no blame would be attached to the physician if they occurred.

Rather than recording lists of symptoms, without weight or judgment, Hippocratic physicians looked for characteristic patterns of signs and symptoms in order to chart the course of an illness. Diagnostic signs are characteristics of the disease that are not self-evident, but must be specially detected. Only a skillful physician could detect the obscure signs betrayed by abnormal colors, sounds, heat, hardness, and swellings. If further information was needed, the physician could prescribe cathartics and emetics, which were meant to restore balance as well as provide further evidence of the state of the patient's humors.

For Hippocrates, disease was not a localized phenomenon, but a disturbance affecting the whole person through some imbalance in the four humors—blood, phlegm, black bile, and yellow bile. The four humors and the four associated qualities—hot, cold, moist, and dry—in the *microcosm* or small world of the human body corresponded to the four elements—earth, air, fire, and water—that make up the *macrocosm* or universe. Various texts in the Hippocratic collection offer observations and theoretical rationalizations concerning the relationship between health and disease and the humors, qualities, and elements, but these explanations are sometimes obscure and inconsistent.

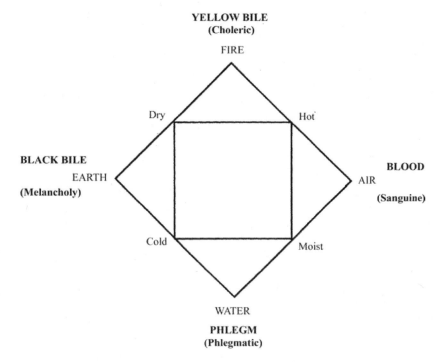

**The four humors and the four elements.**

The humoral doctrine explains health as the result of the harmonious balance and blending of the four humors. An excess of one of the humors results in a *dyscrasia*, or abnormal mixture. Particular *temperaments* were associated with a relative abundance of each humor. The sanguine, phlegmatic, choleric (or bilious), and melancholic temperaments are roughly equivalent to different personality types, and suggest vulnerability to characteristic disorders.

Although the four humors are theoretically related to the four elements, the physician could also justify their existence in terms of certain commonplace observations. Until very recent times, the only "analytic laboratory" available to the physician was that made up of the five senses. In other words, the nose and tongue served as the first analytical chemists. Thus, to understand the nature of the patient's disease, all excretions, secretions, and effluvia had to be analyzed directly in terms of sense perceptions. When examining blood in terms of the senses and the theory of the four humors, blood undergoing the clotting process might seem to reveal the "unmixing" of the four humors. The darkest part of the clot would correspond to black bile, the serum above the clot is apparently yellow bile, and the light material at the top is phlegm. Alternatively, phlegm might be equivalent to nasal mucus, yellow bile could be the bitter fluid stored in the gall bladder, and black bile might be the dark material sometimes found in vomit, urine, and excrement (a sign of internal bleeding).

According to Hippocratic theory, the processes by which the body fought off disease were essentially exaggerated forms of normal physiological functions. Disease was a state in which the organism experienced a greater degree of difficulty in mastering the environment. Restoration of humoral equilibrium proceeded through stages in which the crude or morbid matter in the humors ripened sufficiently to be eliminated through secretions, excretions, or hemorrhages during a *crisis*, which might end in recovery or death. In acute diseases, the elimination of morbid matter generally occurred on certain *critical days*. Charting the course of a disease by means of the critical days and characteristic patterns of signs and symptoms, the physician could expedite the process with proper treatment.

Humoral pathology provided a natural explanation for even the most feared and dreaded mental as well as physical illnesses. Indeed, no treatise in the Hippocratic collection provides a more powerful and timeless attack on ignorance and superstition than *On the Sacred Disease*. Hippocrates declared that even the sacred disease, which we know as epilepsy, was no more sacred or divine than any other illness; like any other disease, it arose from a natural cause. But, frightened by the specter of recurrent, unpredictable seizures in otherwise healthy individuals, ignorant people attributed the disease to the gods. Those who "cured" the disease by magical means supported the false belief in its "sacred" nature. Prescribing purifications, incantations, and bizarre rituals, quacks were quick to claim credit when the patient seemed to recover. When the patient relapsed or died, they blamed their failures on the gods or the patient. The Hippocratic physician regarded such deceptive practices as impious and sacrilegious.

While despising magical practices, Hippocrates did not ignore dreams. Most patients regarded dreams with superstitious awe, but Hippocrates tried to relate dreams to the patient's physiological state. Some dreams might be regarded as precognitive "divine" dreams, but others were obvious cases of wish-fulfillment. The dreams of most interest to the physician were those which expressed some morbid state in symbolic form because they might offer guidance in treatment.

Humoral pathology could explain epilepsy, just as it explained any other disease. (Indeed, one of the problems with humoral theory is the ease with which it explains *everything*, and thus, ultimately, explains nothing at all.) Hippocrates suggested that a child might be born with epilepsy if both father and mother were phlegmatic, because excess phlegm might accumulate during gestation and injure the fetal brain. Many ancient philosophers considered the heart to be the seat of consciousness, but Hippocrates assigned that role to the brain. Therefore, it followed that afflictions of the brain produced the most dangerous diseases.

Attitudes towards epilepsy can been seen as a sort of litmus test for the achievement of enlightened attitudes towards the sick. Unfortunately, Hippocratic medicine was no match for the prejudice surrounding epilepsy, madness, and other supposedly mysterious afflictions. Throughout history, remedies for epilepsy have included magical and superstitious practices, as well as dangerous and futile treatments ranging from bleeding and cauterization to trephination and hysterectomy. By the end of the twentieth century, the problem of defining epilepsy was considered so complex that physicians often spoke of "epilepsies" as a means of distancing their diagnostic struggle from previous views of epilepsy as a unitary pathological entity. Despite centuries of inquiry, the etiology of epilepsy remained obscure, prognosis uncertain, and accepted treatments may have caused more harm than good.

Humoral theory rationalized a therapeutic regimen designed to assist the natural healing tendency by bleeding, purging, and regulating the diet in order to remove morbid humors and prevent the formation of additional bad humors. Given the dangers thought to lurk in most foods, the physician might allow no foods stronger than barley water, hydromel (honey and water), or oxymel (vinegar, honey, and water). Indeed, in order to assist the body's natural healing tendency, the physician might "reduce" the patient's diet almost to the point of starvation.

Despite the Hippocratic preference for mild and simple remedies, Greek physicians could prescribe a wide array of drugs, which were administered in many forms, including poultices, ointments, pessaries, pills, and suppositories. Most components came from local plants, but some were imported from India and Egypt. Remedies might contain pleasant ingredients like cinnamon, cardamom, and saffron. On the other hand, a well-known diuretic for dropsical patients included cantharides beetles, minus the heads, feet, and wings. ("Blistering beetle" or "Spanish fly" has long been used in dried and powdered form as a diuretic or putative aphrodisiac when taken internally, and as a skin irritant when applied externally.)

Some cases, however, called for stronger methods such as cupping, scarification, venesection, cauterization, and other forms of surgery. According to one of the aphorisms that guided Hippocratic medical practice, "What drugs will not cure, the knife will; what the knife will not cure, the cautery will; what the cautery will not cure must be considered incurable." For the most part, "surgery" meant the treatment of wounds, fractures, dislocations, and other traumatic injuries. In such cases, the practitioner's experience and acquired skills were all important because Hippocratic physicians did not perform postmortems or carry out systematic programs of animal dissection. Thus, only chance observations on injured patients and general knowledge of animal anatomy illuminated the "black box" that was the human body.

In managing wounds and ulcers, simple remedies and cleanliness allowed healing to proceed with a minimum of inflammation and pus. Various kinds of herbs, boiled in water or mixed with wine, were used as cleansing agents and wound dressings. Remedies containing certain minerals, such as salts or oxides of copper and lead, were used to dry and soothe wounds. Bandaging wounds and fractures was an art form in which the physician could demonstrate speed, skill, and elegance.

When necessary, the physician could suture wounds, trephine the skull, perform artificial pneumothorax (collapsing the lung), and insert tents and tubes into the chest cavity to drain pus, as recorded in various case histories presented in *On Disease* and *On Wounds*. However, when wounds became gangrenous, the physician was reluctant to intervene, because amputation could lead to death from shock and bleeding. Similarly, the physician preferred to treat abscesses with medicines that would encourage spontaneous rupture and the discharge of pus, rather than opening the abscesses with the knife. Hippocrates urged his followers to cure by selecting the least harmful method. In a Hippocratic text called *On Head Wounds*, the author described the structure of the skull and the relationship between the seriousness of head injuries and the possibility of survival. Practitioners were urged to conduct a careful examination of the wound and evaluate the patient's initial reaction to the injury. The physician was advised to look for signs that predicted death, such as fever, suppuration, discoloration of the bone, delirium, and convulsions. If the patient could survive, treatment options ranged from poulticing and bandaging to trephination.

Whatever success the Hippocratic physician may have had in caring for individual patients, the plague that struck Athens in 430 B.C.E. during the Peloponnesian War demonstrated that his skills were no match for epidemic disease. Hippocrates reputedly warned that in the event of plague the best course of action was "*cito, longe, tarde*," which is usually translated as "go fast, go far, return slowly." The most vivid portrait of the plague was recorded not by a physician, but by the Greek historian Thucydides. Having survived his own battle with the disease and witnessed many tragic cases, Thucydides felt well qualified to write about the plague.

After a year relatively free of disease, the plague attacked Athens so suddenly that at first the people thought that all their wells had been poisoned. Healthy people were seized with headaches, sneezing, hoarseness, pain in the chest, coughing, vomiting, and violent spasms. Although the body was not very hot to the touch, it became reddish and livid, with the eruption of blisters and ulcers. Death usually occurred on the seventh or ninth day, but in those who lingered on, the disease descended into the bowels, where it led to ulceration and diarrhea. Some patients lost their fingers, toes, or eyes. Others suffered from mental confusion so severe they could not remember their own name or recognize their closest relatives. Priests and physicians were helpless against the plague and often fell victim to the disease themselves.

The most terrible feature of the disease, according to Thucydides, was the depression that fell upon the afflicted and the general abandonment of morality and custom by almost the whole population. Fear of the gods and the law was forgotten; no one expected to live long enough to pay the penalty for any transgressions. Only those who had survived an attack of the disease were willing to nurse the sick, because the same person was never stricken twice. Despite Thucydides' vivid description of the epidemic, the exact nature of the disease is obscure. Among the diagnoses that have been offered are typhus, scarlet fever, bubonic plague, smallpox, measles, and anthrax. Whatever this pestilence may have been, it provides a striking example of the recurrent theme of social disintegration linked to war and epidemic disease.

Physicians were also challenged by endemic diseases such as malaria that insidiously attacked the Mediterranean region. The causative agent and the mechanism of transmission for malaria were not discovered until the late nineteenth century, but the association between marshes and malarial fevers was suspected by the time of Hippocrates. When first introduced into a region, malaria may cause deadly epidemics, but the disease generally becomes stubbornly endemic. Instead of killing or immunizing its victims, malaria makes them more susceptible to further attacks and to other diseases. People learn to associate seasonal activities and all forms of exertion with attacks of fever. The chronic loss of agricultural productivity in communities weakened by malaria leads to malnutrition, famine, and increased susceptibility to disease. Malaria has been called the greatest killer in all of human history and a major factor in the decline of Greek science, art, and literature.

## THE CULT OF ASCLEPIUS, GOD OF MEDICINE

Although Hippocrates is the dominant figure in modern accounts of Greek medicine, in antiquity the good doctor shared the stage with the healer who began his career as the "blameless physician" in the *Ilaid*. It was during the age of Hippocrates, not the age of Homer, that Asclepius was elevated to the status of a god. This was a time of extraordinary tension between intellectual freedom and intolerance. Impiety and "godlessness" were crimes that could be punished by death or banishment. Excessive interest in the nature of the universe could even be regarded as a sign of madness, as in the case of Democritus of Abdera, the founder of atomic theory. When Democritus began a series of

dissections as a means of understanding structure and function in animals, his neighbors interpreted these anatomies as signs of madness,
outside the acceptable range of scholarly eccentricity. According to tradition, Hippocrates was called upon to cure the philosopher, but having
spoken at length with Democritus, the physician told the people of
Abdera that they were more likely to be mad than Democritus, who
was both rational and wise.

As demonstrated in the history of other civilizations, what is now
called modern scientific medicine has not totally displaced traditional,
folk, or religious approaches to healing. Thus, it should not be surprising that Hippocratic medicine did not totally displace religious medicine
in the ancient world. For chronic, episodic, and unpredictable conditions, such as arthritis, gout, migraine headache, epilepsy, impotence,
infertility, and malaria, when patients felt that the physician was ineffective, magicians and priests could always offer hope and even the illusion
of cure during the intervals between attacks. Some historians believe
that the increase in magical and superstitious medicine during the age
of Hippocrates may have been due, in part, to the growing burden of
malaria. Still, despite the differences between Hippocratic medicine
and religious medicine, Asclepius and Hippocrates shared certain basic
assumptions about the best approach to healing. "First the word,"
Asclepius taught, "then the herb, lastly the knife."

Over the course of several centuries, the cult of Asclepius spread
throughout the Greek world, established itself in Rome, and only
gradually gave ground to Christianity as arbiter of the meaning of disease and healing. Legendary accounts of the life and times of Asclepius
agree that he was the son of Apollo, but there were disagreements about
the place and manner of his birth. His mother was either a nymph or a
woman named Coronis who was killed by Apollo's sister Artemis. With
poor Coronis on her funeral pyre, Apollo decided to bring his son to the
home of Chiron the centaur, who had tutored many great heroes.
According to Homer, Chiron taught Achilles and Asclepius the secret
of drugs that relieve pain and stop bleeding. Thanks to his mentor,
Asclepius mastered the use of the knife and learned the secret virtues
of herbs. When in addition to curing the sick, Asclepius took to restoring
the dead to life, Pluto, god of the underworld, complained to Zeus. Afraid
that mortals would ignore the gods if they felt that human healers
could save them, Zeus struck down the son of Apollo. Eventually,
Asclepius became the god of medicine and was worshipped in magnificent temples, served by priests who called themselves Asclepiads
(descendants of Asclepius).

Asclepian temples were built at Cos, Cnidus, Epidaurus, and other
sites blessed with springs of pure water and magnificent views. In temple
illustrations, the god was often portrayed with his daughters, Hygeia
and Panacea, and Telesphorus, the god of convalescence. Like Lourdes

and other modern healing shrines, the temples of Asclepius became places for hopeful pilgrimages and miraculous cures. Information about temple medicine has come from studies of archaeological remains, votive tablets that record the stories of satisfied patients, models depicting the organs healed at the temple, and references to temple magic in literary sources. But even in ancient Greece there were skeptics who ridiculed the testimonies as deliberate forgeries or the ravings of hypochondriacs and insisted that there would have been many more tablets if those who were not cured had made declarations.

Among the ruins of the temple at Epidaurus is a shrine dedicated to Hygeia, who may have been the original Greek goddess of health. Like the Chinese sages who would not treat the sick, Hygeia taught people to achieve health and longevity by proper behavior. Her independent cult was eventually subsumed by that of Asclepius and her status was reduced from independent practitioner to physician's assistant. Asclepius also enjoyed the help of holy dogs and sacred snakes. In contrast to the Mesopotamian hero Gilgamesh, who lost the herb of healing to a snake, Asclepius received the precious herb from a sacred serpent. Thus, Asclepius was often portrayed with a snake coiled about his staff. The caduceus, the sign of the modern physician, which contains two snakes intertwined on a winged staff, seems to suggest increased snake-power, but it is actually closer to the magic wand of Mercury, the messenger of the gods and the patron of thieves and merchants.

The Asclepiads boasted that all who entered the temple sanctuary were cured. Presumably, they achieved a perfect record by carefully selecting their patients. Temporary remissions and spontaneous recovery from psychosomatic complaints and self-limited diseases provide all medical systems with a large measure of success. Nevertheless, in Plato's *Republic* Socrates says that Asclepius did not attempt to cure bodies thoroughly wracked by disease. Even the healing god would not lengthen lives that were plainly not worth saving, or allow weak fathers to beget even weaker sons.

The most important part of temple medicine was called "incubation," or temple sleep. Incubation was part of the ancient practice of seeking divine dreams of guidance as the culmination of a series of preliminary rites which might include fasting, prolonged isolation, self-mutilation, and hallucinogenic potions. Sleeping on animal skins in front of an image of Asclepius was a rather mild form of this nearly universal ritual. Some patients reported instantaneous cures after being touched by the god, or licked by the sacred snakes and holy dogs that guarded the temple. Fortunate patients reported that Asclepius himself came to them during therapeutic dreams. Sometimes the god recommended simple remedies, such as vegetables for constipation, but Asclepius might also direct the patient to smear his eyes with blood or swim in icy rivers. For some conditions, cure or improvement might indeed result from the combination of rest, fresh air, good diet, hope, and suggestion encountered at the temples of Asclepius. Religious rituals and the release of tension and anxiety occasioned by following the commands of the god might have cured many psychosomatic complaints, and comforted many patients, even if a specific cure was impossible.

Women were not allowed to give birth within the grounds of the temple, but Asclepius accepted various gynecological and obstetric challenges, especially infertility. Many barren women reported that they became pregnant after visiting the temples. However, as demonstrated by the testimonial of Ithmonice, who asked the god if she could become pregnant with a daughter, supplicants had to be very careful in framing their requests. Hinting at the complications that might occur, Asclepius asked Ithmonice whether she wanted anything else, but she could not imagine wanting more. After carrying the child in her womb for three years, Ithmonice sought another favor from the god. Asclepius reminded Ithmonice that she had only requested conception and had not mentioned delivery, but the god graciously granted her new request. As soon as Ithmonice left the sacred precincts her daughter was born.

According to the testimonies, grateful patients praised the god for curing headaches, paralysis, general debility, and blindness. A man who claimed to have swallowed leeches and a woman who thought she had a worm in her belly testified to being opened up by the god, who removed the infestation and stitched up the incision. Even relatively minor problems might receive the god's attention. One man came to the temple for help because his neighbors made fun of his bald head. During temple sleep, the god anointed his head with a drug that caused the growth of thick black hair.

## ALEXANDRIAN SCIENCE AND MEDICINE

In the ancient world, Alexandria, the city in Egypt named for Alexander the Great (356–323 B.C.E.), represented wealth and stability, a fusion of the ancient lore of Egypt and the most dynamic elements of Greek civilization. Among the greatest treasures of the city were its museum and library. The scholars who worked at the museum and library, under the sponsorship of the rulers of Alexandria, participated in an unprecedented intellectual experiment. According to some estimates, the Alexandrian library contained more than 700,000 scrolls. The librarians collected, confiscated, copied, and edited many manuscripts, including the texts now known as the Hippocratic collection. In discussing the authenticity of various works in the Hippocratic collection, Galen of Pergamum claimed that the rulers of Alexandria were so eager to enhance the library that they confiscated all books found on ships entering the harbor. Galen warned that many forgeries had been created to satisfy the Alexandrian passion for book collecting. The magnificent facilities of the museum are said to have included zoological and botanical gardens, lecture halls, and rooms for research and teaching. To encourage the exchange of ideas, the scholars took their meals together in the great hall of the museum; the meals were free and the salary of the professors was tax exempt. Unfortunately, no contemporary accounts of the famous museum have survived and the evidence concerning the medical research conducted at the museum is ambiguous.

Many sciences flourished at Alexandria, although research was primarily oriented towards fields with practical applications, such as medicine and engineering. Medical experts were expected to supervise city and army sanitation and train military doctors. Most importantly, for a brief and rare interval, the practice of human dissection was not only tolerated, but actively encouraged. Perhaps the Egyptian tradition of cutting open the body and removing certain organs as part of the embalming ritual helped overcome traditional Greek antipathy to the mutilation of corpses. Alexandrian scientists helped establish two of the major themes of Western medical theory: first, that systematic dissection provides essential information about structure and function; second, that this knowledge is valuable in and of itself, even if it provides little or nothing of immediate practical value to clinical medicine, patient care, or public health.

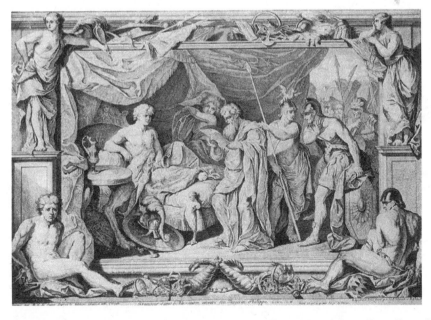

**Alexander the Great and his physicians. As he died, Alexander allegedly said, "I am dying with the help of too many physicians."**

For medical science, the Hellenistic period (roughly the time
between the death of Alexander to about 30 B.C.E., when the Romans
annexed Egypt) is most notable for the work of its most famous, or
infamous, anatomists—Herophilus (ca. 330/320–260/250 B.C.E.) and
Erasistratus (ca. 310–250 B.C.E.). Unfortunately, so little direct information about the Alexandrian era has been preserved that the exact
relationship between these anatomists and the city of Alexandria remains
obscure. Historians agree that both Herophilus and Erasistratus were
skillful anatomists who eagerly exploited the opportunity to conduct
studies of human bodies, but it is not clear whether anatomists of this
era performed some of their studies on living human beings or confined
themselves to postmortems. Anatomists might also have used their
patients and students as experimental subjects for less invasive research.
When Christian theologians such as Tertullian and St. Augustine wanted
evidence of the heinous acts committed by the pagans, they pointed to
the notorious Herophilus and accused him of torturing six hundred
human beings to death. The Roman encyclopedist Celsus charged
Herophilus and Erasistratus with performing vivisection on condemned
criminals awarded to them by the rulers of Alexandria. While these
accusers were obviously not eyewitnesses, some historians have accepted
their allegations; others remain skeptical.

The extent or even the existence of the practice of human vivisection during the Alexandrian era remains controversial because the
writings of Herophilus and Erasistratus have not survived and are known
only through the diatribes of their enemies. Accusations made hundreds
of years later cannot be taken as definitive proof, but there is no particular reason to believe that the authorities would have prohibited human
vivisection, especially if the victims were criminals or prisoners of war.
Certainly, the well-documented atrocities committed in the twentieth
century suggest that there is no limit to the human capacity for depravity, whether individual or state-sponsored. Nor have the events that
marked the beginning of the new millennium challenged such pessimistic
conclusions. Even though conditions during the Hellenistic era made
systematic anatomical research possible, human dissection was still
offensive to prevailing sentiments, evoked superstitious dread, and
created an evil reputation for Herophilus and Erasistratus.

Herophilus, Erasistratus, and their colleagues were engaged in
constructing an entirely new science of human beings rather than an
abstract philosophical system. The argument that Herophilus would
not have made certain errors if he had done vivisections fails to allow
for the influence of pre-existing concepts on perception and interpretation, and the intrinsic difficulty of innovative anatomical studies.
Whatever conditions made the work of Herophilus and Erasistratus
possible did not last long. Human dissection was probably discontinued
by the end of the second century B.C.E., but Alexandrian anatomists

probably continued to use human skeletons for research and teaching even after they were forced to confine dissection and vivisection to other animal species.

In his investigation of the circulatory system, Herophilus noted the difference between the arteries, with their strong pulsating walls, and the veins, with their relatively weak walls. Contrary to the prevailing assumption that the veins carried blood and the arteries carried air, Herophilus stated that both kinds of vessels carried blood. Intrigued by changes in the pulse that correlated with health and disease, Herophilus tried to measure the beat of the pulse using a water clock that had been developed in Alexandria.

Apparently known as a chronic skeptic, Herophilus regarded all physiological and pathological theories as hypothetical and provisional, including Hippocratic humoralism. While he probably did not totally reject humoral pathology, he seems to have preferred a theory of four life-guiding faculties that governed the body: a nourishing faculty in the liver and digestive organs, a warming power in the heart, a sensitive or perceptive faculty in the nerves, and a rational force in the brain. In clinical practice, Herophilus seems to have favored more active intervention than that recommended by Hippocrates and he may have used the concept of hot–cold, moist–dry qualities as a guide to therapeutic decisions. Vigorous bloodletting and a system of complex pharmaceuticals became associated with Herophilean medicine, but the anatomist appears to have urged his students to familiarize themselves with dietetics, medicine, surgery, and obstetrics.

Little is known about Herophilus, except that he probably studied with the physician Praxagoras of Cos, and was said to be the author of more than fifty books, including *On Anatomy, On the Eyes*, and a handbook for midwives, but only a few excerpts of his writings have survived. There is no direct evidence that Herophilus was a member of the faculty of the Alexandrian museum, or that he ever carried out any human vivisections or dissections at that institution. Nevertheless, his access to human cadavers, and perhaps live prisoners, was said to be the result of governmental support.

As a result of his extensive studies of the nervous system, including the connection between the brain, spinal cord and nerves, Herophilus rejected Aristotle's claim that the heart was the most important organ of the body and the seat of intelligence. Herophilus argued that the brain was the center of the nervous system. He also described the digestive system, called attention to the variability in the shape of the liver, and differentiated between tendons and nerves.

For Herophilus, health was the greatest good. The aphorism, "Wisdom and art, strength and wealth, all are useless without health," is attributed to him. He is also credited with the saying: "The best physician is the one who is able to differentiate the possible from the impossible." He urged physicians to be familiar with dietetics, gymnastics, drugs, surgery, and obstetrics. As practitioners, his followers were known to favor bleeding and the aggressive use of complex drug mixtures.

According to a story often dismissed as a myth, an Athenian woman named Agnodice was one of the students affiliated with Herophilus. Distressed by the suffering of women who would rather die than be examined by a male physician, Agnodice disguised herself as a man in order to study medicine. Agnodice won the gratitude of her female patients, but when her subterfuge was discovered, she was prosecuted for violating laws that prohibited women from studying medicine. Her loyal patients are said to have warned her male prosecutors that they would be seen as the cruel enemies of womankind if they condemned to death their only female physician. Agnodice's story has been used for hundreds of years to rally support for the education of medical women. Indeed, in writing about the diseases of women, Hippocrates had pointed to the problem epitomized in the story of Agnodice. Women were often so reluctant to discuss their problems with male physicians that simple illnesses became incurable.

When scholars of the Renaissance sought to challenge the stifling authority of the ancients, especially that of Galen, the long neglected and much vilified Herophilus was lauded as the "Vesalius of antiquity." The title could also have applied to Erasistratus, another intriguing and rather shadowy figure, who was attacked by Galen for the unforgivable heresy of rejecting the Hippocratic philosophy of medicine. Galen wrote two books against Erasistratus and criticized his ideas whenever possible. Galen claimed that Erasistratus and Herophilus were contemporaries, but Erasistratus may have been at least thirty years younger than Herophilus. According to one biographical tradition, when Erasistratus diagnosed his own illness as an incurable cancer he committed suicide rather than suffer inexorable decline.

Like Hippocrates, Erasistratus was born into a medical family. Little is known about his life, other than his decision to give up medical practice to devote himself to the study of anatomy and physiology. In a fragment preserved by Galen, Erasistratus spoke of the joys of research and how it made the investigator ready to devote day and night to solving every aspect of a scientific problem. Ancient sources credit Erasistratus with over fifty books, including specialized texts on fevers, bloodletting, paralysis, drugs, poisons, and dietetics. Erasistratus may have carried out his research at the court of Antiochus in Seleucia, rather than at Alexandria, but the research interests of Herophilus and Erasistratus were strikingly similar. There is, however, some indication that Erasistratus was more interested in the remote and obscure causes of disease than Herophilus. Galen accused Erasistratus of rejecting the Hippocratic philosophy of medicine and following the teachings of Aristotle. Like Herophilus,

Erasistratus probably tried to replace humoral theory with a new doctrine. In the case of Erasistratus, this seems to have developed into a pathology of solids that perhaps did more to guide his anatomical research than his approach to therapeutics.

Erasistratus is said to have been a gifted practitioner who rejected the idea that a general knowledge of the body and its functioning in health was necessary to the practicing physician. Many problems, he argued, could be prevented or treated with simple remedies and hygienic living. Nevertheless, he believed in studying pathological anatomy as a key to localized causes of disease. He was particularly interested in the possibility that disease and inflammation were caused by the accumulation of a localized plethora of blood that forced blood to pass from the veins into the arteries. Skeptical of many standard therapeutic methods and Hippocratic humorology, Erasistratus invoked a mechanical, localized concept of physiological and pathological phenomena based on the atomic theory of Democritus. Like the founder of atomic theory, Erasistratus was apparently willing to speculate about the existence of unseen entities. Having traced the veins, arteries, and nerves to the finest subdivisions visible to the naked eye, Erasistratus postulated further ramifications beyond the limits of vision. The invisible fabric of the body, according to Erasistratus, was made up of a threefold network composed of veins, arteries, and nerves. To complete his picture of the fine structure of the body, Erasistratus proposed the existence of *parenchyma* (material poured in between the network of vessels).

Perhaps because of his theory that disease was caused by a local excess of blood, Erasistratus paid particular attention to the heart, veins, and arteries. In his lost treatises, he apparently gave a detailed description of the heart, including the semilunar, tricuspid, and bicuspid valves. Mechanical analogies, dissections, and perhaps vivisection experiments suggested to Erasistratus that the heart could be seen as a pump in which certain "membranes" served as the flap valves. Using a combination of logic, intuition, and imagination, Erasistratus traced the veins, arteries, and nerves to the finest subdivisions visible to the naked eye and speculated about further subdivisions beyond the limits of vision. He also gave a detailed description of the liver and gallbladder, and initiated a study of the lacteals that was not improved upon until the work of Gasparo Aselli (1581–1626).

Erasistratus accepted the traditional idea that the function of the arteries was to carry *pneuma* (air) rather than blood. The veins, which supposedly arose from the liver, and the arteries, which were thought to arise from the heart, were generally thought of as independent systems of dead-end canals through which blood and *pneuma* seeped slowly to the periphery of the body so that each part of the body could draw out its proper nourishment. He realized, however, that anatomists had to account for the fact that blood, which was supposed to be carried by the veins, spurted out of torn arteries. In order to rationalize the inconsistencies in this system, Erasistratus argued that although the veins and arteries were functionally separate in healthy, intact individuals, there were tiny collapsed or closed connections between the two kinds of vessels. When an artery was damaged, air escaped and venous blood was forced through the connections between the veins and arteries, because—as Aristotle taught—nature abhorred a vacuum. In other words, the presence of blood in the arteries was the result of an injury or some other pathological condition. Observations of engorged veins and collapsed arteries in the cadaver would appear to support these ideas.

Erasistratus concluded that disease was due to *plethora*, that is, an excess of blood from undigested foods that tended to become putrid. When local excesses of blood accumulated in the veins, the overburdened vessels were damaged and blood spilled over from the veins into the arteries. When this occurred, the flow of pneuma, or vital spirit, which was supposed to be distributed by the arteries, would be obstructed. Given this theoretical framework, the logical objective of therapy was to diminish the plethora of blood. One way to accomplish this was to interrupt the production of blood at its point of origin by eliminating the supply of food. In addition to emetics, diuretics, massage, hot baths, and general starvation, Erasistratus ingeniously induced a form of "local starvation" by tying tight bandages around the limbs to trap blood in the extremities until the diseased part of the body had used up its plethora. The use of the ligature to stop the flow of blood from torn vessels was also ascribed to Erasistratus.

Although Erasistratus was sometimes called a materialist, atomist, or rationalist, he did not reject the concept of animating spirits. Apparently he believed that life processes were dependent on blood and pneuma, which was constantly replenished by respiration. Two kinds of pneuma were found in the body: the vital pneuma was carried in the arteries and regulated vegetative processes. Some of the vital pneuma got to the brain and was changed into animal spirits. Animal spirits were responsible for movement and sensation and were carried by the nerves, a system of hollow tubes. When animal spirits rushed into muscles, they caused distension that resulted in shortening of the muscle and thus movement. Perhaps inspired by the experimental approach of Strato (one of Aristotle's favorite students), Erasistratus is said to have attempted to provide quantitative solutions for physiological problems. In one experiment, Erasistratus put a bird into a pot and kept a record of the weight of the bird and its excrement. He found a progressive weight loss between feedings, which led him to conclude that some invisible emanation was lost by vital processes.

A story concerning Erasistratus as a medical practitioner demonstrates his powers of observation and insight into the relationship between afflictions of mind and body. When Seleucus, one of Alexander's generals, married a woman named Stratonice, his son Antiochus fell in love with his stepmother. Desperately trying to hide his feelings, the young man fell ill and seemed close to death. Many physicians had failed to help him when Erasistratus determined that an affliction of the mind had weakened the body through sympathetic relationships. While carefully assessing his patient's physiological reactions to the people who visited him, Erasistratus discovered the stammering, blushing, palpitations, and pallor that followed each visit by Stratonice. Erasistratus reasoned that although we can consciously conceal our thoughts, their influence on the body cannot be controlled. This story was retold many times for its literary merit, but the medical insights were largely ignored. Similar incidents appear in the biographies of other great physicians, including Galen and Avicenna, and were often cited in the extensive medieval and Renaissance literature concerning love-sickness.

For two hundred years, the museum of Alexandria supported a high level of creativity in science, technology, and medicine, and trained numerous physicians, engineers, geographers, astronomers, and mathematicians. Although it is difficult to assess the vitality of such a complex institution, there is some evidence that medical science was already slipping into a state of decline during the time of Herophilus and Erasistratus. The tension that always exists in medicine between disinterested scientific research and the immediate needs of the sick grew and disrupted the ancient search for harmony and balance between the scientist and the healer. Critics of anatomical research charged that such pursuits distracted physicians from caring for patients. Much of the deterioration of scientific research at Alexandria can be blamed on the tumultuous political climate, but scientists and scholars seem to have been undermining the structural supports of their own houses of learning by attacking rival schools of thought, or by leaving Alexandria to established new schools elsewhere. Later writers satirized the museum as a place where large numbers of scholars were kept like birds in a henhouse, endlessly squawking and bickering. Finally, the worst of fates fell upon the Alexandrian scientists; they were persecuted, their grants were cut off, and they had to turn to teaching to eke out a living in new places.

The decline of the Alexandrian tradition was not limited to medical science. Little of the work of the museum or library has survived. The first major episode in the destruction of the library occurred in 48 B.C.E. during the riots sparked by the arrival of Julius Caesar and some three thousand legionnaires. After Caesar conquered Egypt, Alexandria was reduced to the status of a provincial town in the great Roman Empire. Later, Christian leaders encouraged the destruction of the Temple of Muses and other pagan institutions. According to tradition, in 395, the last scholar at the museum, a female philosopher and mathematician named Hypatia, was dragged out of the museum by

Christian mobs and beaten to death. The Muslim conquest of the city in the seventh century (642–646) resulted in the final destruction of the library and the loss of its precious manuscripts.

## MEDICINE IN THE ROMAN WORLD

The Roman Empire was a complex and vigorous combination of Greek and Roman cultural elements, forged through centuries of war. Originally a republic of yeoman farmers, rather than merchants and adventurers like the Greeks, Roman citizens retained a preference for the practical over the abstract and a tendency to idealize the pastoral life even as they constructed cities unprecedented in size and complexity. They excelled in the arts of warfare and administration, as well as architecture, engineering, public health, and hygiene. Roman writers boasted that their ancestors had lived without physicians, though not without medicine, being well endowed with folk remedies, healing deities, and diviners. Presumably, the remarkable sanitary engineering achievements that are associated with Republican and Imperial Rome played an important role in maintaining public health.

When comparing Rome to Greece, critics characterized the Romans as a people without art, literature, science, or philosophy. However, they certainly could not be called a people without gods. Like the Egyptians, the Romans accumulated deities for all major organs and functions of the body. Nevertheless, they still had room in their hearts for new deities, especially when the old ones seemed unwilling or unable to do their duty. In 293 B.C.E., when their traditional gods were unable to stop a pestilence that was decimating Rome, the elders consulted Asclepius at the Temple of Epidaurus. While the Asclepiads conferred with the Roman delegation, a sacred snake emerged from the temple and boarded the Roman ship; this was taken as an omen that the Greek god of medicine intended to help Rome. A temple for Asclepius was constructed at a site selected by the snake, the epidemic ended, and the cult of Asclepius was established in Rome. Greek physicians were as eager to come to the aid of Rome as the sacred snake, but the reception they received was not always quite as warm as that awarded to Asclepius.

Originally, Romans were very skeptical of professional physicians. They did not condemn the practice of medicine per se, but they considered it was unethical to charge fees for treating the sick. Cato the Elder (234–149 B.C.E.) denounced Greek physicians as the worst enemies of Rome and accused them of poisoning and murdering their clients. Indeed, some of the most ambitious practitioners were actually greedy quacks, incompetents, and adventurers who used their knowledge to mislead patients, manufacture poisons, and enter into conspiracies.

Cato was fighting a losing battle, for Rome had been increasingly susceptible to Greek influences since the fourth-century B.C.E.. The introduction of the cult of Asclepius and the influx of Greek physicians were indicative of this trend.

Traditionally, the head of the Roman household was expected to supervise the medical affairs of his family, slaves, and animals. The actual practice of medicine, however, was regarded as a menial task suitable only for slaves and women. Most Romans relied on a combination of magic and folklore to fight disease. Each home had its special shrine and stock of herbal remedies. Appropriate rituals accompanied the administration of all drugs and the performance of any operation. It was an economical arrangement in which the same remedies, charms, and prayers served both man and beast. Cato, for example, was aware of many traditional remedies, but his favorite was cabbage, which might even be superior to chicken soup because, in addition to being harmless, it is a good source of vitamin C. In any case, Cato lived to the ripe old age of 84 during an era when the average life expectancy was about 25 years.

The writings of other Romans, almost by definition nonphysicians, reflect valuable insights into problems of hygiene, sanitation, and public health, especially the importance of water supplies and sewage disposal. Rome obtained its water from a variety of supply systems, but the aqueducts that were bringing millions of gallons of water into Rome by the second century B.C.E. are generally thought of as the quintessentially Roman solution to one of the major problems faced by urban planners. Lower quality water was considered acceptable for the bathing establishments found in every Roman city and almost every town. Admission fees for the public baths were generally minimal, but the Romans should be credited with the establishment of the pay toilet. While public latrines were generally incorporated into the bathing establishments, independent public latrines were usually sited in the busiest sections of cities and towns.

An admirable concern for the purity of water and the sanitary location of dwelling places is found in the text *On Achitecture* (ca. 27 B.C.E.) by the Roman architect and engineer Vitruvius. Also of interest is the suggestion by Marcus Terentius Varro (117–27 B.C.E.) that swampy places might be inhabited by extremely minute animals that could enter the body through the mouth and nose and cause serious illnesses. While wealthy Romans could take advantage of the architectural and engineering skills for which Roman civilization is justly famous, and retreat to peaceful, quiet country villas, most people lived in crowded, unsanitary houses lacking proper kitchens and heating systems, piped water, private baths, or latrines.

Despite Cato's warnings, as Roman society became more refined and prosperous, or, as critics might say, less virtuous and self-sufficient,

Roman citizens were soon eagerly consulting Greek physicians who offered them a medical regimen more sophisticated than cabbages and incantations. The career of Asclepiades (ca. 124–50 B.C.E.) provides an instructive example of how Greek medicine was adapted to a Roman clientele. Originally Asclepiades came to Rome as a rhetorician, but he quickly realized that the practice of medicine offered better prospects. Asclepiades offered treatments that were guaranteed to work "swiftly, safely, and sweetly." While his theoretical approach was mechanistic, in practice Asclepiades advised a sensible regimen, with individualized attention to diet, rest, and exercise, along with simple remedies, such as wine, water, and cold baths, rather than bleeding and purging. Although Asclepiades provided a form of medical practice that could be successful in the framework of Roman expectations, suspicion and skepticism remained, as seen in the writings of Pliny the Elder (23–79).

Like Cato before him, Pliny the Elder, exemplary Roman gentleman and author of one of the major encyclopedic works of antiquity, was suspicious of professional physicians. According to Pliny, physicians were incompetent, greedy, superfluous, and dangerous. Greek physicians, he warned, had seduced Roman citizens away from their traditional herbal remedies and had contributed to the decay of Roman society. Pliny complained that physicians learned their craft by experimenting on patients and denounced them as the only men who could kill with impunity and then blame death on the victim for having failed to obey professional advice.

Pliny's *Natural History* provides an invaluable, far-ranging, if unsystematic survey of science, medicine, agriculture, industry, and the arts of the late republic and early empire. In lauding the virtues of Rome's traditional herbal remedies, Pliny claimed that everything had been created for the sake of man, making the whole world an apothecary shop for those who understood nature's simple prescriptions, such as wound dressings made of wine, vinegar, eggs, honey, powdered earthworms, and pig dung, and ferns used in the treatment of parasitic worms. Among the remedies suggested by Pliny are some that contain pharmacologically active components, such as ephedron for asthma, cough, and hemorrhage.

A more systematic approach to the search for remedies can be found in the work of Dioscorides (ca. 40–80), compiler of the text now known as *De materia medica (The Materials of Medicine)*, one of the first Western herbals. Dioscorides exemplifies the generalization that Roman medicine was usually carried out by Greek physicians. Little is known about his life, except that he may have studied at Alexandria before serving as *medicus* to Nero's armies. "Military doctor" is probably too modern a translation for this term, because it is unlikely that an organized medical or surgical staff accompanied the Roman legions of this period. The Roman army may have had more formal provisions for the care of sick horses than sick soldiers. Nevertheless, throughout the existence of the Roman Empire, the activities of its armies and its medical personnel diffused Greco-Roman medicine throughout Europe, North Africa, and the eastern Mediterranean world.

Serving the Roman legions gave Dioscorides the opportunity to travel widely and study many novel plant species, hundreds of which were not known to Hippocrates. An acute observer and keen naturalist, Dioscorides provided valuable information about medically useful plants, their place of origin, habitat, growth characteristics, and proper uses. He also described remedies made from minerals and animals. Pharmacologists who have examined the text have found recipes for valuable therapeutic agents, including analgesics, antiseptics, emetics, laxatives, strong purgatives, and so forth.

Many of the herbal remedies identified and classified by Dioscorides can be found on the spice shelf of the average modern kitchen. The medical properties assigned to various herbs and spices would, however, surprise modern cooks. For example, cinnamon and cassia were said to be valuable in the treatment of internal inflammations, venomous bites, poisons, runny noses, and menstrual disorders. When properly prepared, such herbs and spices were said to induce abortion. A decoction made from asparagus was recommended as a means of inducing sterility; wearing the stalk as an amulet was said to increase the effectiveness of this prescription. Victims of bites by mad dogs might try a remedy made from river crabs, Gentian root, and wine. Then, to prevent complications, the patient should eat the liver of the dog in question and wear its tooth as an amulet. *De materia medica* includes many bizarre and unpleasant recipes, such as a remedy for malaria made of bedbugs mixed with meat and beans, but recent studies of the text suggest that Dioscorides classified his remedies according to subtle and sophisticated criteria. That is, Dioscorides appears to have based his classification on a drug affinity system rather than on traditional methods such as plant morphology or habitat. This required precise knowledge of growth characteristics of the plants, proper harvesting and preparation, and the effect that particular medicinal herbs exerted when given to a significant number of patients.

In contrast to the herbal text of Dioscorides, which was frequently copied and widely used, the writings of Aulus Cornelius Celsus (ca. 14–37) were essentially forgotten until the rediscovery of his *De re medicina (On Medicine)* in 1426 presented Renaissance scholars with a source of pure classical Latin. *De medicina* became one of the first medical texts to be reproduced by Europe's new printing presses. Celsus had undertaken an ambitious encyclopedic work in four parts: agriculture, medicine, rhetoric, and warfare, but *On Medicine* is the only part that survived. Almost nothing is known about the life of Celsus except for the fact that

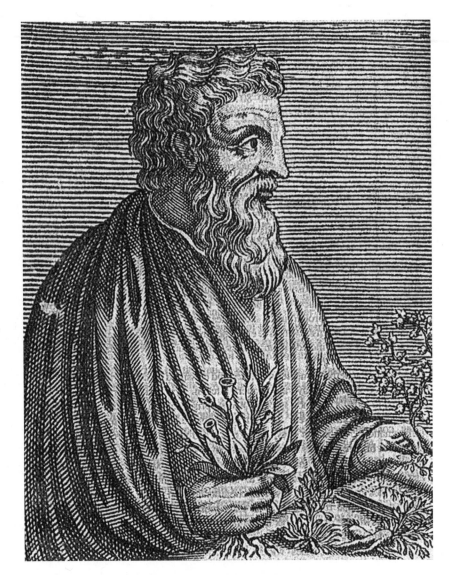

**Dioscorides examining medicinal plants.**

his contemporaries considered him a man of only mediocre intellect. Although Celsus was clearly a master of organization, clarity, and style, the question of whether he composed, compiled, or plagiarized *On Medicine* remains obscure.

In his historical introduction to the discussion of medicine, Celsus noted that the Greeks had cultivated the art of medicine more than any other people. The ancient Romans had enjoyed natural health, without medicine, he asserted, because of their good habits. When they turned to lives of indolence and luxury, presumably under the malign influence of Greek culture, illness appeared and medicine became a necessity.

After the death of Hippocrates, Greek medicine, which was never a monolithic enterprise, fragmented into various disputatious sects, some named after individuals and others, such as the Dogmatists, Empiricists, and Methodists, for their special approach to medical theory. Much about the origins, members, and practices of these sects remains unclear, but, thanks to Celsus, a fairly good account of the medical sects that flourished in his time can be reconstructed.

The Dogmatists emphasized the study of anatomy and claimed Erasistratus, Herophilus, and Hippocrates as their ancestors. Seeing medicine as a composite of practice, theory, and philosophy, the Dogmatists taught that physicians must study anatomy and physiology as well as the evident, immediate, and obscure causes of disease. Members of other sects might differ about many points, but they generally agreed that the Dogmatists were guilty of undue attention to speculative theories and a neglect of the practical goals of medicine.

Holding a more limited or more pragmatic view of the domain of medicine, the Empiricists believed it was necessary to understand evident or immediate causes, but that inquiry into obscure or ultimate causes was superfluous, because nature was ultimately incomprehensible to human beings. In medicine, the physicians should be guided only by the test of experience as it answered the question: does the patient get well? Some Empiricists claimed that the study of anatomy was totally useless for understanding living beings. They regarded human vivisection with horror and held it a crime to cause death in the name of the healing art. However, their emphasis on action was reflected in the excellent reputation of Empiric surgeons.

The Methodists believed that the body was composed of atoms and pores. Disease was the result of abnormal states of the pores due to excess tension or relaxation. Thus, knowledge of the three common conditions of the human body—the constricted, the lax, and the mixed—provided all the guidance the physician needed to treat his patients. Appropriate remedies relaxed or tightened the pores as needed. The Methodists claimed that, because their system was so complete, no further research into the causes of disease and therapeutics was necessary. But Juvenal, a Roman satirist, said that Methodist practitioners had killed more patients than they could count.

Celsus concluded that no sect was wholly right or wrong. In seeking impartially for the truth, it was necessary to recognize that some things that were not strictly pertinent to medical practice were valuable in stimulating and improving the mind of the practitioner. In dealing with cattle, horses, foreigners, and in the aftermath of disasters, it was sometimes necessary to look only at the simplest characteristics of disease. Under normal conditions, a superior physician had to consider geography, climate, and the unique reactions of different patients.

Properly considered, the art of medicine could be divided into three parts: cure by diet (which in this context might better be translated by the term "lifestyle"); cure by medications; and cure by surgery. Experience taught the physician that standard medical practices were not equally appropriate to all patients. The art of medicine should be rational, Celsus concluded, and based on immediate causes, but ultimately medicine was an art that entailed a great deal of informed guesswork. Anatomy was an important part of medical knowledge, but Celsus declared that vivisection was cruel and unnecessary. Students of medicine could learn about the positions and relations of the internal organs from dead bodies, but the practitioner should be alert to the possibility of gaining anatomical knowledge when "windows of opportunity" occurred during the treatment of wounds.

Even though he rejected the Greek concept of the physician as a necessary guide to proper regimen throughout life, Celsus considered it essential for every individual to acquire an understanding of the relationship between disease and the stages of life. Moreover, in explaining this relationship, he offered as much advice as any modern guru of "lifestyles." Acute illnesses, those that "finish a man quickly, or finish quickly themselves," were the greatest threat to the young. The elderly were most threatened by chronic diseases. The middle years were the safest, but disease could strike human beings at any age, in any season. Little could be added to Celsus' conclusion that the best prescription for a healthy life was one of variety and balance, proper rest and exercise, and avoidance of a self-indulgent obsession with medical advice.

Surgery, according to Celsus, should be the most satisfying field for the practitioner, because it brought results that were more certain than treatment by drugs and diets. Physicians knew that some patients recovered without medicine, while some were not cured by the best medical treatment. In contrast, a cure brought about by surgery was clearly the result of skill, not the result of supernatural forces or luck. A surgeon must be filled with the desire to cure his patient and strong enough to perform his necessary work in spite of the patient's pain and suffering. After surgery, the physician must be ready to protect his patient from hemorrhage and the infections associated with the four cardinal signs of inflammation—*calor, rubor, dolor,* and *tumor* (heat, redness, pain, and swelling). The Roman surgeon had mastered tools and techniques that were unknown to his Hippocratic predecessors, such as the use of the ligature for torn blood vessels and special spoons and dilators to remove barbed arrows from wounds. Roman surgeons could perform amputations and plastic surgery, as well as operations for bladder stones, goiter, hernia, cataract, and snakebites.

*De medicina* provides a valuable survey of the medical and surgical practices of first-century Rome. However, during the European Middle Ages, Celsus and all the medical writers of antiquity, except Hippocrates, were eclipsed by the works of the great Galen of Pergamum (130–200 or 210).

## ON GALEN AND GALENISM

No other figure in the history of medicine has influenced concepts of anatomy, physiology, therapeutics, and philosophy as much as Galen, the physician known as the Medical Pope of the Middle Ages and the mentor of Renaissance anatomists and physiologists. Galen left voluminous writings that touch on all the major medical, scientific, philosophical, and religious issues of his time. Contemporary admirers, including his patron the emperor Marcus Aurelius, called him the "First of Physicians and Philosophers." His critics preferred titles like "mule head" and called him a vain, arrogant "windbag." In attempting to sum up his work and thought, scholars have said that, as a physician, Galen was essentially a Hippocratic, but as a philosopher, he was generally an Aristotelian.

Galen was born in Pergamum, a city in Asia Minor that claimed to be the cultural equal of Alexandria. When describing himself, Galen asserted that he had emulated the excellent character of his father, Aelius Nikon, a wealthy architect, known for his amiable and benevolent nature. Although he tried to dissociate himself from the example set by his mother, a bad-tempered woman, perpetually shouting at his father, provoking quarrels, and biting the servants, these efforts may not have been completely successful. By the time he was 14, Galen had mastered mathematics and philosophy. About two years later, Asclepius came to Nikon in a dream and told him that his son was destined to become a physician. While still a student of medicine at the famous sanctuary of Asclepius in Pergamum, Galen composed at least three books. Later, in his advice to medical students and teachers, Galen emphasized the importance of fostering a love of truth in the young that would inspire them to work day and night to learn all that had been written by the Ancients and to find ways of testing and proving such knowledge.

After the death of Nikon, Galen left Pergamum to continue his medical education in Smyrna, Corinth, and Alexandria. On returning to Pergamum after years of study and travel, Galen was appointed physician to the gladiators. Although he also worked at the Temple of Asclepius and established a flourishing private practice, within a few years, he became restless again. In 161, he arrived in Rome where through good fortune, brilliant diagnoses, and miraculous cures he soon attracted many

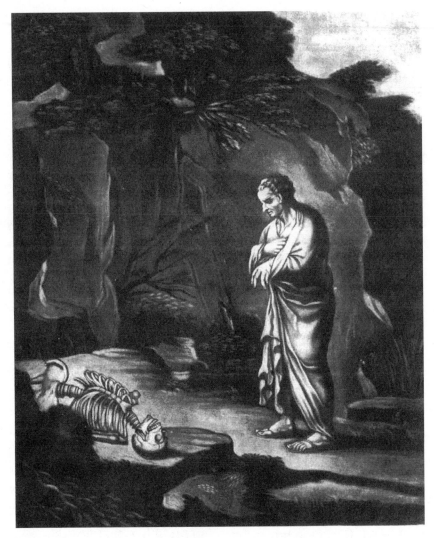

**Galen, contemplating a human skeleton.**

influential patients, patrons, and admirers. During this period, Galen engaged in public anatomical lectures, demonstrations, and disputes, and composed some of his major anatomical and physiological texts. Five years later, Galen returned to Pergamum, claiming that the hostility of other physicians had driven him from Rome. His critics noted that his abrupt departure coincided with the outbreak of an epidemic that had entered the city along with soldiers returning from the Parthian War. Not long afterwards, honoring a request from Emperor Marcus Aurelius, Galen returned to Rome and settled there permanently. Although strictly speaking, Galen was not a "court physician," he did enjoy the friendship and protection of the emperors Marcus Aurelius, Commodus, Septimius Severus, and other prominent figures.

Late in life, troubled by evidence that careless copyists, shameless impostors, and plagiarists were corrupting his writings, Galen composed a guide for the cautious reader called *On His Own Books*, which described the genuine works of Galen, as well as a reading program for physicians. Works for beginners were necessary, Galen complained, because many students lacked a good, classical education and most "physicians" were pretenders who could barely read. Galen's medical, philosophical, and philological writings discussed almost every aspect of medical theory and practice of Greek and Roman times, as well as his own studies of anatomy, physiology, dietetics, and therapeutics. Unfortunately, a fire in the Temple of Peace in 191 destroyed many of his manuscripts. Nevertheless, his surviving works fill about twenty volumes in Greek. Some of his works survived in Arabic and medieval Latin editions.

Galen taught that the best physician was also a philosopher. Therefore, the true physician must master the three branches of philosophy: *logic*, the science of how to think; *physics*, the science of nature; and *ethics*, the science of what to do. With such knowledge, the physician could gain his patient's obedience and the admiration due to a god. Ideally, the physician would practice medicine for the love of mankind, not for profit, because the pursuit of science and money were mutually exclusive. In his writings, Galen portrayed himself as a scholar who realized that it was impossible to discover all that he passionately wished to know despite his persistent search for truth.

The essential features of Galen's system are a view of nature as purposeful and craftsman-like and the principle of balance among the four qualities and the four humors. For Galen, anatomical research was the source of a "perfect theology" when approached as the study of form and function in terms of the "usefulness" of the parts. Instead of sacrificing bulls and incense, the anatomist demonstrated reverence for the Creator by discovering his wisdom, power, and goodness through anatomical investigations. The dissection of any animal revealed a little universe fashioned by the wisdom and skill of the Creator. Assuming that nature acts with perfect wisdom and does nothing in vain, Galen argued that every structure was crafted for its proper function.

## GALEN ON ANATOMICAL PROCEDURES

Dissection might be a religious experience for Galen, but most practitioners studied anatomy for guidance in surgical operations, the treatment of traumatic injuries, ulcers, fistulae, and abscesses. Systematic

dissection was essential preparation for the surgeon, because a practitioner without anatomical knowledge could inadvertently or negli-
gently injure his patients. Where the surgeon could choose the site of
incision, knowledge of anatomy would allow him to do the least damage
possible. On the other hand, if the surgeon had to sever muscles to treat
an abscess, his anatomical knowledge would allow him to predict
subsequent damage and thus escape blame.

Anatomy could also be used to settle larger philosophical issues,
such as the controversy about the seat of reason in the human body.
Aristotelians placed reason in the heart, while others placed it in the
head. One Aristotelian argument was that the voice, which is the instrument of reason, came from the chest. Thus, Galen's demonstration that
the recurrent laryngeal nerves control the voice vindicated those who
argued for control by the brain and explained what happened when surgeons accidentally severed these nerves. Galen thought that it was
unnecessary to justify research by tenuous links to practical benefits,
but, of course, he did not have to prepare grant proposals or yearly
progress reports.

Until the sixteenth century, Galen was generally accepted as the
ultimate authority on anatomical and physiological questions despite
the fact that, because of Roman prohibitions on human dissections, his
"human anatomy" was based on dissection of other species. Often critical of his predecessors, especially Erasistratus and Herophilus, Galen
obviously envied their resources and privileges. Certainly, Galen did
not conceal the fact that his work was based on studies of other animals,
including pigs, elephants, or that "ridiculous imitation of man," the
Barbary ape.

While Galen could not do systematic human anatomies, this does
not mean that he never studied human cadavers. His extensive anatomical experience made it possible for him to put fortuitous opportunities
to good advantage. On one occasion, a flood washed a corpse out of its
grave and deposited the body on the bank of the river; the flesh rotted
away, but the bones were still closely attached to each other. The
enthusiasm with which Galen described such events suggests their rarity,
but some scholars believe that certain passages in *On Anatomical Procedures* suggest that human dissection may have been performed on
criminals left unburied and exposed infants. As Celsus had suggested,
a physician could learn a good deal about the form and functions of
the internal organs by exploiting the wounds and injuries of his patients
as "windows" into the body. Certainly, Galen would have taken full
advantage of the opportunities he had enjoyed while binding up the
gruesome wounds of the gladiators. Indeed, Galen told his readers that
when observing wounds, physicians who had prepared themselves by
systematic dissection of animals knew "what to expect, but the ignorant
learn nothing thereby."

## GALEN ON PHYSIOLOGY: BLOOD, BREATH, PNEUMA, AND SPIRITS

Never satisfied with purely anatomical description, Galen constantly struggled to find ways of proceeding from structure to function, from pure anatomy to experimental physiology. It is rare to encounter a problem in what might be called classical physiology that Galen did not attempt to cope with either by experiment or speculation. By extending medical research from anatomy to physiology, Galen established the foundations of a program that would transform the Hippocratic *art* of medicine into the *science* of medicine.

In formulating his physiological principles, Galen was sometimes misled by preconceived and erroneous ideas and hindered by the technical difficulties inherent in such investigations. Given the magnitude of his self-imposed task, and the voluminous and prolix nature of his writings, the totality of his work has been more honored than understood. His errors, which ultimately stimulated revolutions in anatomy and physiology in the sixteenth and seventeenth centuries, tend to be overemphasized. It is important, therefore, to balance the merits and the defects in the powerful Galenic synthesis that was to satisfy the needs of scholars and physicians for hundreds of years.

Galen's system of physiology encompassed concepts of blood formation, respiration, the heartbeat, the arterial pulse, digestion, nerve function, embryology, growth, nutrition, and assimilation. Galenic physiology rested on the Platonic doctrine of a threefold division of the soul. This provided a means of dividing vital functions into processes governed by vegetative, animal, and rational "souls" or "spirits." Within the human body, *pneuma* (air), which was the breath of the cosmos, was subject to modifications brought about by the innate faculties of the three principle organs—the liver, heart, and brain—and distributed by three types of vessels—veins, arteries, and nerves. The Galenic system is complex and often obscure. Moreover, it is difficult and perhaps counterproductive to attempt absolute distinctions between what Galen actually said and the way in which his doctrines were understood and handed down by later interpreters. In any event, Galen sometimes said different things in different texts and, since not all of his writings have survived, it is possible that interpretations made by particular commentators could have been based on manuscripts that have been lost.

In essence, according to Galen's system, pneuma was modified by the liver so that it became the nutritive soul or natural spirits that supported the vegetative functions of growth and nutrition; this nutritive soul was distributed by the veins. The heart and arteries were responsible for the maintenance and distribution of innate heat and pneuma or vital spirits to warm and vivify the parts of the body. The third adaptation, which occurred in the brain, produced the animal spirits required for sensation and muscular movement; the animal spirits were distributed through the nerves. Sometimes Galen's arguments concerning particular problems suggest reservations about the functions of the spirits, but he was certain that animal life is only possible because of the existence of pneuma within the body.

Because of the central role theories of the motion of the heart and blood have played in the history of Western medical science, Galen's views on this topic have been the subject of considerable attention and controversy. Part of the difficulty in reconstructing a simplified version of Galen's concept of this problem resides in the fact that respiration and the movement of the blood are so intimately linked in Galen's system that it is difficult to unravel the threads of each problem, or consider them apart from his doctrines concerning the elaboration and distribution of pneuma and spirits. Respiration, which was thought to be involved in cooling the excess heat of the heart, was obviously necessary for life. Therefore, vital spirit is necessarily associated with the organs of respiration, which in Galen's system included the heart and arteries as well as the lungs. *If* the natural spirit exists, Galen thought it would be contained in the liver and the veins. Attempting to simplify Galen's prolix arguments, his followers often transformed tentative "if there are" hypotheses into dogmatic "there are" certainties.

In Galen's physiological scheme, blood was continuously synthesized from ingested foods. The useful part of the food was transported as *chyle* from the intestines via the portal vein to the liver, where, by virtue of the innate faculty of the liver, it was transformed into dark venous blood. Tissues could then suck up the nutriments they needed from the blood by virtue of their faculty for specific selection. The useless part of the food was converted into black bile by the spleen. Even Galen could not come to grips with the precise means by which such transformations—all the complex phenomena now subsumed by the term *metabolism*—might be effected.

Like Erasistratus, Galen assumed that there must be connections between the veins (which arose from the liver) and the arteries (which arose from the heart) because bleeding from any vessel could drain the whole system. But Galen ingeniously refuted the idea that, under normal conditions, the arteries contain only air. His arguments and experimental proof were set forth in a brief work entitled *Whether Blood Is Contained in the Arteries in Nature*. If the artery of a living animal is exposed and tied it off at two points, the section of the vessel between the ligatures is full of blood. Moreover, when the chest of a living animal is opened, blood is found in the left ventricle of the heart. According to Galen's scheme, the arterial pulse was generated by the heart. During the diastole of the heart, the dilation of the arteries drew in air through the pores in the skin and blood from the veins. Thus, the arteries served the function of nourishing the innate heat throughout the body. This concept could be demonstrated by tying a ligature around a limb so that it was tight enough to cut off the arterial pulse. Below the ligature, the limb would become cold and pale, because the arteries were no longer able to supply the innate heat.

Although Galen gave a good description of the heart, its chambers and valves, his preconceived concepts led to ambiguities, misinterpretations, and even misrepresentations of anatomical observations. For Galen's system to work, blood had to pass from the right ventricle to the left ventricle. Therefore, he assumed that blood in the right side of the heart could follow various paths. Some of the blood carried impurities, or "sooty vapors," for discharge by the lungs via the artery-like vein (pulmonary artery). Blood could also pass from the right side to the left side of the heart by means of pores in the septum. The pores themselves were not visible, but Galen assumed that the pits found in the septum were the mouths of the pores. The idea that the blood tended to ebb and flow like the tide was long associated with Galenic physiology although this seems to be a misinterpretation of Galen's generally vague statements about the movement of blood within the vessels. However, the system seems to depend on an obscure two-way movement of blood through certain vessels.

After appropriate "digestion" in the lungs, inhaled air was brought to the heart by the pulmonary vein. The modified air was further acted on in the heart and transported to other parts of the body by the arteries. Arterial blood was especially fine and vaporous so that it could nourish the vital spirit. Further refinement was accomplished in the arteries that formed the *rete mirabile*—a network of vessels found at the base of the brain of oxen and other animals, but not in humans. The transformation of arterial blood into animal spirits in the brain and their distribution via the nerves completed the threefold system of spirits.

Clearly, the concept of blood circulation is incompatible with a scheme in which blood is constantly synthesized by the liver to be assimilated or consumed as it ebbs and flows in the blood vessels. Of course the nature of the Galenic system is so complex that "clearly" is hardly an appropriate word to use in a brief description of it. Rather than throw any further obscurity on the subject, let us consider Galen's ideas about the treatment of diseases.

## GALEN ON THERAPEUTICS AND THE CAUSES OF DISEASE

When writing about the nature of therapeutics, Galen argued that scientific knowledge of the causes of disease was essential for successful treatment. For prognosis, Galen relied on traditional tools, such as the examination of the pulse and the urine, and a rather rigid version of the Hippocratic doctrine of the "critical days." Like Hippocrates,

Galen was an excellent clinician and a brilliant diagnostician who believed that the physician must explain disease in terms of natural causes. "Do not inquire from the gods how to discover by divination," he warned his readers, "but take your instruction from some anatomy teacher." All diseases might have a natural cause, but Galen was willing to accept medical advice offered by Asclepius, the god of healing. When Galen was suffering from a painful abscess, Asclepius appeared in a dream and told him to open an artery in his right hand. A complete and speedy recovery followed this treatment.

Humoralism, as embodied in Galenism, apparently was capable of explaining the genesis and essence of all diseases and rationalizing all clinical findings. According to Galen, the humors were formed when nutriments were altered by the *innate heat* that was produced by the slow combustion taking place in the heart. Foods of a warmer nature tend to produce bile, while those of a colder nature produced an excess of phlegm. An excess of bile caused "warm diseases" and an excess of phlegm resulted in "cold diseases." Several Galenic texts dealt with food, the humors, and the relationship between food and the humors. These text included *On the Humors, On Black Bile, On Barley Soup*, and *On the Power of Foods*.

Averting disease by rigid adherence to the principles of Galenic hygiene required continuous guidance by a competent physician, as set forth in Galen's *On Hygiene*. In contrast to Celsus, who believed that the temperate Roman had little need for medical advice, Galen argued that a highly individualized regimen was essential "for Greeks and those who, though born barbarians by nature, yet emulate the culture of the Greeks." The individualized health-promoting regimen prescribed by the physician required constant attention to the "six non-naturals," a confusing Galenic term for factors that, unlike geography, weather, season, and age, could be brought under the patient's control. Today's health and fitness experts would refer to the non-naturals as lifestyle choices, that is, food and drink, sleeping and waking, exercise and rest, "regularity," and "mental attitude." Eventually, in the hands of less gifted practitioners, Galen's program for a sophisticated individualized approach to the prevention and treatment of disease degenerated into a system of bleeding, purging, cupping, blistering, starvation diets, and large doses of complex mixtures of drugs.

Despite his reverence for Hippocrates, when confronted by disease, Galen was not willing to stand by passively, *doing no harm*, while waiting for nature to heal the patient. A major work called *Method of Healing* and many other texts make this preference for action abundantly clear. Galen regarded bleeding as the proper treatment for almost every disorder, including hemorrhage and fatigue. Great skill was needed to determine how much blood should be taken, which vein should be incised, and the proper time for the operation. For certain conditions,

Galen recommended two brisk bleedings per day. The first bleeding should be stopped just before the patient fainted. But the physician should not be afraid to provoke unconsciousness with the second bleed-ing, because patients who survived the first operation would not be harmed by the second. Galen was so enthusiastic about the benefits of venesection that he wrote three books about it.

As proof that nature prevented disease by ridding the body of excess blood, Galen argued that many diseases that attacked men did not affect women, because their superfluous blood was eliminated by menstruation or lactation. Women with normal menstrual cycles supposedly enjoyed immunity to gout, arthritis, epilepsy, melancholy, apoplexy, and so forth. Men who frequently eliminated excess blood through hemorrhoids or nosebleeds could also expect to enjoy freedom from such diseases.

In terms of humoral doctrine, bleeding accomplished the ther-apeutic goals shared by patient and physician by apparently ridding the body of putrid, corrupt, and harmful materials. Some scientists suggest that bleeding might actually have benefited some patients by suppressing the clinical manifestations of certain diseases, such as malaria, by lowering the availability of iron in the blood. Generally speaking, anemia is not a desirable condition, but the availability of iron in the blood may determine the ability of certain pathogens to grow and multiply. Bleeding would also affect the body's response to disease by lowering the viscosity of the blood and increasing its ability to flow through the capillary bed. Bleeding to the point of fainting would force the patient along the path to rest and tranquility. Given the importance of good nursing and a supportive environment, it should also be noted that when a feverish, delirious, and difficult patient is "depleted" to the point of fainting, the caretakers might also enjoy a period of rest and recuperation.

Famous for his knowledge of drugs, Galen investigated the proper-ties of simple medicines, complex concoctions, and exotics from distant places, such as "Balm of Gilead" from Palestine, copper from Cyprus, and Lemnian Earths from the island of Lemnos. Lemnian Earths, or "Seals," were packets of specially prepared clay (much like Kaopectate) with the seal of the goddess stamped on them. Galen recommended these packets of clay for use against poisons, bites of serpents, and putrid ulcers. Various kinds of "earths" have been used as medicines for hundreds of years. Obviously, adding the image of the goddess to packets of Kaopectate would do no harm, but the consumption of some forms of clay and similar impure materials could be dangerous.

Complex drug mixtures were later called Galenicals and the sign of "Galen's Head" above the door identified apothecary shops. Some Galenicals were pleasant enough to be used as beauty aids by wealthy Roman matrons. *Unguentum refrigerans,* an emulsion of water in almond oil, with white wax and rose perfume, is similar to modern cold cream. The Prince of Physicians also prescribed some rather nauseating remedies, such as bile from bulls, spiders' webs, skin shed by snakes, and a digestive oil compounded from cooked foxes and hyenas. As explained in one of Galen's minor works, physicians were often involved in detecting malingerers and may have used noxious remedies to test slaves who did not wish to work, or citizens and soldiers trying to escape political and military duties.

Galen also developed elaborate speculative concepts about the way in which medical preparations worked and provided rationalizations for the positive medicinal value of amulets and excrements. Anecdotes about the accidental discovery of the medical virtues of various noxious agents were also put to good use. For example, in *On Simples*, Galen provided a lively account of the way in which a miserable old man suffering from a horrible skin disease was cured after drinking a jug of wine in which a poisonous snake had drowned.

Throughout the Roman Empire, the rich and powerful lived in fear of encountering poison at the banquet table, while poisonous plants and venomous creatures were constant threats to farmers, travelers, and soldiers. Galen was interested in the bites of apes, dogs, snakes, various wild animals, and (perhaps remembering his mother) human beings, all of which were presumed to be poisonous. Given the universal fear of poisons and venoms, the invention of bizarre antidotes was to be expected. Recipes for antidotes included herbs, minerals, and animal parts or products, such as dried locusts and viper's flesh. Roman recipes for theriacs, or antidotes, can be traced back to Mithridates (132–63 B.C.E.), King of Pontus in Asia Minor.

Famous for his knowledge of medicinal herbs, poisons, and antidotes, Mithridates demonstrated the value of his recipes by means of human experimentation. When exchanging recipes for antidotes with other researchers, Mithridates is said to have sent along a condemned prisoner to serve as a guinea pig. By taking a daily dose of his best antidotes, Mithridates supposedly became immune to all poisons. In 66 B.C.E., trapped in his fortress by the Roman army, Mithridates poisoned all his wives, concubines, and daughters, but no poison could kill Mithridates. According to Galen, Nero's physician Andromachus used Mithradates' poison lore to prepare the ultimate antidote, a formidable concoction containing some 64 ingredients, including opium and viper's flesh. Andromachus claimed that his theriac was a health tonic as well as a universal antidote.

Galen's skill and integrity were so highly regarded by his patrons that three Roman emperors entrusted the preparation of their theriac to him. Because others faced the danger of encountering inferior or counterfeit products, Galen suggested that purchasers test the strength of theriacs by taking a drug that induced mild purging. If the alleged theriac prevented the normal effect of the drug, it might be genuine. Authentic theriac must be made with ingredients of the highest quality. Although the pounding, mixing, heating, and stirring of the final preparation could be accomplished in about 40 days, some authorities thought that a maturation period of 5 to 12 years was essential. During the Middle Ages, theriac became an important trade item for cities such as Venice, Milan, Genoa, Padua, Bologna, and Cairo. In some cities, the production of theriac became a major public event. Theriac, viper's flesh and all, was still found in French and German pharmacopoeias at the end of the nineteenth century. In England, a degenerate form of the universal antidote became the candy known as treacle.

Highly respected as a physician and philosopher, Galen was apparently as skillful in the art of medicine as in the science. Aware of the bad repute brought to the profession by displays of ambition, contentiousness, and greed, Galen emphasized skill, dignity, and a disdainful attitude towards money. He urged physicians to cultivate the art of eliciting clues about the patient's condition even before entering the sickroom. One way was to casually question the messenger who called for the physician, as well as the patient's friends and family. A secret examination of the contents of all basins removed from the sickroom on their way to the dung heap and the medicines already in use could provide further clues. The pulse, casually examined while observing the patient, was another valuable source of information. To escape blame for failures and to win universal admiration, the physician must cultivate the art of making his diagnoses and prognoses seem like acts of divination. A clever application of this tactic was to predict the worst possible outcome while reluctantly agreeing to accept the case. If the patient died, the physician's prediction was vindicated; if the patient recovered, the physician appeared to be a miracle worker.

In many ways, Galen was truly a miracle worker; his contemporaries acknowledged the remarkable quantity and quality of his work. Even those who had engaged in bitter disputes with Galen respected his intelligence, productivity, and the passion with which he defended his doctrines. Yet, despite his brilliance in disputations, public lectures, and demonstrations, Galen seems to have had no students or disciples. Perhaps the personality traits that captivated Roman emperors and high government officials repelled colleagues and potential students. While some of his voluminous writings were lost in the centuries after his death and many were neglected, excerpts of his writings, commentaries, and translations of his texts were to form a major component of the medical curriculum and learned literature of late antiquity and the Middle Ages.

A simplified, transmuted, and partially digested version of his work known as Galenism dominated medical learning throughout the Middle Ages of Europe and the Golden Age of Islam. Galen's authority was not seriously challenged until the introduction of printing and a revival of interest in the true classics of antiquity made the genuine works of Galen and Hippocrates widely available. When Galen's anatomical and physiological doctrines were finally subjected to serious challenges in the sixteenth and seventeenth centuries, the physicians now remembered as reformers and revolutionaries began their work as Galenists. Perhaps their attacks on Galenism should be regarded as the triumph of the true spirit of Galen, physician, philosopher, and scientist.

## SUGGESTED READINGS

Brain, P. (1986). *Galen on Bloodletting.* New York: Cambridge University Press.

Cantor, D., ed. (2001). *Reinventing Hippocrates.* Burlington, VT: Ashgate.

Celsus (1960–1961). *De Medicina.* 3 Vols. (Trans. by W. G. Spencer). Cambridge, MA: Harvard University Press.

Dioscorides (1959). *The Greek Herbal of Dioscorides* (Illus. by a Byzantine in 512 A.D., Englished by John Goodyear, 1655 A.D.). Edited by R. T. Gunther. New York: Hafner.

Edelstein, E. J., and Edelstein, L. (1998). *Asclepius: Collection and Interpretation of the Testimonies.* 2 Vols. New Introduction by G. B. Ferngren. Baltimore, MD: Johns Hopkins University Press.

Flemming, R. (2001). *Medicine and the Making of Roman Women: Gender, Nature, and Authority from Celsus to Galen.* New York: Oxford University Press.

French, R. (2000). *Ancients and Moderns in the Medical Sciences: From Hippocrates to Harvey.* Burlington, VT: Ashgate.

Galen (1997). *Selected Works.* Trans., introduction, and notes by P. N. Singer. New York: Oxford University Press.

Galen (1999). *On My Own Opinions.* Edited, translation, commentary by Vivian Nutton. Berlin: Akademie Verlag.

García-Ballester, L. (2002). *Galen and Galenism: Theory and Medical Practice from Antiquity to the European Renaissance.* Burlington, VT: Ashgate.

Grant, M. (2000). *Galen on Food and Diet.* London: Routledge.

Grmek, M. D. (1991). *Diseases in the Ancient Greek World.* Baltimore, MD: Johns Hopkins University Press.

Hippocrates (1957–1959). *Hippocrates.* 4 Vols. (Trans. by W. H. S. Jones and E. T. Withington). Loeb Classical Library. Cambridge, MA: Harvard University Press.

Jouanna, J. (2001). *Hippocrates.* Baltimore, MD: Johns Hopkins University Press.

King, H. (1998). *Hippocrates' Woman: Reading the Female Body in Ancient Greece.* New York: Routledge.

Kudlien, F., and Durling, R. J., eds. (1990). *Galen's Method of Healing. Proceedings of the 2nd International Galen Symposium.* New York: E.J. Brill.

Laskaris, J. (2002). *The Art is Long: On the Sacred Disease and the Scientific Tradition.* Leiden: Brill.

Lloyd, G. E. R. (1987). *Revolutions of Wisdom. Studies in the Claims and Practice of Ancient Greek Science.* Berkeley, CA: University of California Press.

Longrigg, J. (1998). *Greek Medicine: From the Heroic to the Hellenistic Age: A Source Book.* New York: Routledge.

Nutton, V., ed. (1981). *Galen: Problems and Prospects.* London: Wellcome Institute for the History of Medicine.

Pinault, J. R. (1992). *Hippocratic Lives and Legends.* Leiden: E.J. Brill.

Riddle, J. M. (1985). *Dioscorides on Pharmacy and Medicine.* Austin, TX: University Texas Press.

Rocca, J. (2003). *Galen on the Brain: Anatomical Knowledge and Physiological Speculation in the Second Century A.D.* Leiden: Brill.

Sallares, R. (2002). *Malaria and Rome: A History of Malaria in Ancient Italy.* Oxford: Oxford University Press.

von Staden, H. (1989). *Herophilus: The Art of Medicine in Early Alexandria.* New York: Cambridge University Press.

Temkin, O. (1971). *The Falling Sickness: A History of Epilepsy from the Greeks to the Beginnings of Modern Neurology.* Baltimore, MD: Johns Hopkins University Press.

Temkin, O. (1973). *Galenism: Rise and Decline of a Medical Philosophy.* Ithaca, NY: Cornell University Press.

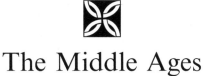

# 5

# The Middle Ages

No simple characterization can describe the state of medical theory and practice in the European Middle Ages, a period from about 500 to 1500. However, it certainly can be said that this was an era in which ideas about the nature of the physical universe, the nature of human beings and their proper place in the universe, and, above all, their relationship to their Creator underwent profound changes and dislocations. The formerly all-powerful Roman Empire, whose borders had encompassed the civilized Western world during the second century, had undergone its well-known ordeal of decline and fall after centuries of anarchy, turmoil, and warfare. Weakened by corruption, misgovernment, and insurrection, the city of Rome lost its role as undisputed political center of its crumbling Empire. In 330, Emperor Constantine established Byzantium (Constantinople) as his capital. By the end of the fourth century, the division of the empire between East and West had become permanent. The East was to become the Byzantine Empire and the West was to enter the era popularly known as the Dark Ages (a term fervently rejected by those who specialize in the study of medieval history). Historians generally described the Renaissance as a revolutionary period in the arts and sciences, which finally ended hundreds of years of intellectual stagnation. Medievalists, however, have rejected the concept of the medieval "Dark Ages" and claim that significant changes in economic, political, and social organizations were already occurring somewhere between 1000 and 1250.

Within this disputed historical context, medieval medicine has been described as everything from a pathological aberration to the dawn of a new chapter in the evolution of the medical profession. In recent years, the literature on medieval medicine has become vastly richer and more sophisticated, particularly with respect to its relationships with religion, education, professional organizations, alternative practitioners, patterns of morbidity and mortality, and the persistence of the classical tradition. The Middle Ages served as a stage for many remarkable scholars, doctors, and diseases, making this period both unique and instructive.

The transition from Greco-Roman culture to medieval Christianity irrevocably transformed the status of the healing art. The Hippocratic tradition based on love of the art, intellectual curiosity, glorification of the healthy body, and the passionate pursuit of physical well-being were foreign to the spirit of the medieval Christian world. Indeed, powerful theologians like Tertullian (160?–230?) could explain pestilence, famine, wars, and natural disasters as God's benevolent means of pruning the insolence of the human race. As a branch of learning, medicine, like all forms of secular learning, was considered inferior to and subordinate to theology. However, the actual state of medicine as the necessary healing art, rather than a branch of learning and a profession, is a more complex problem. If it were true that all sickness was the inexorable consequence of sin, or a test of faith, suffering through such trials and tribulations might well be the theoretically appropriate response.

For the ancient Greeks, the pursuit of health was a worthy objective, but seeking health became problematic within Christian doctrine. The Greeks venerated health and regarded the human body as beautiful and essentially god-like. Christians were taught to despise the flesh and its desires, but as the body housed the soul, or was a temple of God, it deserved some measure of care and respect. Healing was good as an act of love; yet being healed, except by God and His servants, was not necessarily good. Nevertheless, religious healing and secular healing would have to coexist. Theologians could explain disease as a form of punishment or a test of faith, but the majority of people were not saints or ascetics. Medicine, therefore, continued to be a part of normal life. With or without theological rationalizations, the laity never abandoned the quest for health and healing, nor did physicians and scholars wholly abandon the secular Hippocratic tradition.

Hippocratic medicine won varying degrees of acceptance in Europe and Byzantium. Although episodes of hostility and repression can be discovered, examples of accommodation and even respect can also be documented. Followers of Hippocratic medicine found ways to accommodate their art, with varying degrees of success, to the world of Christian beliefs. For their part, theologians found ways to justify the worthiness of healing and health, and the study of the authoritative texts that contained the ancient, secular knowledge essential to the practice of medicine. Setting aside major theological concerns regarding body and soul, it could be argued that medicine was an art, like agriculture, architecture, and weaving, that God had given to humankind. Moreover, the Hippocratic dietetic tradition could be rationalized as another means of the self-discipline essential to Christian life. As a hardworking craftsman, motivated by love of humankind, the legendary Hippocrates was not objectionable. He was anathema to Christian dogma if he was revered as a healing god descended from Asclepius and Apollo or as a savior who could perform miracles of healing independent of God and His representatives. The medieval physician could maintain some degree of professional autonomy and continue to honor the traditional wisdom of Hippocrates, but he would have to learn to award ultimate credit for any cures to God.

Theologians divided medicine into two parts: religious medicine, concerned with "heavenly things," and human medicine, concerned with "earthly things." Human medicine relied on empirical methods such as dietary management, drugs, bleeding, and simple surgical operations. Religious medicine involved prayers, penitence, exorcism, holy relics, charms, and incantations. The two parts of medicine differed in origin and efficacy: experience had taught physicians about the power of herbs, but Christ, "the author of heavenly medicine," could cure the sick by his word alone and even raise the dead from the grave. Thus, the Church, which acted for Christ, could, presumably, heal without earthly medicine.

Some of the early Church Fathers taught that it was sinful to try to cure bodily ills by earthly medicines and that the spirit of God was not found in healthy bodies. Disease served as a test of faith by forcing a choice between secular medicine and the Church. However, it was also possible to argue that the body should be kept strong because those who were sick and weak might more easily succumb to Satan. Moreover, if disease was the punishment for sin and forgiveness was the province of the Church, healing must be a part of the Church's mission of mercy and charity. In any case, except for those who deliberately chose mortification of the flesh, there is ample evidence that popes, priests, and peasants sought remedies for their pain and disease. As the cynic says, everyone wants to go to heaven, but no one wants to die.

Theologians recorded many miracle tales in which pious men and martyred saints cured the sick after human medicine proved useless. Medieval scholars believed that the universe was governed by general laws that had been assigned by God, but theologians established an important role for miracles. Priests might care for the sick with kindness and recognize the medical virtues of drugs, but every cure was ultimately a miracle. Healing miracles were often ascribed to the direct action of saints or their relics. Strictly speaking, "relic" refers to the mortal remains of a saint, but the term was also used to describe objects that had been in contact with these holy persons.

By the fourth century, the remains of certain saints were the objects of public cults, despite the doubts expressed by some theologians as to the propriety of honoring such objects. Those who argued for the veneration of relics triumphed, and the increasing popularity of this form of worship encouraged the discovery, multiplication, and theft of relics. The display of such obvious frauds as hairs from Noah's beard, drops of the Virgin's milk, and other wonders was enough to provoke the skepticism of a saint. In spite of the veritable flood of relics that washed over Europe during the Crusades, the insatiable demand posed the threat of a relic shortfall. One solution was to make a little bit of relic go a long way: the mortal remains of saints and martyrs were dismembered so that the parts could be shared by several shrines. "Contact relics"—water, cloths, or earth that had been in contact with the remains—could also be venerated. Theoretically, the "fullness" of the saint was present in the tiniest fragment of relic or "contact relic." When the need was acute, some relics were invested with the power of self-reproduction.

Miraculous cures were, of course, not uncommon incidents in the lives of martyrs and saintly kings. For example, when Edward the Confessor washed the neck of a scrofulous, infertile woman, her scrofula disappeared and within a year she gave birth to twins. The diluted blood of St. Thomas of Canterbury was said to cure blindness, insanity, leprosy, and deafness, but like their Egyptian and Roman counterparts, most saints tended to specialize. The martyred brothers Cosmas and Damian, famous for their skill in medicine and their refusal to take payment for their services, became the patron saints of physicians and pharmacists. According to traditional accounts, the twin physicians were martyred during the reign of Roman Emperor Diocletian in the early fourth century. No less an authority than Gregory of Tours (538–593), speaking of the miraculous cures at the shrine of Cosmas and Damian assured the sick that "all who prayed in faith departed healed." Unlike many of the other texts of this genre, the stories dealing with Cosmas and Damian often advised the sick to seek the aid of physicians and healing saints. One of their more spectacular cures involved grafting the leg of a dead pagan onto one of their converts. In another episode, the saints appeared to a physician in a dream and told him how to perform a surgical operation and apply healing drugs to a woman with breast cancer. When the doctor went to the church where the woman had gone to pray to Cosmas and Damian, he found that the operation had been miraculously performed. The saints left the final phase of treatment, the application of healing ointments, to the physician.

Some saints became associated with particular diseases or parts of the body through the manner of their death. Because all her teeth had been knocked out during her martyrdom, St. Apollonia became patron saint of toothache and dentistry. Portraits of St. Lucy, who is associated with eye disorders, show her holding a dish containing the eyes torn out by her persecutors. Pestilential disease became the specialty of St. Sebastian who had been wounded but not killed by Diocletian's archers. Sebastian's recovery from the attempted execution suggested that he was immune to the arrows of death. In portraits of the saint, arrows pierce his body at the sites where plague buboes usually appear. An arrow in the heart symbolized the sudden death that often claimed plague victims. He was later sentenced to death by flogging. Women in labor could appeal to Saint Magaret, who entered the world through the mouth of a dragon. Because of her miraculous birth, Margaret was the patron saint of women in childbirth.

Just as the pagan gods were replaced by Christian saints, the rituals of Asclepius were absorbed into Christian practice. Temples were transformed into churches where the worship of Christ the Healer, or his healing saints, provided a familiar setting for medical miracles. In contrast to the Asclepiads who excluded the incurable from the sanctuary, the Church took on the nursing of hopeless cases and promised relief in the next world if faith failed to effect an immediate cure.

Theologians generally mentioned secular physicians only to show how relics and prayers were effective after earthy medicine failed. Given the bias of these authors, such stories can be looked upon as proof that the sick often turned to lay healers. Medieval writings contain many complaints about the physician's love of "filthy lucre" and the high cost of medical care. John of Salisbury, for example, said that physicians were invariably guided by two maxims: "Never mind the poor; never refuse money from the rich." On the other hand, biographies of medieval kings, nobles, and clergymen also refer to dedicated physicians who won the respect and friendship of their patrons.

In making his diagnosis, the medieval physician relied primarily on the patient's narrative of symptoms, but many healers were regarded as masters of the art of uroscopy, that is, inspection of urine. Using a specially marked flask, the physician studied the color of the urine and the distribution of clouds, precipitates, and particles at various levels of the flask in order to determine the nature of the illness and the condition of the patient. A story about the Duke of Bavaria indicates that even in the tenth century, some patients were skeptics. To test his physician, the Duke substituted the urine of a pregnant woman for his own. After making his inspection, the physician solemnly announced that God was about to bring about a great event: the Duke would soon give birth to a child.

The influence of the Church on medical thought is only one aspect of the way in which the Church attained a virtual monopoly on all forms of learning during the Middle Ages. The task of translating Greek medical texts into Latin had begun by the fifth century. For the most part, the study of ancient texts and the preparation of extracts and compilations in the monasteries reflect interest in logic and philology rather than science, but there is evidence that medical manuscripts were consulted for practical purposes. Indeed, the marginal comments found on medical manuscripts provide evidence of interest in applied medicine and pharmacology.

The writings of certain theologians, such as Isidore, Bishop of Seville (ca. 560–636), provide a good example of informed interest in medical matters. Isidore believed that it was possible to use pagan writings to prepare useful encyclopedic texts that would conform to Christian faith and morals. Such studies supported the idea that medicine embraced all the other liberal disciplines of study. Medicine was the art of protecting, preserving, and restoring health to the body by means of diet, hygiene, and the treatment of wounds and diseases. However, medicine was also a "second philosophy," which cured the body, just as the first philosophy cured the soul. Thus the physician had to be well grounded in literature, grammar, rhetoric, and dialectic in order to understand and explain difficult texts and study the causes and cures of infirmities in the light of reason.

Many medical manuscripts were written in the form of a dialogue—the format used in medieval teaching, but medicine was last, and generally least, of the traditional four faculties of the medieval universities: theology, philosophy, law, and medicine. Dialogues usually began with a simple question, such as: "What is medicine?" Students were expected to memorize standard answers and the teacher's exposition of the texts. By the ninth century, medieval scholars had established the concept that medical studies were an integral part of Christian wisdom. If all learning, including the science of health, came from God, the religious need not fear a conflict between the study of the medical literature and theology. Medical knowledge could be enjoyed as an intellectual ornament, an area of serious study, and a potentially useful technique. Of course, it was possible to acknowledge the value of classical medical texts while insisting that health could not be restored by herbs alone. The sick and their attendants must place their faith in God, even as they attempted to find the proper remedy.

Hospitals have been called the greatest medical innovation of the Middle Ages, but because the modern hospital is so closely associated with advances in research, medical education, and surgery, the term "hospital" conjures up images that are inappropriate to earlier time periods. Certainly, medieval hospitals played an important social role, but their primary goals were religious, not scientific. On the other hand, the tendency to dismiss this era as the "Dark Ages" has created the false impression that the medieval hospital was invariably a terrible pest house where the sick only went to die. Some medieval hospitals apparently provided comfort, nursing, and medical care as well as charity.

Confusion about the origins and development of the medieval hospital reflects the paradoxes and tensions of this complex era. Many hospitals were no more than cottages, but in the major towns relatively large institutions served as infirmaries, almshouses, hostels, and leper houses. Of course, the number and nature of these charitable enterprises changed throughout the Middle Ages. During the fourteenth century, some hospitals were trying to discharge the sick poor and replace them with paying clients, whereas others became so intolerable that patients rebelled and demolished them.

## MONASTERIES AND UNIVERSITIES

One of the major innovations of the Middle Ages was the formal establishment of university education in medicine during the twelfth and thirteenth centuries. However, only a tiny fraction of all medical practitioners had any university training. The influence of the faculties of medicine was more closely related to the establishment of a regular curriculum, authoritative texts, technical knowledge, and a medical elite than to the absolute number of university-trained physicians.

The creation and distribution of universities and faculties of medicine throughout Europe were very uneven. Students often had to undertake long journeys in search of suitable mentors. Moreover, the universities of the Middle Ages were very different from both the ancient centers of learning and their modern counterparts, especially in terms of the relationships among students, faculty, and administrators. The exact origins of some of the major universities are obscure. Indeed, "university" was originally a rather vague term that referred to any corporate status or association of persons. Eventually, the term was formally associated with institutions of higher learning. Some historians believe that the "age of reason" began in the universities of the late Middle Ages, with the institutionalization of a curriculum that demanded the exploration of logic, natural philosophy, theology, medicine, and law. Large numbers of students, all of whom shared Latin as the language of learning, were drawn to universities to study with teachers known for particular areas of excellence. Many students entered the universities at the age of 14 or 15 years after securing the rudiments of the seven liberal arts: grammar, rhetoric, logic, arithmetic, geometry, astronomy, and music.

The medical texts available for use by the time medical faculties were established included many translations from Greek and Arabic manuscripts, as well as new Latin collections and commentaries. However, before the fifteenth century, students and professors lacked access to many of the surviving works of Hippocrates, Galen, and other ancient writers. Some of Galen's most important texts, including *On Anatomical Procedures*, were not translated into Latin until the sixteenth century. Some manuscripts were extremely rare and many of the Latin texts attributed to Hippocrates and Galen were spurious.

Although the rise of the university as a center for training physicians is an important aspect of the history of medieval medicine, for much of this period learned medicine was still firmly associated with the church and the monastery. With its library, infirmary, hospital, and herb gardens, the monastery was a natural center for medical study and practice. On the other hand, charitable impulses towards the sick were sometimes obliterated by an all-consuming concern for the soul, coupled with contempt for the flesh. Some ascetics refused to make allowances for the "indulgence" of the flesh, even for sick flesh. St. Bernard of Clairvaux (1091–1153), a mystic who engaged in harsh, self-imposed penances, expected his monks to live and die simply. Building infirmaries, taking medicines, or visiting a physician were forbidden. St. Bernard thought it "unbefitting religion and contrary to simplicity of life" to allow such activities.

Many exemplary stories about the lives of saints and ascetics suggested that a regimen of self-imposed privations led to health, longevity, and peace of mind. Ascetics might fast several days a week, eat nothing but bread, salt, and water, stay awake all night in prayer, and give up bathing and exercise (some saints were famous for sitting on pillars for years at a time). However, the reactions of saints and ascetics to diseases and accidents that were not self-inflicted might be quite different. Here the stories vary widely. Some ascetics accepted medical or surgical treatment for disorders such as cancer and dropsy, whereas others categorically refused to accept drugs or doctors. Some were fortunate enough to be cured in a rather Asclepian fashion by ministering angels who appeared in dreams to wash their wounds and anoint their bruises.

The founders of some religious orders took a more temperate view of the needs of the sick, and infirmaries and hospitals were established as adjuncts to monasteries in order to provide charity and care for the sick. Within many religious orders, the rules of St. Benedict (ca. 480–547) provided reasonable guidelines for care of the sick. Although the monastic routine called for hard work, special allowances were to be made for the sick, infirm, and aged. The care of the sick was such an important duty that those caring for them were enjoined to act as if they served Christ directly. There is suggestive evidence that monks with some medical knowledge were chosen to care for the sick.

By the eleventh century, some monasteries were training their own physicians. Ideally, such physicians would uphold the Christianized ideal of the healer who offered mercy and charity towards all patients, whatever their status and prognosis might be. The gap between the ideal and the real is suggested by evidence of numerous complaints about the pursuit of "filthy lucre" by priest-physicians. When such physicians gained permission to practice outside the monastery and offered their services to wealthy nobles, complaints about luxurious living and the decline of monastic discipline were raised.

The ostensibly simple question of whether medieval clergymen were or were not forbidden to practice medicine and surgery has been the subject of considerable controversy. Only excessive naiveté would lead us to expect that official records and documents are a realistic reflection of the status of forbidden practices. The official Church position was made explicit in numerous declarations and complaints about the study and practice of medicine and surgery by clergymen. Several twelfth-century papal decisions expressed a desire to restrict the practice of medicine by monks. The declarations of the Council of Clermont (1130), the Council of Rheims (1131), and the Second Lateran Council (1139) all contain the statement: "Monks and canons regular are not to study jurisprudence and medicine for the sake of temporal gain." This statement referred specifically to the pursuit of money, not to the study and practice of medicine or law. Obviously, the need for so many official prohibitions indicates how difficult it was to make practice accord with policy.

Another myth about medieval medicine is the assumption that the Church's opposition to "shedding human blood" prohibited surgery. This prohibition was based on opposition to shedding blood because of hatred and war, not to surgery in general, and certainly not to venesection (therapeutic bloodletting). The idea that this position had any medical significance was essentially an eighteenth-century hoax. Venesection was actually a fairly common procedure, performed both prophylactically and therapeutically. When carrying out this important surgical procedure, the doctor had to consider complicated rules that related the patient's condition to the site selected, as well as the season of the year, phase of the moon, and the most propitious time of day. Some guidance was offered by simple illustrations depicting commonly used phlebotomy sites, but these pictures were highly stylized and very schematic.

## MEDICAL EDUCATION AND PRACTICE

The processes that led to the establishment of medicine as a profession based upon a formal education, standardized curriculum, licensing, and legal regulation were set in motion in the Middle Ages. Of course, laws differed from place to place, as did enforcement and the balance of power between unofficial healing and legally sanctioned medicine. Law codes might specify the nature of the contract between patient and doctor and the penalties and fines for particular errors. Physicians could be fined for public criticism of other doctors, failure to consult other physicians in cases of serious illness, or for treating a female patient in the absence of proper witnesses. The law might even require giving more weight to the patient's spiritual welfare than his physical well being. The law could compel the doctor to advise the patient to seek confession, even though the fear inspired by this warning might be dangerous in itself.

Despite some unwelcome constraints, the doctor achieved the benefits of a legally defined status. As a consequence, healers who practiced
without a state-approved license became subject to criminal prosecution
and fines. Professional physicians argued that standards of practice
would be raised by eradicating unfit practitioners, generally identified
as "empirics, fools, and women." However, formal requirements also
excluded many skilled healers. Another unfortunate consequence of
medieval legal codes was the tendency to separate medicine from surgery
and diminish the status of the surgeon.

Not all medical practitioners were either highly educated priest-
physicians or illiterate empirics. For example, the Anglo-Saxon medical
books, known as leechbooks, provide some insights into the concerns
of practitioners and patients outside the realm of the "high medical
culture" of the learned centers of Europe. Little is known about the
education and practice of the typical medieval English physician, but
both monastic physicians and secular healers appeared in illustrations
and paintings. Early English leechbooks were generally compilations
of ancient texts, unique only in that many were written in Old English,
rather than Latin. Presumably, most English doctors—often referred to
as leeches—were literate, at least in the vernacular. By the fourteenth
century, monastic centers of learning were producing scholars with little
tolerance for the Anglo-Saxon leechbooks. Considering the fact that
parchment was a valuable and usable resource, it is rather surprising
that any of the early English medical texts did survive.

Fortunately, the nineteenth-century revival of interest in folklore
inspired the Rev. Thomas Oswald Cockayne (1807–1873) to rescue surviving Anglo-Saxon medical texts and prepare a three-volume collection
with the wonderful title *Leechdoms, Wortcunning and Starcraft of Early
England, Illustrating the History of Science in This Country Before the
Norman Conquest*. The leechbooks describe surgical techniques, herbal
remedies, rituals, and charms to prevent a host of diseases, including
sudden illness caused by "flying venom" and "elf-shot." Descriptions
of "Devil-sickness" and "fiend-sickness" presumably referred to various
forms of mental illness and strange seizures. Many chronic diseases were
attributed to "the worm," a term applied to all manner of worms, insects,
snakes, and dragons. Some rather colorful descriptions of "worms" were
probably inspired by observations of the very real pests that live on
human beings and domesticated animals. Bits of tissue and mucous
in excretions, vomit, blood, or maggots in putrid wounds could also
provide evidence of worms.

Anglo-Saxon leechbooks reflect the mingling of Greek, Roman, Teu-
tonic, Celtic, and Christian concepts of medicine and magic. According
to such texts, healers could variously cure diseases by invoking the names
of the saints, exorcism, or by transferring them to plants, animals, earth,
or running water. The preparation of almost every remedy required the

recitation of some prayer or charm, along with the number magic of the pagan "nines" and the Christian "threes." Despite condemnation of amulets as magical objects, Christianized versions of these highly popular protective devices were discussed in the texts and apparently widely used.

The prescriptions in the leechbooks suggest the common disorders endured by medieval people, such as arthritis, eye diseases, burns and scalds, unwanted pregnancies, impotence, and infertility. A wealth of recipes testify to the universal presence of the louse. Iatrogenic disorders (those caused by medical treatment) such as complications resulting from venesection were not unknown. In retrospect, it would not be surprising to find infection or tetanus among patients whose venesection wounds were dressed with "horses tords." Remedies and charms to regulate the menses, prevent miscarriage, ensure male offspring, and ease the pains of childbirth were discussed at great length.

Skeptics might argue that the remedies in the leechbooks acted only through the power of suggestion, but the leech confidently ascribed great virtues to herbal remedies. Medicinal herbs included lupine, henbane, belladonna, and mandrake. Birthwort was said to cure external cancers, nasturtium juice cured baldness, wolf's comb was used for liver ailments, and swallowwort provided a remedy for hemorrhoids if nine paternosters were recited while the plant was harvested. Patients were well advised to follow instructions carefully, or the results could be disastrous. For example, a son would be born if both man and wife drank a charm prepared from a hare's uterus, but if only the wife drank this preparation, she would give birth to a hermaphrodite.

Scholars and pharmacologists who have re-examined medieval medicine have concluded that some medical practices and recipes were probably practical and effective. For example, lupine, one of the most frequently prescribed herbs in the leechbooks, was recommended for lung disease, seizures, insanity, as an antidote for venom, and for diseases caused by elves, "night-goers," and the devil. Modern researchers suggest that, because manganese deficiency has been linked to recurrent seizures, lupine seeds (which are high in manganese) might be effective in the treatment of epilepsy. Henbane, belladonna, mandrake, and other plants in the *Datura* genus are known to contain potent alkaloids such as scopolamine and hyoscyamine. Depending on preparation and dosage, extracts of such plants could, therefore, have powerful neurological effects when used as drugs, poisons, and hallucinogens.

Given the importance of domestic animals to the medieval economy, the use of many of the same remedies for man and beast is not surprising, but the religious aspects of medieval veterinary medicine are another matter. Whatever beneficial psychological effects holy water and prayers, might have on humans, it is difficult to imagine that religious rites would greatly impress sheep, pigs, and bees. The use of pagan and magical rituals to protect domestic animals was as much condemned as their use in treating humans, with much the same results. Some of the "cures" must have tormented the animals more than the disease. For example, one ritual for horses required cutting crosses on their forehead and limbs with a knife whose haft had been made from the horn of an ox. After pricking a hole in the horse's left ear and inscribing a Latin charm on the haft of the knife, the healer declared the beast cured.

English medicine from a somewhat later period is represented by the work of John of Gaddesden (1280–1361), physician to Edward II. Primarily remembered as the author of *The Rose of England, the Practice of Medicine from the Head to the Feet*, John might have been the model for Chaucer's Doctor of Physic. According to Chaucer, the *Rosa Anglica* was invariably a part of the typical physician's library. John immodestly claimed that his treatise was so well organized and detailed that surgeons and physicians would need no other book. Remedies are suggested for both rich and poor patients. For example, physicians should prescribe expensive diuretic remedies for wealthy patients suffering from chronic dropsy, but poor patients should be told to drink their own urine every morning.

One of the most famous recommendations in the *Rosa Anglica* was the "red therapy" for smallpox, which involved surrounding a victim of smallpox with red things to expedite healing and prevent the formation of scars. In addition to some sound medical advice and acute observations on disease, John discussed traditional charms and rituals, such as wearing the head of a cuckoo around the neck to prevent epileptic seizures. This approach was especially useful in treating young children who would not take medicines. A brief section on surgery includes methods of draining fluid from a patient with dropsy, reduction of dislocations, and the treatment of wounds. Some passages advise the physician to take a particular interest in the treatment of the diseases that would bring him the greatest rewards.

Texts known by the Latin term *regimen sanitatis*, which served as practical guides to health and its preservation, were originally written for wealthy individuals in order to teach them the fundamentals of the concepts used by physicians to justify their therapeutic practices. These health handbooks explicated the Galenic threefold organization of medicine into the following: the naturals (such as the humors and so forth); the contranaturals (diseases and symptoms); the non-naturals (things that affect the body). Guided by the physician, an individual would adopt an appropriate regimen, that is, an elaborate plan, for managing the six non-naturals (air and environment, motion and rest, food and drink, sleep and waking, evacuation and repletion, and affections of the soul). When physicians wrote guides for a wider audience, they placed more emphasis on drugs and other simple ways of preserving health and preventing disease.

## SURGERY IN THE MIDDLE AGES

One problem exacerbated during the Middle Ages was the separation between surgery and medicine. Although the leech of the early medieval period was both physician and surgeon, his surgery was generally limited to simple emergency measures, such as phlebotomy (therapeutic bloodletting), cupping (applying evacuated glass cups to intact or scarified skin in order to draw blood towards the surface), cauterization, and simple emergency measures for coping with the usual run of burns, bruises, wounds, ulcers, sprains, dislocations, toothaches, and broken bones. A few more daring practitioners had the special skills needed for couching cataracts, tooth extraction, and lithotomy (the surgical removal of stones in the urinary bladder).

Modern specialists might be surprised to find their medieval counterparts among the lowly oculists, bone setters, tooth extractors, cutters of the stone, and other empirics, rather than in the company of learned physicians. Nevertheless, during the Middle Ages, ambitious surgeons were trying to win a more respectable professional status for surgery as a branch of knowledge with its own body of technical writings, as well as an eminently useful occupation. The specialized literature of surgery was growing by the thirteenth century, but glimpses of earlier surgical traditions have survived in epic poetry and mythology.

Because the need for surgeons is a common byproduct of warfare, semilegendary stories of great heroes and battles may reflect the conditions of battlefield surgical practice with more immediacy than learned texts. According to Scandinavian epic poets, if professional doctors were not available, the men with the softest hands were assigned to care for the wounded. Many famous physicians were said to have descended from warriors with gentle hands. Truly heroic warriors bound up their own wounds and returned to the battle. Sometimes women cared for the wounded in a special tent or house near the battlefield. One saga described a woman who cleaned wounds with warm water and extracted arrows with tongs. When the woman could not find the tip of the arrow, she made the patient eat boiled leeks. Then, the hidden wound could be located because it smelled of leeks.

Although epic heroes apparently emerged from crude battlefield surgery completely healed and eager to fight, the subjects of more mundane operations often succumbed to bleeding, shock, and infection. Despite their familiarity with the soporific effects of poppy, henbane, and mandrake, surgeons did not routinely use these drugs before an operation. Potions made of wine, eggs, honey, and beer were used to wash and dress wounds. A dressing for burns might be as gentle as a mixture of egg whites, fats, and herbs, or it might be strengthened by the addition of goat droppings.

Despite the low status of most medieval surgeons, some distinguished practitioners deplored the separation between medicine and surgery. The learned doctors of Salerno, the most famous Western medical school of the Middle Ages, maintained high standards of surgery and taught anatomy and surgical technique by dissections of animals. Medieval authors created simplified Latin texts by fusing the work of doctors at Salerno with excerpts from the Arabic literature. A treatise on surgery, based on the lectures of Roger Frugard, who taught and practiced surgery at Parma in northern Italy, was prepared about 1180 by his colleague Guido Arezzo, the Younger. Roger's influential and often copied *Surgery* described methods of wound closure, trephination, and lithotomy and recommended mercury for skin diseases and seaweed for goiter.

In the mid-thirteenth century, Roland of Parma produced an important new edition of Roger's surgical treatise that became known as the *Rolandina*. Roland, who taught at the new medical center in Bologna, based his teaching and practice on Roger's methods. Even as late as the sixteenth century, after newer Latin texts and translations of Galenic and Arabic texts became available, Roger's treatise was still respectfully studied. By the beginning of the fourteenth century, texts for surgeons who were literate but had not mastered Latin were appearing in vernacular languages. These simplified texts provided practical information on medicine and surgery and collections of remedies.

Hugh of Lucca (ca. 1160–1257), town surgeon of Bologna, and his son Theodoric, Bishop of Cervia (1210–1298), may have been the most ingenious of medieval surgeons. Theodoric is said to have attacked the two great enemies of surgery—infection and pain—and rejected the idea that the formation of pus was a natural and necessary stage in the healing of wounds. Indeed, Theodoric realized that the generation of pus, sometimes deliberately provoked by surgeons, actually obstructed wound healing. He also objected to the use of complex and noxious wound dressings.

To overcome the pain caused by surgery, Theodoric attempted to induce narcosis by the use of a "soporific sponge" containing drugs known to produce a sleep-like state. Just how effective his methods were in practice is unclear. Sponges were prepared by soaking them in a mixture of extracts from mandrake, poppy, henbane, and other herbs. Before surgery began, dried sponges were soaked in hot water and the patient was allowed to chew on the sponge and inhale the vapors. If the process was successful, the patient would fall asleep and remember nothing of the operation—if he woke up again.

Sometime in the early fourteenth century, Henri de Mondeville, surgeon to Philip the Fair of France, began writing a major treatise on surgery. The text was still unfinished when Henri died. Moreover, Henri's text was polemical in style, highly argumentative, and hostile to the medical authorities. Proud of his skills and accomplishments as a surgeon, Henri protested the disastrous results of separating surgery from medicine. By the end of the century, the physicians comprising the Faculty of Medicine in Paris were demanding that graduates take an oath that they would not perform any surgical procedures. Henri's work was gradually forgotten and his text was not printed until 1892. Eventually, the title "father of French surgery" was bestowed on Henri's student Guy de Chauliac (ca. 1298–1368), eminent physician and surgeon and author of a treatise on surgery that was still in use in the eighteenth century. Guy's treatise, composed about 1363, is generally considered the most valuable surgical text of its time. For at least two centuries, most of the Latin and vernacular texts on surgery produced in Europe were based on the work of Roger Frugard and Guy de Chauliac.

## WOMEN AND MEDICINE

Apart from a few exceptional women who achieved recognition for their mastery of the medical literature either in convents or the University of Salerno, women were generally excluded from formal medical education and thus from the legal and lucrative professional practice of the art. Nevertheless, it is possible to find women practitioners among all the ranks of the medieval medical community—physicians, surgeons, barber-surgeons, apothecaries, leeches, and assorted empirics. As in the modern university or corporation, their distribution would tend to include much larger numbers at the bottom of the hierarchy than at the top. Although medieval practitioners battled fiercely for control over the paid practice of medicine, there is little doubt that much of the routine, unpaid care of the sick took place in the home and was carried out by women.

With a few rare exceptions, women as practitioners and patients were largely invisible in Western histories of medicine. Although women presumably suffered from most of the diseases and disasters that afflicted men, "women's complaints" were generally discussed only in terms of pregnancy, childbirth, lactation, and menstrual disorders. Women practitioners were assumed to be midwives, nurses, or elderly "wise women." Since the 1970s, historians specializing in women's studies, gender studies, and social history have helped to correct this picture and enrich our knowledge of medical practice and medical care during the Middle Ages. In addition to retrieving the work and lives of exceptional and accomplished women who, nevertheless, became "lost" to history, scholars have become aware of the ways in which surviving documents and conventional methodologies have biased our view of history in terms of gender. Rather than study only the world of the

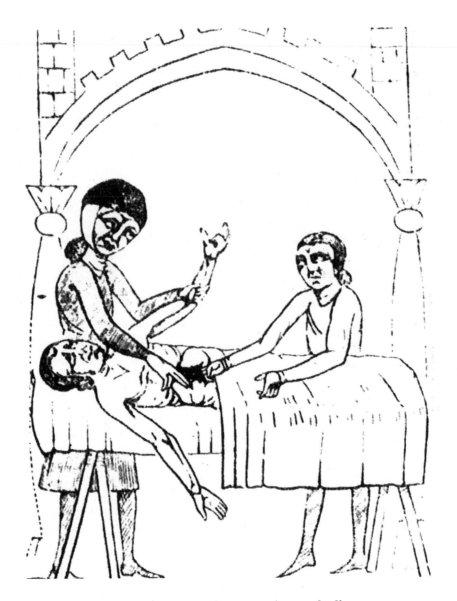

**Medieval depiction of an operation on the liver.**

"elites" of the medical profession, historians have looked more broadly at the world of health-care practitioners and gender issues related to health and disease.

Just as women practitioners were not restricted to the role of midwife, women patients did not restrict their choice of medical advisor to members of their own sex, even if their "complaint" involved sensitive issues, such as fertility. Literacy was quite low during this period, but some women owned and used books, including medical texts. Historians have achieved insights into women's grasp of written medical information by studying the ownership of specific books.

Most of the ordinary women practitioners left no trace in the historical records, but studies of the life and work of Hildegard of Bingen (1098–1179) provide a vivid portrait of one of the twelfth century's most remarkable writers on cosmological and medical questions. Widely known and respected as a writer, composer, and healer during her lifetime, she was soon all but forgotten, except in her native Germany. St. Hildegard has been called a mystic, a visionary, and a prophet, but her writings suggest practical experience and boundless curiosity about the wonders of nature. A revival of interest in St. Hildegard during the twentieth century brought her to the attention of scholars, feminists, musicians, poets, herbalists, and homeopathic practitioners.

As the tenth child of a noble family, Hildegard was offered to God as a tithe and entered a life of religious seclusion at the age of eight years. She took her monastic vows in her teens and was chosen abbess of her Benedictine convent in 1136. At about 15 years of age, Hildegard, who had been having visions since childhood, began receiving revelations about the nature of the cosmos and humankind. The visions were explained to her in Latin by a voice from heaven. In 1141, a divine call commanded her to record and explain her visions. When she began writing, Hildegard thought that she was the first woman to embark on such a mission. After a papal inquiry into the nature of her revelations, Hildegard became a veritable celebrity and was officially encouraged to continue her work. Popes, kings, and scholars sought her advice. At the age of sixty years, Hildegard focused her energies on the need for monastic and clerical reform.

Hildegard's *Physica, The Book of Simple Medicine, or Nine Books on the Subtleties of Different Kinds of Creatures*, is probably the first book by a female author to discuss the elements and the therapeutic virtues of plants, animals, and metals. It was also the first book on natural history composed in Germany. The text includes much traditional medical lore concerning the medical uses or toxic properties of many herbs, trees, mammals, reptiles, fishes, birds, minerals, gems, and metals. Hildegard's other major work, the *Book of Compound Medicine, or Causes and Cures*, discusses the nature, forms, causes, and treatment of disease, human physiology and sexuality, astrology, and so forth. Interestingly, the two books on medicine made no claims to divine inspiration.

Relying primarily on traditional humoral theory, Hildegard usually suggested treatments based on the principle of opposites. Foods, drugs, and precious stones were prescribed to prevent and cure disease. For example, sapphire was recommended for the eyes and as an antiaphrodisiac, which made it an appropriate gem to have in a convent or monastery. Remedies calling for parts from exotic animals, such as unicorn liver and lion heart, were recommended for dreaded diseases like leprosy.

In exploring mental as well as physical diseases, Hildegard discussed frenzy, insanity, obsession, and idiocy. According to Hildegard, even the most bizarre mental states could have natural causes. Thus, people might think a man was possessed by a demon when the real problem might be a simultaneous attack of headache, migraine, and vertigo. Hildegard probably had a special interest in these disorders. Indeed, modern medical detectives have diagnosed her visions as classical examples of migraine.

Most of the women healers who practiced medicine and midwifery during the Middle Ages left no traces of their activities in the written records. Certainly, coming to the attention of the authorities and directly competing with licensed practitioners was dangerous for those forced to live at the margins of society. Thus, although few women were able to attain the learning and influence reached by St. Hildegard in her safely cloistered position, many other medieval women served as nurses, herbalists, and healers in hospitals and infirmaries in Europe and the Holy Land. For example, St. Walpurga (d. 779) was an English princess who studied medicine and founded a convent in Germany. She was often depicted holding a flask of urine in one hand and bandages in the other.

One of the most popular medieval works on women's medicine, a text generally known as the *Trotula*, is attributed to a woman who might have been a member of a remarkable group of women medical practitioners associated directly or indirectly with Salernitan medical culture during the eleventh and twelfth centuries. There is some evidence that women were allowed to study and teach medicine at some Italian universities from the twelfth to the fourteenth centuries. At the University of Salerno, the subject of "women's diseases" fell within the province of women professors. According to some sources, Trotula (also known as Trocta or Trotta) taught, wrote, and practiced medicine during the twelfth century. Nevertheless, Trotula and other medieval medical women have often been dismissed as myths. Indeed, until confronted by recent scholarship on medieval women, many people were more likely to believe in unicorns and alien abductions than the existence of female healers, female medical writers, female professors, or even female readers. Since the 1990s, however, scholars have found evidence that literacy in medieval Europe, including female literacy, was more prevalent than previously assumed. However, the oral transmission of knowledge was still important even with increasing literacy, especially for therapeutic knowledge and techniques. Some scholars assumed that a male physician wrote the text based on the work of a Salernitan female healer and then named the resulting treatise the *Trotula*, in her honor. Perhaps, the putative male author thought of these writings as "women's secrets" which should be attributed to a female writer, rather than a significant medical treatise.

At least in part, the confusion about Trotula as a medical writer illustrates the general problem of establishing the authorship of medieval manuscripts. Many manuscripts were copies that did not name the original author. When printed editions of texts were produced in the fifteenth and sixteenth centuries, assumptions were made about the authors, often without sufficient evidence. If recent scholarship concerning the *Trotula* tradition has not solved the riddle of the text and its author, it has thrown some light on the transmission and corruption of the earlier versions of the manuscripts. Apparently, three different twelfth-century Salernitan manuscripts on women's medicine became fused and evolved into a treatise known as the *Trotula*. Trotula may have written one or more of the original manuscripts, but her name was probably attached to other texts, just as other works were erroneously attributed to Hippocrates or Galen. During the sixteenth century, the manuscripts that now comprise the *Trotula* were edited, rearranged, and printed, thus establishing the final text and serving as the source of several vernacular translations.

The *Trotula* includes discussions of gynecology, obstetrics, the diseases of women, and cosmetics. In addition to more serious aspects of women's medicine, the text includes recipes for perfuming hair, clothes, and breath, cosmetics to whiten the face, hands, and teeth, creams to remove the blemishes that occur after childbirth, preparations that color and thicken the hair, unguents, and stain removers for linens. Recipes for depilatories are accompanied by a very sensible preliminary test that is performed on a feather to make sure the mixture will not burn the skin. The text provides advice about feminine hygiene, menstrual problems, infertility, pessaries for widows and nuns, methods of restoring virginity, drugs to regulate the menses, emmenagogues, and so forth. Trotula seems to have strongly believed that menstruation was crucial to women's health. If that is true, then many recipes that were said to "bring on the menses" may have been prescribed to promote regular menstrual periods, although the same phrase might have been a euphemism for abortifacients. The text discussed the proper regimen for pregnant women, signs of pregnancy, difficult births, removal of the afterbirth, postpartum care, lactation, and breast problems. The discussion of the care and feeding of infants included advice on choosing a wet nurse, remedies for impetigo, infantile worms, vomiting, swelling of the throat, whooping cough, and pain.

Medieval ideas about women's health and physiology were apparently influenced by the Salernitan medical texts that were later printed as the *Trotula*. Perhaps, the lasting impact of the *Trotula* correlates well with recent findings that the Trotula manuscripts were almost invariable owned and used by male practitioners. Historians have suggested that this pattern of ownership indicates that during the Middle Ages, male physicians were already attempting to expand the range of their services to include gynecology. Indeed, some historians believe that essentially all of the medieval gynecological literature was written by men for the use of male practitioners. These findings have challenged previous assumptions that during the Middle Ages, women would only consult female healers about issues such as menstruation, fertility, pregnancy, and childbirth. Women were likely to consult midwives for "female complaints" as well as for childbirth, but determining the scope of medieval midwifery practice is difficult because midwives were not organized into guilds or other formal associations. For the most part, regulations pertaining to midwifery did not appear until the fifteenth century and licensing rules generally dealt with moral character rather than medical skills.

In contrast to common assumptions about female medical practitioners in medieval Europe, recent scholarship suggests that women practiced general medicine and surgery as well as midwifery. For example, in some parts of France, women could practice medicine or surgery if they passed an examination. However, as medical faculties and professional organizations gained prestige and power, laws governing medical practice became increasingly restrictive throughout Europe. Unlicensed practitioners were prosecuted, fined, or excommunicated for disregarding these laws. Many of those who cared for the sick remain nameless, except when they became targets of the battle waged by physicians for control of the medical marketplace. As indicated by the case of Jacoba (or Jacquéline) Felicie in Paris in 1322, the lack of a formal education did not necessarily mean a lack of skill and experience.

The Dean and Faculty of Medicine of the University of Paris charged Jacoba with illegally visiting the sick, examining their pulse, urine, bodies, and limbs, prescribing drugs, collecting fees, and, worse yet, *curing* her patients. Not only did Jacoba feel competent to practice medicine, but also she thought herself capable of pleading her own case. Patients called to testify praised her skill; some noted that she had cured them after regular physicians had failed. Jacoba argued that the intent of the law was to forbid the practice of medicine by ignorant and incompetent quacks. She argued that, because she was both knowledgeable and skillful, the law did not apply to her. Moreover, natural modesty about the "secret nature" of female diseases created a need for women practitioners.

The Dean and Faculty of Medicine who prosecuted Jacoba did not deny her skill, but they argued that medicine was a science transmitted by texts, not a craft to be learned empirically. Actually, the larger goal of the Parisian faculty of medicine was to control the medical practice of surgeons, barbers, and empirics, whether male or female. Thus, trials of unlicensed practitioners provide glimpses into the lives of otherwise invisible practitioners and the relationship between marginal practitioners and the elite medical community. In response to the case against Jacoba, the Court agreed with the interpretation of the statutes put forth by the Faculty of Medicine. Nevertheless, modern ideas about professionalization and the legal status of medical practitioners are very different from those that prevailed during the Middle Ages. Indeed, throughout history, most medical practitioners, whether male or female, were unlicensed and only a tiny minority had university degrees. Competition among many different kinds of medical practitioners was, however, already a factor in the medieval medical marketplace—physicians, surgeons, apothecaries, and empirics.

Medieval documents pertaining to women practitioners are rare, but historians have found a few examples of women who specialized in the treatment of gout and eye disorders and a woman physician who held the title "master" (*magistra*). Between the thirteenth and the fifteenth centuries, some women were granted licenses to practice medicine or surgery, although sometimes their practice was specifically limited to female patients, or conditions that affected the breasts and reproductive organs. For example, a fourteenth-century Spanish law prohibited women from practicing medicine or prescribing drugs, but the law made an exception for the care for women and children. In the absence of formal educational criteria for most occupations, medieval women and men may have worked at different full- or part-time occupations during the course of their lives. Thus, various aspects of healing, including midwifery, herbalism, nursing, and surgery, might have been practiced informally and intermittently. Those who enjoyed some success in such ventures might well be considered healers by family, friends, and neighbors, despite the lack of any specific training or formal licensing. Women were likely to be active participants in the work performed by their father or husband, because there was little or no separation between household and workshop, or caring for family members and supervising apprentices. Very few women appeared in the rolls of medieval guilds, but it is likely that many of the women who asked for permission to practice medicine or surgery when their husbands or fathers died had already been performing the tasks associated with those occupations.

Licensed women doctors essentially vanished by the sixteenth century, but hordes of quacks were busily peddling herbs, amulets, and charms. This army of marginal practitioners included barber-surgeons, herbalists, nurses, and midwives. As the medical profession assumed more power and prestige, the position of women healers became ever more precarious. Whatever the relative merits of scholars, priests, physicians, midwives, and empirics might have been, probably the best physicians of the Middle Ages were those recommended in the popular health handbook known as the *Regimen of Salerno*: doctors Quiet, Rest, Diet, and Merryman. Unfortunately, these doctors were

unlikely to be on the staff of the typical hospital or to make housecalls
at the hovels of the poor.


## EPIDEMIC DISEASES OF THE MIDDLE AGES

Many of the afflictions described in medieval texts are still common
today, but, in popular imagination, the most feared of all pestilential
diseases, leprosy and bubonic plague, still color our perceptions of this
era. Historians might argue that plague and leprosy should not be classified as "medieval diseases." Epidemics of bubonic plague continued into
the nineteenth century and both plague and leprosy remained as significant public health threats in certain parts of the globe at the end of the
twentieth century. On the other hand, it could also be argued that two
of the most devastating pandemics the world has ever experienced—the
Plague of Justinian and the Black Death—seem to provide an appropriate frame for the medical history of the Middle Ages.

When attempting to understand the impact of AIDS, the disease
that emerged in the 1980s to become the great modern pandemic, historians and physicians most often turned to bubonic plague and leprosy as
the most significant historical models of devastating epidemic diseases. If
we can indeed look into the Middle Ages as a "distant mirror," we may
be able to think more clearly about the impact of catastrophic diseases
on society and the human psyche. Plague and leprosy stand out among
the myriad perils and adversities of the Middle Ages, much as AIDS
emerged as the pestilence emblematic of the last decades of the twentieth
century. Many aspects of the origin, impact, and present and future
threat of AIDS are unclear, just as there are many uncertainties about
the historical meaning of leprosy and plague. However, it is not
unreasonable to hope that scientific knowledge concerning pathology
and epidemiology, as well as historical research illuminating the social
context in which particular diseases loomed so large, will eventually
allow us to ask more meaningful questions about the ways in which
people assess and respond to the threat of catastrophic disease.


## BUBONIC PLAGUE

Astrologers blamed the Black Death on a malign conjunction of Saturn,
Jupiter, and Mars. Epidemiologists have traced the cause of epidemic
plague to a catastrophic conjunction of *Yersinia pestis*, fleas, and rats.
A brief overview of the complex ecological relationships of microbes,
fleas, rodents, and human beings will help us understand the medieval
pandemics, the waves of plague that continued well into the seventeenth

century, and the status of plague today. Studying the components of this web of relationships should help dispel the notion that discovering the "cause" of epidemic disease is a simple matter of finding a specific microbial agent. Even if a specific pathogen can be linked to epidemic disease, that microbe is only one strand in the complex web of life, along with fleas, mosquitoes, lice, ticks, wild animals, domesticated animals, and human beings. Moreover, the relationship between human beings and epidemic disease is affected by many factors: biological, climatic, social, cultural, political, economic, and so forth. The magnitude of the plague pandemics provides a striking demonstration of just how powerful a force disease can be in history. Such reminders are essential now that molecular biologists are able to identify, isolate, and manipulate the genetic factors responsible for the awesome virulence of the microbes that cause bubonic plague and other epidemic diseases.

Bacteriologists and epidemiologists have examined historical accounts of plague and laboratory studies of recent outbreaks in order to determine the natural history of plague and its clinical pattern of signs and symptoms. Attempts to compare modern clinical and laboratory descriptions of bubonic plague with eyewitness accounts of ancient and medieval epidemics reveal the difficulties inherent in attaching modern diagnoses to ancient diseases. Historical accounts of devastating epidemics are often vague, confusing, and highly stylized in terms of the signs and symptoms that physicians and laymen considered significant. Fourteenth-century accounts of the Black Death describe horrific symptoms that included painfully swollen lymph nodes, gangrenous organs, bleeding from the nose, bloody sputum, and hemorrhaging blood vessels, which caused splotches and discoloration of the skin.

To add to the confusion, bubonic plague provides an interesting example of the way in which a specific microbe can cause different clinical patterns. In this case, the major forms of illness are known as *bubonic* plague and *pneumonic* plague; a rare form of the disease is known as *septicemic* plague. In the absence of appropriate antibiotics, the mortality rate for bubonic plague may exceed 50 percent; pneumonic plague and septicemic plague are almost invariably fatal. Even today, despite streptomycin, tetracycline, and chloramphenicol, many plague victims succumb to the disease.

If *Y. pestis*, the plague bacillus, enters the body via the bite of an infected flea, the disease follows the pattern known as bubonic. After an incubation period that may last for two to six days, during which the bacteria multiply in the lymph nodes, victims suddenly experience fever, headache, pains in the chest, coughing, difficulty in breathing, vomiting of blood, and dark splotches on the skin. The most characteristic signs of bubonic plague are the painful swellings called *buboes* that appear in the lymph nodes, usually in the groin, armpits, and neck. Other

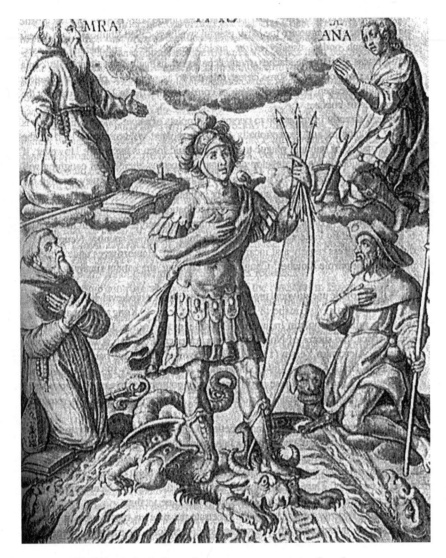

**Religious depiction of proper responses to the plague.**

symptoms include restlessness, anxiety, mental confusion, hallucinations, and coma. Certain bacterial proteins inhibit the immune responses that would otherwise block the multiplication and dissemination of the bacteria. Plague bacteria also release a toxin that may result in shock, circulatory collapse, widespread organ failure, and, finally, death. In septicemic plague, the bacteria spread rapidly throughout the bloodstream, damaging internal organs and blood vessels, leading to gangrene, internal hemorrhaging, bleeding from the nose and ears, delirium, or coma. Death occurs within one to three days, without the appearance of buboes.

Spread directly from person to person by droplets of saliva, pneumonic plague is highly contagious and exceptionally lethal. Just what circumstances lead to widespread transformation of bubonic plague to the pneumonic form is uncertain. When large numbers of bacteria spread to the lungs of patients with bubonic plague, resulting in pulmonary abscesses, fits of coughing and sneezing release droplets of sputum containing hordes of bacteria. When inhaled into the respiratory system of new hosts, plague bacteria multiply rapidly, resulting in the highly contagious condition known as primary pneumonic plague. The incubation period for pneumonic plague is usually only one to three days and the onset of symptoms is very abrupt. Pain in the chest is accompanied by violent coughing that brings up bloody sputum. Neurological disorders progress rapidly and incapacitate the victim. Hemorrhages under the skin produce dark-purple blotches. Coughing and choking, the patient finally suffocates and dies. Patients with this very lethal form of the disease experience high fever, chills, and a fatal pneumonia.

In 2001, researchers succeeded in decoding the genome and plasmids of a strain of *Y. pestis* taken from a Colorado veterinarian who had died of pneumonic plague in 1992. (The infection was contracted from the sneeze of a cat.) On the basis of studies of the DNA sequence, microbiologists suggested that *Y. pestis* probably evolved about 20,000 years ago from *Yersinia pseudotuberculosis*, a minor human intestinal pathogen. Molecular biologists believe that *Y. pestis* became a virulent pathogen by acquiring new genes, losing or silencing certain *Y. pseudotuberculosis* genes, and establishing a remarkable pattern of chromosomal rearrangements that make its genome unusually dynamic. By acquiring genes from other bacteria, *Y. pestis* was able to colonize new environments. One of these genes apparently codes for an enzyme that allows the bacteria to survive in the gut of a flea, which transforms the flea into a vector of the disease.

Some scientists warned that genomic sequence data could be used to create more deadly forms of pathogens for use as biological weapons, perhaps more readily than genetic information could be used to develop preventive vaccines. Although the strain of *Y. pestis* that was sequenced was already capable of causing death within 48 hours, experts in biological warfare point out that it might be possible to add genes that would create variants that are resistant to antibiotics and any potential vaccines.

Many aspects of the natural history of pandemic plague were finally clarified in the 1890s when successive outbreaks attacked Canton, Hong Kong, Bombay, Java, Japan, Asia Minor, South Africa, North and South America, Portugal, Austria, and parts of Russia. Some historical epidemiologists estimate that the plague epidemics of the 1890s killed more than 12 million people, but others believe that over 10 million people in India alone were killed by plague in the late nineteenth and early twentieth centuries. In 1894, Alexandre Yersin (1863–1943) isolated the plague bacillus from the buboes of cadavers during an outbreak in Hong Kong. Using the sample that Yersin sent to the Pasteur Institute in Paris, Émil Roux (1853–1933) prepared the first anti-plague serum. Yersin called the microbe *Pasteurella pestis*, in honor of his mentor, Louis Pasteur. Shibasaburo Kitasato (1852–1931), who is best known for his studies of tetanus and diphtheria, independently identified the plague bacillus while studying the 1894 Hong Kong plague outbreak for the Japanese government.

In 1971, the plague bacillus was renamed *Y. pestis*, in honor of Alexandre Yersin. At least three naturally occurring varieties of *Y. pestis* are known today. All three varieties cause virulent infections in humans and most mammals. The microbe can remain viable for many months in the congenial microclimate of rodent warrens. Its life span in putrefying corpses is limited to a few days, but it may survive for years in frozen cadavers. Thus, local outbreaks depend on the state of rodent communities and the means used to dispose of the bodies of plague victims. During the 1980s and 1990s, the World Health Organization recorded more than 18,000 cases of plague in 24 countries; more than half were in Africa. In the United States, the disease was reported in 13 states. By the end of the 1990s, epidemiologists were warning that cases of plague were actually increasing throughout the world and that the disease should be classified as a re-emerging disease. Until the late 1990s, the plague bacillus was universally responsive to antibiotics. Plague treated with antibiotics had a mortality rate of about 15 percent, in contrast to estimates of 50 to 90 percent for untreated plague. Worse yet, a strain of plague bacilli recently discovered by researchers at the Pasteur Institute of Madagascar is resistant to streptomycin, chloramphenicol, tetracycline, and sulfonamides. If the genes for antibiotic resistance become widely disseminated among other strains of the bacillus, bubonic plague could again emerge as a very serious threat.

Although *Y. pestis* can easily penetrate mucous membranes, it cannot enter the body through healthy, unbroken skin. Therefore, the microbe is generally dependent on the flea to reach new hosts. In the 1890s, scientists reported finding the plague bacillus in the stomach of fleas taken from infected rats, but the "flea theory" was greeted with such skepticism that members of the British Plague Commission in Bombay carried out experiments to prove that fleas *did not* transmit plague. They "proved" their hypothesis because they assumed that "a flea is a flea is a flea." Further progress in "fleaology" revealed that all fleas are not created equal.

Out of some two thousand different kinds of fleas, the black rat's flea, *Xenophylla cheopsis*, deserves first place honors as the most efficient vector of plague, but at least eight species of fleas can transmit the microbe to humans. Depending on host, heat, and humidity, fleas may live for only a few days or as long as a year. An infected flea actually becomes a victim of the rapidly multiplying plague bacillus. Eventually, the flea's stomach becomes blocked by a plug of bacteria. When the starving flea bites a new victim, the ingested blood comes in contact with this plug and mixes with the bacteria. Part of the ingested material, containing tens of thousands of bacilli, is regurgitated into the wound, leading to multiplication of plague bacteria in the lymph glands nearest the bite. Fleas are usually fairly loyal to their primary host species. Unfortunately, *X. cheopsis* finds human beings an acceptable substitute for rats. *Pulex irritans*, the human flea, cannot approach the infective power of the rat flea, but under appropriate conditions quantity can make up for quality. Despite the flea's role as ubiquitous nuisance and vector of disease, Thomas Moffet (1553–1604), father of Little Miss Moffet, noted that, in contrast to being lousy, it was not a disgrace to have fleas.

Once the connection between rats and plague was elucidated, many authorities believed that the black rat, *Rattus rattus*, was the only source of plague epidemics. However, almost two hundred species of rodents have been identified as possible reservoirs of plague. The concept of "sylvatic plague" acknowledges the ecological significance of *Y. pestis* among various species of wild animals.

There is some controversy about the status of the black rat in Europe during the early Middle Ages. Adding to the confusion is the fact that ancient chroniclers did not distinguish between rats and mice when they spoke of "vermin" and the strange behaviors that were considered omens of disaster. Medieval physicians and laymen rightly feared that when rats, mice, moles, and other animals that normally lived underground escaped to the surface, acted as if drunk, and died in great multitudes, pestilential disease would follow. These strange portents were, however, easily reconciled with the idea that noxious vapors generated deep within the earth could escape into the atmosphere where they produced deadly *miasmata* (poisonous vapors).

Sometime during the Middle Ages, the black rat made its way to Europe, found excellent accommodations in its towns and villages, and took up permanent residence. The medieval town may seem picturesque through the misty lens of nostalgia, but it was a filthy, unhealthy place of narrow, winding alleys, not unlike rodent warrens, surrounded by haphazard accumulations of garden plots, pig pens, dung heaps, shops, houses, and hovels shared by humans and animals. Perhaps, it is not just a coincidence that a marked decline in the incidence of European plague occurred at about the same time that the black rat was being driven out by a newcomer, the large brown rat, *Rattus norvegicus*.

Although epidemic bubonic plague may have occurred in very ancient periods, early descriptions of "plagues and pestilences" are too vague to provide specific diagnoses. Thus, the Plague of Justinian in 540 is generally regarded as the first plague epidemic in Europe.

Further waves of plague can be charted over the next several centuries. Eventually, the disease seemingly died out in the West, but it was periodically reintroduced from Mediterranean ports.

According to the historian Procopius (ca. 500–562), the plague began in Egypt in 540 and soon spread over the entire earth, killing men, women, and children in every nation. While the disease always seemed to spread inland from coastal regions, no human habitation, no matter how remote, was spared. Many people saw phantoms before they were attacked by the disease, some collapsed in the streets as if struck by lightning; others locked themselves into their houses for safety, but phantoms appeared in their dreams and they too succumbed to disease. Panic and terror mounted with the death toll as civil life ceased; only the corpse-bearers made their way through streets littered with rotting bodies. As the daily toll reached into the thousands, graves and gravediggers became so scarce that ships were filled with corpses and abandoned at sea. Those who survived were not attacked again, but depravity and licentiousness seemed to consume those who had witnessed and survived the horrors of the plague.

The sick were the objects of great fear, but Procopius noted that the disease was not necessarily contagious, because nurses, gravediggers, and even physicians who examined the bodies of the dead and opened plague buboes at postmortems might be spared. Physicians could not predict which cases would be mild and which would be fatal, but they came to believe that survival was most common in cases where the plague bubo grew large, ripened, and suppurated. St. Gregory of Tours (538–594), an influential bishop and historian, left an account of the plague that is vague in medical details but vivid in conveying the sense of universal despair. Confused and terrified, the people knew of no appropriate response to the plague other than prayer and flight. According to Gregory, large numbers of people threw themselves off the cliffs into the sea "preferring a swift death to perishing by lingering torments."

There are many gaps in our knowledge of the early waves of plague, but there is no lack of speculation. Some argue that the death and disorder caused by the plague led to the decline of the Byzantine Empire. A shift of power in Europe from south to north, Mediterranean to North Sea, may have been the consequence of the failure of plague to penetrate the British Isles, northern Gaul, and Germania. Establishing the death toll is virtually impossible. Overwhelmed by panic and fear, witnesses resorted to symbolic or exaggerated figures to convey the enormity of the disaster. Many accounts of medieval pestilence state that mortality was so great that there were not enough of the living to bury the dead.

Surviving records are essentially silent about the status of plague between the ninth century and its catastrophic return in the fourteenth century. Of course, the absence of specific references to bubonic plague does not prove that the disease did not occur during that period. For the medieval chroniclers, the causes of all great "perils and adversities"—earthquakes, floods, famines, pestilential diseases—were beyond human comprehension or control, and so common that only the most dramatic were worth recording.

During the twelfth and thirteenth centuries, Europe attained a level of prosperity unknown since the fall of Rome. Population growth began to accelerate in the eleventh century and reached its peak by the fourteenth century. Europe remained a largely agricultural society, but the growth of towns and cities reflected a demographic and economic revolution. Nevertheless, even before the outbreak of plague, conditions were apparently deteriorating. Famines had followed bad harvests in the years 1257 and 1258. By about 1300, Europe could no longer bring more land into use or significantly improve the yield of land already under cultivation. Wet and chilly weather led to disastrous harvests from 1315 to 1317. Food prices soared and malnutrition was more prevalent.

Famines, associated with human and animal sickness, occurred intermittently from 1315 to 1322. Contemporary observers said that clergymen and nobles fasted and prayed for a pestilence that would reduce the lower class population so that others could live in more comfort. If this is true, the fourteenth-century pandemic is an awesome testimonial to the power of prayer. The pandemic that was known as the Black Death, the Great Pestilence, or the Great Dying surpassed all previous pestilences as a remedy for overpopulation, while creating more havoc, misery, and fear than any protagonist on the stage of history before the twentieth century.

Exactly where or how the Black Death began is obscure, but many plague outbreaks apparently originated in the urban centers of the Near and Middle East. From these foci of infection, plague spread by ship and caravan trade routes. There are many uncertainties about the route taken by the plague and the rapidity of its progress; however, the outline of its journey by ship via the major ports of the Mediterranean and along the overland trade routes has been charted. The ships of the Italian city-states probably carried the plague to western Europe in 1347 via the Crimean ports on the Black Sea. Within two years, the Great Plague had spread throughout Europe, reaching even Greenland. Some scholars have argued that the speed with which the Black Death spread indicates that the great pandemic was not bubonic plague, which usually spreads relatively slowly, but a form of anthrax, typhus, tuberculosis, or a viral hemorrhagic fever. Others have no candidates for the disease itself, but insist that the pandemic was not caused by *Y. pestis.*

Survivors of the plague years predicted that those who had not experienced the great pestilence would never be able to comprehend the magnitude of the disaster. Indeed, the dispassionate analytic accounts of historians attempting to confirm or disconfirm some hypothesis about cause and effect relationships between the plague and subsequent events make a grim contrast to eyewitness accounts of the pandemic. Some historians see the Black Death as the event that ended the Middle Ages and destroyed medieval social, economic, and political arrangements. Others warn against confusing sequential relationships with cause and effect. Even the mortality caused by the plague remains a matter of controversy. In some areas, the death rate may have been about 12 percent, whereas in others it exceeded 50 percent. Estimates of the numbers killed in Europe alone range from 20 to 25 million; throughout the world, more than 42 million people may have died of the plague. Repopulation after the Black Death seems to have been quite rapid, but repeated outbreaks of plague, along with other disasters, kept total population levels from rising significantly until the eighteenth century.

The plague years provided a significant turning point for the medical profession and the clergy. Many contemporary accounts speak of the lack of physicians, but it is not always clear whether this was due to a high mortality rate among practitioners or because they had hidden themselves away for fear of contagion. The effect of the plague on the Church was undeniably profound, if also ambiguous. Mortality among the clergy seems to have reached 50 percent between 1348 and 1349. Mortality in the Pope's court at Avignon was about 25 percent. In some areas, monasteries, churches, and whole villages were abandoned. Many writers complained that deaths among clergymen led to the ordination of men of lower qualifications and demoralization within the ranks. On the other hand, fear of death among the general populace increased the level of bequests to the Church.

With many fourteenth-century physicians convinced that a catastrophic new disease had appeared, hundreds of plague tractates (treatises devoted to explanations of the disease and suggestions for its prevention and treatment) were written. Perhaps, the most compelling account of the ravages of the plague appears in Giovanni Boccaccio's (1313–1375) introduction to the *Decameron*, a collection of stories supposedly told by ten young men and women who left Florence in an attempt to escape the plague. According to Boccaccio, who had survived an attack of the disease, Florence became a city of corpses as half of Italy succumbed to the plague. Very few of the sick recovered, with or without medical aid, and most died within three days.

Many died not from the severity of their disease, but from want of care and nursing. The poor were the most pitiable. Unable to escape the city, they died by the thousands and the stench of rotting corpses overwhelmed the city. Every morning, the streets were filled with bodies beyond number. Customary funeral rites were abandoned; corpses were dumped into trenches and covered with a little dirt. Famine followed plague, because peasants were too demoralized to care for their crops or their animals. Worse than the disease itself, Boccacio lamented, was the barbarous behavior it unleashed. The healthy refused to aid friends, relatives, or even their own children. A few believed that asceticism would avert the plague, but others took the threat of death as an excuse for satisfying every base appetite. Criminal and immoral acts could be carried out with impunity for there was no one left to enforce the laws of man or God.

A surprisingly cheerful and optimistic view of the great pestilence was recorded by French cleric and master of theology, Jean de Venette. According to de Venette, during the epidemic, no matter how suddenly men were stricken by the plague, God saw to it that they died "joyfully" after confessing their sins. Moreover, the survivors hastened to marry and women commonly produced twins and triplets. Pope Clement VI graciously granted absolution to all plague victims who left their worldly goods to the Church. The Pope sought to win God's mercy and end the plague with an Easter pilgrimage to Rome in 1348. The power of faith proved to be no match for the power of pestilence. Prayers, processions, and appeals to all the patron saints were as useless as any medicine prescribed by doctors and quacks.

Guy de Chauliac, physician to Pope Clement VI, confessed that doctors felt useless and ashamed because the plague was unresponsive to medical treatment. He noted that the disease appeared in two forms, one of which caused buboes and another that attacked the lungs. Physicians, knowing the futility of medical intervention, were afraid to visit the sick for fear of becoming infected themselves. Worse yet, if they did take care of plague victims they could not expect to collect their fees because patients almost always died and escaped their debts. Guy did not join the physicians who fled from Avignon; he contracted the disease, but recovered. Pope Clement VI was more fortunate than his physician. The Pope remained shut up in his innermost chambers, between two great protective fires, and refused to see anyone.

Physicians could not cure the plague, but they could offer advice, much of it contradictory, on how to avoid contracting the disease. Abandoning the affected area was often advised, but opinions varied about the relative safety of potential retreats. If flight was impossible, another option was to turn one's home into the medieval version of a fall-out shelter. To reduce contact with tainted air, doctors suggested moving about slowly while inhaling through aromatic sponges or "smelling apples" containing exotic and expensive ingredients such as amber and sandalwood, strong smelling herbs, or garlic, the traditional theriac of the poor. Bathing was regarded as a dangerous procedure because baths opened the pores and allowed corrupt air to penetrate the outer defenses. Physicians eventually developed elaborate protective costumes, featuring long robes, gloves, boots, and "bird-beaked" masks containing a sponge that had been steeped in aromatic herbs. In response to the plague of 1348, many eminent physicians wrote texts called *plague regimina* to express their ideas about preserving health in dangerous times. Such texts introduced readers to broader ideas about health, including the importance of health as a public good, the importance of policies governing the sanitary situation of towns and cities, and the purity of water, food, and air.

Those fortunate enough to secure medical attention before being stricken were fortified by theriac and dietary regimens designed to remove impurities and bad humors. Once symptoms of the disease appeared, physicians prescribed bleeding and purging and attempted to hasten the maturation of buboes by scarification, cupping, cauterization, poultices, and plasters, which might contain pig fat or pigeon dung. Some physicians advocated a direct attack on the plague bubo, but a surgeon or barber-surgeon carried out the actual operation. For example, regulations promulgated by the Health Board of Florence in 1630 directed the surgeon to apply cupping vessels to the buboes or open them with a razor, dress them with Venice treacle, and cover the surrounding area with pomegranate juice.

During later outbreaks of plague, secular and clerical authorities attempted to limit the spread of the disaster with prayers and quarantine regulations. By the fifteenth century, Venice, Florence, and other Italian cities had developed detailed public health measures. Less advanced states throughout Europe used the Italian system as a model for dealing with epidemic disease. Unfortunately, the well-meaning officials who formulated quarantine rules did not understand the natural history of plague. Some measures, such as the massacre of dogs and cats, must have been counterproductive. Long periods of quarantine—originally a forty-day period of isolation—for those suspected of carrying the contagion caused unnecessary hardships and promoted willful disobedience. Modern authorities generally consider a seven-day quarantine adequate evidence that potential carriers are not infected.

Antiplague measures eventually included mandatory reporting of illness, isolation of the sick, burning the bedding of plague victims, closing schools and markets during epidemics, virtual house arrest of off-duty gravediggers, and laws forbidding physicians from leaving infected areas. Plague rules meant extra taxes, destruction of property, restriction of commerce, privation, pest houses, and unemployment. Quarantined families were supposed to receive food and medicine, but, as always, poor relief funds were inadequate. Public health officials were supposed to have absolute authority in matters pertaining to control of the plague, but they often encountered noncompliance from members of the clergy. During epidemics, the secular authorities could close schools, prohibit festivals, games, parties, and dances, but they were generally unable to stop religious assemblies and processions.

Perhaps, the combination of faith and quarantine, along with more subtle changes in plague ecology, eventually mitigated the effects of further waves of plague, at least in the countryside. During the fifteenth century, the rich could expect to escape the plague by fleeing from the city. Eventually, the general pattern of mortality convinced the elite that plague was a contagious disease of the poor. However, historical studies of plague mortality are complicated by diagnostic confusion between true bubonic plague and other infectious diseases. In the absence of specific diagnostic tests, public health authorities preferred to err on the side of caution and were likely to suspect plague given the slightest provocation. Much "plague legislation" after the Black Death was more concerned with protecting the personal safety and property of the elite than with control of plague itself. However, the concept of granting authority to secular public health officials was established. Epidemic plague essentially disappeared from the western Mediterranean by the eighteenth century. Plague remained a threat in the eastern Mediterranean area well into the nineteenth century, but later outbreaks never achieved the prevalence or virulence of the Black Death.

Plague is still enzootic among wild animals throughout the world, including Russia, the Middle East, China, Southwest and Southeast Asia, Africa, North and South America, resulting in sporadic human cases. Animal reservoirs in the Americas include many different species, but rats, mice, marmots, rabbits, and squirrels are the best known. In Andean countries, guinea pigs raised indoors for food have infected humans. Epidemiologists studying emerging and re-emerging diseases warn that unforeseen changes in the ecology of a plague area could trigger outbreaks among animals and humans. For example, the movement of rapidly expanding human populations into previously wild areas raises the risk that plague and other emerging rodent-borne diseases will cause sporadic cases or even epidemics. Scientists have also speculated about the possibility that plague could be used as a biological weapon. However, they generally agree that only aerosolized pneumonic plague could serve as an effective agent.

In the first decade of the twentieth century, while California politicians and merchants acted as if bad publicity was more dangerous than bubonic plague, the disease escaped from San Francisco and established itself as an enzootic disease among the rodents of the western United States. Plague was first officially reported in San Francisco in 1900. When plague bacilli were isolated from the body of a Chinese laborer found dead in a Chinatown hotel, the Board of Health imposed a total quarantine on Chinatown, in response to both fear of disease and racism. Even though 22 plague deaths were officially recorded in 1900, and additional cases occurred in 1904 and 1907, leading citizens continued to deny the existence of plague. Critics argued that the city and the state put business interests ahead of public health concerns. Finally, afraid that the city would experience further outbreaks of plague and, worse yet, a national boycott, the San Francisco Citizens' Health Committee declared war on rats. Unfortunately, by the time the war had claimed the lives of one million city rats, rodents in the surrounding areas had already become a new reservoir of plague bacteria.

Prairie dog colonies in Colorado provide a large reservoir of plague, but New Mexico has had the largest number of human cases. The extent of plague transmission between rural and urban animals is unknown, but the danger is not negligible. People have been infected by domestic cats, bobcats, coyotes, and rabbits. Because human plague is rare and unexpected, sporadic cases are often misdiagnosed. If appropriate treatment is not begun soon enough, the proper diagnosis may not be made until the autopsy. Almost 20 percent of the cases reported in the United States between 1949 and 1980 were fatal. Whereas only 5 percent of the cases identified between 1949 and 1974 were of the pneumonic form, between 1975 and 1980 this highly virulent form accounted for about 25 percent of New Mexico's plague cases. In the United States, about 10 to 40 cases of plague are reported each year, mainly in New Mexico, Colorado, Arizona, California, Oregon, and Nevada.

Given the speed of modern transportation, it is possible for people who have contracted bubonic plague to travel to areas where the disease is unknown well before the end of the two to seven-day incubation period. One example of the epidemiological cliché that residents of any city are just a plane ride away from diseases peculiar to any point on the globe occurred in 2002 when New York City health officials reported two confirmed cases of bubonic plague. The victims had apparently contracted the illness in New Mexico, before they left for a vacation in New York. They went to an emergency room complaining of flu-like symptoms, high fever, headache, joint pain, and swollen lymph nodes.

The World Health Organization reports one thousand to three thousand cases of plague per year around the world. In some areas, perhaps because of better surveillance or of actual increases in the number of cases, the numbers of suspected and confirmed cases increased during the 1990s. The island nation of Madagascar, for example, reported significant increases in the number of plague cases. Bubonic plague first came to Madagascar via steamboats from India in the 1890s. Although the disease had been brought under control in the 1950s, *Y. pestis* remained widely distributed among the island's rats and their fleas. Public health officials discovered that by the 1990s new variants of *Y. pestis* had emerged, including a multiple antibiotic-resistant strain.

Some historians argue that the pandemic known as the Black Death could not have been caused by *Y. pestis*, because the fourteenth-century disease spread too quickly and was too deadly, and the signs and symptoms were unlike those of modern bubonic plague. Some argue that a bubo or swelling in the lymph glands is not a significant diagnostic sign, because it may occur in filariasis, lymphogranuloma inguinale, glandular fever, relapsing fever, malaria, typhoid, typhus, and other tropical diseases. Some historians contend that chronicles of the plague do not mention major rat deaths and that Europe lacked rodent species that could serve as a plague reservoir between outbreaks. There are, however, Arabic sources that describe the deaths of wild and domesticated animals before the epidemic spread to humans. In any case, studies of rats and other pestiferous rodents suggest that it is always wrong to underestimate their numbers, persistence, fertility, and adaptability.

Plague "revisionists" have suggested that the Black Death was caused by an unknown microbe that no longer exists, anthrax, typhus, tuberculosis, influenza, a filovirus, an unnamed viral hemorrhagic fever, or Ebola fever. Some historians have suggested that the high, but variable mortality rates reported for the Great Dying might have been associated with immunosuppression caused by mold toxins. Mycotoxins could affect rats as well as people, which would account for rat deaths. Advocates of the "Ebola hypothesis" argue that the most significant signs of the Black Death were red spots on the chest, rather than the buboes in the lymph nodes. As further evidence, they argue that the 40-day quarantine adopted by public health authorities corresponds to the latency and infectious period of a hemorrhagic virus. The disappearance of the disease in Europe during the "little ice age" of the late seventeenth and early eighteenth centuries has been attributed to a decrease in the infectivity of the virus caused by the cold, or a mutation in the virus. In addition to putative changes in the hemorrhagic virus, they suggest that a possible genetic mutation could have made 40 to 50 percent of Europeans less susceptible to the hemorrhagic fever virus. Despite uncertainties about the rapid dissemination of the medieval pandemic and the nature of the European rat population, the Ebola hypothesis itself seems to demand an excessive multiplication of possibilities; it also requires faith in the idea that a lethal tropical disease achieved global distribution during the plague years and persisted in some unknown reservoir even in northern regions of the world between outbreaks.

Most epidemiologists believe that *Y. pestis* was the cause of the disease that medieval observers called the plague. Because the same agent is transmitted in different ways and can cause different clinical patterns in people, the disease caused by *Y. pestis* does not seem inconsistent with historical accounts of plague. Many factors have, of course, changed since the fourteenth century, but, even in wealthy nations, untreated bubonic plague has a high mortality rate and victims of pneumonic plague have died within 48 hours of exposure to the disease. A comparison of modern medical photographs with historical and artistic depictions of plague victims suggests that medieval images of plague victims, saints, and martyrs are not inconsistent with modern bubonic plague. Paintings of St. Roche typically show buboes in the groin. Artists, however, were often more interested in achieving an aesthetic goal rather than a realistic clinical likeness. Medieval authors refer to buboes, pustules, or spots, which appeared on the neck or in the armpit and groin. During modern outbreaks, the buboes usually appear in the groin. This seems to correlate with the fact that fleabites in modern homes are generally no higher than the ankles. Of course, people in the Middle Ages lived and interacted with animals and pests far differently, and the pattern of fleabites might have been quite different. Similarly, differences between medieval and modern homes, towns, and cities suggest that plague would not spread in the same manner.

Interesting evidence of the existence of bubonic plague in medieval Europe was reported in 2000 by researchers who identified *Y. pestis* DNA in the remains of bodies buried in France in the fourteenth century. Critics who insist that the Black Death was not caused by *Y. pestis* responded by arguing that such findings only prove that *some* cases of plague occurred in Europe, but the countless other victims of the Black Death died of Ebola or some unknown disease. However, the tests that proved positive for *Y. pestis* did not find evidence of other possible causes of the Black Death in bodies from the mass grave. Attempts to exonerate rats, fleas, and *Y. pestis* have encouraged more sophisticated analyses of the history of plague but have not been compelling in their support for alternative hypotheses.

Even after the publication of the genome of *Y. pestis* and the warning that such information would be of interest to bioterrorists, perhaps the most dangerous characteristic of bubonic plague today is its ability to camouflage itself as a "medieval plague" of no possible significance to modern societies. Much about the disappearance of plague from the ranks of the major epidemic diseases is obscure, but we can say with a fair degree of certainty that medical breakthroughs had little to do with it. In its animal reservoirs, the plague is very much alive and presumably quite capable of taking advantage of any disaster that would significantly alter the ecological relationships among rodents, fleas, microbes, and human beings.

## FROM LEPROSY TO HANSEN'S DISEASE

More than any other disease, leprosy demonstrates the difference between the biological nature of illness and the attributes ascribed to the sick. Indeed, it is fair to say that leprosy and Hansen's disease (the modern name for true leprosy) stand for different *ideas* more than different *diseases*. The word *leper* is still commonly used to mean one who is hated and shunned by society.

Medieval attitudes towards the leper were based on biblical passages pertaining to "leprosy," a vague term applied to various chronic, progressive skin afflictions, from leprosy and vitiligo to psoriasis and skin cancer. The leper, according to medieval interpretations of the Bible, was "unclean" and, therefore, a dangerous source of physical and moral pollution. Biblical rules governing leprosy demanded that persons and things with suspicious signs of leprosy must be brought to the priests for examination. Leprosy was said to dwell not only in human beings, but also in garments of wool or linen, objects made of skins, and even in houses. Diagnostic signs included a scaly eruption, boil, scab, or bright spot. When the signs were ambiguous, the priest shut the suspect away for as long as two weeks for further observations. When a final judgment had been reached, the leper was instructed to dwell in isolation and call out as a warning to those who might approach him, "unclean, unclean."

Islamic teachings also reflected fear of leprosy. "Fly from the leper," warned the Prophet Muhammad, "as you would fly from a lion." According to Islamic law and custom, people suffering from leprosy were not allowed to visit the baths. It was said that foods touched by a leper could transmit the disease and that no plants would grow in soil touched by the bare feet of a leper.

A brief survey of modern findings about this disease may help us understand the ambiguities and complexities of the medieval literature concerning leprosy. *Mycobacterium leprae*, the bacillus that causes the disease, was discovered in 1874 by the Norwegian physician Gerhard Hansen (1841–1912). Hansen had observed leprosy bacilli as early as 1871, but it was very difficult to prove that the bacteria found in skin scrapings of patients actually caused the disease. No animal model was available and the putative leprosy bacillus refused to grow in artificial media. It took almost one hundred years for scientists to overcome these obstacles. To honor Gerhard Hansen and avoid the stigma associated with the term leper, the disease was renamed Hansen's disease.

What is most surprising about Hansen's disease is the fact that it is only slightly contagious. Many people having extended and intimate contact with lepers, such as spouses, nurses, and doctors, do not contract the disease, whereas others with little contact become infected. Where leprosy remains endemic, almost all people have been exposed to the infectious agent, but only a small percent actually contract the disease. Those who do seem to have a deficiency in their immune system that makes them unusually susceptible to *M. leprae*. Evidence of the limited degree of contagiousness of leprosy today does not, of course, prove that the disease was not more contagious in the past. Nevertheless, leprosy could not have been as contagious as medieval writers assumed. Religious and medical authorities argued that leprosy could be spread

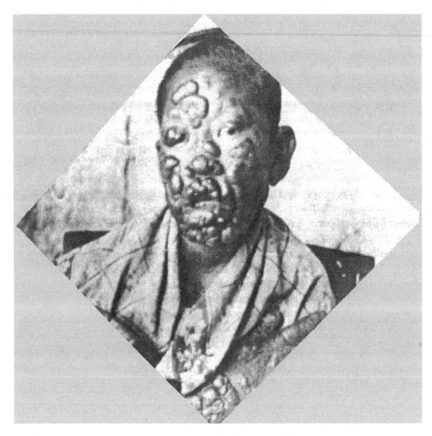

**A man with leprosy (photographed in Manila in 1899).**

by the glance of a leper or an unseen leper standing upwind of healthy people.

Various indeterminate patterns exist between the two polar forms of Hansen's disease, known as tuberculoid and lepromatous. If infected people mount a partial immune response, the disease will assume the tuberculoid form, which is not infectious or dangerous to others. The early symptoms of tuberculoid leprosy include skin lesions and loss of sensation in the affected areas. Unfortunately, the loss of sensation and the weak immune response may eventually result in damage to tissues. About 80 percent of all cases take this form. Patients with the tuberculoid form mount a partially effective cell-mediated immune response to the infection, although this does not eliminate the bacteria. Individuals with the more severe lepromatous form have essentially no immune response. The bacteria multiply freely and large numbers of bacteria are discharged in the nasal secretions. The lepromatous form is characterized by skin lesions consisting of raised blotches, nodules, and lumps. Eventually, the thickening of the skin of the forehead and face, exaggeration of natural lines, and loss of facial hair produce the so-called "lion face." As the disease progresses, ulcerating skin lesions lead to destruction of cartilage and bone. About 30 percent of all victims of Hansen's disease eventually develop crippling deformities due to damaged joints, paralysis of muscles, and loss of soft tissue and bone, especially the fingers and toes. Loss of sensitivity caused by nerve damage results in repeated injuries and infections.

Leprosy seems to have been rare in Europe before the fall of Rome. Although the disease was creeping into the Mediterranean arena by the sixth century, the Crusades of the eleventh and twelfth centuries created ideal conditions for a major invasion. Indeed, there are estimates that by the end of the twelfth century one out of every two hundred Europeans was infected with leprosy. The high incidence of leprosy among pious persons, especially Crusaders and pilgrims returning from the Holy Land, was a potential source of embarrassment to the Church. The Crusades were part of massive movements of human populations that broke down ancient barriers and carried infectious diseases to new populations. However, after reaching its peak in the thirteenth century, leprosy all but disappeared from Europe.

Priests, doctors, and lepers were involved in the examination of alleged medieval lepers. If incriminating signs of leprosy were found—bright spots, depigmented patches, sores, thickened skin, hoarse voice, and "lion face"—the accused was found guilty. A funeral service, rather than an execution, followed the verdict. Although the rites of exclusion could be held in a church, performing them in a cemetery with the leper standing in a grave made the symbolic death and burial more dramatic. Having sprinkled earth on the leper's head, the priest declared him dead to the world, but reborn to God. Although hated by all men, the leper was said to be loved by God and could, therefore, look forward to compensation in the next world. The rules governing lepers and marriage reflect the ambiguity of the leper's status. Despite the leper's symbolic death, leprosy was not necessarily accepted as a cause for the dissolution of marriage. Indeed, the Church decreed that a man with leprosy could require a healthy wife to continue sexual relations.

Feared by all and condemned to live in isolation, lepers were also the conspicuous targets of religious charity. Thousands of leper houses were established by various religious orders throughout Europe. Where lepers were granted the special privilege of begging for alms, other impoverished people apparently pretended to be lepers in order to receive alms or be admitted to leper houses. Miserable as these places might be by modern standards, they were presumably better than the alternatives.

Sometimes lepers were the objects of "heroic charity," such as that of Queen Mathilda, who expressed her piety by bringing lepers into her own rooms where she fed them and washed their feet. On finding her so

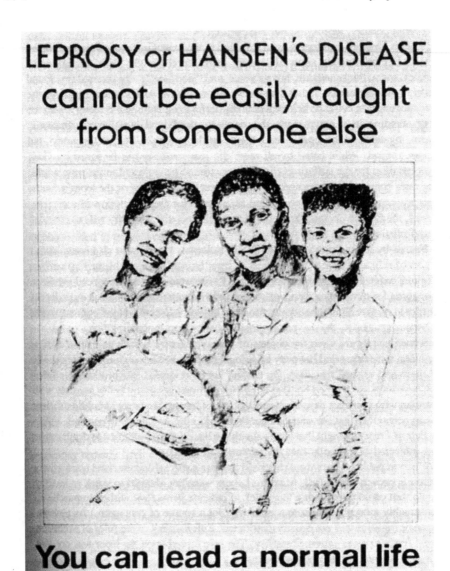

# LEPROSY or HANSEN'S DISEASE cannot be easily caught from someone else

## You can lead a normal life

**Leprosy is now known as Hansen's disease.**

occupied, her brother was filled with revulsion and warned her that King Henry might not enjoy being intimate with a woman who spent her days washing the feet of lepers. Mathilda's piety was, however, so contagious that she soon had her brother kissing the lepers. In contrast, Philip the Fair of France, thought that lepers should be buried alive or burned to death rather than subjected to merely symbolic rites of isolation and burial.

When in public, lepers were supposed to wear a special costume and warn others of their approach with a bell, or rattle. Lepers were not allowed to speak to healthy people, but could point with a long stick to indicate items they wished to purchase. (Presumably, money taken from a leper was not a troublesome source of contagion.) As always, justice or injustice was not equally distributed. Enforcement of the rules of exclusion varied from benign neglect to extreme brutality. The role forced upon the leper was not that of a sick person, but that of a scapegoat for all of medieval society. Perhaps, there were also economic motives at both the state and the family level for the persecution of lepers, who often lost their right to property and inheritance.

Given the ambiguity of the early signs of leprosy, how was it possible to "discover" lepers? Theoretically, lepers were supposed to report their disease to the authorities, but "closet lepers" were probably detected and exposed by suspicious neighbors. Medieval descriptions of all diseases contain highly stylized and speculative material expressed in terms of humoral pathology. The divergence between modern and medieval observations is, however, more striking in the case of leprosy than for other diseases. In the absence of immunological and bacteriological tests, even the most skillful modern diagnostician may find it difficult to distinguish leprosy from other diseases that produce chronic, progressive skin lesions. Although some changes in clinical patterns may occur over time, it seems likely that medieval authors, whether physicians or priests, often described what they expected to see rather than what they actually saw.

Many medical authorities assumed that leprosy was caused or transmitted by improper sexual acts, such as intercourse with a menstruating woman, or contact with a healthy woman who had previously had intercourse with a leper. The presumption of a link between leprosy and "moral defilement," specifically lechery, persisted into the twentieth century. However, sex and sin were not the only causes of leprosy recognized by medieval physicians. The disease could be inherited from a leprous ancestor or acquired from the bite of a poisonous worm, rotten meat, unclean wine, infected air, and corrupt milk from a leprous wet nurse. Various diets were commonly recommended to prevent or cure leprosy; almost every food fell under suspicion at one time or other. Indeed, many years of research convinced Sir Jonathan Hutchinson (1828–1913) that eating rotten fish caused leprosy.

Although the only useful medieval response to leprosy was the isolation of the afflicted, physicians, quacks, and the Bible offered hope of miraculous cures. According to Matthew, Jesus healed a leper simply by touching him and saying "be thou clean." In contrast to this instantaneous cure, Naaman, who was cured by the Prophet Elisha, had to wash himself in the Jordan River seven times. Bartolomeus Anglicus (fl. 1250) admitted that leprosy was hard to cure, except of course by the help of God, but he did suggest a remedy made from the flesh of a black snake cooked in an earthen pot with pepper, salt, vinegar, oil, water, and a special "bouquet garni." Because this powerful snake soup would make the patient dizzy and cause his body to swell, theriac was needed to counteract undesirable side effects. Eventually, the patient's flesh would peel and his hair would fall out, but these problems would subside. An equally promising remedy from a fifteenth-century leech-book combined a bushel of barley and half a bushel of toads in a lead cauldron. The mixture was simmered until the flesh of the toads fell from the bones. The barley brew was dried in the sun and then fed to newly hatched chicks. The chicks were roasted or boiled and fed to the leper.

Driven by fear and hope, desperate lepers might attempt even the most gruesome of cures, be it eating human gall bladders or bathing in blood. Because many transient skin lesions were probably mistaken for Hansen's disease, appeals to saints, baths, bizarre potions, and strange diets were sometimes followed by miraculous cures of the *post hoc ergo propter hoc* variety. This well-known logical fallacy, in which sequence is confused with cause, has all too often secured the reputation of useless remedies and healers.

Perhaps, the most surprising aspect of medieval leprosy is the virtual disappearance of the disease from Europe by the fourteenth century. Obviously, this change was not the result of any medical break-through. Even the cruel measures taken to isolate lepers were of dubious efficacy in breaking the chain of transmission because the disease has a long latent period during which susceptible individuals may be exposed to infection. Changing patterns of commerce, warfare, and pilgrimages may have broken the chain of contagion by which leprosy reached Europe from areas where the disease remained, and still remains, endemic.

If leprosy all but vanished from Europe with minimal medical or public health advances, could it not be totally eradicated today through deliberate efforts? There are good reasons to consider Hansen's disease a logical candidate for a global eradication campaign. Unlike bubonic plague, leprosy does not seem to have a natural animal reservoir. There-fore, breaking the chain of person-to-person transmission should eventually eliminate the disease. Leprosy was one of six infectious dis-eases that the World Health Organization selected as targets of a world-wide public health campaign launched in 1975. However, malaria, schistosomiasis, filariasis, leishmaniasis, trypanosomiasis, and leprosy do not present a major threat to wealthy nations or individuals. Thus, they do not receive the attention that has been awarded to smallpox, poliomyelitis, measles, and other preventable infectious diseases.

Because the early symptoms of Hansen's disease are similar to many other ailments, its victims may be misdiagnosed and subjected to inappropriate treatments for long periods of time. The drugs most frequently used to treat leprosy are dapsone, rifampicin, and clofazi-mine; often all three drugs are given as a multidrug regimen for six months to two years. Despite the appearance of strains of *M. leprae* resistant to each of these drugs, public health authorities argue that if a partial course of therapy were instituted for all lepers, the disease could be eradicated. Even if the afflicted individual is not completely cured, drug treatment renders the patient noninfectious and breaks the chain of transmission. Unless resources are allocated for a major assault on leprosy, the worldwide incidence of the disease will inevitably increase and multidrug resistant Hansen's disease will become more difficult to treat.

The World Health Organization estimates that more than one hundred years after the discovery of the causative agent for leprosy, about 15 million people are still suffering from the disease. The number could actually be much higher because Hansen's disease is often misdiagnosed or unreported. Many patients still think of the diagnosis as a curse. About 90 percent of all cases were found in ten countries: India, Indonesia, Brazil, Democratic Republic of the Congo, Guinea, Madagascar, Mozambique, Myanmar, Nepal, and Tanzania, but Hansen's disease remains a significant public health problem in other impoverished areas. For example, in Somalia, during the floods that affected over sixty villages and over one hundred thousand people in 2000, hundreds of leprosy victims were among those forced out of their homes and villages. Some lepers were so debilitated by the disease that they had to be carried in wheelbarrows and carts pulled by donkeys. Most of those suffering from leprosy had been living in perpetual quarantine since the 1980s when they were exiled to two remote villages. Villagers and the authorities in nearby towns quickly expressed concern about the sudden influx of leprosy victims.

The Kalaupapa Peninsula, on the island of Molokai, Hawaii, was once a place of permanent exile for thousands of victims of Hansen's disease. About eight thousand people have been exiled to Kalaupapa since 1865 when King Kamehameha V signed an act to prevent the spread of leprosy. Mandatory exile, as well as all admissions to Kalaupapa, ended in 1969. By 2003, only about 40 elderly patients remained. The survivors were too disabled or disfigured by the disease to leave a place that once was little more than a prison. The former leper colony became a National Historical Park. Another well-known American leper hospital was founded in Carville, Louisiana, in 1913. Facing strict, life-long isolation, patients described Carville as more like a prison or "living cemetery" than a hospital. By the late twentieth century, almost all cases of Hansen's disease in the United States were found in immigrants who had contracted the disease in areas where it remains endemic.

Politics and poverty account for much of the difficulty in mounting a global campaign against leprosy, but research on Hansen's disease has also been hindered by the reluctance of *M. leprae* to multiply and be fruitful in laboratory animals and artificial media. Research has been facilitated by the discovery that the bacilli will multiply in the nine-banded armadillo, the footpads of mice, and several nonhuman primates.

## ISLAMIC MEDICINE

The period known as the Middle Ages in European history roughly corresponds to the Golden Age of Islam. Contacts between the Islamic world and the Western world began with conflict and misunderstanding and have generally persisted in this pattern ever since. Indeed, some scholars have called the concept of a historic Golden Age of Islam a myth used to create the illusion of a peaceful, multicultural Muslim world of learning, culture, and intellectual achievement. Ignorance of Islamic culture is obviously a perpetual source of danger in the modern world where about one in every five people is a Muslim, that is, a follower of Islam. Islam, the religion founded by Muhammad (570–632), literally means "to submit to God's will or law." When Muhammad was about 40 years old, he received the call to Prophethood and a series of visions in which the Koran (Qu'ran) was revealed to him. By the time of his death, practically all of Arabia had accepted Islam and a century later Muslims had conquered half of Byzantine Asia, all of Persia, Egypt, North Africa, and Spain.

Early Western accounts of "Arabian medicine" reflected the legacy of conflict rather than an analysis of Islamic medicine as a component of a system of faith and a means of dealing with the universal problem of illness. For many European scholars, Arabian medicine was significant only in terms of the role it played in preserving Greek literature during the European Dark Ages. Above all, Arabic texts and translation were credited with making Aristotle known in Christian Europe. Arabian medicine was understood as synonymous with Arabic medicine—Arabic being the language of learning throughout areas of the world under Islamic control. Thus, Arabic texts need not have Arab authors; Persians, Jews, and Christians took part in the development of the Arabic medical literature.

Written sources for the study of classical Islamic medicine come from a geographic area stretching from Spain to India and a time span of some nine hundred years. Just as the term Chinese medicine is broadly used with respect to medical practice in the countries that came within the sphere of China's influence, the term "Islamic medicine" is used to designate the system of ideas and practices that was widely transmitted with the Arab conquests. Islamic medicine was introduced into Arab countries in the ninth century and reached its peak during the European Middle Ages. Like Chinese medicine and Ayurvedic medicine, Islamic medicine, also known as *yunani medicine* (Greek-Islamic medicine), is a living system still respectfully studied and practiced by traditional healers.

Discussions of Arab achievements in science, medicine, and philosophy once focused on a single question: were the Arabs merely the transmitters of Greek achievements or did they make any original contributions? The question of originality is now regarded as essentially inappropriate when applied to a period in which the quest for empirical scientific knowledge was virtually unknown. During the Golden Age of Islamic medicine, physicians, philosophers, and other scholars accepted the writings of the ancients as truth, example, and authority, to be analyzed, developed, and preserved. Having no attachment to the doctrine of the primacy of originality and progress, medieval scholars saw tradition as a treasure chest, not as a burden or obstacle. Like their counterparts in the Christian West, scholars in the Islamic world had to find a means of peaceful coexistence with powerful religious leaders who took the position that knowledge could come only through the Prophet Muhammad, his immediate followers, and the Koran.

## PROPHETIC MEDICINE

References to the importance of health and well-being can be found in the Koran and other teachings associated with Muhammad. Muslims were taught that the Koran was given to believers as "a guide and a medicine" and the restorer of both spiritual and physical health. In a literal sense, the Koran could actually be taken as a medicine by writing a passage from the sacred book on a cloth, washing out the ink, and drinking the wash water. Fragments concerning medical lore culled from the Koran and the "sayings and doings" (*Hadith*) of the Prophet were gathered together as the "medicine of the Prophet." These sayings reflect Muhammad's general approval of traditional Arab medicine, but later commentators apparently supplied additional maxims. Some of the medical maxims encouraged care of the sick and suggested broad principles of health, whereas others referred to particular diseases and health problems and medical or spiritual treatments.

One of the most widely quoted sayings of the Prophet is: "God has sent down a treatment for every ailment." Muhammad was also quoted as saying that valid knowledge was of only two kinds: "knowledge of faith and knowledge of the body." The idea that stress induces diseases seems to be inherent in the saying that "excessive worry makes for physical illness in a person." The sayings of the Prophet provided guidance on medical ethics and tradition, consolation of the sick, the evil eye, magic, amulets, and protective prayers. Some orthodox Muslims considered the medicine of the Prophet superior to secular medicine in providing care for the soul and the body.

Many of the Prophet's medical sayings dealt with sensible eating and drinking to prevent disease. Others referred to the relationship between suffering and sin. "A believer will suffer no sickness nor even a thorn to pierce his skin," Muhammad declared, "without expiating one of his sins." However, there was also the promise that sickness and suffering could confer religious merit, because Muhammad promised that "He who dies on a sickbed, dies the death of a martyr." Another saying promised that a woman who died in childbirth gained the rank of a martyr.

Muhammad referred to natural causes of illness, the natural effects of medical treatments, and divine or supernatural aspects of illness. When God sent misfortune or disease as a test, the faithful could gain religious merit by bearing the trial patiently. Several passages suggest that the sick should bear their sufferings and call for a doctor only when the situation became unbearable. Thus, while natural medicine was not prohibited, some religious leaders were hostile and intolerant of secular studies, in general, and medicine, in particular. Traditionalists who wanted to preserve indigenous customs fought the infiltration of Greek ideas by attributing traditional beliefs to the Prophet. While Arab medicine during Muhammad's lifetime was essentially Bedouin folk medicine, a few scholar-physicians of that period were already familiar with the principles of Greek and Indian medicine and may have successfully prescribed such remedies for Muhammad.

Some theologians justified the acceptance of Greek medicine by reminding the faithful that the Prophet had come to teach only the Sacred Law and not medicine or other practical matters. His allusions to medicine, therefore, were not part of divine revelation, but spontaneous references to traditional folk remedies, such as henna for gout, camel urine for stomach problems, and antimony for eye disorders. Such folklore predated Islam and was neither religious nor scientific. On the other hand, if Muslims used a traditional remedy like honey, it could have a positive effect through the power of faith because Muhammad called honey a health-restoring food.

Although the Prophet unquestionably recommended cupping and the use of honey in treating certain illnesses, his position on cauterization was ambiguous. On some occasions, Muhammad ordered the use of the cautery and even treated some of his wounded followers by cauterization, but after admitting that cauterization could restore health, he reportedly prohibited its use. To rationalize the use of the cautery, commentators argued that the prohibition was only intended to stop practitioners from boasting that the cautery was a totally effective measure. Healers were expected to confess that *all* remedies worked only by God's will. Muhammad forbade the use amulets that invoked supernatural agents, but he allowed the use of those whose contents were in keeping with the teachings of the Koran.

Over the years, books of "Prophetic medicine" were compiled by theologians and religious leaders who hoped to counter the growing influence of Greek medicine. Nevertheless, Greek philosophy, science,

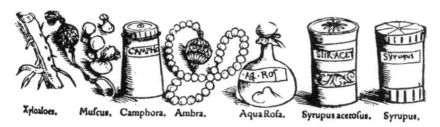

Xyloaloes.　Mufcus.　Camphora.　Ambra.　AquaRofa.　Syrupus acetofus.　Syrupus.

**Pharmaceutical Preparations.**

and medicine eventually captivated Arab physicians and scholars, resulting in the formation of the modified Greco-Arabic medical system that continues to flourish as *yunani medicine*. Finding a means of justifying a scientific, even secular approach to medicine was a challenge to Muslim scholars, much as it had been to Christians. While the value of medicine was generally accepted, some theologians accused doctors of confusing the priorities of the common people by encouraging them to place physical health before religious values. However, Prophetic medicine, whatever the uncertainties of interpretation, clearly taught that "after faith, the art and practice of medicine is the most meritorious service in God's sight." Medical writers justified the study and practice of medicine as a form of religious service that was pleasing to God, as long as it relieved human suffering while acknowledging the primacy of faith.

By the end of the seventh century, under the leadership of the first four *caliphs* (successors to the Prophet), the Arabs had completed the conquest of Syria, Persia, and Egypt, and the process of assimilating Greek philosophy, science, and medicine into Islamic culture began. Thus, many sources of learning were available to Arab scholars. Muhammad had said: "Seek knowledge, even in China," but it was originally the Persian city of Jundi Shapur that served as an intellectual magnet for Muslim scholars. The ancient city of Jundi Shapur provided a uniquely tolerant and peaceful meeting point for the study of the philosophical and medical traditions of Persians, Indians, Nestorians, Zoroastrians, Jews, and Greeks. The scholars of Jundi Shapur began the monumental task of assembling and translating Greek texts, including those of Hippocrates and Galen.

After the triumph of the Abbasid caliphs in 750 and the establishment of Baghdad as the capital of the Islamic Empire, the Hellenization of Islamic culture accelerated rapidly. Baghdad and Cairo developed into independent centers of scholarship. The library established in Cairo in 988 was said to house well over one hundred thousand volumes. In 1258, the Mongols conquered Baghdad and its great libraries were destroyed. So, many manuscripts were thrown into the river that, according to one observer, the Tigris ran black, red, and green with ink. Another chronicler said that the river was so thick with manuscripts that one could walk across it.

At the school for translation established during the reign of the Caliph Al-Ma'mun (813–833), many of Galen's medical and philosophical works were translated into Arabic. One of the most important translators was Hunayn Ibn Ishaq (809–875), a scholar who was often heard reciting Homer in Greek as he walked the streets of Baghdad. Hunayn translated works by Galen, Hippocrates, Dioscorides and composed summaries, commentaries, and study guides for medical students. The ancient version of the ever-popular student "cram book" was a popular genre among Arab scholars; hundreds have survived.

## HOSPITALS AND CLINICAL MEDICINE

Certain elements in Islamic theology, especially the call for total resignation to the will of God, might have inhibited the faithful from actively pursuing public-health initiatives. On the other hand, Muhammad made it a point to visit the sick in order to bring comfort, hope, and advice. This exemplary behavior was cited as the inspiration for the establishment of charitable institutions, such as hospitals, hospices, religious centers, and educational institutions. Financial support was encouraged, or demanded, by religious law. Little is known about the earliest Islamic hospitals, but there is general agreement that such institutions were founded in the early eighth century. Some were apparently modeled on the hospital and school of Jundi Shapur, but others served more specific roles, such as isolating lepers or caring for the blind and disabled. Other charitable enterprises included the organization of teams of physicians and female medical personnel to visit the sick in prisons and mobile dispensaries that served rural areas.

Detailed records were compiled by clinicians at many Muslim hospitals in a format that became known as "treatments based on repeated experience." Such records were important in allowing the larger hospitals to assume much of the task of medical education and clinical research. It was the reputation of individual sages and masters of medicine rather than that of the hospital per se that attracted students. Moreover, the teacher, rather than the institution, granted the student a certificate indicating achievements in medical theory and clinical experience. A truly dedicated student might travel to several different cities to study special areas of medicine with famous masters. Women, trained separately by private tutors, could serve as nurses, midwives, and gynecologists.

A scandal concerning the death of a patient in a Baghdad hospital in 931 is said to have been the stimulus for the establishment of a more formal system of testing doctors. Reports on the impact of testing say that 160 out of 860 medical practitioners in Baghdad failed the examination. Formal testing of pharmacists began in the ninth century. Rules and regulations varied considerably with time and place throughout the Muslim world. In response to the perceived lack of "quality control" for practitioners, handbooks for laymen offered advice on "How to Test a Doctor" in order to distinguish a true physician from a quack. Stories about how patients tested their doctors seem to have universal appeal. One famous example involved a man who presented his physician with the urine of a mule and claimed it was that of a favorite slave girl. The wise physician responded that the girl must have been bewitched, because only a mule would pass such urine. When the doctor recommended a good feed of barley as the appropriate remedy, he was appointed chief personal physician to the caliph.

As institutions of religious learning known as *madrasas* developed, the medical sciences became an optional part of the curriculum. By the thirteenth century, students at some of these institutions could specialize in either religion or natural science. Many physicians complained that standards of medical education and practice deteriorated as teaching hospitals were displaced by religious institutions where theology and religious law overshadowed medicine and science.

Some doctors were known for the huge fortunes they had acquired, whereas a few were remembered for establishing hospitals and charitable clinics. Most experts in medical ethics argued that it was appropriate to charge fees for treating the sick. The physician needed to earn enough to marry and educate his children, without having to engage in work that would interfere with the study of science. Thus, it was important for the rich to pay large fees so that the doctor could care for the poor without charge. Dressed in his white shirt and cloak, distinctive doctor's turban, carrying a silver-headed stick, perfumed with rose-water, camphor, and sandalwood, the physician was an impressive figure. However, despite the honors accorded to scholar-physicians, skepticism about medical practitioners remained strong. In many popular stories, the Devil appears disguised as a physician, or the physician kills his patient through ignorance or treachery. In one such story, a physician murdered his patient by poisoning the lancet used for venesection. Months later, the physician himself needed bleeding; by accident, he used the poisoned lancet. Another eminent physician proved he had a fool for a patient when he treated himself for elephantiasis by allowing starving vipers to bite him. The venom drove out the elephantiasis, but it induced leprosy, deafness, and loss of vision. The persistence of this attitude towards physicians is apparent in the autobiography of Jehangir, son of the great Mogul emperor Akbar (1542–1605). After describing how the treatment that the aged Akbar had endured turned diarrhea into dysentery, dysentery into constipation, and constipation into diarrhea and death, Jehangir concluded that, except for God's decree and doctors' mistakes, no one would ever die.

## THE GREAT SAGES OF ISLAMIC MEDICINE

Although medieval physicians, whether Muslims, Jews, or Christians, generally assumed that Galenism was a complete and perfect system, the great sages of Islamic medicine are of interest in their own right, not just in terms of their role in preserving classical medicine. Latin translations of the works of a few authors, including Rhazes, Avicenna, Albucasis, and Averroes, were most influential in Europe, but the Arabic works of many other scholars held a place in the Muslim world that had no parallel in the West. Some Muslim physicians, such as the mysterious Geber (Jabir ibn Hayyan, 721–ca. 815) became better known as alchemists or philosophers. Averroes (1126–1198; Abu'al-Walid Muhammad ibn Ahmad ibn Muhammad ibn Rushd) was best known for his commentaries on Aristotle, and his interests included medicine and jurisprudence. His reputation for rationalism and piety was based on his ideas about the nature of human intellect and the relationship between philosophy and religion.

Rhazes (ca. 864–ca. 925; al-Razi; Abu Bakr Muhammad 'ibn Zakariya ya-Razi) has been called the greatest physician of the Islamic world. His biographers said that when Rhazes became director of the first great hospital in Baghdad, he selected the most healthful location by hanging pieces of meat at likely sites and finding the one where there was the least putrefaction. The indefatigable Rhazes was the author of at least two hundred medical and philosophical treatises, including his unfinished masterpiece the *Continens, or Comprehensive Book of Medicine*. The *Continens* was translated into Latin by the Jewish physician Faraj ibn Salim (known as Farragut, in Latin) for King Charles of Anjou. The text was completed in 1279 and finally printed in 1486. The printed volumes weighed more than 20 pounds.

Insights into the tension between orthodoxy and philosophy in the Muslim world can be found in *The Conduct of a Philosopher*, a book Rhazes wrote to rebut attacks on his personal conduct. In answer to charges that he had overindulged in life's pleasures, Rhazes answered that he had always been moderate in everything except acquiring knowledge and writing books. By his own reckoning, he had written more than 20,000 pages in one year. Although Rhazes taught that a middle road between extreme asceticism and overindulgence was the most healthful, he confessed that his devotion to his work and his writing had caused grave damage to his eyes and hands. All biographical accounts agree that Rhazes became blind near the end of his life and that he refused treatment because he was weary of seeing the world and unwilling to undergo the ordeal of surgery. Eventually, biographers adopted the spurious but irresistible story that Rhazes lost his sight because his patron al-Mansur had beaten him on the head with one of his books as punishment for the failure of an alchemical demonstration. Presumably, the text used in the beating was a minor treatise on alchemy; if the massive *Continens* had been used, the beating would have been fatal.

The case histories compiled by Rhazes provide insight into the range of complaints for which his contemporaries consulted physicians, which signs and symptoms the physician thought significant, the kinds of treatment used, the occupations and family background of his patients, and the relationship between patient and physician. Just as physicians had ethical obligations to patients, patients had an ethical duty to trust and co-operate with their physicians. It was most important, according to Rhazes, for people to follow the doctor's advice. "With a learned physician and an obedient patient," Rhazes promised, "sickness soon disappears." Unfortunately, not all patients were obedient and not all physicians were learned or even competent. Rhazes had seen impostors who claimed to cure epilepsy by making a cut at the back of the head and then pretending to remove stones or blood clots. Other quacks pretended to draw snakes through the patient's nose, worms from the ears or teeth, frogs from under the tongue, and bones from wounds and ulcers.

In dealing with wealthy and powerful patients, Rhazes was generally ingenious and sometimes daring. Before initiating treatment when al-Mansur seemed to be suffering from an incurable crippling ailment, Rhazes asked the patient for his best horse and mule. The next day Rhazes had al-Mansur take a hot bath while he administered various remedies. Suddenly, Rhazes threatened his patient with a knife and shouted insults at him. In a frenzy, al-Mansur scrambled from the bath, but Rhazes ran outside where his servant waited with the horse and mule. Later, Rhazes sent al-Mansur a letter explaining that he had provoked him in order to use fear and anger as a means of increasing his innate heat and obtaining an instantaneous cure. Having recovered from both his ill health and his anger, al-Mansur showered his physician with gifts.

One of Rhazes' case histories appears to be the first written description of "rose-fever," to use the term adopted in the nineteenth century. Rhazes noticed that one of his patients seemed to suffer from a kind of catarrh (runny nose) or cold every spring. Convinced that the problem was caused by the scent of roses, Rhazes advised his patient to avoid aromatic things such as roses, herbs, onions, and garlic. If the symptoms became particularly troublesome, he recommended cupping on the neck and bleeding from arteries of the temples.

Rhazes' book *On Smallpox and Measles* provides valuable information about diagnosis, therapy, and concepts of diseases. Among the ancients, diseases were generally defined in terms of symptoms such as fever, diarrhea, skin lesions, and so forth. Therefore, Rhazes' treatise on smallpox and measles is a major landmark in establishing the concept of specific disease entities. According to Rhazes, smallpox was caused by the acquisition of impurities from the maternal blood during gestation. When the child reached puberty, these impurities tended to boil up in a manner analogous to the fermentation of wine. The problem was essentially universal, and children rarely escaped the disease. Measles, which Rhazes recognized as a separate disease, was caused by very bilious blood, but even an experienced physician might have trouble distinguishing smallpox from measles. To protect his reputation, the physician should wait until the nature of the illness was clear before announcing his diagnosis. Proper management before the onset of smallpox might lessen its virulence and prevent blindness, but once the disease began the physician should encourage eruption of the pox by wrapping, rubbing, steaming, purging, and bleeding and by taking special precautions to prevent blindness. According to Rhazes, pustules that became hard and warty, instead of ripening properly, indicated that the patient would die. Various recipes were supposed to remove pockmarks, but the nearly universal presence of smallpox scars suggests that these remedies—which included sheep's dung, vinegar, sesame oil, and the liquid found in the hoof of a roasted ram—were about as useful as modern antiwrinkle creams. In reality, once smallpox appeared, medicine did little to alter the course of the disease, except to make it worse, but an elaborate regimen gave the physician and the patient a sense of control, comfort, and hope.

Islam's "Prince of Physicians," Avicenna (980–1037; Abu Ali Hysayn ibn Abdullah ibn Sina), was the first scholar to create a complete philosophical system in Arabic. Critics complained that his influence inhibited further developments, because no physician was willing to challenge the master of philosophy, natural science, and medicine. According to Avicenna's autobiography, when he was only 10 years old, he amazed his father and teachers by mastering the Koran. After surpassing his teachers in jurisprudence and philosophy, the young scholar turned to the natural sciences and was soon teaching medicine to established physicians. However, when Avicenna began to study clinical medicine, he realized that some things could be learned only from experience and not from books. Thereafter, Avicenna spent his days catering to his wealthy patrons and devoted his nights to lecturing his students, dictating his books, and drinking wine. Temperance was certainly not one of Avicenna's virtues. Eventually, wine, women, and work wrecked his constitution. Unwilling to wait for gradual improvement, he attempted a drastic cure by taking medicated enemas eight times per day. This regimen caused ulcers, seizures, colic, and extreme weakness. When his strength was all but gone, he abandoned all forms of treatment and died. Some of his rivals said that he actually died of an accidental, self-administered overdose of opium. His enemies exulted that his medicine could not save his life and that his metaphysics could not save his soul.

Avicenna's great medical treatise, the *Canon*, was written for physicians, but the abridgment called the *Poem on Medicine* served as a layman's introduction to medical theory. With Avicenna's *Canon* as their guide, traditional healers still diagnose illness by feeling the pulse and inspecting urine, cure diseases that Western medicine cannot name, comfort their patients with satisfying explanations of their conditions, and care for patients who do not accept and cannot afford modern psychiatric methods. Followers of Avicenna learned to find diagnostic clues in the size, strength, speed, elasticity, fullness, regularity, and rhythm of the pulse and the color, density, transparency, turbidity, sediments, quantity, odor, and frothiness of urine samples. Having made his diagnosis, the physician could find much practical advice in the works of Avicenna for treating illness and maintaining the health of his patients under different conditions. For example, to provide partial relief from lice, the traveler should rub his body with a woolen ribbon that had been dipped in mercury and wear the ribbon around his neck—rather like a flea collar—until a thorough attack on the pests was possible.

Establishing an appropriate regimen in infancy provided the foundation of a life-long plan for the preservation of health. Much of Avicenna's advice on infant care seems quite sensible, but his remedies for deficient lactation include a daily dose of white ants or dried earthworms in barley water. Elderly patients required a regimen emphasizing moistening and warming measures, such as soothing olive oil baths. Boiling a fox or lizard in the oil made it more effective when treating severe joint pain. The physician had to be adept at assessing the quality of water, because bad water caused a host of disorders, including enlargement of the spleen, constipation, hemorrhoids, diarrhea, and insanity. Waters containing metallic substances and those infested with leeches were dangerous, but Avicenna noted that water containing iron strengthened the internal organs, stopped diarrhea, and stimulated the sexual organs.

Elegant expositions of the philosophical principles of medicine and the relationship between mind and body are woven into Avicenna's case histories. Like Erasistratus, Avicenna demonstrated how physiological phenomena betray our hidden thoughts by using the pulse as a lie detector. In treating a case of love-sickness, Avicenna unobtrusively kept his finger on the patient's wrist and detected the irregularity of the pulse that corresponded to mention of the lover's name. Another challenging case involved a young man who suffered from melancholy and the delusion that he was a cow. The man mooed loudly, refused to eat, and begged to be killed and made into stew. The patient cheered up immediately when Avicenna sent word that the butcher would soon come to slaughter him. Avicenna came into the sickroom with a butcher's knife and asked for the cow. Mooing happily, the young man was bound hand and foot, but after a thorough examination Avicenna declared that the cow was too thin to be butchered. The patient ate so eagerly that he soon recovered his strength and was cured of his delusion.

Avicenna expected the physician to master surgical techniques for treating a wide variety of wounds and injuries. Although the doctor might prescribe drugs to relieve pain before the operation, the patient still had to be bound and restrained by the surgeon's assistants. After the operation, the wound was washed with warm water, vinegar, or wine. Nevertheless, postsurgical infection was so common that the same Persian word meant both wound and pus.

A more specialized guide to Arab surgery was provided by Albucasis (936–1013; Abu 'l-Qasim Khalaf ibn 'Abbas al-Zahrawi), an ascetic man who devoted much of his time to working among the poor. Nevertheless, Albucasis offered harsh and practical advice to fellow physicians. According to Albucasis, a wise physician would guard his reputation by recognizing incurable conditions and leaving such cases to divine providence. As demonstrated by his choice of subject matter, however, Albucasis was willing to deal with dangerous conditions. His *On Surgery and Surgical Instruments* is one of the first comprehensive illustrated treatises on this important subject. Bleeding, cupping, and cauterization constituted the major forms of surgical practice at the time. *On Surgery* and Rhazes' treatise on smallpox were among the earliest classical Arabic texts to be printed in England. In discussing the uses of cauterization from "head to heel," Albucasis praised the cautery as an instrument with "universal application" for almost every disorder, organic or functional. Despite his piety, Albucasis was obviously not inhibited by the uncertainties surrounding the Prophet's position on the use of the cautery. He prescribed cauterization to arrest hemorrhage, prevent the spread of destructive lesions, strengthen organs that became cold in temperament, and remove putrefactive matter. By counteracting excessive humidity and coldness of the brain, cauterization cured disorders such as headache, epilepsy, lethargy, and apoplexy. To perform the operation on the patient's shaved head, the surgeon placed his hand on the root of the nose between the eyes and applied the cautery to the spot marked by his middle finger. If the bone was exposed when the sizzling stopped, cauterization was complete; if not, the operation should be repeated. Some surgeons believed in keeping the wound open, but Albucasis advised readers that it was safer to avoid further interventions. If the cautery failed to cure chronic migraine or acute catarrh, Albucasis suggested bleeding from the arteries.

Both Albucasis and Avicenna provided detailed discussions of the theory and practice of bloodletting. In all but the very old and very young, venesection was valuable for both the preservation of health and the treatment of disease. Drugs assisted the body in the elimination of noxious humors through purging, vomiting, and diuresis, but venesection immediately removed excess humors in the same proportion as they were present in the blood vessels. As stipulated by Galen, venesection was even useful in the treatment of hemorrhages because it diverted blood to the opposite side of the body. Doctors commonly selected from about 30 sites for venesection: 16 of these were in the head, 5 in the arms and hands, and 3 in the legs and feet. Despite the danger of damage to nerves, the elbow veins were frequently used in the treatment of disorders of the chest, abdomen, and eyes.

The patient's strength and the color of the blood determined the amount to be taken. If the blood was initially black, the doctor should continue bleeding until it became red; if the blood was thick, he should bleed until it became thin. Bleeding could be carried out in several small installments for a weak patient, but a person with hot, sharp, abundant blood and fever should be bled until he fainted. Albucasis warned the doctor to keep his finger on the pulse during bleeding to avoid the possibility that the patient might die rather than faint. For some conditions, leeches, cupping, and cauterization were preferable to venesection. Cupping, with or without scarification, was considered less debilitating than venesection, but leeches were sometimes more appropriate because the creatures could be applied to parts of the body beyond the reach of cupping vessels. Leeches were excellent for drawing blood from deep tissues, but they had to be carefully selected. Large-headed leeches that were black, gray, or green, or had hairy bodies with blue stripes, were said to cause inflammation, hemorrhage, fever, fainting, and paralysis. Albucasis described techniques for removing a leech stuck in the throat, but did not explain how the leech got there.

Female patients presented special difficulties because a chaste woman would not expose her body to a male doctor. If a woman required surgery, Albucasis suggested calling for a competent woman doctor, a eunuch, or an experienced midwife. The midwife should know the signs and manner of normal delivery, have wisdom and dexterity, and be skillful in dealing with abnormal presentations, prolonged labor, and the extraction of a dead fetus. It is interesting that Albucasis said that women doctors were "uncommon," rather than nonexistent. The reference to eunuchs is also notable because castration was forbidden by Moslem law. Nevertheless, after apologizing for mentioning this operation, Albucasis described it in some detail.

Pharmacology, alchemy, and optics were also of great interest to Arab scientists. Arabic treatises on medicinal plants and drugs played a large role in shaping the development of pharmacy as an independent profession. The medical formulary of al-Kindi (ca. 801–ca. 866; Abu Yusuf Yaqub ibn-Ishaq al-Kindi) served as a model for Arabic treatises on pharmacology, botany, zoology, and mineralogy. Persian and Indian drugs that were unknown to Hippocrates and Galen appeared in such formularies, as did new kinds of drug preparations. Linguistic analysis of the medical materials discussed by al-Kindi indicates that 33 percent of the drugs came from Mesopotamian and Semitic traditions, 23 percent from Greek sources, 18 percent from Persian, 13 percent from Indian, 5 percent from Arabic, and 3 percent from ancient Egyptian sources. Unfortunately, many of al-Kindi's other writings—some 270 treatises in logic, philosophy, physics, mathematics, music, astrology, natural history, and medicine—were lost. al-Kindi's interest in theories of vision and practical ophthalmology was probably stimulated by the high frequency of eye diseases in the Middle East. Many Arabic works deal specifically with the anatomy of the eye, its role in vision, and the treatment of eye diseases. Although the theory of vision might seem a rather esoteric branch of knowledge, al-Kindi argued that it would prove to be the key to the discovery of nature's most fundamental secrets. The Latin version of his work on optics, *De aspectibus*, was very influential among Western scientists and philosophers.

## THE STRANGE CASE OF IBN AN-NAFIS

Western scholars long maintained that the major contribution of Arabian medicine was the preservation of ancient Greek wisdom and that medieval Arabic writers produced nothing original. Because the Arabic manuscripts thought worthy of translation were those that most closely followed the Greek originals (all others being dismissed as corruptions), the original premise—lack of originality—was confirmed. The strange story of Ibn an-Nafis (1210–1280; Ala ad-Din Abu al-'Ala 'Ali ibn Abi al-Haram al-Qurayshi-ad-Dimashqi Ibn an-Nafis) and the pulmonary circulation demonstrates the unsoundness of previous assumptions about the Arabic literature. The writings of Ibn an-Nafis were essentially ignored until 1924 when Dr. Muhyi ad-Din at-Tatawi, an Egyptian physician, presented his doctoral thesis to the Medical Faculty of Freiburg, Germany. If a copy of Tatawi's thesis had not come to the attention of the historian Max Meyerhof, Ibn an-Nafis' discovery of the pulmonary circulation might have been forgotten again. Some texts by Ibn an-Nafis that were thought to be lost were rediscovered in the 1950s.

Honored by his contemporaries as a learned physician, skillful surgeon, and ingenious investigator, Ibn an-Nafis was described as a tireless writer and a pious man. His writings included the *Comprehensive Book on the Art of Medicine*, the *Well Arranged Book on Ophthalmology*, and a *Commentary on the Canon of Ibn Sina*. According to biographers, while serving as Chief of Physicians in Egypt, Ibn an-Nafis became seriously ill. His colleagues advised him to take wine as a medicine, but he refused because he did not wish to meet his Creator with alcohol in his blood.

It is not clear how Ibn an-Nafis reached his theory of the pulmonary circulation, but he was known to be critical of Galenic dogma. Like Galen, Ibn an-Nafis could not conduct human dissection. In his *Commentary*, Ibn an-Nafis explained that religious law prohibited human dissection, because mutilation of a cadaver was considered an insult to human dignity. In the pre-Islamic Arab wars, victors sometimes deliberately mutilated the bodies of their enemies. Islamic law prohibited this ritualistic mutilation, and orthodox legal experts argued that scientific dissection was essentially the same violation of the dignity of the human body. It seems quite unlikely that the physician who refused to take wine to save his life would have acted against religious law and the dictates of his own conscience to satisfy scientific curiosity. During the twentieth century, some Muslim theologians reasserted this prohibition on the mutilation of cadavers in response to advances in organ transplantation. The general population seemed eager to accept organ transplants, but some religious authorities tried to forbid such procedures.

In the midst of a fairly conventional discussion of the structure and function of the heart, Ibn an-Nafis departed from the accepted explanation of the movement of the blood. His description of the two ventricles of the heart accepts the Galenic doctrine that the right ventricle is filled with blood and the left ventricle with vital spirit. His next statement, however, boldly contradicted Galen's teachings on the pores in the septum. Ibn an-Nafis insisted that there were no passages, visible or invisible, between the two ventricles and argued that the septum between the two ventricles was thicker than other parts of the heart in order to prevent the harmful and inappropriate passage of blood or spirit between them. Thus, to explain the path taken by the blood, Ibn an-Nafis reasoned that after the blood had been refined in the right ventricle, it was transmitted to the lungs where it was rarefied and mixed with air. The finest part of this blood was then clarified and transmitted from the lungs to the left ventricle. Therefore, the blood can only get into the left ventricle by way of the lungs.

Perhaps, some still obscure Arabic, Persian, or Hebrew manuscript contains a commentary on the curious doctrines of Ibn an-Nafis, but there is as yet no evidence that later authors were interested in these anti-Galenic speculations. Thus, although Ibn an-Nafis did not influence later writers, the fact that his concept was so boldly stated in the thirteenth century should lead us to question our assumptions about progress and originality in the history of science. As only a small percentage of the pertinent manuscripts have been analyzed, the questions may go unanswered for quite some time.

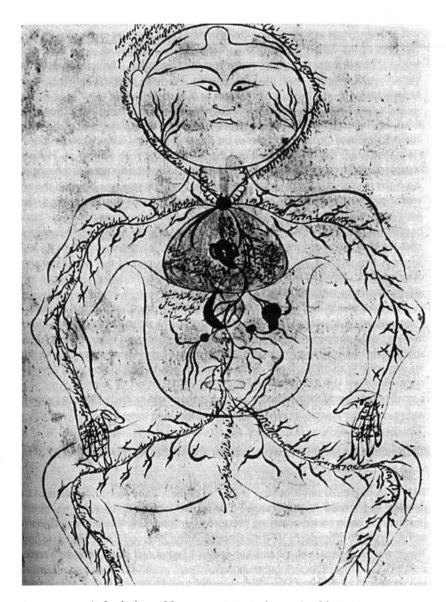

**A depiction of human anatomy in an Arabic text.**

## THE SURVIVAL OF GRECO-ISLAMIC MEDICINE

Islamic medicine (also known as yunani medicine) did not disappear at
the end of the Middle Ages but continued to develop and spread to
other areas. During the nineteenth century, traditional practitioners came
under increasing pressure from competing Western-style doctors and

government officials. In 1838, the Ottoman Sultan, Muhammad II, established the first Western-style medical school and hospital in Istanbul and staffed it with French doctors. The Sultan asserted that traditional Islamic medicine had become stagnant and sterile. Many other Muslim countries eventually followed this example and tried to ban the practice of traditional medicine.

Even where twentieth century laws regulating medical practice drove traditional practitioners underground, diligent explorers could still find them. For example, in French-ruled Algeria, traditional healers and their patients were reluctant to talk to outsiders because it was illegal for people without the proper French qualifications to perform surgery. Nevertheless, yunani doctors performed eye surgery, tooth extractions, cupping, cautery, bloodletting, and assisted in difficult births. Although anesthetic drugs were available, most traditional practitioners did not use them before surgery. Some healers claimed that their methods were so gentle that the patient did not suffer, but strong assistants were invariably needed to restrain the patient. Many people treated themselves with yunani drugs and cauterization in order to avoid the costs of seeing a doctor and because of their faith in such remedies.

Under British rule of the Indian subcontinent, both Muslim and Hindu traditional systems survived. In the 1960s, the Pakistani government ordered the registration, licensing, and utilization of *hakims* (traditional scholar-physicians), because Western medicine was too expensive and rarely available to the rural population. Western-style doctors strenuously objected to this official recognition of their rivals. With official recognition by the governments of Pakistan and India and regulations administered through the Ministries of Health, male and female yunani practitioners, known as *tabibs* and *tabibas*, respectively, flourished in urban and rural settings. Many practitioners learned the art as apprentices, but others enrolled in yunani medical colleges where the curriculum includes the *Canon* of Avicenna and the standard components of modern medicine. Yunani doctors still diagnose illness by inspecting the pulse, urine, stools, and tongue and prescribe traditional drugs and diets. Scientific analyses of yunani remedies have confirmed the value of many medicinal plants, but hundreds of traditional drugs have not been investigated. In general, however, modern Muslim societies have not succeeded in establishing the complete acculturation of modern medicine into Islam, despite the fact that medieval Islam successfully assimilated Greek, Persian, and Indian medical traditions. Despite the explosive revival of Islamic fundamentalism in the 1980s, India and Pakistan appear to be the only nations where a serious effort is being made to incorporate Greco-Islamic medical traditions into modern health care planning.

## SUGGESTED READINGS

Aberth, J. (2000). *From the Brink of the Apocalypse: Confronting Famine, War, Plague, and Death in the Later Middle Ages.* New York: Routledge.

Albucasis (1973). *Albucasis on Surgery and Instruments.* Edited by M. S. Spink and G. L. Lewis. Berkeley, CA: University California Press.

Arnaldez, R. (2000). *Averroes: A Rationalist in Islam* (Trans. by D. Streight). Notre Dame, IN: University of Notre Dame Press.

Van Arsdall, A., trans. (2002). *Medieval Herbal Remedies: The Old English Herbarium and Anglo-Saxon Medicine.* New York: Routledge.

Avicenna (1930). *A Treatise on the Canon of Medicine of Avicenna Incorporating a Translation of the First Book* (Trans. by O. C. Gruner). London: Luzac.

Avicenna (1974). *The Life of Ibn Sina* (Trans. by W. E. Gohlman). New York: State University of New York Press.

Berger, M. (1999). *Hildegard of Bingen: On Natural Philosophy and Medicine: Selections from Cause et Cure.* Rochester, NY: D. S. Brewer.

Boeckl, C. M. (2000). *Images of Plague and Pestilence: Iconography and Iconology.* Kirksville, MO: Truman State University Press.

Brody, S. N. (1974). *The Disease of the Soul; Leprosy in Medieval Literature.* Ithaca, NY: Cornell University Press.

Brown, P. (1980). *The Cult of the Saints. Its Rise and Function in Latin Christianity.* Chicago, IL: University Chicago Press.

Bullough, V. L. (2004). *Universities, Medicine and Science in the Medieval West.* Burlington, VT: Ashgate.

Cadden, J. (1993). *Meanings of Sex Differences in the Middle Ages: Medicine, Science and Culture.* Cambridge: Cambridge University Press.

Cameron, M. L. (1993). *Anglo-Saxon Medicine.* Cambridge: Cambridge University Press.

Carmichael, A. G. (1986). *Plague and the Poor in Renaissance Florence.* New York: Cambridge University Press.

Cockayne, T. O. (1864–1866). *Leechdoms, Wortcunning and Starcraft of Early England. The History of Science Before the Norman Conquest.* Collected and edited by the Rev. T. O. Cockayne (1807–1873). 3 Volumes. Bristol, UK: Thoemmes Press, 2001.

Cohn, S. K., Jr. (2002). *The Black Death Transformed. Disease and Culture in Early Renaissance Europe.* Oxford: Oxford University Press.

Fakhry, M. (2001). *Averroes (Ibn Rushd): His Life, Works and Influence.* Great Islamic Thinkers Series. Oxford: Oneworld Publications.

French, R., Arrizabalaga, J., Cunningham, A., and García-Ballester, L., eds. (1998). *Medicine from the Black Death to the French Disease.* Brookfield, VT: Ashgate.

García-Ballester, L. (2001). *Medicine in a Multicultural Society: Christian, Jewish and Muslim Practitioners in the Spanish Kingdoms, 1222–1610.* Burlington, VT: Ashgate.

García-Ballester, L. (2002). *Galen and Galenism: Theory and Medical Practice from Antiquity to the European Renaissance.* Burlington, VT: Ashgate.

García-Ballester, L., French, R., Arrizabalaga, J., and Cunningham, A., eds. (1994). *Practical Medicine from Salerno to the Black Death.* Cambridge: Cambridge University Press.

Getz, F. (1998). *In: Medicine in the English Middle Ages.* Princeton, NJ: Princeton University Press.

Gottfried, R. S. (1986). *Doctors and Medicine in Medieval England, 1340–1530.* Princeton, NJ: Princeton University Press.

Green, M. H. (2002). *The Trotula: An English Translation of the Medieval Compendium of Women's Medicine.* Philadelphia, PA: University of Pennsylvania Press.

Green, M. H. (2000). *Women's Healthcare in the Medieval West: Texts and Contexts.* Burlington, VT: Ashgate/Variorum.

Herlihy, D. (1997). *The Black Death and the Transformation of the West.* Cambridge, MA: Harvard University Press.

Khan, M. S. (1986). *Islamic Medicine.* London: Routledge & Kegan Paul.

Kreuger, H. C. (1963). *Avicenna's Poem on Medicine.* Springfield, IL: Thomas.

Matossian, M. K. (1989). *Poisons of the Past. Molds, Epidemics, and History.* New Haven, CT: Yale University Press.

McNeill, W. H. (1989). *Plagues and Peoples.* New York: Anchor Books.

Moore, R. I. (2000). *The First European Revolution, c. 970–1215. The Making of Europe.* New York: Blackwell Publishers.

Rhazes (1948). *A Treatise on the Smallpox and Measles* (Trans. from the original Arabic by W. A. Greenhill). London: Sydenham Society.

Scott, S, and Duncan, C. J. (2001). *Biology of Plagues: Evidence from Historical Populations.* New York: Cambridge University Press.

Siraisi, N. G. (1990). *Medieval and Early Renaissance Medicine: An Introduction to Knowledge and Practice.* Chicago, IL: University of Chicago Press.

Stannard, J. (1999). *Herbs and Herbalism in the Middle Ages and Renaissance.* Edited by K. E. Stannard and R. Kay. Brookfield, VT: Ashgate.

Stannard, J. (1999). *Pristina Medicamenta: Ancient and Medieval Medical Botany.* Edited by K. E. Stannard and R. Kay. Brookfield, VT: Ashgate.

Ullman, M. (1978). *Islamic Medicine.* Edinburg: Edinburg University Press.

Voights, L. E., and McVaugh, M. R. (1984). *A Latin Technical Phlebotomy and Its Middle English Translation.* Philadelphia, PA: American Philosophical Society.

# 6

# The Renaissance and the Scientific Revolution

The term Renaissance designates the rebirth of the arts and sciences that accompanied the complex and often painful economic, social, political, and intellectual transformations that took place in Europe between about 1300 and 1650. The Renaissance was a new age of exploration of the word, the world, the mind, and the human body. The Renaissance era may have ultimately transformed European culture in a profound and permanent way that led to the modern world, but it was also a period in which superstition, mysticism, intolerance, and epidemic disease flourished. During this period, Europe experienced the disintegration of medieval economic, social, and religious patterns, the expansion of commerce, cities, and trade, and the growth of the modern state. While such a profound transformation might seem to imply a sharp break with the past, in many ways the Renaissance was the natural culmination of the Middle Ages. Scholars have argued that the Renaissance was not yet an age of individualism, as indicated by the importance of kinship ties and the growth of religious and professional associations. For the most part, towns and cities were urban islands surrounded by traditional rural life. Moreover, medievalists have argued that the outlines of modern society were already being formed between the late tenth century and the early thirteenth.

As an era of scientific and philosophical interest, if not therapeutic advances, the Renaissance was a time of special importance for medicine. The death rate circa 1500 was about three times the present level, and life expectancy was perhaps half that of modern Europe. War, famine, and epidemic disease appeared so often that fears of the imminent end of the world were widespread. However, the exact relationship between the Renaissance and the renaissance of medicine is extremely complicated. It is possible to speak of a long medical renaissance that began in the twelfth century, a distinct medical renaissance of the sixteenth century, and a medical revolution of the seventeenth century.

## INVENTIONS THAT CHANGED THE WORLD

Francis Bacon (1561–1639), England's premier philosopher of science and Lord High Chancellor, said that if we considered the "force, effect, and consequences" of all the products of human ingenuity, the three most important inventions were printing, gunpowder, and the compass. It was especially significant, Bacon noted, that the three inventions that had changed the appearance and state of the world were unknown to the ancients.

The first European book printed with movable type appeared in 1454, which was about four years after printing began in Europe. The establishment of printing presses throughout Europe in the 1460s launched a communications revolution that might, at least in part, account for the permanence of the Renaissance. Texts printed with movable type before 1501 are known as *incunabula*, a term coming from the Latin word for cradle, to indicate that such texts represent the infancy of the printed book.

The print revolution accelerated the trend towards literacy, the diffusion of ideas, and the establishment of a vernacular literature, and transformed a scribal and image culture into a print culture. Interest in educational problems was not limited to higher learning and university curricula, but included reform programs for elementary education. In contrast to centuries of laboriously hand-copied manuscripts, within a few decades, millions of books had been reproduced. By the end of the fifteenth century, printing presses had been established in some three hundred European cities and towns. While scholars praised printing as "the art that preserved all other arts," advocates of literacy could say "shame on those who cannot read." Censorship rules were a serious threat to printers in many countries, because publishing heretical materials could be punished by imprisonment or death.

The role of the printing press in the Renaissance and the Scientific Revolution has, however, been a matter of debate among scholars. Theological, legal, and classical texts generally preceded works on science and medicine. Jean Charlier de Gerson's writings on self-abuse, *De pollutione nocturna*, printed in Cologne about 1466, may have been the first printed medical book. Some historians emphasize the importance of the printing press in standardizing and preserving texts, as well as increasing the numbers of texts available. Of course, careless and ignorant printers could introduce errors and multiply errors more rapidly than scribes could corrupt hand-made books. But copy editors, proofreaders ("correctors"), and skillful editors understood the danger of introducing errors. Errors in the text or the illustrations and captions could be particularly dangerous in medical and surgical books. When editing medical texts for a printer in Lyon, the French humanist François Rabelais (1490?–1553), who is best known for his satirical attacks on superstition and scholasticism, allegedly said: "One wrong word may now kill thousands of men!"

An avalanche of advice literature, especially texts dealing with health and diet, was a major product of the print revolution. Popular texts in the vernacular told people what foods, drugs, and spices were "good" or "bad" for their health, explaining proper food choices in terms of humoral and medical theories. Advice on hygiene still discussed the Galenic rules of health or regimen in terms of the six non-naturals: food and drink, air or the environment, exercise and rest, sleep and waking, evacuation and repletion, and the passions of the soul or the emotions. Similar formats were adopted by texts that gave advice to wealthy readers about sex, clothing, cosmetics, health, family life, managing pregnancy and childbirth, wet-nursing, child rearing, and so forth. Medical writers had to find ways of adapting medical theories to New World plants—such as tomatoes, potatoes, and tobacco—that were being used as foods and drugs. Written advice could get very detailed without causing embarrassment to the advisor or the patient. Of course, the advice literature was probably consulted more often by those who were ill than by those who might learn to preserve their health by actually following lifestyle advice. The authors of advice literature often complained that people only worried about diet and proper regimen when they were already sick.

Despite the inevitable grumbling about the vulgarity of printed books as compared to manuscripts and the fear that an excess of literacy might be subversive, scholars and an increasingly literate populace were generally more concerned with acquiring the new treasures than in complaining about the end of scribal culture. Once in print, a text could speak to students directly, rather than through the professor or keeper of manuscripts. The mass-produced book made it possible for the young to study, and perhaps even learn, by reading on their own. Without the art of papermaking, which originated in China, the knowledge revolution launched by the printing press would have been impossible. Johannes Gutenberg's Bible, one of the few early books to be printed on parchment, required the skins of three hundred sheep. Europeans would have run out of sheep before printers ran out of orders for books. Although printed books were not as difficult to obtain as manuscripts, they were still very expensive and had to be chained to library shelves to discourage theft.

Gunpowder weapons have an important place in the history of medicine because they forced surgeons to deal with problems unknown to Hippocrates and Galen. The Chinese probably invented gunpowder and the compass, but others have claimed prior or independent invention. As Europeans followed the compass around the world, they brought back new plants, animals, and remedies and left in their wake a series of ecological and demographic catastrophes that transformed the world.

## THE MEDICAL HUMANISTS

The Scientific Revolution is generally thought of as the great transformation of the physical sciences that occurred during the sixteenth and seventeenth centuries, and is primarily associated with Nicolaus Copernicus (1472–1543), Johannes Kepler (1571–1630), Galileo Galilei (1564–1642), and Isaac Newton (1642–1727). Some scholars have tried to explore the question of why the Scientific Revolution occurred in Europe in the seventeenth century, rather than in China or Islamic areas, which reached a sophisticated level in science and technology centuries earlier. Other scholars have dealt with the questions by arguing that there was no such thing as a European Scientific Revolution. After all, during the alleged Scientific Revolution, interest in astrology, alchemy, magic, religion, and theory persisted. Yet other scholars see the Scientific Revolution as a valid metaphor for the transition from a pre-modern to a modern worldview, in which science is at the very core of life and thought. Writers who lived through the era traditionally called the Renaissance often expressed an awed awareness of changing ideas, such as the Copernican Theory. John Donne (1572–1631), English poet and clergyman, thought that the sun-centered image of the cosmos might well be true, but he lamented that the new philosophy "calls all in doubt." Truly, the world had lost its traditional "coherence." Men no longer knew where to find the sun, the earth, and the planets. Yet poets and the human mind can eventually adjust even to the displacement of earth and sun. Alexander Pope (1688–1744), in his *Essay on Man* (1734), saw the new vision as exciting rather than frightening, and hoped new ideas about the universe might tell us "why Heaven has made us as we are."

Thus, just as the Renaissance transformed the arts, the Scientific Revolution ultimately transformed ideas about the nature of the universe and the nature of man. During the period from about 1450 to 1700, medieval scholasticism was replaced by a new approach to understanding the natural world. Applying this new mode of thought to anatomy, physiology, and medical education would have been impossible without the work of the humanist scholars. Like the scholastics of the Middle Ages, the humanists were devoted to words and books and the difficult task of integrating experience and practice with classical learning. While the intellectual ferment and scholarly enthusiasms of this period were unique, religion still permeated Renaissance life and the way in which scholars, artists, explorers, and natural philosophers saw the world, even the New World. Even if humanism was indicative of a new state of mind, half of the books printed during this era dealt with religious subject matter.

A good case can be made that humanism and humanists at universities throughout Western Europe played a key role in transforming the scholastic medieval curriculum. University faculties fought about funding, arrogant celebrity scholars, full-time and adjunct positions, pensions, and dress codes, and complained about town and gown tensions, while students attempted to censure professors for what they considered inadequate teaching. In other words, much about the academic environment has remained the same. Despite the persistence of many aspects of the medieval intellectual tradition, humanist scholars, especially those at Italian universities, fomented a real intellectual revolution. But, for many reasons, the Italian universities were in decline in the seventeenth century as universities in other regions offered strong competition for students and faculty.

While the humanist scholars were generally more concerned with art and literature than science, their new perspective served the needs of the medical sciences as well. As staunch supporters of the newly purified Galenic texts, humanist scholars rejected corrupt medieval translations. Nevertheless, their excessive respect for ancient authorities made them skeptical of attempts to create a new medical science that would be independent of the ancient Greeks. The work of Thomas Linacre (1460?–1524) and John Caius (1510–1573), outstanding English medical humanists, exemplifies the nature of scholarship and medical education during this period.

Thomas Linacre studied Greek in Florence and Rome before receiving the degree of Doctor of Medicine from the University of Padua in 1496. In addition to his scholarly work, he maintained a lucrative private medical practice, taught Greek, and served as personal physician to King Henry VII. Linacre edited and translated Galen's writings on hygiene, therapeutics, disease symptoms, the pulse, and so forth. He was also highly regarded as a grammarian. His last book, a study of Latin syntax, was published posthumously. As founder and guiding light of the College of Physicians, Linacre helped to mold the character of the English medical profession. He and other elite English physicians gained the power to determine who could legally practice medicine in the Greater London area. The Royal College of Physicians had the power to fine and imprison unlicensed medical practitioners. Graduates of Cambridge and Oxford, which Linacre himself had attended, were exempted from these harsh penalties. Under the leadership of Linacre's devoted disciple John Caius, the College of Physicians grew in power and prestige, taking control of medical licensing away from religious authorities, and using strict regulations to enhance the status of approved physicians. Nevertheless, Caius was troubled by what he saw as a decline in English medical humanism.

In terms of the development of institutions of higher learning, England lagged behind the universities and professional schools of the continent. Thus, like other English scholars, Caius had to pursue his studies abroad. After abandoning his theological studies, Caius became a medical student at the University of Padua, where he met Andreas Vesalius (1514–1564), the rising star of Renaissance anatomy. Both men were involved in editing and publishing new Latin versions of Galenic texts, but their reactions to discrepancies between Galenic anatomy and the human cadaver were quite different. While Vesalius insisted on returning to the "true book of the human body," Caius was confident that once all the writings of Galen were critically edited, medical knowledge would be virtually complete.

In 1546, Caius was appointed anatomical demonstrator to the United Company of Barbers and Surgeons. Since 1540, the Company of Barbers and Surgeons had been allotted the bodies of four convicted felons per year for anatomical demonstrations. After considerable lobbying by Caius and other elite physicians, the College of Physicians received a similar bequest in 1565. Whereas other presidents of the College of Physicians had generally ignored unqualified practitioners, especially outside London, Caius wanted to control medical licensing for all of England. Although his goal of raising standards for medical education and practice was laudable, efforts to limit the number of practitioners by dictating their credentials had adverse effects, especially for women and the poor. Obviously, the needs of the common people could not be met by the small numbers of physicians who belonged to the medical aristocracy, which was not necessarily a meritocracy. Because women were not admitted to the universities, female practitioners were easy targets for licensing reforms. In addition to his campaigns against unlicensed practitioners, quackery, witchcraft, and superstition, Caius challenged those who dared to criticize Galen.

Respect for the ancients did not blunt Caius' ability to observe and describe new phenomena, as shown in his account of an illness known as the English sweating sickness. His remarkable *Boke or Counseill against the Disease Called the Sweate* (1522) was the first original description of disease to be written in England in English. In all probability, Caius would be distressed to know that his vernacular description of the "sweats" is now regarded as his most important medical work. At least five severe outbreaks of Sudor Britanica, or *sudor anglicus*, apparently occurred between 1480 and 1580. The disease was characterized by copious sweat, fever, nausea, headache, cramps, pain in the back and extremities, delirium, hallucinations, and a profound stupor. Within about 24 hours the disease reached a critical stage, when either the disease or the patient came to an abrupt end. Even among strong, healthy men, the mortality rate was extremely high. Many victims lapsed into coma and died within 24 to 48 hours. Moreover, the disease seemed to seek out Englishmen even if potential Scottish, Irish, and Welsh victims were available.

According to Caius, a stricken town was fortunate if only half of all souls were claimed by the disease. After carefully evaluating the clinical pattern and natural history of the disease, he concluded that the sweating sickness was a new disease. Some historians believe that the disease was brought to London in 1485 when Henry VII's mercenaries returned from France and Flanders. The disease might have been a virulent form of influenza, ergotism (a reaction to fungal toxins), food poisoning, or a totally unknown and extinct disease, but the exact nature of these epidemics and the reason for their peculiar geographical distribution are still obscure.

## AUTOPSIES, ART, AND ANATOMY

While the artists and anatomists of the Renaissance are inextricably associated with the reform of anatomy, the study of human anatomy—from bodies, as well as from books—had not been entirely neglected since the death of Galen. During the Middle Ages, human dissection was not pursued with the freedom and intensity so briefly enjoyed by Herophilus and Erasistratus, but it had not been absolutely forbidden or abandoned. Interest in dissection and vivisection increased slowly between the twelfth and the seventeenth centuries, but medieval autopsies were normally conducted to investigate suspicious deaths or outbreaks of plague, or even to search for special signs inside the bodies of purported saints. Such postmortems were probably about as informative as the rituals conducted in some primitive tribes to determine whether death was due to witchcraft.

Human dissection was practiced to a limited extent during the thirteenth and fourteenth centuries in those universities in southern Europe having medical faculties. Statutes of the University of Bologna dating back to 1405 recognized the practice of dissection. In 1442, the city of Bologna authorized the provision of two cadavers each year to the university for dissection. During the fifteenth century, similar provisions were made for most of the major European universities. Thus, medical students were able to observe a limited number of human dissections. However, they knew that examinations and dissertations required knowledge of accepted texts, not the ability to perform practical demonstrations. Students pragmatically attended dissections to confirm their readings of the ancient authorities and to prepare for examinations. Medieval and Renaissance students were probably not too different from students running a typical "cookbook" experiment today. Such experiments are performed to teach a standard technique or confirm some accepted fact, not to make novel observations.

Anatomical demonstrations throughout Europe varied considerably, but the typical public anatomy featured the corpse of a criminal guilty of a crime heinous enough to merit the sentence of "execution and dissection." After acknowledgment of the Papal Indulgence for the ceremony, a learned professor would read a great oration on the structure of the human body while a barber-surgeon attacked the cadaver. Generally, the debates between the Galenists of the medical faculty and the Aristotelians of the faculty of philosophy drew more attention than the mutilated corpse. Anatomical demonstrations continue to provide public education and entertainment, as indicated by public displays of transparent anatomical models. Transparent organs were on display at the First International Hygiene Exhibition (1911). Museums in Europe and the United States were exhibiting various Transparent Men and Transparent Women in the 1930s.

By about 1400, human dissection was part of the curriculum of most medical schools. Anatomies were also performed in some hospitals. However, well into the sixteenth century, medical students were in little danger of being forced to confront radically new ideas about the nature of the human body. The medical curriculum of the Renaissance university reflected a heavy commitment to the ancient authorities. Students were expected to master texts by Avicenna, Galen, and Hippocrates. The number of medical students was rather small, especially in northern Europe. Throughout the sixteenth century, the annual number of candidates for the degree of Bachelor of Medicine in Paris was less than 20.

For teachers as well as students, the purpose of dissection was to supplement the study of Galenic texts, but because of the complexity of Galen's writings, simplified guides were needed. One of the best-known early dissection manuals was the *Anatomy* (1316) of Mondino de Luzzi (ca. 1275–1326), who served as public lecturer at the University of Bologna from 1314 to 1324. Mondino's *Anatomy* was practical and succinct. The first printed edition of the popular text appeared in 1478 and was followed by at least 40 editions. But medical humanists rejected the work, and turned to newly restored editions of anatomical works by Galen, especially *On the Use of the Parts* and *On Anatomical Procedures*. Some of the early texts included simple diagrams, but these images did little to illuminate anatomical principles. Mastery of the principles of artistic perspective in the fifteenth century made the new art of anatomical illustration possible.

The development of a special relationship with the sciences, especially anatomy, mathematics, and optics, as well as the inspiration of classical Greek ideals, gave Renaissance art much of its distinctive character. Both artists and physicians sought accurate anatomical knowledge. Artists placed a new emphasis on accurately representing animals and plants, scientific use of perspective, and above all the idea that the human body was beautiful and worthy of study. To make their art true to life and to death, artists attended public anatomies and executions and studied intact and flayed bodies in order to see how the muscles and bones worked.

While many Renaissance painters and sculptors turned to dissection, none exceeded Leonardo da Vinci (1452–1519)—painter, architect, anatomist, engineer, and inventor—in terms of artistic and scientific imagination. Leonardo's notebooks present a man of formidable genius and insatiable intellectual curiosity; they also reveal the problem of situating Leonardo within the history of science and medicine. His notebooks are full of brilliant projects, observations, and hypotheses about human beings, animals, light, mechanics, and more. Freud, who "psychoanalyzed" Leonardo, called the artist "the forerunner...of Bacon and Copernicus." But the grand projects were never completed, and thousands of pages of notes and sketches went unpublished. The secretive, left-handed artist kept his notebooks in code, a kind of mirror writing. It is tempting to speculate that if Leonardo had systematically completed his ambitious projects and conscientiously published and publicized his work, he might have revolutionized several scientific disciplines. Instead, Leonardo's legacy has been assessed as "the epitome of greatness in failure," because that which is unknown, incomplete, and disorganized cannot be considered a contribution to science. To regard Leonardo as typical of his era is of course unrealistic, although he had many brilliant contemporaries. Nevertheless, Leonardo's work indicates the scope of the ideas and work that a person of genius might achieve with the materials available in the fifteenth century.

Leonardo, who was the illegitimate son of a peasant woman and a Florentine lawyer, grew up in his father's house. At 14 years of age, Leonardo was apprenticed to Andrea del Verrochio (1435–1488), painter, sculptor, and the foremost teacher of art in Florence. Verrochio insisted that all his pupils learn anatomy. Within 10 years, Leonardo was recognized as a distinguished artist and had acquired wealthy and powerful patrons. Despite these advantages, Leonardo led a restless and adventurous life, serving various patrons, prosecuted on charges of homosexuality, beginning and discarding numerous projects for machines, statues, and books. It was art that first led Leonardo to dissection, but he pursued anatomical studies of animals and humans with almost morbid fascination for nearly 50 years, dissecting pigs, oxen, horses, monkeys, insects, and so forth. Granted permission to study cadavers at a hospital in Florence, the artist spent many sleepless nights surrounded by corpses. While planning a revolutionary anatomical treatise, Leonardo dissected about thirty bodies, including a seven-month fetus and a very elderly man.

Studies of the superficial anatomy of the human body had inexorably led Leonardo to an exploration of general anatomy, comparative anatomy, and physiological experiments. Through dissection and experimentation, Leonardo believed he would uncover the mechanisms that governed movement and even life itself. Leonardo constructed models to study the mechanism of action of muscles and the heart valves and carried out vivisections to gain insight into the heartbeat. For example, he drilled through the thoracic wall of a pig and, keeping the incision open with pins, observed the motion of the heart. Although he realized that the heart was actually a very powerful muscle, he generally accepted Galen's views on the movement and distribution of the blood, including the imaginary pores in the septum. Like so many of his projects, Leonardo's great book on the anatomy of "natural man" was left unfinished. When he died, his manuscripts were scattered among various libraries, and some were probably lost.

Convinced that all problems could be reduced to mechanics and mathematics, Leonardo was contemptuous of astrology and alchemy and distrustful of medicine. Indeed, he believed that preserving one's health was most easily accomplished by avoiding doctors and their drugs. Like Cato and Pliny, he denounced physicians as "the destroyers of life," who lusted after wealth despite their inability to make an informed diagnosis. Leonardo's notebooks, however, contain prescriptions as bizarre as any Galenical remedy, such as a mixture of nutshells, fruit pits, and chickpeas to break up stones in the bladder.

## ANDREAS VESALIUS ON THE FABRIC OF THE HUMAN BODY

Just as Copernicus and Galileo revolutionized ideas about the motions of the earth and the heavens, Andreas Vesalius (1514–1564) transformed Western concepts of the structure of the human body. Vesalius' great treatise, *The Fabric of the Human Body* (*De humani corporis fabrica*), appeared in 1543, the year in which Nicolaus Copernicus (1473–1543) published the text that placed the sun, rather than the earth, at the center of the universe (*On the Revolutions of the Heavenly Spheres*). Vesalius was heir to the humanist medical tradition that had rediscovered the original writings of Hippocrates and Galen. He was a member of the first generation of scholars to enjoy access to the complete works of Galen. The *Fabrica*, which is considered the first anatomical treatise based on direct observation of the human body, is still regarded as a milestone in the history of anatomy. In honor of its place in the history of Western medicine, in 1998, scholars began publishing a five-volume English translation of the first edition of the *Fabrica*.

Given the scope of his work, Vesalius can be considered a classical scholar and humanist, as well as a physician, anatomist, and artist. Unlike Linacre and Caius, however, Vesalius was able to renounce

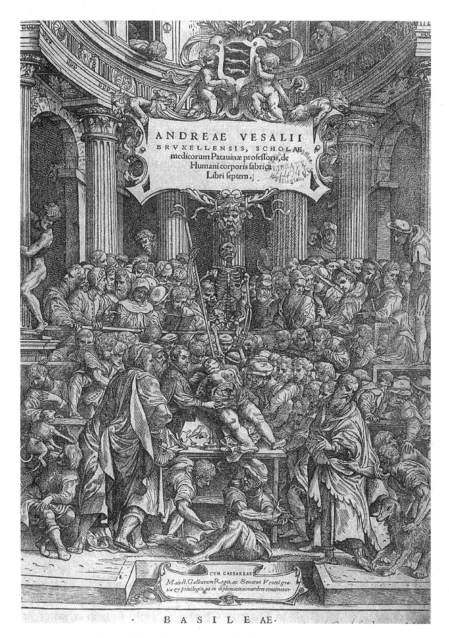

**Andreas Vesalius, on the fabric of the human body.**

the errors of the ancients clearly and publicly. Through his scholarship and his own observations, he came to realize that human anatomy must be read from the "book of the human body," not from the pages of Galen. With all due modesty, Vesalius regarded his work as the first real advance in anatomical knowledge since the time of Galen.

A horoscope cast by Girolamo Cardano, a Milanese physician, fixes the birth of Andreas Vesalius in Brussels, Belgium, on December 31, 1514, at 5:45 a.m. Vesalius was born into a world of physicians, pharmacists, and royal patronage. His father was imperial pharmacist to Charles V and often accompanied the Emperor on his travels. As a youth, Vesalius began to teach himself anatomy by dissecting mice and other small animals. Although he studied at both the University of Paris and Louvain, institutions notable for their extreme conservatism, his innate curiosity was not destroyed by the benefits of higher education.

While a student at the University of Paris, Vesalius served as assistant to Jacobus Sylvius (1478–1555), an archconservative who saw human dissection only as a means of pursuing Galenic studies. Unfortunately, the atmosphere in Paris became so threatening that Vesalius found it necessary to leave without a degree. In the fall of 1537, he enrolled in the medical school of the University of Padua, a venerable, but relatively enlightened institution. He was awarded the M.D. in December 1537, and appointed lecturer-demonstrator in anatomy and surgery. Abandoning the traditional professorial role, Vesalius lectured and dissected simultaneously. These dissection-lectures occupied the anatomist and his audience from morning to night for three weeks at a time. To minimize the problem of putrefaction, anatomies were scheduled for the winter term. Several bodies were used simultaneously so that different parts could be clearly demonstrated. Anatomies began with a study of the skeleton, and then proceeded to the muscles, blood vessels, nerves, organs of the abdomen and chest, and the brain.

By 1538, Vesalius was beginning to recognize differences between Galenic anatomy and his own observations, but when the young anatomist publicly challenged Galen, Sylvius denounced his former student as "Vesanus" (madman), purveyor of filth and sewage, pimp, liar, and various epithets unprintable even in our own permissive era. Vesalius in turn told his students that they could learn more at a butcher shop than at the lectures of certain blockhead professors. Referring to the dissection skills of his former teacher, Vesalius said that Sylvius and his knife were more at home at the banquet table than the dissecting room. In 1539, Marcantonio Contarini, a judge in Padua's criminal court, became so interested in Vesalius's work that he awarded the bodies of executed criminals to the university and obligingly set the time of execution to suit the anatomist's convenience.

Finally, to mark his independence from Galen, Vesalius arranged a public dissection lecture in which he demonstrated over two hundred differences between the skeletons of apes and humans, while reminding his audience that Galen's work was based on the dissection of apes. Hostile reactions from outraged Galenists were inevitable. Vesalian anatomists were vilified as the "Lutherans of Physic" on the grounds that the heresies of such medical innovators were as dangerous as Martin Luther's

(1483–1546) effect on religion. Tired of the controversy, Vesalius became court physician to Charles V, Holy Roman Emperor and King of Spain, to whom he dedicated the *Fabrica*. Soon Vesalius discovered that imperial service was almost as unpleasant as the stormy academic world.

The patronage of a king, pope, or wealthy nobleman might allow a scientist to continue his research, but such patrons were often difficult and demanding patients. Charles V suffered from gout, asthma, and a variety of vague complaints exacerbated by his predilection for quack remedies. Moreover, kings often loaned their physicians to other royal courts. Thus, when Henry II of France was injured while jousting, Vesalius and the French surgeon Ambroise Paré were among the medical consultants. Using the heads of four recently decapitated criminals, Paré and Vesalius carried out experiments to ascertain the nature of the injuries. They correctly predicted that the wound would be fatal. According to a doubtful, but persistent tradition, Vesalius went on a pilgrimage to the Holy Land to extricate himself from the Emperor's service, or as a penance for initiating a premature autopsy. Vesalius may have used the excuse of a pilgrimage to explore the possibility of returning to a professorship at Padua. Unfortunately, he died on the return voyage.

Despite being steeped in the conservative academic scholarship of his time, Vesalius confronted and rejected Galen's authority and demanded that anatomists study only the "completely trustworthy book of man." Vesalius attributed his own disillusionment with Galen to his discovery that Galen had never dissected the human body. However, a minor work, known as the "Bloodletting Letter," suggests that practical problems concerning venesection forced Vesalius to question Galenic dogma. Venesection was the subject of violent controversy among sixteenth-century physicians. No one suggested abandoning bloodletting; rather, the medical humanists attacked what they called corrupt Arabist methods and demanded a return to the pure teachings of Hippocrates and Galen.

Unfortunately, even after "purification," Galen's teachings on the venous system remained ambiguous. When Hippocratic texts contradicted each other and Galen, which authority could tell the physician how to select the site for venesection, how much blood to take, how rapidly bleeding should proceed, and how often to repeat the procedure? Struggling with these questions, Vesalius began to ask whether facts established by anatomical investigation could be used to test the validity of hypotheses. Unable to ignore the implications of his anatomical studies and clinical experience, Vesalius became increasingly critical of the medical humanists. He could not tolerate the way they ignored the true workings of the human body while they debated "horse-feathers and trifles."

*The Fabric of the Human Body* was a revolutionary attempt to describe the human body as it really is without deferring to Galen when the truth could be learned through dissection. Vesalius also demonstrated how well anatomical truths could be conveyed in words and illustrations. About 250 woodblocks were painstakingly prepared and incorporation into the text where their placement complemented and clarified matters described in the text. Ironically, critics of Vesalian anatomy attacked the *Fabrica* on the grounds that the illustrations were false and misleading and would seduce students away from direct observation. Actually, the importance of dissection is emphasized throughout the text and careful instructions were given on the preparation of bodies for dissection and the instruments needed for precise work on specific anatomical materials.

The *Fabrica* was intended for serious anatomists, but Vesalius also prepared a shorter, less expensive text, known as the *Epitome*, so that even medical students could appreciate the "harmony of the human body." The *Epitome* contained eleven plates showing the bones, muscles, external parts, nerves, veins, and arteries, and pictures of organs that were meant to be traced, cut out, and assembled by the reader. The Vesalian texts and illustrations were widely plagiarized and disseminated, often in the form of inferior translations and abstracts that failed to credit the originals.

In response to his critics, Vesalius denounced the "self-styled Prometheans" who claimed that Galen was always right and argued that the alleged errors in his works were proof that the human body had degenerated since the classical era. Galenists, Vesalius declared, could not distinguish between the fourth carpal bone and a chickpea, but they wanted to destroy his work just as their predecessors had destroyed the works of Herophilus and Erasistratus. Recalling how he had once been under Galen's influence, Vesalius admitted that he used to keep the head of an ox handy to demonstrate the *rete mirabile*, a network of blood vessels that Galen had placed at the base of the human brain. Unable to find the *rete mirabile* in human cadavers, anatomists rationalized this inconsistency by asserting that, in humans, the structure disappeared very soon after death. When Vesalius finally came to terms with Galen's fallibility, he openly declared that such a network was not present in humans.

In contrast to his revolutionary treatment of anatomy, Vesalius did not go much further than Galen and Aristotle in physiology and embryology. He gave an exhaustive description of the structure of the heart, arteries, and veins, and was skeptical of the Galenic claim that the blood moved from right heart to left heart through pores in the septum, but the motion of the blood remained obscure. Thus, while Galen was challenged on anatomical details, his overall anatomical and physiological doctrines remained intact. For example, having ruled out the presence of the *rete mirabile* in humans, Vesalius had to find an alternative site for the generation of the animal spirits. By interpreting Galen's various

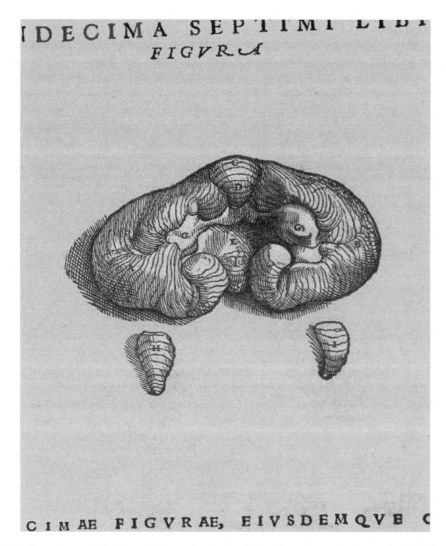

**Inferior view of the cerebellum as depicted in *De Humani Corporis Fabrica*, 1543.**

accounts of the process that generated them, Vesalius concluded that Galen thought that only part of this process occurred in the *rete mirabile*; the final modifications may have involved the brain and its ventricles. Vesalius could, therefore, ascribe the function of the nonexistent *rete mirabile* to the general vicinity of the cerebral arteries.

Historians generally agree that anatomical research has been the cornerstone of Western medicine since the sixteenth century. Inspired by the new Vesalian anatomy, physicians focused on direct observation of the body as the only means of generating valid anatomical knowledge. But anatomical knowledge and the right to perform human dissection also served as a means of establishing a unique professional identity and asserting power over life and death. The emphasis on human dissection as an essential aspect of medical education, however, led to increasing tension between the apparently insatiable need for cadavers and the widespread prejudice against human dissection. Until recent times, anatomists were often forced into dangerous and illegal methods of obtaining human bodies. As a medical student in Paris, Vesalius fought off savage dogs while collecting human bones from the Cemetery of the Innocents. In Louvain, he stole the remains of a robber chained to the gallows and brought the bones back into the city hidden under his coat. Grave-robbing incidents were reported wherever Vesalius conducted his famous lecture-demonstrations. One ingenious group of medical students reportedly obtained a corpse, dressed it, and walked their prize into the dissecting room as if it were just another drunken student being dragged into class. Despite anecdotes that feature the bravado of enterprising anatomists, being associated in the popular mind with hangmen and grave robbers was humiliating and dangerous to anatomists. When anatomists were fortunate enough to obtain cadavers, they faced grave dangers during routine dissections, because even the smallest cut could result in a fatal infection.

Long after most European nations had made legal provisions for anatomical studies, body snatching provided the bulk of the teaching material for gross anatomy in Great Britain, Canada, and the United States. Anatomists too timid to obtain cadavers themselves turned to entrepreneurs known as "Resurrectionists" or "Sack-Em-Up Men," who procured bodies by grave robbing, extortion, and murder. In England, under the Murder Act of George II, the bodies of criminals considered vile enough to be worthy of death and dissection were awarded to the Royal College of Surgeons as a "peculiar mark of Infamy added to the Punishment." When England's 1832 Anatomy Act allowed the state to give the unclaimed bodies of paupers to medical schools, poverty became virtually as deeply stigmatized as criminality. It is interesting to note that the Visible Human Project began with the use of a 39-year-old criminal executed by lethal injection in 1993. The body was frozen, sectioned, and transformed into the first fully digitized human being. Today, the National Library of Medicine's Visible Human Project provides invaluable radiological scans and digitalized photographs of cross-sections of a male and a female cadaver.

American physicians also attempted to establish a professional identity through anatomical knowledge. This created an infamous black market for cadavers. Following the example set in England, physicians successfully lobbied for laws that allocated paupers' bodies to medical schools. But scandalous stories of body snatching and dissection-room pranks continued to inflame the public. Advocates of improved medical and surgical training were obliged to remind legislators and laymen that if doctors did not practice on cadavers, they would have to learn the art at the expense of their patients. The Latin motto used by Medical Examiners and Pathology Departments around the world—"*Hic locus est ubi mors gaudet succurrere vitae*" (This is the place where death delights to help the living)—stresses the insights physicians and researchers gain through human dissection.

By the beginning of the twentieth century, gross anatomy had become an essential part of the curriculum at every American medical school. By the end of that century, the hours devoted to formal anatomy training had sharply declined and the shortage of instructors had become more significant than the problem of obtaining cadavers. Many medical educators argued that computerized scans and three-dimensional representations of the human body provided better teaching tools than traditional dissections, although standardizing models ignores the variability of human anatomy. Others insist that human dissection is an essential aspect of conveying the lesson of human mortality and the meaning of being a doctor. The French anatomist Marie François Xavier Bichat (1771–1802) stressed the importance of conducting autopsies. "Open up a few corpses," he wrote, "you will dissipate at once the darkness that observation alone could not dissipate."

## MEDICINE AND SURGERY

On at least one important point Galen and Vesalius were in full agreement. Both argued that medicine and anatomy had degenerated because physicians had given up the practice of surgery and dissection. During the Middle Ages, the distinction between theoretical and practical medicine had been exaggerated by learned physicians, and power plays within university faculties exacerbated this tension. To enhance the dignity of the medical faculty, theoretical, logical, and universal ideas concerning the nature of human beings were emphasized at the expense of empirical and mechanical aspects of the healing art. While the Scientific Revolution produced little change in medical practice, even the most highly educated physician was becoming susceptible to the germs of skepticism. Instead of admitting their limitations, physicians tried to maintain the illusion of the infallibility of the rules and principles of medicine, while blaming failures on errors made by patients and apothecaries.

During this period, however, patients could still select specific kinds of practitioners out of a diverse field in order to fit their budget and their own perception of their medical condition. There is evidence that patients expected the healers they hired to produce significant results. The records of the Protomedicato, the judicial arm of the College of Medicine in Bologna, for example, contain cases where patients sued practitioners for breach of contract. That is, healers entered into contracts that promised to cure patients within a specific time. However, when the healers were actually physicians, the courts endorsed payment for services rather than for results, because physicians were professionals rather than craftsmen.

Physicians might have been engaged in increasingly sophisticated debates about the nature and cause of disease, but their therapeutics lagged far behind their most novel theories. Wise or cynical laymen noted that life and death appeared to be unaffected by medical treatment. A king might have the best physicians in the world, but when ill, his chances of recovery were not really any better than those of a poor peasant with no doctor at all. When therapeutics was the weakest link in medicine, psychological comfort was the practitioner's major contribution. Under these conditions, the quack might provide more comfort, at lower cost.

Although surgery and medicine could not be totally disentangled, traditions and laws delineated the territorial rights of practitioners. As a general rule, surgeons were expected to deal with the *exterior* of the body and physicians dealt with its *interior*. Surgeons dealt with wounds, fractures, dislocations, bladder stones, amputations, skin diseases, and syphilis. They performed bleedings under the direction of physicians, but were expected to defer to physicians in the prescription of postoperative care. Surgical practice was itself divided into separate areas of status, competence, and privilege among surgeons, barber-surgeons, and barbers.

University-trained physicians were a tiny minority of those who professed knowledge of the healing arts, but they were especially concerned with the status of the medical profession. Physicians considered themselves men of letters. Still echoing Galen, physicians contended: "He that would be an excellent physician must first be a philosopher." Physicians argued that medicine was a science that must be learned from classical texts, not a craft to be learned by experience. Elite physicians could command a salary many times greater than that of surgeons. The status differential between physicians and surgeons is also apparent in the services they were willing to provide. For example, judiciously appraising service in plague pesthouses as a potential death sentence, physicians remained outside and shouted advice to the surgeons, who examined and treated the patients. Despite such hazardous duty, surgeons were poorly paid. For example, a young surgical apprentice appointed to a pesthouse in 1631 (after two surgeons died of the plague) was later awarded just enough money to buy new clothing so that he could burn the clothes he had worn for eight months while in the pesthouse. If the sick could not afford physicians or surgeons they could consult apothecaries, practitioners who had secured the right to a monopoly on preparing and selling drugs.

In many areas, a license to practice medicine could be obtained on the basis of education or by an examination measuring practical skills. Learned physicians saw the latter form of licensing as a loophole through which their unlettered, ignorant competitors gained legal recognition. This "loophole"—the demonstration of skill and experience—was especially important to women, because they were denied access to a university degree. Most women practitioners seem to have been the widows of physicians or surgeons, but some were licensed for their skill in treating particular problems. Female practitioners were occasionally recruited by the public health authorities to care for female patients quarantined in pesthouses during plague outbreaks.

Today, specialization is regarded as a sign of maturity in the evolution of a profession. However, in premodern times, "specialists" such as oculists, bonesetters, and cutters of the stone were more likely to be uneducated empirics than learned physicians. Licensed physicians constantly complained about competition from great hordes of ignorant empirics. Not all educated laymen agreed with the physicians' assessment of the distinction between physicians and the empirics. In particular, the plague years convinced many observers that much that had been written by learned doctors produced "much smoke" but "little light."

## AMBROISE PARÉ AND THE ART OF SURGERY

Of course, the education, training, status, and legal standing of surgeons and physicians varied considerably throughout Europe. But almost everywhere, warfare provided golden opportunities for enterprising surgeons; the battlefield has always been known as the ultimate medical school. In such an environment, it was possible for Ambroise Paré (1510–1590), an "unlettered" barber-surgeon, to think his own thoughts, learn by experience, and bring pride and dignity to the art of surgery. To Paré surgery was a divine calling, despite the lowly status of its practitioners. Described by his contemporaries as independent, gentle, impetuous, and ambitious, Paré was honest enough to admit that his major contributions to surgery were simple and not necessarily original. Nevertheless, his willingness to break with tradition and courageously follow methods suggested by his own observations pointed the way towards a general renaissance in surgery. Unlike previous generations of innovative craftsmen, Paré and his peers could emerge from obscurity because the printing press allowed them to publish popular texts in the vernacular. Paré's writings were collected and reprinted many times during his lifetime and translated into Latin, German, English, Dutch, and Japanese. Always willing to learn from ancient authorities, contemporary physicians and surgeons, or even quacks with

a promising remedy, Paré was a deeply religious man, who acknowledged only one final authority.

Little is known about Paré's background and early life. Even the
date of his birth and his religion are uncertain. Paré rarely discussed
his training and apprenticeship, other than the fact that he had lived
in Paris for three years during the nine or ten years he had studied surgery. Although apprenticeship was ostensibly a time for learning, pupils
were all too often exploited by cruel masters who neglected their obligation to teach. To obtain more practical experience, Paré worked at
the Hôtel Dieu, a hospital that provided examples of a great variety
of disorders, as well as opportunities to participate in autopsies and anatomical demonstrations. Conditions at the hospital were so miserable
that during one winter, four patients had the tips of their noses frozen
and Paré had to amputate them.

Paré's surgical texts provide vivid and moving accounts of the
horrors of war, as well as accounts of the kinds of wounds caused by
weapons unknown to Hippocrates and Galen. After a battle, the stench
of rotting corpses seemed to poison the air; wounds became putrid,
corrupt, and full of worms. All too often, injured soldiers died from
lack of food and attention, or from the economy measures used to treat
them. For example, surgeons believed that mild contusions were best
treated with bed rest, bleeding, wet cupping, and sweat-inducing drugs.
Such gentle and time-consuming treatments were fine for officers and
nobles, but a common soldier was more likely to be wrapped in a cloth,
covered with a little hay, and buried in manure up to his neck to
encourage sweating.

Gunpowder weapons were, as Francis Bacon noted, among the
world-shaking inventions unknown to the ancients. Although gunpowder was referred to in Europe as early as the thirteenth century, it
was not until the fourteenth century that pictures of primitive cannons
appeared. Thus, to rationalize the treatment of gunpowder wounds,
physicians had to argue from analogies. John of Vigo (1460–1525),
one of the first to write specifically on the surgical problems of the
new warfare, argued that wounds made by firearms were poisoned. Traditionally, poisoned wounds, such as snakebites, were neutralized by
cauterization. To assure that deep, penetrating gunpowder wounds were
thoroughly cauterized, Vigo recommended the use of boiling oil. When
Paré began his career in military surgery, he followed Vigo's methods
until his supply of oil was exhausted and he was forced to treat the rest
of his patients with a wound dressing made of eggs, oil of roses, and turpentine. In comparing the outcome of these treatments, Paré discovered
that the patients who had received the mild dressing healed better than
those cauterized with boiling oil. Based on these observations, Paré
promised himself that he would never again rely on books when he

could learn from experience. In his writings, Paré urged other surgeons to follow his example.

When cauterization was necessary, Paré preferred the "actual cautery" (red hot irons) to the "potential cautery" (strong acids or bases, boiling oil). To aid the healing of burned flesh, Paré recommended a dressing of raw onions and salt. An elderly female healer taught Paré about the use of raw chopped onion in the treatment of burns. After conducting his own tests, Paré determined that the remedy was effective. In the 1950s, scientists reported that onions contain a mild antimicrobial agent. Thus, in the absence of modern antibiotics, onion might be valuable in preventing bacterial superinfection of burns. In some cases, however, Paré recommended the use of his famous puppy oil balm. He had procured the secret recipe for puppy oil at great trouble and expense, but he openly published it for the benefit of all surgeons and patients. To prepare puppy oil dressing, the surgeon began by cooking two newborn puppies in oil of lilies until the bones dissolved. The oil was mixed with turpentine and a pound of earthworms, and then cooked over a slow fire. Paré was convinced that puppy oil soothed pain and promoted healing.

When the Faculty of Physicians challenged Paré to explain why so many men died of minor gunpowder wounds, Paré examined the components of gunpowder to see whether the ingredients contained a special venom or fire. He concluded that there was neither fire nor venom in gunpowder. Indeed, soldiers, blessedly ignorant of medical theory, drank gunpowder in wine to stimulate healing, or applied gunpowder to wounds as a drying agent. Quoting Hippocrates' *On Airs, Places, and Waters*, Paré argued that the noxious air of the battlefield corrupted the blood and humors so that after a battle even small wounds became putrid and deadly. Finally, Paré suggested that many of these deaths were due to the will of God. If it seems unfair for Paré to blame wound infection on God, it should be remembered that when a patient recovered, Paré invariably said that he dressed the wound, but God healed the patient.

Battlefield surgery often included the amputation of arms or legs, an operation that could lead to death from hemorrhage. Many patients died after amputations because cauterization destroyed the flaps of skin needed to cover the amputation site and increased the danger of infection. The use of the ligature for the repair of torn blood vessels was an old but neglected technique when Paré brought it to the attention of his contemporaries and demonstrated its value in amputations. If the surgeon had performed his task with skill, wealthy patients could be fitted with ingenious and beautifully ornamented prosthetic devices that allowed for various degrees of movement. Paré also devised wooden legs suitable for the poor.

When Paré suffered a compound fracture of the leg, he was fortunate to avoid the usual treatment, which was amputation. (In a simple fracture, there is no external wound. Compound fractures involve a break in the skin; the existence of this external wound often leads to complications.) In 1561, Paré was kicked by his horse; two bones in his left leg were broken. Afraid of being kicked again, he stepped back and fell to the ground, causing the fractured bones to break through flesh, hose, and boot. The only medicaments that could be found in the village—egg whites, wheat flour, oven soot, and melted butter—did nothing to assuage the excruciating pain, which Paré suffered with quiet dignity. Knowing the usual course of such injuries, Paré feared that he must lose his leg to save his life, but the fracture was reduced, the wound was bandaged, the leg was splinted, and rose ointment was applied until the abscess drained.

Despite Paré's reputation for kindness, he had a consuming curiosity that made him willing to use human beings as experimental subjects. When Charles IX praised the virtues of a bezoar stone (a hard indigestible mass found in the stomach or intestinal tract of animals) he had received as a gift, Paré argued that such stones were not really effective antidotes to poisons. To settle the argument, one of the king's cooks, who was about to be hanged for stealing two silver plates, was allowed to participate in Paré's experiment. The condemned man was given the bezoar stone and a poison provided by the court apothecary. Unfortunately for the cook, Paré was correct about the uselessness of bezoar stones, as well as many other widely prescribed and fearfully expensive remedies and antidotes, such as unicorn horn and mummy powder. Noblemen drank from vessels made of unicorn horn and carried unicorn horn with them when traveling in order to ward off illness, much as modern tourists rely on quinine, Dramamine, and Kaopectate. True unicorn horn was very expensive because the bashful creature could only be captured by a beautiful virgin, but the major sources of unicorn horns were the rhinoceros and the narwhale.

Expressing skepticism about the existence of the unicorn, Paré conducted a series of experiments on alleged unicorn horns, such as examining the effect of unicorn preparations on the behavior and survival of venomous spiders, toads, scorpions, and poisoned pigeons. In no case did unicorn horn demonstrate any medicinal virtues. Despite Paré's work and the questions raised by other skeptics, apothecaries vigorously defended the virtues of "true" (high quality, high price) unicorn horn. On aesthetic and medical grounds, Paré rejected the use of mummy powder; he said it was shameful for Christians to consume remedies allegedly derived from the dead bodies of pagans. Ever skeptical, Paré revealed that expensive preparations sold as the mummies of ancient Egyptians were actually fabricated in France from bodies that had been dried in a furnace and dipped in pitch. But some physicians recommended mummy in the treatment of bruises and contusions, because of its alleged power to prevent blood from coagulating in the body. Advocates of mummy as a medicine urged physicians to select high quality, shiny black preparations, because inferior products that were full of bone and dirt, and gave off an offensive odor, were not effective. Well into the seventeenth century, physicians were still prescribing a variety of disgusting remedies, including mummy preparations, bezoar, powdered vipers, dried animal parts, human placentas, the entrails of moles, and filings or moss from an unburied human skull. Such remedies were also found in various editions of the London Pharmacopoeia.

Opposing the use of established remedies required courage and independence. When Paré published his studies of poisons and anti- dotes, physicians and apothecaries attacked him for trespassing on their territory. One critic claimed that one must believe in the medical virtues of unicorn horn because all the authorities had proclaimed its efficacy. Paré replied that he would rather be right, even if that required standing all alone, than join with others in their errors. Ideas that had been accepted for long periods of time were not necessarily true, he argued, because they were often founded upon opinions rather than facts.

Although Ambroise Paré was the exemplar of sixteenth-century French medicine, thanks to Louis XIV's (1638–1715) fistula-in-ano, Charles-François Félix (1635?–1703) had a rare opportunity to demon- strate the efficacy of the art of the surgery. For many months, physi- cians had subjected the king to emetics, purges, leeches, bleedings, and other futile and dangerous remedies. The king's distress was caused by a seed or fecalith that had lodged itself in the royal rectum, causing inflammation, abscesses, and a fistula. On November 18, 1686, the desperate king turned from medicine to surgery. According to Félix's enemies, the surgeon had been practicing for the operation in a Parisian hospital. Some of his human guinea pigs did not survive, but their deaths were attributed to poisoning and the corpses were disposed of secretly. In any case, the operation on the king was entirely successful. A much relieved and grateful monarch granted royal rewards and favors to the surgeons, much to the displeasure of the physicians.

## THE OCCULT SCIENCES: ASTROLOGY AND ALCHEMY

Scientists and scholars once looked at the sixteenth and seventeenth centuries as the period in which "rationalism" began to replace magical and even religious thinking, or at least push occultism to the periphery. Since the 1970s, many historians have labored mightily to find evidence that the great figures once regarded as founders of a rational, experi- mental, scientific method were actually more interested in astrology, alchemy, and other forms of mysticism and occult phenomena. To be historically accurate, it is anachronistic to use the terms "science" and "scientist" for this time period, but historians note that astrology and natural magic could be considered proper examples of "applied science."

Historians once emphasized the artistic and scientific triumphs of the Renaissance, but recently scholars have focused on the many ways in which superstition and the occult sciences flourished. Medicine, along with the other arts and sciences, remained entangled with astrology, alchemy, and other varieties of mysticism. Out of this mixture of art, science, and magic arose new challenges to medical theory, philosophy, and practice. One form of prognosis known as astrological medicine was based on the assumption that the motions of the heavenly bodies influenced human affairs and health. More broadly, astrology was a form of divination. In practice, astrological medicine required knowing the exact time at which the patient became ill. With this information and a study of the heavens, the physician could prognosticate the course of illness with mathematical precision and avoid dangerous tendencies. In therapeutics, astrological considerations determined the nature and timing of treatments, the selection of drugs, and the use of charms. For example, the sun ruled the chronic diseases, Saturn was blamed for melancholy, and the moon, which governed the tides and the flow of blood in the veins, influenced the outcome of surgery, bloodletting, purging, and acute illness. The putative relationships between the heavenly bodies and the human body were so complex, numerous, and contradictory that in practice it was impossible to carry out any operation without breaking some rule. While medical astrology occupies a prominent place in the Renaissance, it can be seen as a continuity of popular medieval doctrines that were not necessarily linked to scholarly medical theory. Physicians may have continued to study and utilize medical astrology, but many Renaissance medical treatises ignored or even explicitly condemned astrology.

Even in the twenty-first century, a quick survey of shelves in most major bookstores indicates that astrology attracts many more readers than astronomy. Chemists, secure in their knowledge that alchemy has few devotees today, have long been amused at the continuous battle against superstition waged by astronomers. Alchemists, however, occupy an ambiguous position in the history of medicine and science, praised as pioneers of modern chemistry, damned as charlatans, or treated reverently as purveyors of an alternative way of knowing the universe.

It is generally assumed that the primary goal of alchemy was to transform base metals into gold, but alchemy is a term that encompasses a broad range of doctrines and practices. Particularly in Chinese medicine, alchemy encompassed the search for the elixirs of health, longevity, and immortality. In Western history, the idea that the task of alchemy was not to make gold or silver, but to prepare medicines, can be found in the writings of Philippus Aureolus Theophrastus Bombastus von Hohenheim (1493–1541), alchemist, physician, and pharmacologist. Fortunately, he is generally referred to as Paracelsus (higher than Celsus), the term adopted by the Paracelsians of the seventeenth century, who believed that therapeutics could be revolutionized by the development of chemical or spagyric drugs. (Spagyric comes from the Greek words meaning "to separate" and "to assemble.") Little is known with any certainty about his early life and education. Although he left behind a large, if disorganized, collection of writings in medicine, natural philosophy, astrology, and theology, only one authentic portrait exists. His place in the history of medicine is ambiguous, but in modern German history, Paracelsus served as a major cultural icon during the Nazi era.

After a brief period as a student at the University of Basel, Paracelsus became tired of academic dogmatism and immersed himself in the study of alchemy. Instead of consulting scholars and professors, Paracelsus sought out the secret alchemical lore of astrologers, gypsies, magicians, miners, peasants, and alchemists. Although there is no evidence that he ever earned a formal academic degree, Paracelsus bestowed upon himself the title "double doctor," presumably for honors conferred on him by God and nature. Nevertheless, Paracelsus secured an appointment as Professor of Medicine and city physician of Basel. Despite his new academic credentials, he seemed more interested in staging scenes that would now be called media events. To show his contempt for ancient dogma, he burned the works of Avicenna and Galen while denouncing orthodox pharmacists and physicians as a "misbegotten crew of approved asses." Wearing the alchemist's leather apron rather than academic robes, he lectured in the vernacular instead of Latin. Although these public displays enraged his learned colleagues, it was a dispute over a fee for medical services that forced him to flee from Basel. His enemies happily noted that he died suddenly in a mysterious, but certainly unnatural, fashion when only 48, while Hippocrates and Galen, founders of the medical system he rejected, had lived long, productive lives.

In opposition to the concept of humoral pathology, especially the doctrines of Galen and Avicenna, Paracelsus attempted to substitute the doctrine that the body was essentially a chemical laboratory, in which the vital functions were governed by a mysterious force called the *archaeus*, a sort of internal alchemist. Disease was, therefore, the result of derangements in the chemical functions of the body rather than a humoral disequilibrium. Physicians should, therefore, study the chemical anatomy of disease rather than gross anatomy. Anatomical research itself was, therefore, irrelevant to understanding the most profound questions about the vital functions of the human body. Because life

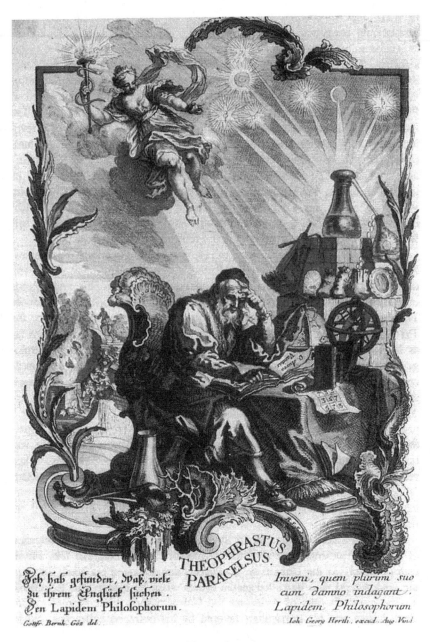

Jch hab gefunden, Was viele
zu ihrem Unglück suchen.
Den Lapidem Philosophorum.

*Gottfr. Bernh. Göz del.*

*Inveni, quem plurimi suo
cum damno indagant.
Lapidem Philosophorum*

*Joh. Georg Hertli. excud. Aug Vind.*

**Paracelsus.**

and disease were chemical phenomena, specific chemical substances must serve as remedies. The specific healing virtue of a remedy would depend on its chemical properties, not on the qualities of moistness, dryness, and so forth associated with humoral theory.

In a burst of optimism, Paracelsus declared that all diseases could be cured when, through alchemy, one came to understand the essence of life and death. The challenge of finding a specific remedy for each disease seemed overwhelming, not because of a scarcity of medicines, but because nature was one great apothecary shop. Confronting nature's embarrassment of riches, the alchemist could be guided by the method of separation, the Doctrine of Signature, and the astrological correspondences among the seven planets, seven metals, and the parts of the body.

Rejecting the Galenic principle of curing by the use of contraries, Paracelsus favored the concept that like cures like. But, discovering

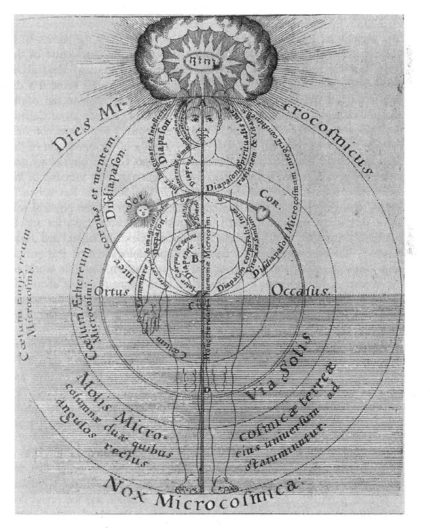

The Microcosm—a seventeenth-century alchemical chart showing the human body as world soul.

the true nature of the remedy, which was traditionally a complex mixture, could only be accomplished by alchemically separating the pure
from the impure, the useful from the useless. Within the vast *materia
medica* already known to sixteenth-century healers, poisons had always
been of particular interest, because they were obviously very powerful
agents. Paracelsus argued that alchemy made it possible to separate out
the curative virtues hidden within these perilous substances. Galenists
denounced Paracelsians as dangerous radicals who used poisons as
remedies. In response to these accusations, Paracelsus ridiculed his critics
for their use of unsafe purgatives, exorbitantly priced theriacs, and noxious mixtures made with mummy powder, dung, and urine. All things
could act as poisons, he declared, but the art of alchemy could "correct"
poisons.

In place of traditional complex herbal preparations, Paracelsus
and his followers favored the use of purified drugs, especially minerals
such as mercury, antimony, iron, arsenic, lead, copper, and their salts,
and sulfur. Determining whether new chemical remedies actually had
specific therapeutic virtues could, obviously, be very risky. Fortunately,
many toxic materials cause such rapid purgation that not enough
would be absorbed to provide a lethal dose. Moreover, in some cases,
the alchemical purification processes probably removed everything
but the solvent. On the other hand, some attempts at purification
produced interesting new substances. For example, attempts to distill
off the essence of wine created "strong liquors" that were made into
medicinal cordials. On occasion, entirely new and interesting drugs
emerged from the chaos of the alchemical laboratory. Of special interest
is the possibility that Paracelsus was one of the first to discover the
narcotic effects of ethyl ether, which was known as "sweet vitriol."
Not all Paracelsian drugs were derivatives of toxic metals; his "laudanum," a preparation used to induce restful sleep and ease pain, was
essentially opium in wine.

Although Paracelsus ridiculed traditional uroscopy, he accepted
the underlying idea that since urine contains wastes collected from the
whole body it must harbor valuable diagnostic clues. Instead of uroscopy by ocular inspection, he proposed diagnosis by chemical analysis,
distillation, and coagulation tests. Given the state of qualitative and
quantitative analysis, however, his chemical dissection was likely to be
about as informative as ocular inspection. In urine analysis, as in studies
of potential remedies, many Paracelsians ignored the important residues
and concentrated all their attention on the distillate. A work attributed
to Paracelsus, but generally regarded as spurious, provided instructions
for the chemical examination of urine by the measurement of volume
and specific gravity, using a measuring cylinder ingeniously designed
as a replica of the human body.

To replace humoral categories of disease, Paracelsus attempted to develop a system based on analogies to chemical processes. While generally obscure and inconsistent, his chemical concepts were peculiarly appropriate to metabolic diseases, dietary disorders, and certain occupational diseases. For example, in classifying gout as a "tartaric disease," he had indeed chosen an example of a metabolic disease in which body chemistry has gone wrong: in gouty individuals, a metabolic product forms local deposits, primarily in the joints, in a manner very roughly analogous to the way in which tartrates sediment out of wine. He also pointed to a relationship between cretinism in children and goiter in adults (disorders caused by a lack of iodine in the diet). According to Paracelsus, miners, smelter workers, and metallurgists exhibited a variety of symptoms because their lungs and skin absorbed dangerous combinations of unwholesome airs and clouds of poisonous dust. This noxious chemical mixture generated internal coagulations, precipitations, and sediments. Such examples can create the impression that Paracelsus had valid reasons for his attack on Galenism and actually held the keys to a new system of therapeutics, but it is easy to read too much into the Paracelsian literature and confuse obscurity with profundity. Nevertheless, later advocates of chemical or Paracelsian medicine were involved in the transformation of pharmacology and physiology, diagnostics, and therapeutics. The Society of Chemical Physicians was founded in 1665. Successful examples of chemical medicines forced even the most conservative physician to think about the limits of Galenism and tempted many orthodox physicians to experiment with the new remedies. Despite the opposition of the College of Physicians and its attempts to suppress the use of the new chemical remedies, the English Paracelsians achieved considerable recognition. By the mid-1670s, even those who rejected Paracelsian philosophy were beginning to accept the new chemical remedies. Moreover, debates about the chemical philosophy of life served as an alternative to the mechanistic systems that invaded the medical sciences in the wake of the Newtonian revolution. Debates between "mechanist physicians" and "chemical physicians" continued into the eighteenth century.

Despite evidence of intellectual continuity, Renaissance scholars seemed to believe that they were making a major break with the medieval and Arabic past, primarily by recapturing and assimilating classic Greek texts. Similarly, many physicians were convinced that medicine was undergoing rapid and significant changes. Physicians and surgeons were acquiring anatomical and pharmacological knowledge and ideas that promoted increasingly sophisticated debates about the nature of the human body and the cause of disease. This did not automatically change the nature or efficacy of their prescriptions and procedures, but it made the search for further knowledge possible and highly desirable.

## SYPHILIS, THE SCOURGE OF THE RENAISSANCE

The changing pattern of epidemic diseases or diagnostic categories characteristic of the Renaissance is almost as striking as the transformation
of art, science, and scholarship. Although leprosy did not entirely disappear, and waves of plague continued to break over Europe, diseases
previously rare, absent, or unrecognized—such as syphilis, typhus,
smallpox, and influenza—became major public health threats. Many
diseases are worthy of a full biography, but none raises more intriguing questions than syphilis, the "Scourge of the Renaissance." Because
syphilis is a sexually transmitted disease, it is a particularly sensitive
tracer of the obscure pathways of human contacts throughout the world,
as well as the intimate links between social and medical concepts.

In mocking tribute to Venus, the Roman goddess of love, the term
*venereal* has long served as a euphemism in matters pertaining to sex.
But in an era that prides itself on having won the sexual revolution,
the more explicit term *sexually transmitted disease* (STD) has been substituted for *venereal disease* (VD). Any disease that can be transmitted
by sexual contact may be considered a venereal disease. A more restrictive definition includes only those diseases that are never, or almost
never, transmitted by any mechanism other than sexual contact. Until
the second half of the twentieth century, syphilis and gonorrhea were
considered the major venereal diseases in the wealthy, industrialized
nations, but the so-called minor venereal diseases—chancroid, lymphogranuloma venereum, and granuloma inguinale—also cause serious
complications. Scabies and crab lice gain membership in the club if
the less rigorous definition of STD is accepted. Additional modern
members of the STD club are genital herpes, trichomoniasis, nongono-
coccal urethritis, and AIDS. Genital herpes was winning its battle to
become the most feared venereal disease in the United States until the
1980s, but since then AIDS has emerged as the great modern plague.

Despite the antiquity of references to venereal diseases, many
Renaissance physicians were convinced that syphilis was unknown in
Europe until the end of the fifteenth century; others argued that there
was one venereal scourge as old as civilization that appeared in many
guises, including those known as gonorrhea and syphilis. The confusion
is not surprising, as a brief overview of the natural history of the major
venereal diseases will indicate. A specific differential diagnosis of
syphilis or gonorrhea cannot be based on symptoms alone. In the
twentieth-century laboratory, a tentative diagnosis of syphilis can be
confirmed by the Wassermann blood test, but for gonorrhea, confirmation requires identification of *Neisseria gonorrhoeae*, a small gram-
negative gonococcus discovered by Albert Neisser (1855–1916) in 1879.

Gonorrhea is generally recognized as the oldest and probably most
common venereal disease. Galen may have given this ancient illness its

common name; gonorrhea actually means "flow of seed." Colloquial names include clap, dose, strain, drip, and hot piss. Symptoms of gonorrhea usually appear about three to five days after infection, but the incubation period may be as long as ten days. Pain, burning, and the discharge of pus from the urethra are usually the first symptoms noticed in males. Eventually, inflammation may obstruct the flow of urine and lead to a life-threatening stricture of the urethra. Surgeons attacked the problem with sounds (curved metal rods) to stretch the narrowed channel and catheters to provide relief from retention of urine. Avicenna introduced medicines into the bladder with a silver syringe, and, for good measure, inserted a louse in the urethra. (If a louse was not available, a flea or bug might do equally well.) Sedatives and opiates provided some relief from pain and anxiety, but for psychological impact, nothing could surpass quack remedies containing various dyes that caused the patient to pass technicolor waters.

In women, gonorrhea is often a silent infection that insidiously attacks the internal organs, leading to peritonitis, endocarditis, arthritis, ectopic pregnancies, spontaneous abortions, stillbirths, chronic pelvic inflammatory disease, and sterility. Infants can acquire gonorrheal infection of the eyes during birth. To prevent this form of blindness, Karl Siegmund Credé, at the Lying-In Hospital in Leipzig, introduced the application of silver nitrate to the eyes of newborns. Less frequent complications—skin lesions and arthritis, conjunctivitis, endocarditis, myocarditis, hepatitis, meningitis—can occur in men and women if the gonococcus becomes widely disseminated via the bloodstream. Many patients treated for arthritis and gout were probably suffering from gonococcal infections.

Public health authorities once thought that penicillin would eradicate gonorrhea, but in the late twentieth century gonorrhea was still the most common venereal disease and the most prevalent bacterial disease on earth. Penicillin-resistant strains have become so common since they were discovered in the 1970s that this antibiotic is no longer used for gonorrhea treatment. Trends in the development of antibiotic-resistant strains of the gonococcus provide no grounds for optimism. New "superstrains" have appeared throughout the world. By 2002, strains of both fluoroquinolone and multidrug resistant gonorrhea migrated from Asia to Hawaii to California. Previously, gonorrhea could be treated with single-dose therapy using fluoroquinolones or cephalosporins. In some regions, 60 to 80 percent of gonorrhea cases are resistant to fluoroquinolones. Treatments that alleviate symptoms without curing the infection are particularly troublesome, because patients who mistakenly think they are cured can easily infect others.

Syphilis, which is caused by a spirochetal bacterium known as *Treponema pallidum*, has been called the great mimic because in the course of its development it simulates many other diseases. Syphilitic lesions can be confused with those of leprosy, tuberculosis, scabies, fungal infections, and various skin cancers. Before the introduction of specific bacteriological and immunological tests, the diagnostic challenge of syphilis was reflected in the saying "Whoever knows all of syphilis knows all of medicine." Untreated syphilis progresses through three stages of increasing severity. A small lesion known as a chancre is the first sign. The chancre may become ulcerated or disappear altogether. The second stage may include fever, headache, sore throat, a localized rash, skin lesions, patchy bald spots, swollen and tender lymph nodes, sore mouth, and inflamed eyes. Symptoms may appear within weeks or months of infection and subside without treatment. During the third stage, chronic obstruction of small blood vessels, abscesses, and inflammation may result in permanent damage to the cardiovascular system and other major organs. Neurosyphilis causes impaired vision, loss of muscular coordination, paralysis, and insanity. A syphilitic woman may experience miscarriages or stillbirths, or bear a child with impaired vision, deafness, mental deficiency, and cardiovascular disease.

If diseases were catalogued in terms of etiological agents instead of means of transmission, syphilis would be described as a member of the treponematosis family. The treponematoses are diseases caused by members of the *Treponema* group of spirochetes (corkscrew-shaped bacteria). Although these microbes grow slowly, once established in a suitable host they multiply with inexorable patience and persistence. Syphilis is one of the four *clinically* distinct human treponematoses; the others are pinta, yaws, and bejel. In terms of microbiological and immunological tests, the causative organisms are virtually identical, but distinct differences are readily revealed in naturally occurring infections.

Some bacteriologists believe that pinta, yaws, bejel, and syphilis are variants of an ancestral spirochete that adapted to different patterns of climate and human behavior. According to what is generally known as the *unitary theory*, the nonvenereal treponematoses are ancient diseases transmitted between children. As people migrated to temperate areas and covered themselves with clothing, nonvenereal transmission was inhibited. Under these conditions, many people reached adulthood without acquiring the immunity common in more primitive times. Pinta, a disease endemic in Mexico and Central America, is characterized by skin eruptions of varying color and severity. Until *Treponema carateum* was discovered, pinta was classified among the fungal skin diseases. Yaws, a disease caused by *Treponema pertenue*, flourishes in hot, moist climates. Like syphilis, yaws leads to destruction of tissue, joints and bone. Bejel, or nonvenereal endemic syphilis, is generally acquired in childhood among rural populations living in warm, arid regions. Like syphilis, bejel has a latent phase, and afflicted individuals may be infectious for many years.

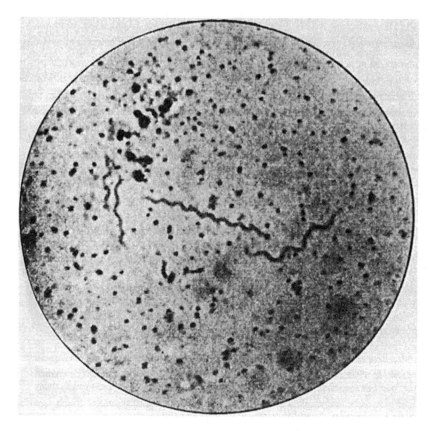

**Syphilis spirochetes as depicted by F. R. Schaudinn and P. E. Hoffmann in 1905.**

Despite advances in understanding the treponematoses, medical historians are no closer to a definitive account of the origin of syphilis than medical authorities are to eradicating STDs. Reliable accounts of syphilis first appear in the sixteenth century, when the affliction that marked its victims with loathsome skin eruptions was known by many names. The French called it the Neapolitan disease, the Italians called it the French disease, and the Portuguese called it the Castilian disease. In India and Japan, it was called the Portuguese disease, and the names Canton disease, great pox, and *lues venereum* were also used. The name used today was invented by Girolamo Fracastoro (Latinized as Fracastorius; 1478–1553), an Italian physician, scientist, mathematician, astronomer, geologist, and poet. In *Syphilis, or the French Disease* (1530), Fracastoro created the story of Syphilis the shepherd, who brought about the first outbreak of the scourge by cursing the sun. To punish men for this blasphemy, the sun shot deadly rays of disease at the earth. Syphilis was the first victim of the new pestilence, but the affliction soon spread to every village and city, even to the king himself.

Examining the historical evidence concerning the origin of syphilis is like entering a labyrinth. If we include the speculations of Fracastoro, his contemporaries, and subsequent medical writers, we come up with many theories but no definitive answer to the question raised in the sixteenth century: What causes presided at the origin of syphilis? Sixteenth-century medical astrologers traced the origin of the new venereal scourge to a malign conjunction of Jupiter, Saturn, and Mars in 1485 that produced a subtle poison that spread throughout the universe, unleashing a terrible plague upon Europe. Followers of astrology might still argue that this theory has never been disproved, but more scientifically plausible theories are still hotly debated.

The so-called Columbus Theory of the origin of syphilis is based on the fact that the New World was the source of plants and animals previously unknown to Europeans. Many Renaissance physicians, therefore, assumed that the great pox was one of the new entities imported from the New World to the Old World by Columbus and his crew. The fifteenth century was a time of great voyages, commercial expansion, and warfare, during which previously isolated peoples were suddenly immersed in a globalized germ pool. Many epidemic diseases flourished under these conditions, but it was syphilis that became known as the "calling card of civilized man."

Much circumstantial evidence supported the Columbus Theory: the timing of the voyages, the dispersal of the crew, their transformation from sailors to soldiers, their presence in areas where the disease was first reported, the testimony of physicians, the subsequent spread of syphilis, and its changing clinical pattern. Indeed, some historians blamed the physical and mental deterioration of Columbus on syphilis, although other explanations are equally plausible. While evidence for the Columbus Theory can be assembled in a fairly convincing package, it is important to remember that *coincidence* must not be confounded with *cause*. Moreover, the diagnostic value of documents designed to link "evil pocks" to immorality, human afflictions, and messages from God is somewhat suspect.

Rodrigo Ruiz Diaz de Isla (1462–1542), a Spanish physician, was probably the first to assert that members of the crew of Columbus had imported syphilis to Europe from the West Indies. In a book not published until 1539, de Isla claimed that in 1493 he had treated several sailors with a strange disease characterized by loathsome skin eruptions. Additional support for the Columbus Theory is found in reports written in 1525 by Gonzalo Hernandez de Oviedo y Valdez, Governor of the West Indies. According to Oviedo, sailors infected in the New World had joined the army of Charles VII at the siege of Naples (1494). When the French army was driven out of Italy in 1495, infected troops and camp followers sparked epidemics throughout Europe.

The Columbus Theory requires, at the very least, conclusive proof of the existence of syphilis in the New World *before* 1492. Unequivocal evidence of syphilis in Europe before the voyages of Columbus would disprove this theory. However, given the difficulties inherent in paleopathology, the diagnostic evidence for syphilis in pre-Columbian America and Europe remains problematic and the debate among historians continues. The problem is compounded by a recent tendency to blur distinctions between syphilis and nonvenereal treponemal infections.

The so-called Leprosy Theory is based on the possibility that syphilis, the great mimic, might have hidden itself among the legions of medieval lepers. References to "venereal leprosy" and "congenital leprosy" in Europe before 1492 are compatible with this theory, but all medieval allusions to a connection between leprosy and sex must be examined cautiously. According to a related sixteenth-century suggestion, the new venereal scourge was a hybrid produced by sexual intercourse between a man with leprosy and a prostitute with gonorrhea. To determine whether some of those who were called lepers were actually suffering from syphilis, scientists have looked for syphilitic lesions in bones found in leper cemeteries. The evidence remains ambiguous.

Another hypothesis known as the African or Yaws Theory essentially reverses the Columbus Theory. According to this theory, syphilis was one of the many disasters Europeans brought to the New World by merging the germ pools of Africa and Europe in the Americas. With Native Americans brought to the verge of extinction by smallpox and other foreign diseases, Europeans were importing African slaves into the New World within 20 years of the first contacts. If Africans taken to Europe and the Americas were infected with yaws, changes in climate and clothing would have inhibited nonvenereal transmission of the spirochete. Under these conditions, yaws could only survive by becoming a venereal disease.

If true, the African Theory would explain the apparent relationship between the appearance of syphilis and the adventures of Columbus and his crew. It would also provide a form of intercontinental microbiological retribution with a fitting lesson about the evils of slavery. However, this theory is based on rather weak and controversial circumstantial evidence. Given the antiquity of interchanges between Europe and Africa, yaws could have been introduced to Egypt, Arabia, Greece, and Rome from Africa centuries before the voyages of Columbus. Therefore, some other spark would be needed to trigger the fifteenth-century conflagration. Partisans of various theories have presented many ingenious arguments, but the evidence does not yet seem totally compelling. The question of the origin of syphilis is further complicated by confusion between gonorrhea and syphilis in the early literature.

Whatever the source of syphilis, Fracastoro believed that in its early stage, the disease could be cured by a carefully controlled regimen, including exercises that provoked prodigious sweats. Once the disease had taken root in the viscera, a cure required remedies almost as vile as the disease. In another flight of fancy, Fracastoro told the story of a peaceful gardener named Ilceus who was stricken with a terrible disease as punishment for killing a deer sacred to the Greek god Apollo and his sister Diana. The gods had sworn that no remedy would be found within their realm, but Ilceus journeyed to a cavern deep within the bowels of the earth. Here, he was cured when the resident nymphs plunged him into a river of pure quicksilver (mercury).

Unlike the nymphs, doctors liked to combine mercury with other agents, such as lard, turpentine, incense, lead, and sulfur. Perhaps the most bizarre prescription was that of Giovanni de Vigo (1450–1525) who added live frogs to his quicksilver ointment. Fracastoro preferred a remedy rich in mercury, black hellebore, and sulfur. Covered with this mixture, the patient was wrapped in wool and kept in bed until the disease was washed out of the body in a flood of sweat and saliva. An alternative method of curing by emaciation involved spartan diets, purges, sudorifics, and salivation induced by mercury. If this 30-day regimen did not cure syphilis, it would certainly do wonders for obesity.

Mercury became so intimately linked to the venereal scourge that quacksalvers used mercury as an operational definition for syphilis; if mercury provided a cure, the patient was syphilitic. The link between syphilis and mercury probably resulted from the belief that mercury cured diseases of the skin. Reasoning by analogy from the effectiveness of mercurial ointments for scabies and other skin disorders, doctors assumed that mercury would also triumph over syphilitic ulcers. In any case, syphilis made it possible for quacksalvers to acquire so many patients they were able to achieve the dream of the alchemists—the transmutation of mercury into gold. Patients undergoing mercury inunction sat in a tub in a hot, closed room where they could be rubbed with mercury ointments several times a day. Those who would rather read Shakespeare than ancient medical texts will find many references to the torments of syphilis and the "tub of infamy." Other references to "rubbing and tubbing" indicate that this form of treatment was very well known. If the association between syphilis and mercury had not been so completely forgotten by the end of the twentieth century, the Moral Majority would certainly have demanded censorship of the Mother Goose rhyme "Rub-a-dub-dub, three men in a tub..."

Unequivocal proof of mercury toxicity is rather recent, but suspicions about the dangers of quicksilver were not uncommon among Renaissance practitioners. Bernardino Ramazzini (1633–1714) devoted a chapter of his great treatise *On the Diseases of Workers* to "diseases of those who give mercurial inunction." As Ramazzini so aptly put it, the lowest class of surgeons performed mercury inunction because the better class of doctors would not practice "a service so disagreeable and a task so full of danger and hazard." Realizing that no fee could compensate for loss of their own health, some quacksalvers made their patients rub each other with mercurial ointments. By the early nineteenth century, some critics of mercurial remedies realized that excessive salivation and ulcers in the mouth were signs of "morbid mercurial irritation," rather than a sign that syphilis had been cured.

Even physicians who regarded mercury as a marvelous remedy were not about to let patients escape their full therapeutic arsenal. Syphilitics were dosed with brisk purgatives, clysters, sudorifics, and tonics, and subjected to bizarre dietary restrictions. Many therapeutic regimens, including that of Fracastoro, emphasized heat, exercise, and sweating. Indeed, "fever therapy," also known as therapeutic hyperthermia, was used for both syphilis and gonorrhea well into the twentieth century. Experiments on therapeutic hyperthermia utilized tuberculin, bacterial vaccines, fever cabinets, and malaria. During the first half of the twentieth century, malaria fever therapy was used in the treatment of patients with advanced neurosyphilis. Paretic patients were given intravenous injections of blood infected with *Plasmodium vivax* or *P. malariae* (the causative agents of relatively benign forms of malaria), resulting in fevers as high as 106 degrees Fahrenheit. After about 12 cycles of fever, some blood would be taken for further use and the patient would receive quinine to cure malaria. Physicians maintained favored strains of malaria by transmitting the infection from patient to patient. Theories of fever have undergone many changes since antiquity, but the significance of fever in disease is still an enigma. The rationale for fever therapy is that high body temperature must be a defense mechanism that destroys or inhibits pathogenic microbes before they kill the host. Elevation of body temperature is, however, not without risk. Not surprisingly, after undergoing therapeutic hyperthermia, many patients suffered from disorientation and other unpleasant side effects.

During the first phase of the syphilis epidemic, the only serious challenge to mercury treatment was a remedy known as guaiac, or Holy Wood. Guaiac was obtained from evergreen trees indigenous to South America and the West Indies. To explain the discovery of this remedy, Fracastoro, who had recommended vigorous exercise, sweating, and mercury, provided an appropriate myth about a group of Spanish sailors who observed natives of the New World curing syphilis with Holy Wood. According to the Doctrine of Signatures, if syphilis originated in the New World, the remedy should be found in the same region. Imported Holy Wood became the remedy of choice for physicians and their wealthy clients, while mercury remained the remedy of the poor. Attacking those who prescribed Holy Wood, Paracelsus complained that wealthy merchants and physicians who were deluding the sick by promoting expensive and useless treatments had suppressed his work on the therapeutic virtues of mercury.

One of the most influential and enthusiastic of the early anti-mercurialists, Ulrich Ritter von Hutten (1488–1523), was a victim of both the venereal disease and the noxious cures prescribed by his physicians. In 1519, von Hutten published a very personal account of guaiac and syphilis. Having suffered through eleven cures by mercury in nine years, von Hutten claimed that guaiac had granted him a complete and painless cure. He urged all victims of the venereal scourge to follow his example. However, he died only a few years after his cure, perhaps from the complications of tertiary syphilis.

Of course there were many minor challenges to mercury and Holy Wood, including preparations based on gold, silver, arsenic, lead, and dozens of botanicals. Holy Wood retained its popularity for little more than a century, but mercury was still used as an antisyphilitic in the 1940s. As humoral pathology gradually gave way to a pathology based on the search for localized internal lesions, copious salivation was no longer interpreted as a sign of therapeutic efficacy, and milder mercurial treatments gained new respect. Because of the unpredictable nature of syphilis, case histories could be found to prove the efficacy of every purported remedy.

Perhaps the long history of the medical use of mercury proves nothing but the strong bond between therapeutic delusions and the almost irresistible compulsion to do something. Quicksilver therapy for syphilis has been summed up as probably the most colossal hoax in the history of medicine. With the medical community and the public convinced that mercury cured syphilis, it was almost impossible to conduct clinical trials in which patients were deprived of this remedy. However, the Inspector General of Hospitals of the Portuguese Army noticed an interesting unplanned "clinical test" during British military operations in Portugal in 1812. Portuguese soldiers with syphilis generally received no treatment at all, while British soldiers were given vigorous mercury therapy. Contrary to medical expectation, the Portuguese soldiers seemed to recover more rapidly and completely than their British counterparts. About a hundred years later, Norwegian investigators provided further support for therapeutic restraint in a study of almost two thousand untreated syphilitics. In 1929, follow-up studies of subjects in the 1891–1910 Oslo Study indicated that at least 60 percent of the untreated syphilitics had experienced fewer long-term problems than patients subjected to mercury treatments.

Evaluating remedies for venereal disease was also complicated by widespread confusion between gonorrhea and syphilis. Many physicians assumed that gonorrhea was essentially one of the symptoms of syphilis and that, therefore, mercury was an appropriate treatment for all patients with venereal disease. In the eighteenth century, eminent British surgeon and anatomist John Hunter (1728–1793) attempted to untangle diagnostic confusion between gonorrhea and syphilis by injecting himself (or, according to a less heroic version of the story, his nephew) with pus taken from a patient with venereal disease. Unfortunately, Hunter's results increased the confusion, because he concluded that gonorrhea was a symptom of syphilis. In retrospect, his results are best explained by assuming that his patient had both syphilis and gonorrhea.

Philippe Ricord (1799–1889), author of *A Practical Treatise on Venereal Diseases: or, Critical and Experimental Researches on Inoculation Applied to the Study of These Affections*, is generally regarded as the first to separate syphilis and gonorrhea. His work brought the term "syphilis" into greater use as a replacement for the nonspecific *lues venerea*. According to Ricord, the primary symptom of syphilis was the chancre and only the primary chancre contained the "contagion" of syphilis. Because he could not find an animal model for syphilis, and he believed that it was unethical to conduct experiments on healthy humans, Ricord tested his doctrine on patients who were already suffering from venereal disease. Using a technique he called "autoinoculation," Ricord took pus from a venereal lesion and inoculated it into another site to see whether the lesion could be transferred. Although Ricord argued that his experiments proved that only pus from a primary syphilitic chancre produced a chancre at the site of inoculation, many other physicians reported that secondary syphilis was contagious.

All lingering doubts as to the distinction between syphilis and other venereal diseases were settled at the beginning of the twentieth century with the discovery of the "germ of syphilis" and the establishment of the Wassermann reaction as a diagnostic test. In 1905, Fritz Richard Schaudinn (1871–1906) and Paul Erich Hoffmann (1868–1959) identified the causal agent of syphilis, *Spirochaeta pallida*, which was later renamed *Treponema pallidum*. Hideyo Noguchi (1876–1928) quickly confirmed the discovery. Diagnostic screening was made possible in 1906 when August von Wassermann (1866–1925) discovered a specific blood test for syphilis. The Wassermann reaction redefined the natural history of syphilis, especially secondary and tertiary stages, and latent and congenital syphilis. Wassermann and his coworkers, who embarked on their research with assumptions that later proved to be incorrect, have been compared to Columbus, because they unexpectedly arrived at a remarkable new destination while searching for something quite different. Use of the Wassermann blood test as a precondition for obtaining a marriage license was widely promoted during the early twentieth century as a means of preventing the transmission of syphilis to children. Advocates of eugenics saw these tests as part of their

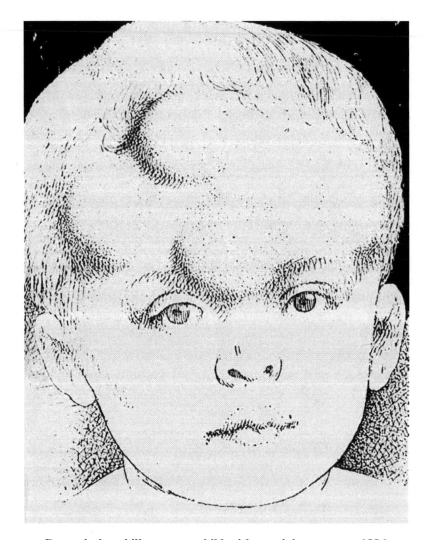

**Congenital syphilis—young child with cranial gummata, 1886.**

campaign to prevent the birth of defective children. When Noguchi demonstrated *T. pallidum* in the brains of paretics (patients suffering from paralytic dementia), the natural history of syphilis was complete, from initial chancre to paralytic insanity and death. At the time that Noguchi established the link between *T. pallidum* and paresis, patients with this form of insanity accounted for about 20 percent of first admissions to the New York State Hospitals for the mentally ill. Such patients generally died within five years.

Shortly after the identification of *Treponema pallidum* and the discovery of a sensitive diagnostic test, new drugs allowed public health officials to launch campaigns dedicated to the eradication of the venereal diseases. Prevention through abstinence or chastity had, of course, always been a possibility, but the "just say no" approach has never prevailed over the STDs. Condoms had been promoted as implements of safety since the seventeenth century, but sophisticated observers ridiculed these devices as "gossamer against disease" and "leaden against love." In 1910, when Paul Ehrlich (1854–1915) introduced the arsenical drug Salvarsan, it became possible to see syphilis as a microbial threat to the public health, rather than divine retribution for illicit sex. Success in finding a specific remedy for syphilis was made possible when Sakahiro Hata (1873–1938) developed a system to test drug activity in rabbits infected with the spirochetes. Paul Ehrlich had been testing a synthetic arsenical compound called atoxyl against the trypanosomes that cause sleeping sickness. Atoxyl destroyed trypanosomes in the test tube, but it caused blindness in human beings. By synthesizing related arsenical compounds, Ehrlich hoped to create one that was lethal to trypanosomes and safe for humans. Derivative number 606, synthesized in 1907, proved to be a "charmed bullet"—it was effective against the spirochetes of syphilis, but relatively safe for people.

Salvarsan helped physicians and patients think of syphilis as a medical rather than a moral problem, but the transition was difficult and slow. Despite advances in treatment, attitudes towards venereal disease had hardly changed since 1872 when Dr. Emil Noeggerath shocked his colleagues at a meeting of the American Gynecological Society by openly declaring that some 90 percent of sterile women were married to men who had suffered from gonorrhea. Presumably the good doctors were shocked by Dr. Noeggerath's direct discussion of venereal disease, not by his statistics. When Salvarsan and other drugs proved effective in curing the major venereal diseases, the righteous worried that God would have to find some other punishment for immorality. According to those who persist in seeing disease as punishment for individual and collective sin, genital herpes and AIDS, viral diseases beyond the reach of antibiotics, were sent to serve this purpose.

The trade name Salvarsan reflected the high hopes the pharmaceutical industry and the medical community had for the new remedy. Moralists, quacks, and those who made fortunes by defrauding victims of venereal diseases denounced Ehrlich's "modified poison." The majority of physicians, however, welcomed Salvarsan along with mercury as "destroyers of spirochetes." Though some physicians optimistically predicted that Salvarsan would eradicate the disease, more cautious or prescient observers warned that syphilis was likely to thwart such therapeutic illusions.

After a significant decline in the incidence of the disease during the 1950s, rates of infection began to climb again in the 1960s. While AIDS hysteria eclipsed other public health problems in the 1980s, the Centers for Disease Control continued to report an increase in primary and secondary syphilis. Certainly, the persistence of gonorrhea and syphilis—despite Salvarsan, penicillin, venereal disease control programs, case finding and tracing of sexual contacts, premarital testing, endless moralizing and preaching, and educational campaigns—does not promote optimism about the control of AIDS, the new "venereal scourge." Both AIDS and syphilis present fascinating biological puzzles that require an understanding of social and environmental forces, as well as microbiology and immunology. Indeed, it is almost impossible to resist drawing parallels between syphilis, with its five hundred year history, and AIDS, which has been known as a diagnostic entity only since the 1980s. Fears, prejudice, and lack of effective or enlightened medical and public responses typify the reaction to both diseases. In particular, the history of the infamous Tuskegee Study is indicative of the way in which deep social and cultural pathologies are revealed through the stigmata of specific diseases.

## SYPHILIS AND HUMAN EXPERIMENTATION

In 1932, the United States Public Health Service initiated a study of the natural history of untreated syphilis, very loosely modeled on the Oslo Study, although the project was not motivated by therapeutic skepticism. Conducted in Macon County, Alabama, with the assistance of personnel at the Tuskegee Institute, the Veterans Administration Hospital in Tuskegee, the Macon County Health Department, and so forth, the experiment became known as the Tuskegee Study, although in the 1970s, the Tuskegee Institute claimed to have had little or no contact with the experiment after the 1930s. Six hundred poor black men were recruited for the study with promises of free medical care and money for burial (after autopsy): four hundred were diagnosed as syphilitic and two hundred were selected to serve as uninfected controls.

Published reports from the Tuskegee Study of Untreated Syphilis in the Negro Male appeared with some regularity from 1936 into the 1960s. Various federal and local officials assisted the investigators when complications arose. For example, R. A. Vonderlehr, Assistant Surgeon General, exerted his influence to make sure that subjects of the Tuskegee Study of Untreated Syphilis did not receive effective treatments from nonparticipating physicians. In 1943, when Vonderlehr was told that the Selective Service Board might compel some of the subjects to be treated for venereal disease, he asked the Board to exclude study participants from the draft. Vonderlehr had no doubt that the Board would cooperate, if researchers described the "scientific importance" of completing the study. Throughout the course of the experiment, the physicians conducting the study deliberately withheld available therapy and deceived the participants by assuring them that they were receiving appropriate medical care for "bad blood." In 1970, an official of the Public Health Service declared that the Tuskegee Study was incompatible with the goal of controlling venereal disease because nothing had been learned in the course of this poorly planned and badly executed experiment that would ever "prevent, find, or cure" a single case of syphilis. But it was not until 1972, when investigative reporters brought the experiment to public attention, that the study was terminated.

Eight survivors of the Tuskegee Study, including 95-year-old Mr. Shaw and Mr. Fred Simmons, who gave his age as about 110 years, were present in 1997 when President Clinton offered an official apology for the infamous Tuskegee Study. The President's goal was to rebuild trust in the nation's biomedical research system by establishing rules that would ensure that all medical research programs would conform to the highest ethical standards and that researchers would work more closely with communities. The Department of Health and Human Services announced plans to establish a Tuskegee center for bioethics training that would serve as a memorial to the victims of the Tuskegee study. The President also extended the charter of the National Bioethics Advisory Commission.

The Tuskegee Study revealed nothing of value about the natural history of syphilis, but told a disturbing story of racism, poverty, and ignorance. Historians who have analyzed the Tuskegee Study concluded that it "revealed more about the pathology of racism than it did about the pathology of syphilis." Official investigations have generally focused on the question of why the study was allowed to continue after the 1940s, when penicillin became the drug of choice in treating the disease. The assumption was often made that withholding treatment during the 1930s was justifiable on the grounds that the treatments then available were both worse than the disease and ineffective. During the 1930s, physicians were no longer praising Salvarsan as a miracle cure for syphilis, but they were subjecting patients to long, expensive, painful treatment programs involving numerous intramuscular injections of Salvarsan in combination with applications of mercury or bismuth ointments. Perhaps ethical questions about the treatment of the well-to-do, as well as the withholding of treatment from the poor are applicable to the time period preceding the introduction of penicillin.

Both the Oslo and the Tuskegee Experiment involved studies of naturally acquired syphilis, but other research on the disease involved the deliberate infection of human subjects. While some researchers used themselves as guinea pigs, experiments carried out by Dr. Camille Gibert (d. 1866) and Dr. Joseph Alexandre Auzias-Turenne (d. 1870) in Paris in 1859 involved the use of hospital patients. Auzias-Turenne called himself the inventor of "syphilization," that is, a series of inoculations with what were said to be successively weaker forms of the "syphilitic virus" taken from patients at different stages of the disease. Auzias-Turenne believed that his experiments would settle the contemporary debate about the symptoms and contagiousness of secondary syphilis. To prove that secondary syphilis was contagious, Auzias-Turenne inoculated four hospitalized patients—who were free of venereal disease—with "purulent matter" taken from a patient with syphilis in the secondary phase. All four patients contracted the disease. For the most part, the medical community condemned these experiments as unethical and unnecessary. In general, doctors and the public objected to experiments that might harm any patient—rich or poor. Nevertheless, Auzias-Turenne felt triumphant because his work forced Ricord to admit that secondary syphilis was contagious.

Laboratory animals, such as rabbits, were eventually used for many studies of *Treponema pallidum*, but researchers argued that some questions could only be answered by experiments on human subjects. For example, in 1916, Udo J. Wile inoculated rabbits with treponemes taken from the brains of paretic patients. These studies were done in order to determine whether neurosyphilis was caused by a specific strain of the agent that causes syphilis. Wile obtained samples of brain tissue by trephining the skulls of patients hospitalized for forms of insanity associated with syphilis. Noguchi and other scientists had studied the relationship between *T. pallidum* in preserved brain sections of paretics or fresh autopsy material, but Wile argued that it was important to demonstrate the existence of active spirochetes in the brains of living paretics. Such findings, he warned, had important implications for the management of patients, because many physicians assumed that paretics could not transmit the disease.

## THE DISCOVERY OF THE CIRCULATION OF THE BLOOD

The Scientific Revolution is generally thought of in terms of the physical sciences, but by shifting the focus of concern from physics and astronomy to medicine and physiology, we can search for new ways of understanding and integrating science and medicine into the context of the political, religious, and social changes of this period. In the sixteenth century, as we have seen, anatomists and alchemists challenged ancient ideas about the nature of the microcosm, the little world of the human body. In the seventeenth century, William Harvey and the new experimental physiology transformed ways of thinking about the meaning of the heartbeat, pulse, and movement of the blood. Revolutionary insights into the microcosm reinforced the shock waves created when Copernicus, Kepler, and Galileo removed the earth from its place at the center of the universe.

Blood has always conjured up mysterious associations far removed from the physiological role of this liquid tissue. Blood has been used in religious rituals, fertility rites, charms, and medicines, and no horror film would be complete without buckets of blood. Strength, courage, and youthful vigor were thought to reside in the blood. Even Renaissance physicians and theologians believed in the medicinal power of youthful blood. The physicians of Pope Innocent VIII (1432–1492) are said to have prescribed human blood as a means of reviving the dying pontiff. How the blood was to be administered is unclear, but the results were predictable. The three young donors died, the Pope died, and his physicians vanished.

With philosophers, physicians, and ordinary people sharing a belief in the power of blood, the nearly universal enthusiasm for therapeutic bloodletting seems paradoxical to modern sensibilities. Nevertheless, for hundreds of years, Galenic theory and medical practice demanded and rationalized therapeutic and prophylactic bloodletting as a means of removing corrupt humors from the body. According to the Roman encyclopedist Pliny the Elder (23–79), even wild animals practiced bloodletting. Phlebotomists attacked the sick with arrows, knives, lancets, cupping vessels, and leeches. Indeed, until rather recent times, the surgeon was more commonly employed in spilling blood with leech and lancet than in staunching its flow.

Although Renaissance anatomists rejected many Galenic fallacies concerning the *structure* of the human body, their concepts of *function* had undergone little change. Ancient dogmas served as a defensive perimeter for physicians confronting professional, political, intellectual, and theological minefields. Even Vesalius avoided a direct attack on Galenic physiology and was rather vague about the whole question of the distribution of the blood and spirits. When scientific inquiry led to the brink of heresy, Vesalius found it expedient to cite the ancients and marvel at the ingenuity of the Creator. But, despite the delicate issue of the relationship between the movement of the blood and the distribution of the spirits, other sixteenth-century scientists were able to challenge the Galenic shortcut between the right side and the left side of the heart.

Michael Servetus (1511–1553), the first European physician to describe the pulmonary circulation, was a man who spent his whole life struggling against the dogmatism and intolerance that permeated the Renaissance world. If any man died twice for his beliefs it was Servetus. His attacks on orthodoxy were so broad and blatant that he was burnt in effigy by the Catholics and in the flesh by the Protestants. While challenging religious dogma, Servetus proved that contemporary anatomical information was sufficient to allow a heretic to elucidate the pathway taken by the blood in the minor, or pulmonary circulation.

Servetus left his native Spain to study law, but he soon joined the ranks of wandering scholars and restless spirits destined to spend their lives disturbing the universe. After his first major treatise, *On the Errors*

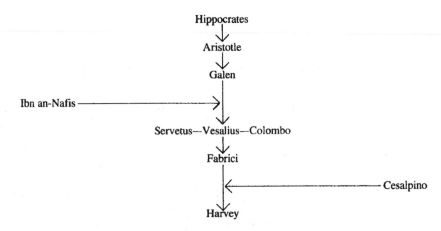

**Discovery of the minor and major circulation.**

*of the Trinity* (1531), was published, both Catholic and Protestant theologians agreed that the author was a heretic of the worst sort. Finding it necessary to go underground, Servetus established a new identity as "Michael Villanovanus." Under this name, he attended the University of Paris before moving to Lyons, where he published a new edition of the *Geographia* of Ptolemy, the Alexandrian astronomer and geographer. Even when editing a classic of such great antiquity, Servetus could not resist the opportunity to express dangerous opinions. While describing France, Servetus referred to the ceremony of the Royal Touch in which the king miraculously cured victims of scrofula (tuberculosis of the lymph nodes of the neck). "I myself have seen the king touch many attacked by this ailment," Servetus wrote, "but I have never seen any cured."

Returning to the University of Paris to study medicine, Servetus supported himself by lecturing on mathematics, geography, and astronomy. When he stepped over the line that Christian doctrine had drawn between acceptable areas of astrology and the forbidden zone of judicial astrology (essentially fortune-telling), he was threatened with excommunication. Attacks on judicial astrology can be traced back to the time of St. Augustine (354–430), but theological opposition and philosophical skepticism seem to have intensified by the end of the fifteenth century. Although his first impulse was to defend his actions, the case was hopeless and Servetus returned to his underground life. The eventual separation between medicine and astrology among the learned circles in France has been attributed to the attack of the medical faculty of Paris on an astrologer named Villanovanus in 1537.

As if looking for more trouble, Servetus entered into a correspondence with John Calvin (1509–1564), the French Protestant reformer

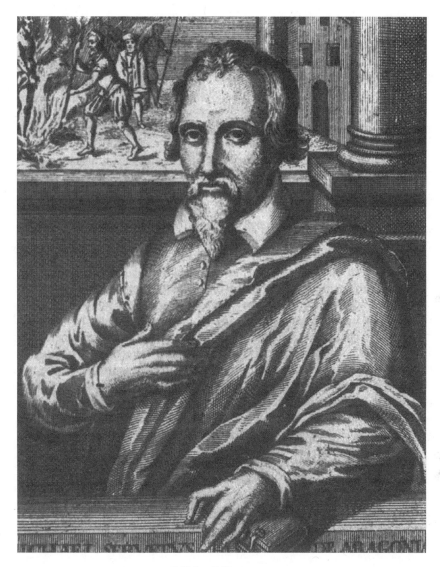

**Michael Servetus.**

who founded a religious system based on the doctrines of predestination and salvation solely by God's grace. In addition to criticizing Calvin's *Institutiones*, Servetus sent him an advance copy of his radical treatise, *On the Restitution of Christianity* (1553). Calvin responded by sending pages torn from the *Restitution* to the Catholic Inquisition with the information that Servetus had printed a book full of scandalous blasphemies. Servetus was arrested and imprisoned, but managed to escape before he was tried, convicted, and burned in effigy. Four months later, Servetus surfaced in Calvin's Geneva, where he was arrested and condemned to burn "without mercy." Attempts to mitigate the sentence to burning "with mercy" (strangulation before immolation) were unsuccessful. Almost all the newly printed copies of the *Restitution* were added to the fire. In 1903, the Calvinist congregation of Geneva expressed regrets and erected a monument to the martyred heretic. Moreover, a review of his case revealed that the death sentence had been illegal, because the proper penalty should have been banishment.

Given the fact that Servetus' account of the pulmonary circulation is buried within the seven hundred page *Restitution*, it is clear that his inspiration and motives were primarily religious, not medical or scientific. According to Servetus, to understand the relationship between God and humanity, and to know the Holy Spirit, one must understand the spirit within the human body. Knowledge of the movement of the blood was especially important, for as stated in Leviticus, "the life of the flesh is in the blood." Disputing Galenic concepts, Servetus argued that the fact that more blood was sent to the lungs than was necessary for their own nourishment indicated that passage of blood through pores in the septum was not the major path by which blood entered the left side of the heart. In Galen's system, aeration was the function of the left ventricle of the heart, but Servetus thought that changes in the color of the blood indicated that aeration took place in the lungs. Then, the bright red blood that had been charged with the vital spirit formed by the mixing of air and blood in the lungs was sent to the left ventricle. Servetus did not go on to consider the possibility of a systemic blood circulation. Apparently, he was satisfied that he had reconciled physiology with his theological convictions concerning the unity of the spirit.

What effect did Servetus have on sixteenth-century science? In retrospect, Servetus seems a heroic figure, but if his contemporaries knew of his work, they were unlikely to admit to being in sympathy with the ill-fated heretic. Moreover, historians believe that only three copies of the *Restitution* survived the flames. It is unlikely that Servetus influenced anatomists any more than Ibn an-Nafis, the Egyptian physician who had described the pulmonary circulation in the thirteenth century. However, there are always many uncertainties about the actual diffusion of information and ideas—especially those that might be considered heretical, dangerous, and subversive—as opposed to the survival of documentary evidence. Whatever influence Servetus did or did not have on sixteenth-century science, his career remains a fascinating revelation of the dark underside of the Renaissance and religious intolerance. His *Restitution* proves that in the sixteenth century, a man with rather limited training in medicine and anatomy could recognize the workings of the pulmonary circulation.

While in no way as colorful a figure as Servetus, Realdo Colombo (Renaldus Columbus; ca. 1510–1559) was a more influential scientist and teacher. Colombo, the son of an apothecary, was apprenticed to an eminent Venetian surgeon for seven years before he began his studies of medicine, surgery, and anatomy at the University of Padua. The records of the university refer to him as an outstanding student of surgery. When Vesalius, who had served as professor of anatomy and surgery since 1537, left the university in 1542 to supervise the publication of the *Fabrica*, Colombo was appointed as his replacement. Colombo was appointed to the professorship on a permanent basis in 1544 after Vesalius resigned. Displaying little reverence for his eminent predecessor, Colombo became one of the most vociferous critics of the *Fabrica* and the former colleagues became bitter enemies. Vesalius described Colombo as a scoundrel and an ignoramus.

From the time of his first public anatomical demonstrations to his death, Colombo drew attention to errors in the work of Vesalius and boasted of his own skills in surgery, autopsy, dissection, and vivisection. However, Colombo's attempt to create an illustrated anatomical treatise that would supercede the *Fabrica* was unsuccessful. In 1545, Colombo left Padua to take a professorship at Pisa. Three years later, he settled permanently in Rome. Later, the anatomist Gabriele Fallopio (1523–1562), who referred to Vesalius as the "divine Vesalius," accused Colombo of plagiarizing discoveries made by him and other anatomists. Fallopio's own *Observationes anatomicae* was primarily a series of commentaries on the *Fabrica*.

Colombo might have been demonstrating the pulmonary circulation as early as 1545, but his anatomical treatise, *De re anatomica*, was not published until 1559. Calling on the reader to confirm his observations by dissection and vivisection, Colombo boasted that he alone had discovered the way in which the lungs serve in the preparation and generation of the vital spirits. Air entered the lungs, where it mixed with blood brought in by the pulmonary artery from the right ventricle of the heart. Blood and air were taken up by the branches of the pulmonary vein and carried to the left ventricle of the heart to be distributed to all parts of the body. Although Ibn an-Nafis and Michael Servetus had also described the pulmonary circulation, Colombo apparently had no knowledge of their work and made the discovery through his own dissections and vivisection experiments. Moreover, because Colombo's formal training was inferior to that of Vesalius, he was apparently less familiar with certain aspects of Galen's writings on the lungs, heart, and blood. Despite his declarations of originality and daring, Colombo was rather conservative in his discussion of the functions of the heart, blood, and respiration. In any case, Galenic dogma was still too firmly entrenched for relatively modest inconsistencies and corrections to cause a significant breach in its defenses.

The difficulty of establishing the relationship between a scientific discovery, or a specific observation, and the conversion of physicians to a new theory is very well illustrated in the case of Andrea Cesalpino

(Andreas Cesalpinus; 1519–1603). Celebrated as the discoverer of both the minor and major circulation by certain admirers, Cesalpino, Professor of Medicine and Botany at the University of Pisa, was a learned man who combined a great reverence for Aristotle with an appreciation of Renaissance innovations. His medical doctrines were based on the Aristotelian philosophical framework established in his *Quaestionum peripateticarum* (1571). While he also wrote several books on practical medicine, his major area of interest was botany.

Certainly, Cesalpino had a gift for choosing words like *circulation* and *capillary vessels* that ring with remarkable prescience in the ears of posterity, at least in translation. His descriptions of the valves of the heart, the blood vessels that link the heart and lungs, and the pathways of the pulmonary circulation were well defined. Cesalpino also spoke of the heart in very lyrical terms as the fountain from which four great blood vessels irrigated the body "like the four rivers that flow out from Paradise." While his contemporaries generally ignored Cesalpino's ideas about the heart, modern champions of Cesalpino have devoted much effort to finding his references to the circulation and arranging these gems into patterns that escape the notice of less devoted readers.

Like Servetus, Cesalpino is worth studying as a reflection of the range of ideas available to anatomists in the sixteenth century. Cesalpino was preoccupied with Aristotelian ideas about the primacy of the heart and the movement of innate heat. As Aristotle's champion, Cesalpino attacked Galenic concepts with philosophic arguments and anatomical evidence. For this work, Cesalpino deserves a place in the history of physiology, but not the place properly occupied by William Harvey.

Because William Harvey suggested that the demonstration of the venous valves by Girolamo Fabrici (Hieronymus Fabricius; 1533–1619), his teacher at the University of Padua, had been a major factor in making him think the blood might travel in a circle, the discovery of these structures occupies an important place in the story of the circulation. Many other anatomists described the venous valves at about the same time, but we shall examine only the work of the man who directly inspired Harvey.

After earning his doctorate at the University of Padua, Fabrici established a lucrative private practice and gave lessons in anatomy. Eventually he replaced Gabriele Fallopio as professor of surgery and anatomy. Teaching anatomy was a difficult and unpleasant task and Fabrici, like Fallopio, seems to have evaded this responsibility whenever possible. Sometimes he disappeared before completing the course, angering students who had come to Padua to learn from the great anatomist. Fabrici saw teaching as drudgery that conflicted with his research and private practice. Students complained that he was obviously bored and indifferent when teaching. Presumably, they thought it more natural for the teacher to be enthusiastic and the students to be bored and indifferent.

*On the Valves of the Veins* was not published until 1603, but Fabrici noted that he had been studying the structure, distribution, and function of the venous valves since 1574. Fabrici assumed that Nature had formed the valves to retard the flow of blood from the heart to the periphery so that all parts of the body could obtain their fair share of nutrients. Arteries did not need valves because the continuous pulsations of their thick walls prevented distention, swelling, and pooling. Calling attention to a common procedure, Fabrici noted that when a ligature was tied around the arm of a living person, in preparation for bloodletting, little knots could be seen along the course of the veins. Careful dissection reveals that these swellings correspond to the location of the valves in the veins. Intrigued by Fabrici's demonstrations of the venous valves, Harvey repeated his simple experiments and observed that when the ligature was in place, it was not possible to push blood past the valves. Fabrici believed that the little structures in the veins acted like the floodgates of a millpond, which regulate volume, rather than valves that regulate direction. Unlike Fabrici, Harvey realized that the venous blood was directed to the heart, not to the periphery.

## WILLIAM HARVEY AND THE CIRCULATION OF THE BLOOD

William Harvey (1578–1657) was the eldest of seven sons born to Thomas Harvey, and the only member of this family of merchants and landowners to become a physician. After earning the Bachelor of Arts degree from Caius College, Cambridge, in 1597, Harvey followed the footsteps of the great English humanist-scholars to Padua. In 1602, Harvey returned to England and established a successful medical practice. His marriage to Elizabeth Browne, the daughter of Lancelot Browne, physician to Queen Elizabeth I and James I, gave him access to the highest court and professional circles. In rapid succession, Harvey was elected Fellow of the College of Physicians, appointed physician to St. Bartholomew's Hospital, Lumleian Lecturer for the College of Physicians, and physician extraordinary to James I. Harvey retained the latter position when Charles I became king in 1625 and was promoted to physician in ordinary in 1631 and senior physician in ordinary in 1639. (As strange as it may seem, *ordinary* in the court medical hierarchy was more prestigious than *extraordinary*.)

As one of the king's physicians, Harvey was charged with some peculiar assignments, such as the diagnosis of witchcraft, an area of considerable interest to James I. Harvey's duties also entailed extensive travels with King Charles I and service during the Civil War. It was at the request of the king that Harvey performed one of his most unusual

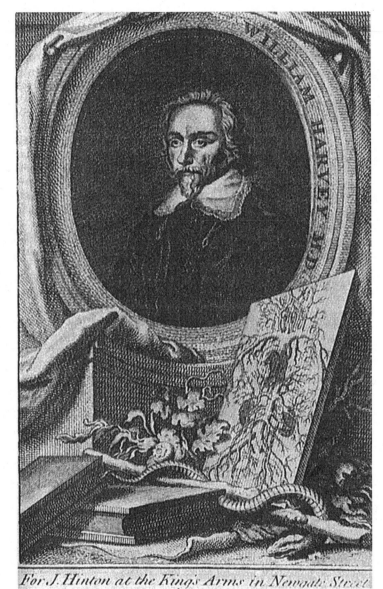

For J. Hinton at the King's Arms in Newgate Street

**William Harvey.**

autopsies, the postmortem of Thomas Parr, who had claimed to be the oldest man in England. Brought to London in 1635, Old Parr was presented to Charles I, and exhibited at the Queen's Head Tavern. Life in London undermined Parr's good health and he soon died, supposedly 152 years old. From the autopsy results, Harvey concluded that pleuropneumonia was the cause of death, but others thought it might have been old age.

Harvey may have inspired a revolutionary approach to experimental biology and human physiology, but professionally and socially he was a man whose conservative demeanor and outward conformity generally protected him from political intrigues and professional rivalries. Throughout the battles between the followers of King Charles I and the parliamentary forces under Oliver Cromwell (1599–1658), Harvey remained loyal to his king. After the Royalists were defeated and King Charles was publicly beheaded in 1649, Harvey retired to live with his brothers in the countryside near London. Tormented by gout and deteriorating health, he apparently became addicted to opium and may have attempted suicide more than once.

Notes for his Lumleian Lectures suggest that Harvey arrived at an understanding of the motion of the heart and blood well before 1628, when *An Anatomical Treatise on the Motion of the Heart and Blood in Animals* (usually referred to as *De motu cordis*) was published. Perhaps Harvey delayed publication because, as he confessed in his book, his views on the motions of the blood were so novel and unprecedented that he was afraid he would "have mankind at large for my enemies."

Considering that Harvey, like all medical students for hundreds of years, had been force-fed a steady diet of Galenism, and that conformity was generally the ticket to success and advancement within an extremely conservative profession, how was it possible for Harvey to free himself from the past? Rather than finding it remarkable that generations of physicians had meekly accepted Galenism, we should be moved to wonder how Harvey was able to realize that the grand and elegant doctrines about the motions and functions of the heart and blood that were universally accepted by his teachers and fellow students were wrong. When reading *De motu cordis*, one is struck most by the thought that *in principle*, Harvey's experiments and observations could have been performed hundreds of years before. During the seventeenth century, new instruments, such as the telescope and microscope, literally opened up new worlds to science and imagination, but Harvey's work was performed without the aid of the microscope.

Like Aristotle, whom he greatly admired, Harvey asked seemingly simple but truly profound questions in the search for final causes. In thinking about the function of the heart and the blood vessels, he moved closer to Aristotle's idea that the heart is the most important organ in the body while he revealed the errors in Galen's scheme. Harvey wanted to know why the two structurally similar ventricles of the right and left heart should have such different functions as the control of the flow of blood and of the vital spirits. Why should the artery-like vein nourish only the lungs, while the vein-like artery had to nourish the whole body? Why should the lungs appear to need so much nourishment for themselves? Why did the right ventricle have to move in addition to the movement

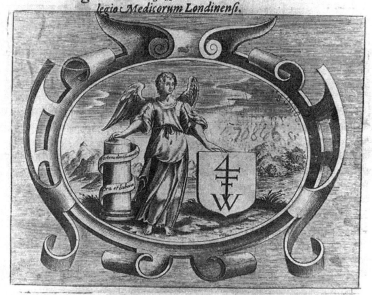

*EXERCITATIO*

# ANATOMICA DE
## MOTV CORDIS ET SAN-
### GVINIS IN ANIMALI-
BVS,

*GVILIELMI HARVEI ANGLI,*
*Medici Regii, & Profeſſoris Anatomiæ in Col-*
*legio: Medicorum Londinenſi.*

*FRANCOFVRTI,*
Sumptibus GVILIELMI FITZERI.
*ANNO M. DC. XXVIII.*

**William Harvey's** *De motu cordis* **(courtesy of the National Library of Medicine).**

of the lungs? If there were two distinct kinds of blood—nutritive blood from the liver distributed by the veins and blood from the heart for the distribution of vital spirits by the arteries—why were the two kinds of blood so similar? Such questions were not unlike those that Harvey's contemporaries were prepared to ask and debate.

Using arguments based on dissection, vivisection, and the works of Aristotle and Galen, Harvey proved that in the adult, all the blood must go through the lungs to get from the right side to the left side of the heart. He proved that the heart is muscular and that its most important movement is contraction, rather than dilation. But his most radical idea was that it was the beat of the heart that produced a continuous circular motion of the blood.

In warm-blooded animals, the systole (contraction) and diastole (expansion) of the heart are so rapid and complex that Harvey at first feared that only God could understand the motion of the heart. He solved this problem by using animals with simpler cardiovascular systems and a slower heartbeat, such as snakes, snails, frogs, and fish. With cold-blooded animals, or dogs bled almost to death, Harvey was able to create model systems that essentially performed in slow motion. When observations and experiments were properly analyzed, it was apparent that the motion of the heart was like that of a piece of machinery in which all the parts seemed to move simultaneously, until one understood the motions of the individual parts.

Harvey also posed a question of child-like simplicity that modern readers find most compelling, because the answer seems to be totally incompatible with Galenic theories. Yet, if this aspect of his work is overemphasized, it tends to remove Harvey from his seventeenth-century context and makes him appear more modern in outlook and approach than is really appropriate. Harvey asked himself: How much blood is sent into the body with each beat of the heart? Even the most cursory calculation proves that the amount of blood pumped out by the human heart per hour exceeds the weight of the entire individual. If the heart pumps out 2 ounces of blood with each beat and beats 72 times per minute, 8640 ounces ($2 \times 72 \times 60$), or 540 pounds, of blood is expelled per hour. Whether calculated for humans, sheep, dogs, or cattle, the amount of blood pumped out of the heart in an hour always exceeds the quantity of blood in the whole animal, as demonstrated by exsanguination. Skeptical readers could go to a butcher shop and watch an experienced butcher exsanguinate an ox. By opening an artery in a live animal, the butcher can rapidly remove all the blood.

It is all too easy to assume that these arguments should have provided an immediate deathblow to the Galenic system. However, the kind of evidence that appears most compelling today did not necessarily appeal to Harvey's contemporaries. Arguing from experimental and quantitative data in biology was remarkable in an era when even physicists were more likely to speculate than to weigh and measure. Moreover, opponents of Harvey's work presented what seemed to be quite logical alternatives, at least in light of accepted Galenic theory. For example, some critics argued that the heart attracted only a small amount of blood from the liver, where sanguification (the formation of blood) occurred. This blood foamed and expanded to such a great extent under the influence of the heat of the heart that the heart and arteries appeared to be full. Furthermore, multiplying the putative volume of blood discharged by the heart by the number of beats per minute was meaningless, because it was not necessary to assume that blood was driven from the heart through the arteries with each heartbeat.

Having solved the mechanical problem of the motion of the heart and blood, and demonstrated the true function of the venous valves, Harvey generally avoided arguments about the generation and distribution of the various kinds of spirits. Harvey had demonstrated the errors in Galen's system and had discovered essentially all that could be known about the structure and function of the cardiovascular system without the use of the microscope. Thus, one of the major gaps in Harvey's work was his inability to identify the structures joining the arterial and the venous system. He was forced to close this gap with hypothetical anastomoses or pores in the flesh. As scientists like Marcello Malpighi (1628–1694) extended the limits of anatomical study with the microscope, the capillary network completed the cardiovascular system.

Also unfinished at the time of Harvey's death was a book he planned to publish about his ideas on disease. The manuscript for this book may have been among those destroyed during the Civil War. Because of this loss, Harvey's concept of how knowledge of the circulation might solve questions about disease and medical practice must be constructed by piecing together comments made in his surviving works. *De motu cordis* promised that the new understanding of the circulation would solve many mysteries in medicine, pathology, and

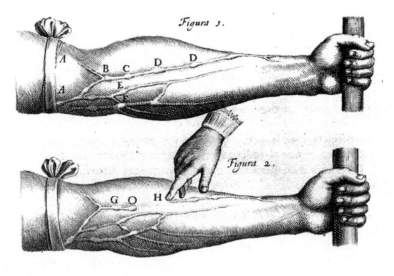

**William Harvey's demonstration of the role of the venous valves in the circulation of the blood.**

therapeutics. In later works, Harvey alluded to his "Medical Observations," but no such book was ever published.

Replacing the Galenic system that had so thoroughly, if incorrectly, explained the *purpose* of the heart, lungs, liver, veins, arteries, and spirits was completely beyond Harvey's technical and theoretical methods and goals. For seventeenth-century physicians, the new theory of the circulation raised more questions than it answered. If Harvey was correct, how could all the vital phenomena that Galenism had dealt with so long and so well be explained? For example, if the tissues did not consume the blood, how did they secure their nourishment? If the blood was not continuously formed from food by the liver, how was it synthesized? If the blood moved in a closed, continuous circle, what was the purpose of the arterial and venous systems and how did the body accomplish the generation and distribution of the vital spirit and the innate heat? If the venous blood did not originate in the liver, which had such a central role in the Galenic system, what was the function of this organ? If vital spirit was not produced by the mixture of air and blood in the lungs or in the left ventricle of the heart, what was the function of respiration? What was the difference between arterial and venous blood if all of the blood was constantly recirculated? If Galen were incorrect about the anatomy and physiology of the human body, what principles would guide medical practice?

Like almost all fundamental discoveries, Harvey's work provoked an avalanche of new questions and a storm of controversy. Many critics were unable or unwilling to understand the implications of Harvey's work. Others found it impossible to give up the old Galenic system that had provided all-encompassing rationalizations for health and disease, diagnosis, and therapeutics. How could medicine be saved if Galen was sacrificed for the sake of Harvey's radical theory? The theory of continuous circulation raised many disturbing questions for which Harvey provided no answers. Such questions stimulated Harvey's admirers to embark on new experimental ventures, while critics denounced his theory as useless, false, impossible, absurd, paradoxical, and harmful.

Well aware of the revolutionary nature of his work, Harvey predicted that no one under 40 would understand it. His work constituted a revolution in science worthy of comparison to that launched by Sir Isaac Newton. Although illness, age, and the loss of precious materials and manuscripts during the Civil War prevented Harvey from accomplishing all his goals, he did live to see his followers establish a new experimental physiology inspired by his ideas and methods. The questions raised by Harvey's work provided the Oxford physiologists—men such as Robert Boyle, Robert Hooke, Richard Lower, John Mayow, and Christopher Wren—with a new research program for attaining a better understanding of the workings of the human body.

## HARVEY'S PARADOXICAL INFLUENCE: THERAPY
## BY LEECH AND LANCET

Harvey's work opened up new fields of research and ignited violent controversies, but it certainly did not threaten the livelihood of phlebotomists. While provoking new arguments about the selection of appropriate sites for venesection, the discovery of the circulation seemed to stimulate interest in bloodletting and other forms of depletion therapy. Not even Harvey seemed to worry about the compatibility, or incompatibility, of therapeutic bloodletting and the concept of a closed, continuous circulation. Indeed, Harvey defended venesection as a major therapeutic tool for the relief of diseases caused by *plethora*. Long after accepting Harvey's theory, physicians praised the health-promoting virtues of bloodletting with as much (if not more) enthusiasm as Galen.

In addition to prescribing the amount of blood to be taken, doctors had to select the optimum site for bleeding. Long-standing arguments about site selection became ever more creative as knowledge of the circulatory system increased. Many physicians insisted on using distant sites on the side opposite the lesion. Others chose a site close to the source of corruption in order to remove putrid blood and attract good blood for repair of the diseased area. Proper site selection was supposed to determine whether the primary effect of bloodletting would be *evacuation* (removal of blood), *derivation* (acceleration of the blood column upstream of the wound), or *revulsion* (acceleration of the blood column downstream of the wound). Debates about the relative effects of revulsion and derivation are at the heart of François Quesnay's (1694–1774) physiocratic system, the first so-called scientific approach to economics. (The term physiocracy refers to the idea that society should allow natural economic laws to prevail.) The debate between Quesnay, Professor of Surgery and physician to Louis XV, and the physician Jean Baptiste Silva (1682–1742) began with conflicting ideas about medical issues involved in bloodletting and culminated in rationalizations of social and economic theories.

Bleeding was recommended in the treatment of inflammation, fevers, a multitude of disease states, and hemorrhage. Patients too weak for the lancet were candidates for milder methods, such as cupping and leeching. Well into the nineteenth century, no apothecary shop could be considered complete without a bowl of live leeches, ready to do battle with afflictions as varied as epilepsy, hemorrhoids, obesity, tuberculosis, and headaches (for very stubborn headaches leeches were applied inside the nostrils). Enthusiasm for leeching reached its peak during the first half of the nineteenth century. By this time, leeches had to be imported because the medicinal leech, *Hirudo medicinalis*, had been hunted almost to extinction throughout Western Europe. François Victor Joseph

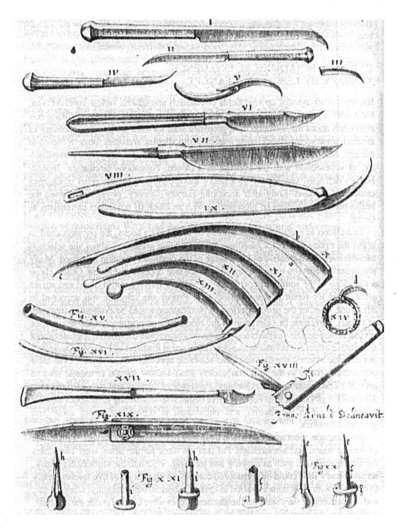

**Bloodletting instruments as depicted in a 1666 text by Johann Schultes (1595–1645).**

Broussais (1722–1838), an influential French physician, was the undisputed champion of medical leeching. Broussais believed that almost all diseases were caused by an inflammation of the digestive tract that could be relieved by leeching. Perhaps the most bizarre use of leeches was the case of a young woman who attempted to commit suicide with the aid of fifty leeches.

Leeches live by sucking blood and will generally attach themselves to almost any available animal, be it fish, frog, or human. On the positive side, leeches are excellent fish bait and they probably control the snail population in lakes and ponds. Moreover, unlike snails (the vector of schistosomiasis, also known as bilharzia or snail fever), leeches do not play a significant role as intermediate hosts of human parasites. The leech became a favorite experimental animal among neurobiologists, who considered its ganglion a thing of beauty.

In comparison to other medical procedures, leeching had the virtue of being essentially painless. The amount of blood taken was controlled by prescribing the appropriate number of leeches. In the 1980s, plastic and reconstructive surgeons rediscovered the usefulness of leeching; the anticoagulant action of leech saliva improves local blood flow and thus aids healing. Leeches were also used as a means of draining blood clots from donor skin flaps in order to increase adhesion to the recipient site. Leeches simply drop off the skin once they are full of blood. The success of leech therapy created a new era of leechmania as scientists gathered together in 1990 to present papers celebrating the Biomedical Horizons of the Leech. Researchers reported that leeches produce a remarkable array of enzymes, anticoagulants, antibiotics, and anesthetics. Moreover, patients, especially children, become fascinated by these living medical instruments. In the not too distant future, the best of the leech products will probably appear as pure and very expensive drugs, synthesized by the powerful new techniques of molecular biology and patented by innovative pharmaceutical companies.

For hundreds of years after the death of Galen, physicians warned their patients about the dangers posed by a plethora of blood. If a plethora of blood caused disease, bloodletting was the obvious remedy. Spontaneous hemorrhages and venesection were, therefore, as natural and helpful to the maintenance of life as the menstrual purgation was in healthy women. Bleeding was a perfectly rational means of treatment within this theoretical framework. To explain the persistence of bloodletting, physicians have tried to find modern explanations for the success stories of their predecessors. For example, in patients with congestive heart failure, bleeding might provide some relief because hypervolemia (an excess of blood) is a component of this condition. But well into the nineteenth century, many physicians believed that a "useless abundance of blood" was a principal cause of all disease.

Vigorous therapeutics, including copious bleeding and massive doses of drugs, formed the basis of the so-called heroic school of American medicine, best exemplified by the death of George Washington in 1799. Under the supervision of three distinguished physicians, Washington was bled, purged, and blistered until he died, about 48 hours after complaining of a sore throat. Across the Atlantic, the eminent Edinburgh surgeon John Brown (1810–1882) treated his own sore throat by applying 6 leeches and a mustard plaster to his neck, 12 leeches behind his ears, and, for good measure, removing 16 ounces of blood by venesection.

Questioning the validity of bloodletting required a large dose of skepticism and courage. Jan Baptista van Helmont (1579–1644), physician and chemical philosopher, was one of the rare individuals who dared to protest against the "bloody Moloch" presiding over medicine. Van Helmont claimed that bloodletting was a dangerous waste of the patient's vital strength. Not only did he reject bloodletting as a medical treatment, he denied the doctrine that plethora was the cause of disease. In answer to attacks on his position launched by orthodox physicians, van Helmont proposed putting the question to a clinical test. To demonstrate that bloodletting was *not* beneficial, van Helmont suggested taking two hundred to five hundred randomly chosen poor people and dividing them into two groups by casting lots. He would cure his allotment of patients without phlebotomy, while his critics could treat the other half with as much bloodletting as they thought appropriate. The number of funerals in each group would be the measure of success, or failure.

Such tests of bloodletting were not carried out until the nineteenth century, when the French physician Pierre Charles Alexandre Louis (1787–1872) used his "numerical system"—the collection of facts from studies of large numbers of hospitalized patients—to evaluate therapeutic methods. Louis's statistical studies of the efficacy of venesection had little impact on the popularity of bloodletting. Critics of the numerical system charged Louis's followers with excessive zeal in the art of diagnosis, and negligence in treating the sick. Many doctors believed that Louis's attempt to evaluate the efficacy of bloodletting was a rash, reckless rejection of the wisdom of the ages. Even admirers of the numerical system were reluctant to modify their therapeutic habits and were skeptical of applying facts obtained in Parisian hospitals to other environments. Louis's studies indicated that bloodletting did not affect the course of pneumonia, a condition in which venesection was thought to be particularly beneficial. Some physicians argued that Louis's data actually proved that venesection was ineffective when performed too conservatively. The controversy inspired tests of multiple bleedings in rapid succession in the treatment of endocarditis, polyarthritis, pneumonia, typhoid fever, and other diseases. Anecdotal evidence of patient survival, not statistical data, was taken as proof of efficacy.

Unconvinced by skeptics or statistics, most physicians continued to believe that bleeding was one of the most powerful therapeutic methods in their time-honored and rational system. Only a learned physician could judge whether to bleed from veins or arteries, by leech, lancet, or cupping. Advocates of bloodletting argued that more patients were lost through timidity than through the loss of blood. Two hundred years after Harvey discovered the circulation of the blood, medical authorities were still instructing their students to treat hemorrhage by bleeding to syncope (fainting, or collapse), because venesection encouraged coagulation of the blood and arrested hemorrhage.

Some doctors have suggested that bloodletting may have remained so widely used in the treatment of human and animal disease, at least in part, because it was actually effective against a wide spectrum of disorders. One hypothesis for the therapeutic value of bloodletting is that iron-binding proteins are part of the body's defense mechanism for coping with infection and neoplasia. Low levels of iron stores seem to correlate with reduced mortality from some infectious diseases, whereas excess iron apparently promotes the growth of certain pathogens and exacerbates the inflammatory response. Modern medicine recognizes the value of venesection as a way to treat certain iron-overload disorders. Of course, severe iron-deficiency anemia is dangerous to health, but it is unclear what the optimum iron levels might be under different physiological conditions and microbial challenges.

It is generally assumed that the practice of therapeutic bloodletting became extinct by the end of the nineteenth century, but according to the 1923 edition of Sir William Osler's *Principles and Practice of Medicine*—the "Bible" of medicine for generations of American doctors—after a period of relative neglect, bleeding was returning to favor in the treatment of cardiac insufficiency and pneumonia. Indeed, a renaissance of bloodletting had begun about 1900, particularly for pneumonia, rheumatic fever, cerebral hemorrhages, arterial aneurysms, and epileptic seizures that were thought to be correlated with menstruation. Bloodletting was said to be effective in relieving pain and difficulty in breathing, and it was important in treating fevers, because it lowered body temperature. Other than doing nothing, which was generally anathema to doctors and patients, the practitioner had few alternatives to offer a febrile patient. From a practical point of view, bleeding convinced doctor, patient, and family that something important, something supported by hundreds of years of learned medical tradition, was being done. Those who have observed the quiet prevailing among blood donors might also consider the fact that a quiet patient, especially one brought to a state close to fainting, will get more rest and be less of a nuisance to caretakers than a restless, delirious, and demanding one.

## BLOOD TRANSFUSION

As a scientist, Harvey demonstrated admirable skepticism towards dogma and superstition, but he was not especially innovative as a practitioner and he does not seem to have considered the possibility of therapeutic blood transfusions. His disciples, however, were soon busily injecting drugs, poisons, nutrients, pigments, and blood itself into animal and human veins. The transfusion and infusion of medicinal substances into the bloodstream did not become part of the standard therapeutic arsenal for many years, but seventeenth-century experimentalists did raise intriguing possibilities. Interest in transfusion was high from 1660 until about 1680, when various countries began to outlaw this dangerous, experimental practice. Many of the early therapeutic experiments based on the theory of circulation appear as paradoxical as the continued enthusiasm for bloodletting.

Although the first transfusion experiments generated great expectations, blood transfusion did not begin to satisfy the four cardinal virtues of a successful medical technique—simplicity, certainty, safety, and efficacy—until after World War I. The immunological mechanisms that guard the body against foreign invaders and distinguish between self and nonself provided the major obstacles to successful blood transfusion. Of course, unlike twentieth-century transplant surgeons, seventeenth-century physicians had no reason to suspect the existence of immunological barriers between different individuals and species. Why should they expect incompatibilities between blood donors and recipients when most wise men believed that four elements and four humors were sufficient to explain the macrocosm and the microcosm?

The avalanche of experiments on blood transfusion that followed acceptance of Harvey's theory led to competing claims for priority. The first significant studies of blood transfusion were performed by Christopher Wren, Richard Lower, and Robert Boyle in England, and by Jean Denis in Paris. According to Thomas Sprat's *History of the Royal Society* (1667), Christopher Wren was the first to carry out experiments on the injection of various materials into the veins of animals. During experiments exhibited at meetings of the Royal Society, animals were purged, intoxicated, killed, or revived by the intravenous injection of various fluids and drugs. Dogs, birds, and other animals were bled almost to death and sometimes revived by the injection of blood from another animal.

Reasoning that the nature of blood must change after it has been removed from the living body, Richard Lower decided to transfer blood between living animals by connecting the artery of the donor to the vein of the recipient. During a demonstration performed at Oxford in February 1666, Lower removed blood from a medium-sized dog until it was close to death. Blood taken via the cervical artery of a larger dog revived the experimental animal. Using additional donors, Lower was able to repeat this procedure several times. When the recipient's jugular vein was sewn up, it ran to its master, apparently none the worse for its bizarre experience. These remarkable experiments led observers to speculate that someday blood transfusions would cure the sick by correcting bad blood with blood from a more robust donor. This approach might even be used to improve temperament, perhaps by injecting the blood of a Quaker into an Archbishop.

At about the same time that Lower was engaged in blood transfusion experiments in animals, Jean Baptiste Denis (or Denys, ca.

1625–1704), Professor of Philosophy and Mathematics at Montpellier and physician to Louis XIV, was already crossing the species barrier in preparation for therapeutic experiments on humans. In March 1667, after 19 successful transfusions from dog to dog, Denis transfused blood from a calf into a dog. Observing no immediate adverse effect, Denis concluded that animal blood could be used to treat human diseases. Denis suggested that animal blood might be a better remedy than human blood, because animal blood would not be corrupted by passion, vice, and other immoral human traits. Humans were well nourished by the flesh of animals; thus, it was reasonable to assume that animal blood could also be well assimilated by human beings. As a practical matter, animal blood could be transfused directly from an artery.

With the help of Paul Emmerez, a surgeon and teacher of anatomy, Denis tested his methods on a 15-year-old boy who had suffered from a stubborn fever. To reduce excessive heat, his doctors had performed twenty therapeutic bleedings in two months. Dull, drowsy, and lethargic from the combined effects of illness and medical attention, the patient had been pronounced incredibly stupid and unfit for anything. On June 15, 1667, Emmerez drew off about 3 ounces of blood from a vein in the boy's arm and Denis injected about 10 ounces of arterial blood from a lamb. The operation caused a marvelous transformation: the boy regained his former wit, cheerfulness, and appetite. The only adverse effect was a sensation of great heat in his arm.

After this happy outcome, Denis injected about 20 ounces of lamb's blood into a healthy 45-year-old paid volunteer. Again, except for a sensation of warmth in the arm, no ill effects were reported. In another experiment, a patient suffering from a frenzy was given a large transfusion of calf's blood. Though cured of his frenzy, the patient experienced pains in the arm and back, rapid and irregular pulse, sweating, vomiting, diarrhea, and bloody urine. Given the poor man's state of health and previous treatments, Denis saw no compelling reason to blame the patient's physical problems on the transfusion. However, the death of another patient effectively ended the first phase of experimental blood transfusions.

A 34-year-old man who had been suffering attacks of insanity for about 8 years improved after 2 transfusions of calf's blood. When the madness reappeared, treatment was resumed, and the patient died. Certainly the death of a patient following the ministrations of a flock of physicians was not without precedent, but this case precipitated a violent controversy and an avalanche of pamphlets. At first, Denis blamed the patient's death on overindulgence in wine, women, and tobacco, but he later suggested that the widow had deliberately poisoned his patient. Although the courts did not convict Denis of malpractice, to all intents and purposes, blood transfusion was found guilty. Denis and Emmerez abandoned experimental medicine and returned to conventional careers, which presumably included the use of orthodox remedies more revolting and dangerous than calf's blood.

English scientists were quite critical of the experiments performed by Denis, but they too were experiencing mixed success in blood transfusions. About six months after Denis's first human transfusion, Richard Lower and his associates hired Arthur Coga, a man described as debauched, frantic, and somewhat cracked in the head, as a test subject. Some of Lower's colleagues were skeptical, but others believed that the transfusion might cool Coga's blood and rid him of his frenzy. After the injection of about 12 ounces of sheep's blood, Coga reported feeling much improved. Unfortunately, after a second transfusion, his condition deteriorated. Rumors circulated that his bad behavior had been deliberately engineered by parties trying to discredit the Royal Society and make the experiment look ridiculous. The learned Fellows of the Royal Society were justified in their fear of ridicule. Their reports provided satirists like Jonathan Swift (1667–1745) and Thomas Shadwell (1641–1692) with ample raw material. In Shadwell's comic play *The Virtuoso*, amateur scientist Sir Nicholas Gimcrack transfuses 64 ounces of sheep's blood into a maniac. After the operation, the patient becomes so wholly sheepish that he bleats perpetually, chews the cud, and sprouts a magnificent coat of wool, while a sheep's tail emerges from his "human fundament." Sir Nicholas plans to transfuse many more lunatics so that he can harvest the wool.

Safe blood transfusions were made possible when the immunologist Karl Landsteiner (1868–1943) demonstrated the existence of distinct human blood group types. In 1930, Landsteiner was awarded the Nobel Prize for his studies of blood group factors. Landsteiner found that all human beings belong to one of four different blood groups, designated O, A, B, and AB. Blood group typing also provided information that was useful in criminal cases, paternity suits, genetics, and anthropology. Indeed, so much information can be gleaned from blood that patients hospitalized for several weeks might begin to think that bloodletting is once again an integral part of medical care.

Despite the fact that blood transfusion has become a routine procedure, myths and superstitions continue to flourish in one form or another, making many people reluctant to donate or accept blood. Of course, not all fears about the safety of blood transfusion are unjustified. Unless blood is properly tested, recipients of blood and blood products are at risk for diseases like syphilis, malaria, hepatitis, AIDS, and even West Nile fever. Infected and contaminated human tissues and organs have caused serious infections in recipients. Many transplants involve soft tissues such as tendons, ligaments, and cartilage obtained from cadavers for use in elective orthopedic surgery. One body can supply enough tissue for thirty orthopedic transplants. Heart valves are also collected and used as replacements. Failure to prevent or detect bacterial or fungal contamination has led to deaths caused by infections. A new hazard of blood transfusions and organ transplants first emerged in 2002 when four patients who received the heart, liver, and kidneys of the same donor were infected with the West Nile virus. This virus is especially dangerous to people with weakened immune systems, such as patients undergoing organ transplants.

Inevitably, the need to detect and exclude unhealthy donors creates conflicts between public health concerns and individual liberty. Denying a person the right to donate blood may not seem a great infringement of personal liberty, but being labeled as a carrier of the hepatitis virus or the AIDS virus may have very serious consequences.

## NEW HEARTS FOR OLD

The emergence of cardiovascular disease as the major cause of death in the industrialized nations is a recent phenomenon, but deaths due to heart attack and stroke have long been of interest to physicians and scientists. Unfortunately, the approaches to the treatment of heart disease that have seized the most media attention—heart transplant surgery and the artificial heart—are methods that are unlikely to have commensurate effects on morbidity and mortality. The first human heart transplant operation was performed by South African surgeon Christiaan Barnard in December 1967. In the wake of Barnard's emergence as a world-class celebrity, other heart surgeons were soon performing equally dramatic operations.

Some of most daring and unsuccessful efforts in the 1960s and 1970s involved the transplantation of the hearts of chimpanzees, baboons, sheep, and artificial hearts into moribund patients. Ten years after Barnard triggered an era of boundless excitement and fierce competition among surgical centers, the heart transplant industry experienced a wave of disappointment and disillusionment. When cyclosporin was introduced in 1980 to suppress rejection after heart transplantation, its success stimulated the development of new cardiac transplantation programs. By the mid-1980s, at least two thousand cardiac transplant operations were being performed in more than one hundred transplant centers in the United States each year.

Organ transplantation has been called the greatest therapeutic advancement of the second half of the twentieth century and also the subject of the most hyperbole. But post-transplantation issues, such as complications arising from immunosuppressive drugs and the recurrence of the initial disease, as well as ethical issues, including the problem of the utilization of scarce resources, persist. The demand for organs has expanded to include people with a wide range of ailments, like hepatitis

C. Although the number of people, living or dead, donating organs has increased each year, the number of people waiting for organs has more than quadrupled. Thus, thousands of people die each year while waiting for organs.

In retrospect, it is clear that the great expectations generated by the first heart transplants were based solely on the boldness of the surgical feat, rather than any rational hopes of long-term success. The same problem that defeated Denis three centuries before—the body's rejection of foreign materials—insured the failure of organ transplantation. Unlike Denis, however, doctors in the 1960s were well aware of the body's immunological barriers. Even with drugs that suppressed the patient's immune system, and attempts to provide some degree of tissue matching, the risk of organ rejection and postsurgical infections were virtually insurmountable obstacles.

Optimistic surgeons pointed out that blood transfusion had once faced seemingly insurmountable obstacles, and they predicted that organ transplants would one day be as commonplace as blood transfusions. Advocates of organ transplantation even managed to ignore the obvious objection that while blood is a renewable resource, hearts are not. Nevertheless, as surgeons proclaimed a new era in which organ transplants would be routine rather than experimental, healthcare prophets warned that in the not too distant future, the supply of money rather than hearts might become the rate-limiting factor. Given the tremendous toll taken by cardiovascular diseases, some analysts contend that prevention rather than treatment is our most pressing need. High-risk, high-cost therapy has been likened to fighting infantile paralysis by developing more sophisticated artificial-lung machines instead of preventive vaccines. Unfortunately, prevention lacks the glamour and excitement of surgical intervention.

## SANTORIO SANTORIO AND THE QUANTITATIVE METHOD

All too often, Harvey's success is simplistically attributed to his ingenious use of quantitative methods within a mechanistic framework. But as the career of Santorio Santorio (Sanctorius, 1561–1636) indicates, allegiance to the mechanical philosophy and the ability to carry out painstaking experiments and perform precise measurements were not enough to provide meaningful answers to very different kinds of questions. Many seventeenth-century scientists welcomed the idea of extending medical knowledge through the quantitative method, but no one transformed this goal into a way of life with the dedication of Santorio, physician and philosopher. In Italy, he is honored as the founder of quantitative experimental physiology. Santorio established a successful private practice after graduating from the University of Padua in 1582.

In 1611, he was appointed to the Chair of Theoretical Medicine at the University, but by 1624, his students were charging him with negligence on the grounds that his private practice often took precedence over his teaching duties. Although he was found innocent, Santorio resigned from the University in 1629 in order to return to Venice.

In addition to medical practice, Santorio became intimately involved in research concerning a phenomenon known as *insensible perspiration*. According to classical theory, a kind of respiration taking place through the skin produced imperceptible exhalations known as insensible perspiration. Santorio believed that he could reduce the problem of insensible perspiration to purely mechanical processes that could be studied by exact measurements. In order to do so, he invented a special balance, a chair suspended from a steelyard, in which he measured his body weight after eating, drinking, sleeping, resting, and exercising, in health and disease, for more than thirty years.

Santorio published his results as a series of aphorisms in a small book entitled *Ars de statica medicina* (*Medical Statics*, 1614). The book went through at least 30 editions and was translated into several languages; the first English translation appeared in 1676. Although each aphorism was presented as a deduction from measurements, Santorio was rather vague about his experimental methods. Nevertheless, he boasted that he had accomplished something new and unprecedented in medicine—the exact measurement of insensible perspiration by means of reasoning and experimentation. Thinking that others might share his dedication to the quantitative lifestyle, Santorio suggested that readers might like to emulate his example and live a life "according to rule." For example, while eating their meals, they could sit on a special balance that would provide a warning when the proper amount of food had been consumed.

Convinced that measuring insensible perspiration was essential to medical progress, Santorio argued that physicians who did not understand quantitative aspects of this phenomenon could not cure their patients. In answer to Santorio's claim that he could measure the amount of insensible perspiration, critics charged that even if the *quantity* of vapors could be measured it was their *quality* that was significant in pathological phenomena.

In his other writings, Santorio revealed that despite his innovative goals, he was still working and thinking in terms of seventeenth-century medicine's Galenic heritage. As a whole, his life and work were devoted to reason, experience, and the study of Hippocrates, Galen, and Avicenna. While accepting the fact that Renaissance anatomists had contradicted Galen on particular points, Santorio did not regard this as a major problem for the theory and practice of medicine. Quantitative studies of metabolism, not unlike those of Santorio, were still being performed in the nineteenth century when the great French physiologist,

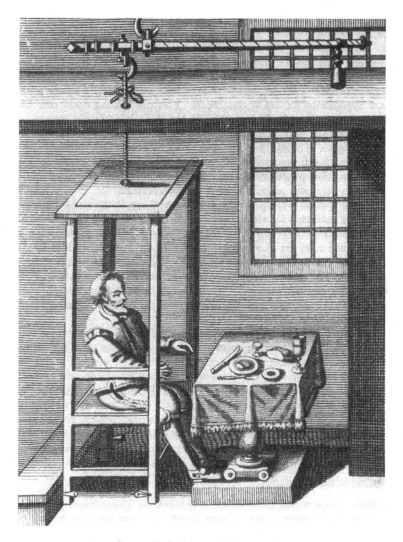

**Santorio in his weighing chair.**

Claude Bernard (1813–1878), denounced such experiments as attempts to understand what occurred in a house by measuring who went in the door and what came out the chimney.

In keeping with the goals expressed in *Medical Statics*, Santorio invented and improved several instruments capable of making measurements useful in medical practice and scientific investigation, including a clinical thermometer, a hygrometer, a pulsimeter, a water bed, specialized tables, beds, baths, chairs, enemas, and various surgical tools. Santorio did not reject the legacy of Hippocrates and Galen, but he was a champion of scientific medicine and an opponent of the superstitious, mystical, and astrological influences so common in his era. The spirit of invention was marvelously developed in this physician, even if his results were not commensurate with the painstaking nature of his investigations. He did not expect his measuring instruments and quantitative experiments to create a break with the past, but rather to provide more certain means of supporting the practice of Galenic medicine. After all, Galen himself had set an example of life-long dedication to observation and experiment.

## SUGGESTED READINGS

Arrizabalaga, J., Henderson, J., and French, R. K. (1997). *The Great Pox: The French Disease in Renaissance Europe.* New Haven, CT: Yale University Press.

Bainton, R. H. (1960). *Hunted Heretic: The Life and Death of Michael Servetus, 1511–1553.* Boston, MA: Beacon Press.

Black, R. (2001). *Humanism and Education in Medieval and Renaissance Italy: Tradition and Innovation in Latin Schools from the Twelfth to the Fifteenth Century.* New York: Cambridge University Press.

Brandt, A. M. (1987). *No Magic Bullet: A Social History of Venereal Disease in the United States Since 1880. With a New Chapter on AIDS.* New York: Oxford University Press.

Bylebyl, J. J., ed. (1979). *William Harvey and His Age. The Professional and Social Context of the Discovery of the Circulation.* Baltimore, MD: Johns Hopkins Press.

Carlino, A. (2000). *Books of the Body: Anatomical Ritual and Renaissance Learning.* Chicago, IL: University of Chicago Press.

Carmichael, A. G. (1986). *Plague and the Poor in Renaissance Florence.* New York: Cambridge University Press.

Cipolla, C. M. (1992). *Miasmas and Disease: Public Health and the Environment in the Pre-Industrial Age* (Trans. by E. Potter). Yale University Press.

Cohen, H. F. (1994). *The Scientific Revolution: A Historiographical Inquiry.* Chicago, IL: University of Chicago Press.

Costantino, M. (1993). *Leonardo: Artist, Inventor, and Scientist.* New York: Crescent.

Crosby, A. W. (1986). *Ecological Imperialism: The Biological Expansion of Europe, 900–1900.* New York: Cambridge University Press.

Cunningham, A. (1997). *The Anatomical Renaissance: The Resurrection of the Anatomical Projects of the Ancients.* Burlington, VT: Ashgate.

Cunningham, A., and Grell, O. P. (2001). *The Four Horsemen of the Apocalypse: War, Famine, Disease and Gospel in Reformation Europe.* New York: Cambridge University Press.

Davis, A. B. (1973). *Circulation Physiology and Medical Chemistry in England 1650–80.* Lawrence, KS: Coronado Press.

Debus, A. G. (2001). *Chemistry and Medical Debate: Van Helmont to Boerhaave.* Nantucket, MA: Science History Publications.

Eisenstein, E. (1983). *The Printing Revolution in Early Modern Europe.* New York: Cambridge University Press.

Field, J. V., and James, F. A. J. L., eds. (1993). *Renaissance and Revolution: Humanists, Scholars, Craftsmen, and Natural Philosophers in Early Modern Europe.* New York: Cambridge University Press.

Fox, R. C., and Swazey, J. P. (1992). *Spare Parts: Organ Replacement in American Society.* New York: Oxford University Press.

Fracastoro, G. (1984). *Fracastoro's "Syphilis"* (Trans. and Intro. by G. Eatough). Liverpool: Francis Cairns.

Frank, R. G., Jr. (1980). *Harvey and the Oxford Physiologists. Scientific Ideas and Social Interactions.* Berkeley, CA: University of California Press.

French, R. (2000). *Ancients and Moderns in the Medical Sciences: From Hippocrates to Harvey.* Burlington, VT: Ashgate.

Fuchs, T., and Grene, M. (2001). *The Mechanization of the Heart: Harvey & Descartes.* Rochester, NY: University of Rochester Press.

Gentilcore, D. (1998). *Healers and Healing in Early Modern Italy.* New York: Manchester University Press.

Goliszek, A. (2003). *In the Name of Science: A History of Secret Programs, Medical Research, and Human Experimentation.* New York: St. Martin's Press.

Grell, O. P., ed. (1998). *Paracelsus: The Man and His Reputation, His Ideas, and Their Transformation.* Leiden: Brill.

Grendler, P. F. (2002). *The Universities of the Italian Renaissance.* Baltimore, MD: Johns Hopkins University Press.

Hakim, N. S., and Papalois, V. E., eds. (2003). *History of Organ and Cell Transplantation.* River Edge, NJ: Imperial College Press.

Harvey, W. (1961). *Lectures on the Whole of Anatomy* (Annotated trans. by C. D. O'Malley, F. N. L. Poynter, and K. F. Russel). Berkeley, CA: University of California Press.

Harvey, W. (1976). *An Anatomical Disputation Concerning the Movement of the Heart and Blood in Living Creatures* (Trans. by G. Whitteridge). Oxford: Blackwell.

Hayden, D. (2003). *Pox: Genius, Madness, and the Mysteries of Syphilis.* New York: Basic Books.

Jacob, J. R. (1999). *The Scientific Revolution: Aspirations and Achievements, 1500–1700.* Humanities Press.

Jones, J. H. (1993). *Bad Blood: The Tuskegee Syphilis Experiment.* New York: The Free Press.

Keele, K. D. (1983). *Leonardo da Vinci's Elements of the Science of Man.* New York: Academic Press.

Lindemann, M. (1999). *Medicine and Society in Early Modern Europe.* Cambridge: Cambridge University Press.

Moreno, J. D. (2000). *Undue Risk: Secret State Experiments on Humans.* New York: Routledge.

Morgani, G. (1984). *The Clinical Consultations of Giambattista Morgani.* Charlottesville, VA: University of Virginia Press.

Newman, W. R., and Grafton, A., eds. (2001). *Secrets of Nature: Astrology and Alchemy in Early Modern Europe.* Cambridge, MA: MIT Press.

O'Malley, C. D. (1964). *Andreas Vesalius of Brussels, 1514–1564.* Berkeley, CA: University of California Press.

O'Malley, C. D. (1965). *English Medical Humanists: Thomas Linacre and John Caius.* Lawrence, KA: University of Kansas Press.

Osler, M. J., ed. (2000). *Rethinking the Scientific Revolution.* New York: Cambridge University Press.

Pagel, W. (1984). *The Smiting Spleen. Paracelsianism in Storm and Stress.* Basel: Karger.

Park, K. (1985). *Doctors and Medicine in Early Renaissance Florence.* Princeton, NJ: Princeton University Press.

Pomata, G. (1998). *Contracting a Cure: Patients, Healers and the Law in Early Modern Bologna.* Baltimore, MD: Johns Hopkins University Press.

Quétel, C. (1990). *History of Syphilis.* Cambridge, UK: Polity Press.

Ramazzini, B. (1940). *De morbis artificum diatriba. Diseases of Workers* (Trans. and notes by W. C. Wright). Chicago, IL: University of Chicago Press.

Reverby, S. M., ed. (2000). *Tuskegee's Truths: Rethinking the Tuskegee Syphilis Study.* Chapel Hill, NC: University of North Carolina Press.

Richardson, R. (2001). *Death, Dissection and the Destitute.* 2nd ed. Chicago, IL: University of Chicago Press.

Saunders, J. B. de C. M., and O'Malley, C. D. (1947). *Andreas Vesalius Bruxellensis: The Bloodletting Letter of 1539.* New York: Henry Schuman.

Shapin, S. (1996). *The Scientific Revolution.* Chicago, IL: University of Chicago Press.

Siraisi, N. G. (1990). *Medieval & Early Renaissance Medicine.* Chicago, IL: University of Chicago Press.

Starr, D. (1998). *Blood: An Epic History of Medicine and Commerce.* New York: Alfred A. Knopf.

Temkin, O. (1973). *Galenism. Rise and Decline of a Medical Philosophy.* Ithaca, NY: Cornell University Press.

Vesalius, A. (1949). *The Epitome of Andreas Vesalius* (Trans. from the Latin, with Introduction and Anatomical Notes by L. R. Lind and C. W. Asling). Cambridge, MA: MIT Press.

Vesalius, A. (1998). *On the Fabric of the Human Body.* Book 1: *The Bones and Cartilages.* (Trans. by W. F. Richardson and J. B. Carman). San Francisco, CA: Norman Publishing.

Vesalius, A. (1999). *On the Fabric of the Human Body*. Book 2: *The Ligaments and Muscles*. (Trans. by W. F. Richardson and J. B. Carman). San Francisco, CA: Norman Publishing.

Vesalius, A. (2002). *On the Fabric of the Human Body*. Book 3: *The Veins and Arteries*. Book 4: *The Nerves*. (Trans. by W. F. Richardson and J. B. Carman). San Francisco, CA: Norman Publishing.

Voights, L. E., and McVaugh, M. R. (1984). *A Latin Technical Phlebotomy and Its Middle English Translation*. Philadelphia, PA: American Philosophical Society.

Wear, A. (2000). *Knowledge and Practice in English Medicine, 1550–1680*. New York: Cambridge University Press.

Webster, C. (2002). *The Great Instauration: Science, Medicine and Reform, 1626–1660*. 2nd ed. Oxford: Peter Lang.

Whitteridge, G. (1971). *William Harvey and the Circulation of the Blood*. New York: American Elsevier.

Williams, G. S., and Gunnoe, C. D., eds. (2002). *Paracelsian Moments: Science, Medicine, & Astrology in Early Modern Europe*. Truman State University Press.

Younger, S. J., Fox, R. C., and O'Connell, L. J., eds. (1996). *Organ Transplantation: Meanings and Realities*. Madison, WI: University of Wisconsin Press.

# 7

# Native Civilizations and Cultures
of the Americas

Initial European reports about the New World spoke of a veritable Eden, populated by healthy, long-lived people, who could cure illness with exotic medicinal plants and did not know the diseases common in other parts of the world. Columbus said he found "Paradise-on-Earth" in the newly discovered Indian Islands. Glowing reports of the idyllic conditions and wealth to be found in the New World could be attributed to ignorance, or to the hyperbole of an advertising campaign designed to attract European settlers and investors. In any case, within decades, the discovery and conquest of the Americas led to an unprecedented interchange of peoples, plants, animals, and pathogens on a global scale. With the demographic catastrophe that overcame Native Americans and the demands of Spanish colonizers for labor, the establishment of the slave trade brought vast numbers of Africans to the New World. Thus, within a few decades, the Americas became the site of the mixing of the peoples and germs of previously separate continents.

By the end of the twentieth century, historians had generally agreed that a new comparative and common history of the Americas was essential. Also necessary was recognition of the fact the so-called New World was only new to Europeans; the Americas had long ago been discovered and settled by ancestors of those now called Native Americans, Indians, or Amerindians. Because the history of the native peoples of America is known primarily through documents produced by European explorers, conquerors, missionaries, and settlers, a Eurocentric bias is probably inevitable. Moreover, except for the earliest accounts of the Spanish conquerors, European reports were composed in the wake of the catastrophic demographic collapse that virtually destroyed the foundations of Native American civilizations and cultures. Scholars are now attempting to transcend the assumptions implicit in such terms as Discovery, New World, and European Expansion in order to understand the history of the Americas before 1492, but given the fragmentary nature of the evidence, the desired grand synthesis of the history of the Americas remains a formidable and unfinished task.

Historians and scientists continue to debate the nature and timing of the earliest migration of humans into the Americas. Some scholars believe that human beings first crossed a land bridge from Siberia to the New World at the end of the last Ice Age, that is, about 10,000 years ago. These migrants might have been skilled nomadic hunters who eventually contributed to the extinction of mastodons, mammoths, horses, camels, and other species of large mammals. Other evidence suggests that human beings might have arrived in the New World about 20,000 years ago, and pursued a way of life in which gathering plants was as important as hunting. Sites in both North and South America have provided evidence of human artifacts that appear to be 15,000 to 20,000 years old, but most early sites are very poorly preserved. The evidence is so fragmentary and ambiguous that each discovery of prehistoric tools and artifacts renews the arguments about migration patterns, the identity of the first people to arrive in the Americas, and their relationship to contemporary American Indians.

Some scientists believe that Ice Age skeletons and DNA tests might settle the debate about the identity of the people who originally arrived in the Americas. By the end of the twentieth century scientists had found genetic evidence that suggested independent waves of migrations of people from Asia, Polynesia, and even Western Europe. Nevertheless, the evidence from artifacts, human remains, and even human DNA remains ambiguous. Whenever humans first came to the Americas, significant waves of immigration from Eurasia presumably ceased when the land bridge linking Alaska and Siberia disappeared, leaving the populations of the Americas isolated from the rest of the world. The relative genetic homogeneity of native Americas might have affected their response to Old World infectious agents. The distribution of blood types in the Americas, for example, is less variable than that found in Eurasia.

Uncertainties about the pattern of early migrations lead to uncertainty about the disease patterns that would have prevailed in the prehistoric New World. Scholars have suggested that the migration through the Bering Strait into America served as a "cold filter" that screened out many pathogens and insects, but that does not mean that pre-Columbian America ever was a disease-free Garden of Eden. Throughout most of the Americas, however, population density was presumably too low to support the endless cycles of epidemic and childhood diseases common in the urban centers of the Old World. There were, of course, dangerous animals, poisonous reptiles and plants, as well as insects and arthropods that could serve as vectors of disease.

Diseases that were almost certainly present in the Americas before 1492 include arthritis, cancer, diseases of the endocrine system, nutritional deficiency diseases, osteoporosis, intestinal parasites, dysentery, bronchitis, pneumonia, tuberculosis, rickettsial and viral fevers, pinta, Carrión's disease (Oroya fever or Verruga Peruana), *uta* (American leishmaniasis), and Chagas' disease. (*Trypanosoma cruzi*, the parasite that causes Chagas' disease, is transmitted by the blood-sucking *barbeiro*, or kissing bug. The clinical course of this incurable disease is quite variable, but the infestation may damage the liver, spleen, and heart. The causative agent and means of transmission were identified by the Brazilian scientist Carlos Chagas (1879–1934). Epidemiologists estimate that about 18 million people in Latin America are infected with Chagas' disease; about 50,000 die of the disease every year.) There is considerable uncertainty about the pre-Columbian prevalence of tuberculosis in the Americas, but studies of Peruvian mummies have revealed evidence of pulmonary tuberculosis, as well as tapeworm, pinworm, and roundworm.

The microorganisms that cause wound infections, boils, sore throats, and food poisoning were probably fairly common. "Fevers" were certainly endemic in the Americas, but the pre-Columbian status of malaria and yellow fever are uncertain. Many regional febrile diseases caused by microbes and parasitic worms were probably transmitted by American mosquitoes, ticks, flies, fleas, and bugs. Rocky Mountain spotted fever, for example, is caused by a peculiar pathogen (*Rickettsia rickettsii*) found only in the Americas. Other American diseases with high mortality rates—including Colorado tick fever, St. Louis encephalitis, Western equine encephalitis, and Eastern equine encephalitis—are caused by arboviruses (viruses transmitted by arthropods, such as mosquitoes and ticks) that find a reservoir in reptiles, birds, and mammals.

Cholera, plague, smallpox, measles, scarlet fever, malaria, typhus fever, typhoid fever, influenza, and probably gonorrhea and leprosy were unknown in the pre-Contact period. There is even uncertainty about the kinds of vermin native to the New World. For many epidemic and endemic diseases, vectors, such as insects, arthropods, and rodents, are critical factors in their distribution and transmission. Ticks, biting ants, mosquitoes, flies, lice, gnats, chiggers, scorpions, spiders, flies, and poisonous snakes were indigenous to the Americas, but Europeans probably brought new species of fleas, roaches, lice, bedbugs, and rats.

Malaria has been a powerful agent in world history, but its pre-Columbian global distribution is uncertain. Even if malaria was originally present in the Americas, more virulent African strains could have been imported in association with the slave trade. Whether or not human malaria was a significant problem in pre-Columbian America, quinine, the drug that made it possible to cure malaria, was found in the New World. Quinine, which is extracted from a plant indigenous to South America, was originally known as cinchona or Peruvian bark.

Native Americans suffering from an epidemic fever allegedly discovered the therapeutic value of cinchona when they drank water from a pond bordered by cinchona trees. Eventually the story of cinchona became linked to that of the Countess of Chinchón, wife of the Viceroy of Peru. Sadly, the story of the feverish Countess and the Native American remedy seems to be a myth used to explain the export of Peruvian bark to Europe in the 1630s. Francesco Torti's (1658–1741) book *Therapeutice specialis* (1712), on pernicious intermittent fevers, was instrumental in establishing the value of cinchona bark therapy.

Although many sixteenth-century physicians considered syphilis a new disease that had been imported from the New World, the pre-Columbian distribution of syphilis is still controversial. There is, however, evidence that other members of the treponematosis family were widely distributed throughout the world; the form known as pinta was present in the Americas. The global epidemics of syphilis that followed 1492 could have been the result of exchanges of previously localized strains of treponemes. Other sexually transmitted diseases presumably existed in the Americas, but gonorrhea was probably absent.

The origin of yellow fever is almost as mysterious and controversial as that of syphilis and concerns the same problem of Old versus New World distribution of disease in pre-Columbian times. Claims that Mayan civilization was destroyed by yellow fever or that epidemics of this disease occurred in Vera Cruz and San Domingo between 1493 and 1496 remain doubtful. Some epidemiologists contend that yellow fever, a viral disease transmitted to humans by mosquitoes, caused epidemics in the Americas long before European contact, but others believe that the disease was imported from Africa.

Unlike the controversy surrounding syphilis and yellow fever, there seems to be general agreement that tuberculosis existed in pre-Contact America. Tuberculosis infections, in communities where the disease is endemic, are usually contracted in early childhood, via the respiratory route. Primary lesions may develop in the lungs and viable bacteria may remain encapsulated, until some kind of stress or stimulus reactivates the infection. Thus, the skeletal lesions characteristic of tuberculosis may occur in only a small percentage of infected individuals.

Human skeletal remains and mummies provide evidence for the presence of certain diseases in pre-Contact America, but there is much uncertainty and difficulty in the interpretation of such materials. As the techniques of molecular biology improve, researchers might gain critical information through studies of DNA recovered from human remains. Some scholars argue that all attempts to attach modern diagnostic names to ancient remains are futile, although the urge to do so seems to be irresistible. Others argue that, social constructionism notwithstanding, diseases should be thought of as true biological entities that persist through time.

Generally, about 15 percent of the skeletons found in typical North American archeological samples show evidence of identifiable conditions like trauma, infection, and arthritis. Of course, the conditions that are recognizable in skeletons were not necessarily the immediate cause of death, because few acute diseases leave a characteristic mark in the bones. Moreover, very different conditions may produce similar lesions. The kinds of acute, viral diseases that probably had the greatest impact on Native Americans after contact with Europeans are unlikely to affect the skeleton, but evidence of injury and death from European weapons can be found in Indian cemeteries.

Where conditions are favorable, biological anthropologists have analyzed the remains of pre- and post-Conquest populations and compared this evidence with European observations about early encounters with Native Americans. Studies of early human remains from the Georgia coastal region, for example, indicate that even prior to contact, the quality of life had deteriorated. By the twelfth century, these coastal people had begun cultivating maize, which resulted in less dietary variety and increases in the frequency of nonspecific bone inflammation and dental caries. Increases in population size were supported by a basically sedentary subsistence economy that included farming, hunting, gathering, and fishing.

Researchers have used the techniques of molecular biology to study DNA recovered from ancient human remains. For example, some of the skeletons recovered from a peat bog in Florida contained intact crania and preserved, but very fragile brain matter. Although the Windover site skeletons had been in the peat bog for about seven thousand years, scientists were able to perform some studies on their mitochondrial DNA.

Estimates of the population of the Americas in 1492, as well as the magnitude and specific causes of the demographic collapse that followed the arrival of Europeans, are controversial and very far from precise. Demographers have attempted to compare archeological evidence concerning settlement patterns, burials, and accumulations of refuse with population estimates recorded by early European explorers. Despite the increasing sophistication of analytic techniques, population estimates for the early encounter period have been characterized as underestimates, overestimates, or even ridiculed as "numbers from nowhere."

Despite universal agreement that Old World diseases had a catastrophic effect on Native Americans, assessing the impact of European contact is not a simple matter. Population change is the result of complex forces and estimates of populations in the past lack precision. Demographers can generally be divided into two schools of thought. "High Counters" argue that there was a very large pre-Contact Native American population and that it was drastically reduced by the epidemic diseases, chaos, and exploitation that followed the Conquest.

"Low Counters" argue that European invaders exaggerated the numbers of people they encountered in order to magnify their victories.

Some scholars argue that the pre-Contact population for the entire New World was probably between 8 and 13 million, but estimates for the population of Mexico in 1492 have ranged from as low as one million to as high as thirty million. Whatever the absolute figures might have been, contact between the Old and New Worlds apparently led to the worst demographic disaster in human history. When Spanish bureaucrats attempted to conduct a census of Mexico in the late 1540s, observers guessed that the population was less than a third of the pre-Conquest level. A census conducted in the 1570s reflected further decreases in the native population due to war, disease, and other hardships. Winning over the demoralized survivors, the conquerors and their priests displaced native shamans, priests, and chiefs and substituted European agriculture and animal husbandry for native systems of production. Environmental damage and social disruption were exacerbated by the introduction of European domesticated animals.

Unfortunately, little direct evidence remains concerning the pre-Columbian medical beliefs and practices of the diverse peoples of the Americas. What is known is often obscured by the difficulties of decoding the meanings of ancient symbols, artifacts, and artwork. Observations made by Europeans compound the problem, because of inevitable misunderstanding and deliberate distortions. By the time Native Americans began using European alphabets to record their own histories and concepts, New World people, plants, and animals had undergone profound dislocations.

The Americas confronted Europeans with an array of new plants, animals, and human beings. In many ways, such discoveries must have been a profound shock to Europeans, but much of the new information was incorporated into biblical and traditional systems of thought. European herbals were soon full of pictures of exotic plants from the New World, accompanied by fabulous accounts of their medical virtues. Indeed some physicians predicted that the medical wealth of the New World would prove more valuable than gold and silver. The Americas offered exotic new foods and medicinal substances, such as cocaine, curare, guaiac, ipecac, jalap, lobelia, Peruvian balsam, sarsaparilla, tobacco, and quinine. Today, about one-third of the world's most important plants can be traced back to the New World. Europeans did, however, bring many plants and animals to the Americas, including wheat, barley, rice, legumes, various fruits, sugarcane, pigs, horses, cows, sheep, donkeys, mules, chickens, and goats. Thus, contact between Europe and the Americas resulted in many changes, both deliberate and accidental, in the distribution of plants and animals throughout the world.

## NATIVE CIVILIZATIONS OF LATIN AMERICA

Centuries before Europeans arrived in the Western hemisphere, cultures that generally satisfied the criteria used to define civilizations had developed, primarily in the regions now known as Mexico, Guatemala, and Peru. It is impossible to know how these civilizations and other indigenous cultures would have evolved, if they had not been conquered and colonized, but studies of the Mayan cities of Copán, Palenque, Chitchén Itzá, and Uxmal, the Aztec city of Tenochtitlán, the Inca cities of Cuzco and Machu Picchu, and others, reflect the evolution of complex social organizations and governments, confederations and empires, art and architecture, writing and record keeping, mathematics, astronomy, and complex calendrical calculations. The written languages of pre-Columbian American civilizations involved hieroglyphic-like glyphs that were pictographic, ideographic, or phonetic in nature. Records were inscribed on stone monuments or recorded on paper or animal hides. Unfortunately, almost all pre-Columbian codices (manuscripts) were destroyed by the Spanish conquerors. Europeans generally denigrated New World cultures, even the Aztec, Maya, and Inca, because they did not use iron, the plow, the arch, or an alphabet. Their rulers might have amassed great empires and wealth, but Europeans considered native religions and governments primitive, savage, and barbaric.

In the Americas, the transition from nomadic hunting and gathering to a sedentary lifestyle probably began in coastal Peru and the Basin of Mexico about 6000 B.C.E. The valleys of Central America and the northwest portion of South America provided the appropriate conditions for agricultural production, rapid population growth, diversification of trade and industry, the establishment of towns and cities, and the emergence of privileged classes of priests, rulers, nobles, and warriors. Mesoamerica was the site of the rise and fall of several remarkable civilizations, including the Olmec, Zapotec, Toltec, Mixtec, Aztec, and Maya. Members of these groups cultivated a variety of important food crops, as well as tobacco and rubber, and produced drugs, poisons, fermented drinks, dyes, cloth, and ceramics. Scientists thought that corn was domesticated much later than other major cereals, such as wheat and rice, but there is evidence of the cultivation of maize in Mexico more than seven thousand years ago. In some regions, the basic diet of corn, beans, potatoes, manioc, yucca, tomatoes, and chilies, was supplemented with turkey, duck, fish, shellfish, and even dogs and guinea pigs.

Studies of the skeletal remains of people who lived in the Western Hemisphere over the last seven thousand years suggest that the general health of Native Americans had been deteriorating for centuries before 1492, but many uncertainties remain. Thousands of skeletons from many sites in North and South America have been analyzed for evidence of infections, malnutrition, degenerative joint disease, dental health, stature, anemia, arrested bone development, and trauma from injuries. Declining health indicators seem to be associated with the rise of agriculture and urban cultures in South and Central America. Archeological evidence also suggests several periods of population growth and decline before European contact. So attributing the total collapse of New World empires to the Conquest might be excessively Eurocentric. On the other hand, the impact of European diseases and military conquest was so profound and sudden that autochthonous patterns of possible development were abruptly transformed or terminated.

Europeans quickly recognized and exploited divisions and hostilities among native peoples who had been harshly treated by warring empires. Internal strife and tribal revolts, as well as European invaders, contributed to the fall of the Aztec and Inca empires. Contact events involving the Aztecs, Mayas, and Incas were especially dramatic, primarily because Mexico and Peru had the highest population densities and the most extensive trade and transport networks in the Americas. Such factors provide ideal conditions for the spread of epidemic diseases. Narratives of the fall of Aztec, Maya, and Inca empires suggest that Europe's most devastating offensive weapons may have been highly contagious eruptive fevers, such as smallpox and measles, and the panic and fear that accompany exceptionally virulent epidemic diseases. Malnutrition, famine, and the breakdown of long-standing social networks would have intensified the impact of infectious diseases.

## AZTEC CIVILIZATION

The Aztec Empire was the last of a succession of indigenous civilizations—Olmec, Mixtec, Zapotec, Toltec, and others—that once flourished in Mesoamerica, the region that now comprises most of modern Mexico, Guatemala, Belize, Honduras, and El Salvador. Despite the upheavals associated with the rise and fall of various early civilizations, the general belief system and traditions of Mesoamerican culture included a sacred calendar and a solar calendar, hieroglyphic writing, a complex pantheon of deities, and blood sacrifices.

After the fall of Toltec civilization, the Aztecs established an empire that dominated the region from the fourteenth to the sixteenth century. Their capital city, Tenochtitlán (now Mexico City), had a population that probably exceeded two hundred thousand. The magnificent garden city of the Aztecs had evolved from marshy islands in a shallow lake. When the Spanish Conquest began in 1519, Hernán Cortés (1485–1547) proved adept at exploiting tribal divisions and tensions within the Aztec Empire. According to Spanish accounts, Tenochtitlán was constructed on a grand scale, as demonstrated by its buildings, temples, pyramids, monuments, roads, aqueducts, fountains, bathhouses, public latrines, and gardens. The Spanish tried to destroy the great temple of Tenochtitlán and all vestiges of Aztec religion, but some ancient ruins remain within the heart of modern Mexico City.

Water management has always been one of the major problems of urban development. Spanish observations and archeological evidence suggest that the drinking water available to residents of Tenochtitlán was better than that of most sixteenth-century European cities. Personal cleanliness was so highly valued that even the common people bathed daily. Steam baths were considered essential for purification, relaxation, and as a means of fighting off fevers and poisons. In keeping with the high value the Aztecs placed on cleanliness, the streets of Tenochtitlán were swept and washed daily by hundreds of street cleaners, who were supervised by health officers and inspectors. Law and customs prohibited dumping refuse into the lake or canals. Night soil (human excrement used as fertilizer) was collected and taken by barge to farms on the mainland. Urine was collected for use in dyeing cotton cloth. Prior to contact with Europeans, strict attention to cleanliness might have mitigated the spread of indigenous diseases. Nevertheless, dysenteries, gastrointestinal disorders, rheumatism, and respiratory infections must have been fairly common, and drawings and pottery figures seem to depict the hunchback characteristic of tuberculosis of the spine.

The Aztecs developed many measures and institutions to promote the health and welfare of the residents of the capital city and distant territories. Shelters or hospitals for warriors, the sick, and needy individuals, staffed by government-supported doctors, were established throughout the Empire. European observers noted that begging, which was so common in Europe, was virtually unknown in the Aztec Empire. The highly centralized government collected tribute from subject nations, in the form of maize, cocoa, and other foods, as well as cotton, rubber, gold, and feathers. A public assistance department distributed maize to the poor and supplied food as needed in times of crop failures. To control contagious diseases, Aztec rulers established a system of strict quarantines and had physicians send patients to isolation centers.

Considering the wealth, power, complexity, and sophistication of the Aztec Empire, it is difficult to comprehend how Hernán Cortés, who came to the New World in 1519 with about six hundred men and a limited supply of horses and gunpowder weapons, was able to capture the Aztec capital in 1521 and dismantle the foundations of a remarkable civilization. Despite the advantages of gunpowder weapons, given the differences in the numbers of Spanish soldiers and Aztec warriors, a purely military confrontation would certainly have been won by the Aztecs. Many other factors, however, favored the invaders, including growing tensions within the Aztec empire. Many scholars argue that smallpox, a highly contagious viral disease previously unknown in the Americas, was the most powerful of Cortés's allies. Although Cortés and his comrades seemed unaware of the devastation caused by a disease so familiar to residents of the Old World, Native American survivors came to see the smallpox epidemic of 1520 as the turning point in their history. Aztec chronicles refer to the time before the arrival of the Spanish as a comparative paradise where the people were free of smallpox and other deadly fevers. When Europeans came, they brought fear and disease wherever they went. Spanish observers said that God had cursed Mexico with plagues of Biblical proportion so that the natives died by the thousands of smallpox, measles, war, famine, slavery, work in the mines, and other forms of oppression.

A Spanish ship apparently brought smallpox to the New World in 1516. Attempting to contain a smallpox epidemic in Santo Domingo in 1519, Spanish officials imposed quarantine regulations. By that time, the disease was already causing outbreaks among Native Americans along the coast of Mexico, as Cortés and his army prepared to attack the Aztec empire. Smallpox quickly spread throughout central Mexico, and migrated north and south through the most densely populated regions of the Americas. Europeans did not directly observe the impact of early epidemics in North America, but when Hernando de Soto (1496?–1542) explored Florida in 1539, he found evidence that many areas had already been depopulated. Just how far the first waves of smallpox traveled is uncertain, although some historians argue that European diseases did not reach northeastern North America until the early seventeenth century. Nevertheless, archeological evidence suggests that disease-induced population declines occurred in some areas of North American as early as the sixteenth century, well before significant direct contact between Native Americans and Europeans. Thus, European reports from the Americas after the smallpox epidemics of 1520 are likely to reflect societies that had already been devastated by epidemic disease.

Some historians suggested that the Conquest was possible because the Aztecs were overcrowded, malnourished, starving, and unable to cope with disease. As proof of this hypothesis, they argue that the Aztecs used human sacrifice to satisfy their need for protein. Others contend that the Aztecs were quite successful up to the time of the Conquest and that human sacrifice served important religious and political purposes unrelated to a quest for dietary protein. Although the Spanish conquerors helped create the image of the Aztecs as followers of a barbaric religion that demanded the sacrifice and consumption of huge numbers of war captives, independent evidence supports the conclusion that human sacrifice and ritual cannibalism were indeed integral aspects of Aztec religion.

According to Aztec beliefs, human beings had to support the essential balance of the universe by offering their own blood to the gods and performing ritual human sacrifices. To make blood sacrifices, the Aztecs slashed their tongues, ear lobes, or sexual organs with obsidian blades, fish spines, stingray spines, or agave thorns. Members of the elite were expected to perform the various rituals, fasts, and autosacrifices even more enthusiastically than the common people, because their blood was especially valuable.

Human sacrifice was not an unusual aspect of ancient cultures, but the magnitude of human sacrifice practiced by the Aztecs was apparently unprecedented. Many of the early Spanish accounts of the horrific extent of cannibalism were, however, based on hearsay evidence from enemies of the Aztecs. In any case, charging the Aztecs with sacrificing and eating thousands of war captives provided a rationale for the Spanish campaign to eradicate Aztec culture and religion.

Some scholars have argued that the economic, social, and nutritional base of the Aztec Empire encouraged human cannibalism. According to the "nutritional cannibalism" hypothesis, the Aztecs had so depleted their resources that the elite class turned to cannibalism as a source of high quality protein. Aztec warfare and sacrifice, therefore, served as a means of coping with population growth, environmental degradation, uncertain harvests, and protein deficiency.

Critics of this hypothesis insist that all classes in Aztec society— nobles, commoners, and slaves—generally consumed sufficient calories and had access to adequate levels of plant and animal proteins. Human sacrifice, therefore, was not a response to famine and population pressure. Moreover, those who engaged in ritual cannibalism held the most privileged place in society and were presumably the least likely to be suffering from protein deficiency. The Aztecs were accused of many atrocities, but they were not typically accused of cannibalizing the bodies of those who died in battle, nor did the practice of cannibalism coincided with times of scarcity. Generally, rites of sacrifice and cannibalism peaked at harvest time, which suggests that they were rituals of thanksgiving. Although the Aztecs were masters of human sacrifice, and conducted rituals in which they removed the heart, flayed the skin, and performed other mutilations of their unfortunate captives, they did not seem to have had an abstract interest in anatomy and dissection.

The Aztec agricultural system provided a diet that was certainly different from, but not necessarily inferior to that of contemporary Europeans. The agricultural techniques used by the Aztecs could feed a large population because of the intensive use of human labor, appropriate crop varieties, recycling of nutrients, efficient use of water resources, and the intercropping of maize, beans, and squash, the traditional Indian food triad. Maize, the basic food plant of the Aztec, Inca, and Maya civilizations, can grow where it is too dry for rice and too wet for wheat. Religious rites, paintings, and ceramic figures acknowledged the importance of maize in Aztec society. Excessive dependence on maize is associated with nutritional deficiencies, such as pellagra, but a diet that combined maize, beans, and squashes provides nutritional balance. Moreover, Native Americans prepared maize in ways that increased the availability of essential nutrients. The Aztec diet also included a variety of vegetables, fruits, algae, and drought-adapted plants, such amaranth, mesquite, and maguey. In comparison to Europeans, the Aztecs had relatively few domesticated animals, but they did keep llamas, dogs, and guinea pigs. They supplemented their basic diet with insects, fish, amphibians, reptiles, wild birds, and small mammals—such as grasshoppers, ants, worms, frogs, tadpoles, salamanders, iguanas, armadillos, weasels, and mice. Although the Spanish considered these Aztec delicacies totally repulsive, many insects and amphibians are actually quite nutritious.

Europeans may not have appreciated the superiority of pre-Conquest Aztec standards of public health, sanitation, and personal hygiene, but they were impressed by the knowledge of Aztec physicians and herbalists. Cortés considered native doctors quite skillful, and especially valued their knowledge of medicinal herbs. Aztec rulers established zoos and botanical gardens in which herbalists cultivated plants from many regions in order to concoct and study potential remedies. Before new remedies were used by members of the elite, they may have been tested on potential sacrificial victims or members of the lower classes. The information herbalists and healers collected might have been included in pre-Conquest codices, but Spanish soldiers and priests destroyed all the Aztec texts that they could find. Eventually some Spanish priests worked with Aztec informants to reconstruct parts of the old medical lore.

Because of their military and economic domination over much of Mexico, Aztec religious and medical practices diffused throughout the region. Thus, the little that is known about Aztec beliefs and practices can probably be generalized to other Mesoamerican cultures. Like most ancient cultures, the Aztecs believed that the agents that caused disease could be supernatural, magical, or natural. Medical practices, therefore, involved a mixture of magic, religion, and empirical science. For illnesses and conditions that did not respond to the usual domestic medicines, people consulted members of the medical community. Although medical practitioners apparently developed specialized knowledge and techniques, healers retained both medical and priestly attributes. Priests, shamans, and other kinds of healers drove out or neutralized the evil spirits that caused disease through the use of prayers, spells, charms, amulets, and other magical devices. Aztec healing rituals included confession, purification rites, massage, and exploration of the body in order to find "object intrusions" that caused serious illnesses.

Healers found diagnostic clues by studying the patient's appearance, behavior, and dreams. After consulting the viscera of an animal oracle, a healer might prescribe amulets and talismans made of shells, crystals, stones, or animal organs. If wearing these protective devices proved unsuccessful, a shaman could help the patient pass the disorder to a new victim. Healing rituals might involve penance, self-mutilation, baths, incantations, inhaling smoke, or eating images of gods made out of amaranth dough. Hallucinogenic agents were essential aspects of the diagnostic and curative procedures for certain illnesses. A shaman might ingest hallucinogens and travel to other worlds to consult supernatural beings and then return with a diagnosis and perhaps a remedy. Rituals that symbolically honored the gods, such as burning various oils and resins to produce an aromatic smoke, might also have practical value in driving away noxious insects.

Aztec priests served a large pantheon of gods and goddesses, including many that were associated with certain kinds of disease, specific remedies, and medical practitioners. Numerous gods ruled over daily life and many of them demanded human and animal sacrifices. The gods could afflict individuals or whole societies as punishment for personal or collective transgressions. There were gods that were linked to medicinal herbs, skin diseases, respiratory diseases, dysentery, sleep and the interpretation of dreams, women's diseases, and childbirth. Diagnosing the cause of supernatural ailments and performing the rites of appeasement required the services of healers who served the appropriate gods. In terms of specialization of functions, Aztec healers might be characterized as phlebotomists, surgeons, or internists who dealt with disorders of the eyes, stomach, bladder, and so forth. Aztec dentists treated inflamed gums, extracted ulcerated teeth, and performed cosmetic procedures. The art of healing could be passed down from father to son, through apprenticeships, or studied at certain temples where priests taught their students about the relationships among gods, diseases, and healing, as well as astrology and the art of casting horoscopes.

Sorcery might be indirectly involved as a cause of traumatic wounds, but the immediate causes of sprains, dislocations, fractures, and poisoning by venomous snakes and insects were usually quite obvious. In the treatment of fractures and sprains, Aztec healers compared favorably with their European counterparts. Razor-sharp obsidian scalpels and blades were used in surgery, bloodletting, and rituals of self-mutilation. Researchers who studied obsidian instruments and weapons suggested that the usefulness of these artifacts might have been one of the reasons pre-Columbian cultures did not develop European-style metallurgy.

A general concern for cleanliness must have been a great advantage in Aztec surgery and obstetrics. Preparations containing narcotic plants and fungi, such as jimson weed, marijuana, mescaline, and peyote, probably contributed to pain relief. Wounds, boils, and abscesses were washed and dressed with various herbs, oils, poultices, and ointments. Surgeons set fractures, using splints and casts, and closed wounds with sutures made of human hair. Aztec and Maya surgeons performed trepanations, although the Inca are best known for this operation. Head wounds were also treated by covering them with protective plasters made of resins, egg white, feathers, blood, and ashes. In addition to medicinal herbs, Aztec remedies contained minerals, such as jade and charcoal, and animal parts and products, such as bile, venom, urine, antlers, pulverized bones, and honey. An elastic gum, later known as India rubber, was used to make enema syringes.

Chronicles by Spanish observers, including physicians and clergymen, provide early glimpses of disease and medical practices in the New World, but such records introduced many distortions. Unable and unwilling to accept unfamiliar doctrines, Europeans attempted to force New World concepts into classical European theories. Although some missionaries were interested in Aztec civilization, their goal in collecting information about pre-Contact customs was primarily to expedite the conversion of the Indians to Christianity. Missionaries wanted to understand Indian religions, deities, and rituals so that they could detect forbidden rituals disguised as Christian worship. Priests even prohibited the use and cultivation of amaranth, a staple Aztec grain that provides high quality protein, because it was used in native healing rites. Typically, images of native gods were made of amaranth dough and eaten during religious festivals. To Spanish priests and conquistadors, this seemed a parody of the Catholic Eucharist. After the Conquest, amaranth became quite rare, but in the 1970s, nutritionists rediscovered its value.

After the Conquest, the establishment of Spanish missions resulted in devastating epidemics of smallpox, measles, and other diseases among Indians removed from their villages and forced to provide labor for their new rulers. Missions were established by Spanish priests to consolidate groups of formerly dispersed natives to in order to facilitate their conversion to Catholicism. Missionized Indians experienced disruption of their traditional social systems, overcrowding, unsanitary conditions, malnutrition caused by an increasingly restricted diet, epidemic diseases, a harsh workload, all of which led to decreases in birthrates and increases in mortality rates. Surveys carried out by colonial authorities in the seventeenth century documented the continuing decline in Indian populations, the increasing demands for tribute and labor, and the breakdown of Native American communities.

Missionaries established colleges in New Spain as early as the 1530s where they trained Aztecs as scribes and translators in order to compile ethnographic information and expedite the conversion of the Indians. Accounts of Aztec drugs have, therefore, been preserved in a few texts written in Nahuatl, the language of the Aztecs, and translated into

Spanish or Latin. Important natural histories of New Spain were also compiled by Spanish physicians. In 1570, King Philip II sent Francisco Hernández (1517–1587) to the New World to gather information about the "natural things" found in the new Spanish empire. Hernández was expected to consult local doctors, medicine men, and herbalists, test the alleged properties of New World herbs, trees, and medicinal plants, and determine which might provide new drugs. Although Hernández generally remained close to Mexico City, native doctors and herbalists gave him information about hundreds of plants and animals that were unknown in Europe. Hernández attempted to confirm the alleged medical virtues of New World species by conducting clinical trials at hospitals in Mexico City. When he returned to Spain, Hernández had hundreds of illustrations and notes in Náhuatl, Spanish, and Latin describing some three thousand plants. Hailed by admirers as the Spanish Pliny, Hernández composed a multivolume natural history of New Spain and a report on the history and customs of the native peoples.

According to Hernández, the Aztecs knew the curative and economic aspects of some 1,200 medicinal plants. In addition to purges, febrifuges, tonics, and so forth, the New World provided novel intoxicating preparations, from which chemists eventually isolated various hallucinogens, psychoactive drugs, anesthetics, analgesics, and narcotics. Although Hernández evaluated Aztec medicinal materials and treatments in terms of classical European humoral theories, he noted the usefulness of Náhuatl taxonomies. To make his work more widely accessible, Hernández had it translated from Latin into Spanish and Náhuatl. Unfortunately, the great treatise he had planned was not published during his lifetime. Other naturalists prepared abstracts and excerpts that were prized by physicians for many generations.

After Mexico fell to the conquistadors in 1521, it became the Spanish Colony of New Spain, along with much of Central America, Texas, California, Arizona, New Mexico, and so forth. By 1523, the Aztec capital had been largely rebuilt with palaces and fortresses for the new military government; churches, hospitals, and schools were constructed on the ruins of Aztec temples and palaces. During some three hundred years of colonial rule, Spanish administrators and settlers attempted to transplant European medical institutions and ideas into a world devastated by military conquest, epidemic disease, and the collapse of the indigenous social structure. With little regard for local conditions, officials attempted to establish in New Spain the same rigid laws, licensing requirements, and institutional structures that governed medical practitioners, pharmacists, and midwives in Spain. Except for herbal lore, indigenous medicine was condemned, suppressed, and virtually extinguished. In time, however, a unique form of medicine evolved that incorporated elements of indigenous practice and Hippocratic traditions.

Although the Spanish destroyed the hierarchy and authority of the Aztec Empire, they could not readily change the folk beliefs of indigenous peoples. Indeed, the most fundamental beliefs of the common people were much older than the Aztec Empire and had survived the rise and fall of previous conquerors. In Mexico today, traditional healers, known as *curanderos* and *brujos*, continue to attract patients. Advocates of modern medicine generally see such traditional healers as obstacles to medical progress and threats to the public health. But the remedies of the curanderos may reflect a mixture of ancient Aztec practices, folklore, and Hippocratic theories.

## MAYAN CIVILIZATION

Europeans may have caught glimpses of the Maya during the last voyage of Columbus in 1502, but they learned almost nothing about this civilization until 1517 when a storm drove three Spanish ships towards the northeastern tip of the Yucatan peninsula. Survivors of this voyage brought back stories of mysterious cities with temples containing great treasures. The encounter between Spaniards and the Maya was recorded by Bernal Diaz del Castillo (ca. 1492–1581), a Spanish soldier who participated in the conquest of Mexico and Diego de Landa (1524–1579), who served as Bishop of Yucatan. Studying the Maya in his attempt to convert them, Diego de Landa collected and destroyed many Mayan codices. After the Conquest, Mayan converts to Christianity recorded historical and religious traditions that had been passed down orally or in hieroglyphic records. Doubts have been raised about the authenticity and reliability of post-Conquest Mayan texts, but some of the stories in these texts seem to be corroborated by inscriptions found in ancient Mayan temples.

Members of the Mayan linguistic and cultural group occupied tropical areas that are now parts of Mexico, Guatemala, Belize, Honduras, and El Salvador. At its height, Mayan civilization could boast of magnificent cities, temples, pyramids, monuments, ceremonial centers, hieroglyphic writings, complex calendrical computations, elaborate irrigation systems, prosperous markets, and an extensive system of paved stone roads. Mayan civilization flourished for almost a thousand years before entering a period of general decline. By the time the Spanish arrived in the early sixteenth century, the ruins of many Mayan cities were lost in the jungles of Guatemala and southern Mexico. Some Mayan communities in remote and inaccessible areas preserved their language and culture long after the Conquest. Anthropologists and historians have gained insights into the history of the Maya by studying the culture of their descendants.

Recent studies of artifacts and carved stone monuments in the ruins of ancient cities have challenged previous ideas about the timing of the early stages of the classic Maya period. For example, the ruins of Cival, an ancient city in Guatemala, revealed all the characteristics of classic Mayan cities: complex architecture, pyramids, palaces, ceramics, and writings inscribed on stone. Surprisingly, Cival was probably occupied by 600 B.C.E. and reached its peak about 150 B.C.E. Archeologists previously assumed that the classic Maya period began about 250 B.C.E. Other cities, once considered preclassic, have also revealed very early evidence of a highly developed culture.

The classic period of Mayan civilization ended in the ninth century with the mysterious collapse of major Mayan cities. Although many factors—overpopulation, malnutrition, epidemics, war, climate change, deforestation, soil erosion, drought, and crop failures—must have contributed to the decline of Mayan civilization, warfare and climatic change were probably especially significant. A century-long succession of severe dry spells began about the seventh century. The presence of numerous human skeletons in cenotes and caves sacred to the Maya suggests that in response to the devastating droughts, the Maya offered more and more sacrifices to the gods as their appeals for rain grew increasingly desperate.

Eighteenth-century explorers imagined the Maya as highly civilized, urban, and peaceful people who were presumably obsessed with art, cosmology, astronomy, mathematics, and complex calendrical calculations. Classic Mayan civilization was thought of as a confederation of peaceful, cooperative city-states dominated by powerful priests and wealthy nobles, supported by hard-working peasants. But as archeologists explored more sites and began to decode Mayan art and inscriptions, a very different portrait of the Mayan Empire emerged. New evidence indicates that the Maya lived in a state of almost constant warfare; captives taken in battle were tortured and sacrificed to the gods.

Most Mayan inscriptions are chronicles of specific rulers, gods, myths, and rituals, but some provide insights into beliefs about health and disease, as well as bloodletting rituals and human sacrifices. As depicted in Mayan artwork, bloodletting was an important part of religious and political ceremonies. Kings and aristocrats were expected to perform the rite of self-sacrifice with the most frequency and enthusiasm, because their blood was particularly prized. Anesthetized by religious enthusiasm, and perhaps drugs, they would pierce their tongue, penis, or earlobe and pull a rope through the wound. The blood was collected and offered to the gods. One carving depicted a ceremonial occasion in which a noblewoman pulled a thorn-studded rope through her tongue, while her blood dripped into a basket at her feet.

Violent rivalry between states might have been reflected in rituals that were apparently enacted against buildings and their inhabitants.

In many ruined temples and palaces throughout Central America, archeologists have found puzzling collections of smashed ceramics, figurines, tools, ornaments, and other artifacts. Scholars suggest that ritualized feasting might have preceded violent "termination rituals" in which buildings and their contents were ceremonially destroyed, presumably to represent the physical and spiritual defeat of an enemy. The debris found in the wreckage of Mayan buildings was previously attributed to squatters and vandals who might have occupied such building after they had been abandoned by kings and nobles. Historians and archeologists are trying to develop a more balanced view of Mayan civilization, presumably somewhere between the discarded myth of a peaceful Mayan world and a new one that might overemphasize cruelty and violence.

Studies of the ethnobiological doctrines of Mayan speaking peoples have provided insights into ancient Mayan life, cultural concepts, and botanical knowledge. Mayan concepts of plant classification have been of particular interest to modern pharmacological scientists. Mayan remedies included the usual array of local medicinal herbs, minerals, and animal parts and products, as well as many concoctions involving tobacco. Europeans first observed a custom they called "tobacco drinking" among the Aztecs, but they discovered even more exotic uses for tobacco among the Maya. One recipe included tobacco and a remarkable extract made by soaking live toads in a herbal liquor. Tobacco was a key component of remedies for pain, flu, colds, sores, toothache, abscesses, fevers, fatigue, and the bites of poisonous snakes. Women took tobacco to prevent miscarriage, to expel the placenta, and so forth.

Tobacco mixed with coca and lime made from burning seashells was used as a stimulant or intoxicant. In addition to fighting fatigue, such preparations were said to offer protection against snakes and other poisonous animals. During healing rituals, shamans and medicine men often consumed large doses of tobacco in order to douse the patient with tobacco-enriched saliva. Tobacco intoxication was said to allow the shaman to see inside the patient. Tobacco, mixed with other herbal intoxicants, was also taken by way of enema syringes, as depicted in Mayan art. Tobacco drinking and tobacco-smoke enemas were soon adopted in Europe. Although some European physicians condemned the use of tobacco, others praised its purgative, soporific, and intoxicating properties.

European physicians were also somewhat ambivalent about cocoa, another interesting product used as a food and a tonic by the Maya. Cocoa powder and chocolate were made from the seeds of the cacao tree (also known as the chocolate tree). Recent studies suggest that the Maya used cocoa in beverages as early as 600 B.C.E., about a thousand years earlier than previously thought. Spanish explorers noted that Mayas liked to pour cocoa mixture from one vessel to another to generate a froth. Cocoa was probably roasted, ground, and mixed with spices and water. This ancient beverage might have been energizing, but it must have been rather bitter. Cacao was exported to Spain in the 1520s, but the exotic new beverage did not become popular in Europe until the seventeenth century. Even though many regarded chocolate with suspicion, others praised its alleged medical virtues.

## INCAN CIVILIZATION

Cuzco in Peru was the heart of the Inca Empire, which once included parts of the regions that are now Argentina, Bolivia, Chile, Colombia, and Ecuador. The Incas had conquered vast territories, encompassing very diverse environments, and subdued people of very different cultures. The remarkable Incan road system, which depended on relay runners and rest houses, allowed the Inca rulers to communicate with officials throughout the empire. The ruins of many agricultural terraces, irrigation canals, and cities in Peru predating the Inca Empire testify to complex societies that once flourished in this region. There is considerable archeological evidence in the region of periods of population growth accompanied by the rise of complex societies, followed by periods of collapse and decline, long before European contact.

Incan civilization lasted only about a hundred years, but it was at its peak when Francisco Pizarro (1475?–1541) and his small band of treasure hunters arrived in 1532. Fortunately for Pizarro, the leadership of the Inca Empire had recently been weakened by a struggle for the throne after the death of the king and other important members of the Inca nobility, possibly from smallpox. Within two years, Pizarro had captured and executed Atahualpa (1502?–1533), whose reign as emperor began in 1525, and destroyed the foundations of the Incan empire. Pizarro's success was apparently aided by the devastating impact of European epidemic diseases that had preceded direct European contact. A catastrophic epidemic, which might have been smallpox, swept the region in the mid-1520s, leaving the Empire vulnerable to Pizarro's plans for the conquest of Peru. Subsequent epidemics, which may have included typhus, influenza, smallpox, and measles, devastated the region by the end of the sixteenth century. In the 1550s, descendants of Incan nobles recited the oral history and traditions of their ancestors for scribes like Juan de Betanzos who transcribed the memoirs that were later published as *Narrative of the Incas*.

Unlike the Mayas and Aztecs, the Incas did not develop a system of writing, but their professional "rememberers" encoded and recorded information by using quipus (or khipus), knotted strings in many colors. Spanish conquerors and missionaries, suspecting that quipus might contain accounts of Inca history and religion, as well as more mundane financial records, burned whole libraries of quipus. Archeologists originally thought of the quipu as a textile abacus or mnemonic device, but some scholars believe that certain complex quipus might contain more than financial records and census data. If quipus recorded words as well as numbers they would represent a unique writing system, but this possibility remains controversial. No Incan "Rosetta Stone" has been discovered and no khipus have been deciphered.

Archeologists are gaining new information about Incan civilization through explorations of recently discovered sacred places and hidden cities, as well as analyses of artifacts and human remains at well-known archeological sites like Machu Picchu. In 1911, Hiram Bingham III discovered Machu Picchu, a city fifty miles from Cuzco. Bingham popularized the expression "lost city" through his influential books, *Machu Picchu: A Citadel of the Incas* and *Lost City of the Incas*. Machu Picchu was probably one of many private estates and country retreats of the Inca nobility. Skeletons examined by physical anthropologists indicate that many families lived and died at Machu Picchu. The simplicity of grave goods, however, suggests that the bodies are those of people who worked at the estate, rather than the nobles who used the site as a retreat. The skeletal remains indicate that the workers were fairly well fed, although their diet was heavily based on corn, and tooth decay was common. Workers apparently came from many different parts of the empire, as indicated by differences in the shapes of their skulls. Different ethnic groups created distinctive cranial deformations by binding the heads of their infants.

The discovery of an ancient cemetery on the outskirts of Lima, Peru, might reveal even more about life, health, disease, and social organization among the Incas than the discovery of another "lost city." The dry soil of the coastal Peruvian desert provided excellent conditions for preservation, even though the bodies were not embalmed. By 2003, archeologists had uncovered the remains of more than two thousand Incas, but the cemetery contains many more graves, as well as priceless artifacts. The mummies represent a wide spectrum of age groups and social classes. In many cases, the hair, skin, and eyes were still intact. Many of the bodies were buried in groups known as mummy bundles, some of which contained as many as seven individuals and weighed about four hundred pounds. These cocoon-like bundles were made by wrapping bodies together in layers of raw cotton and patterned textiles. Some bundles contain adults and children, as well as grave goods including tools, weapons, utensils, pottery, foods, textiles, implements for sewing and weaving, ornaments, and so forth. Some mummies were buried with headdresses that marked them as members of the nobility. "False heads" (large cotton-filled bumps, often covered with wigs), another sign of high social status, were found in about 40 mummy bundles. Well-preserved human mummies have also been found at other sites in Peru and Chile.

Pottery figures found in Peruvian archeological sites indicate that the Incas were quite familiar with Verruga peruana, the eruptive stage of Carrión's disease. Spanish observers described illnesses consistent with both the eruptive skin lesions of Verruga peruana and the acute febrile stage known as Oroya fever. The bacteria that cause Carrión's disease can be found in various small animals in South America. Human beings become infected when the infectious agent is transmitted by the sandfly. Until the 1870s, when thousands of workers died of the acute febrile form of the disease during the construction of a railroad from Lima to Oroya, the disease was one of many obscure fevers and skin disorders found in rural areas. In 1885, Daniel A. Carrión (1859–1885) demonstrated the fundamental identity of Verruga peruana and Oroya fever by inoculating himself with blood from a verruga patient. He died of Oroya fever, which, in the absence of antibiotics, has a very high mortality rate. Ten years later, Ernesto Odriozola (1862–1921) published an account of Carrión's experiments and named the disease in his honor. Leishmaniasis might have been brought to the Americas along with the slave trade, but some Peruvian pottery figures depicted deformities of the lips and nose that represent an indigenous disease known as *uta*, or American leishmaniasis.

Medical knowledge and surgical practice, as well as the organization of the Incan medical community, were apparently highly developed. An elite group of hereditary physicians attended the Inca emperor, but other physicians, surgeons, herbalists, and healers provided care for the general populace. Therapeutic methods included herbal remedies, baths, bleeding, massage, various forms of wound treatment, and so forth. In addition to managing wounds, fractures, and dislocations, Peruvian surgeons performed major operations, such as amputation and trepanation (trephination), perhaps with the help of coca leaves. Thousands of trepanned skulls, found in archeological sites, provide the most dramatic testimony to the surgical skills of Native American healers.

Coca, a shrub that the Incas considered sacred, is the source of cocaine and other alkaloids. Sixteenth-century observers said that the natives of Peru planted coca in the forests of the Andes, gathered the leaves, spread them on cloths, and allowed them to dry in the sun. The dry leaves were mixed with wood ash or unslaked lime and chewed to ward off fatigue, relieve drowsiness, lift the spirits, and make it possible to endure extreme exertion, despite hunger, thirst, and cold. Coca mixed with tobacco and other substances was said to produce a state of intoxication. Modern physiological research supports the traditional belief that Peruvian Indians used coca because it promoted adaptation to hunger, cold, and fatigue at high altitudes.

In the 1860s, an American diplomat visited Cuzco, where he acquired a collection of curiosities that included a trepanned human skull, which he sent to Paul Broca (1824–1880), the French anthropologist. Broca's discussion of the skull at the 1867 meeting of the Anthropological Society of Paris stimulated the search for more examples of prehistoric surgery. Trepanned skulls were eventually found in the Americas, Europe, Africa, and Asia, leading to debates about whether the technique developed in one culture and spread to others, or independently evolved in separate regions. The origins of various forms of trepanation are obscure, but the procedure certainly appeared in both the Americas and the Old World before the voyages of Columbus.

Probably more than half of all ancient trepanned skulls in the world have been found in Peru. Before the operation, both the patient and the surgeon probably chewed coca leaves, which would provide both mood elevation and a coca juice extract that the surgeon could apply to the skull as a local anesthetic. Despite the seriousness of this operation, many patients recovered and went on to live a normal lifespan. Some individuals survived two or three operations, as indicated by skulls with multiple trepanations and evidence of healing. The operation was probably done to treat severe headaches, epilepsy, and head injuries, such as depressed skull fractures caused by close encounters with clubs, sling stones, or the star-headed mace during battles. Trepanation can remove bone fragments and relieve pressure on the brain.

Studies of hundreds of Peruvian trepanned skulls, dated from about 400 B.C.E. to the 1530s, have distinguished four methods of trephination: scraping, rectangular incision, circular incision, and drilling and cutting. Scraping involved wearing away an area of bone until the *dura mater* was reached. Rectangular incision involved cutting four grooves to form a square and lifting out a piece of bone. Circular cutting had the best rate of success and survival. The surgeon rapidly cut circular grooves deeper and deeper into the skull until a piece of bone could be removed. Drilling a series of holes next to each other and then cutting out a piece of skull was quite rare and very dangerous because of the possibility of puncturing the brain.

Researchers find that many elements of traditional medicine have been passed down for more than five hundred years by the inhabitants of the Andean region of Peru and Bolivia. Like most traditional systems, the healing art was based on magic, empiricism, and religion. A rare intermingling of Western medicine and traditional Indian culture occurred during the 1930s in Puno, an isolated, mountainous region in southeastern Peru. At that time, interest in native medical concepts and practices had been encouraged by the emergence of a nationalistic movement called *indigenismo*, which emphasized and celebrated native traditions and culture. The movement stimulated the work of Manuel Nuñez Butrón (1900–1952), a physician who organized an Indian rural sanitary brigade in Puno. The goal of the sanitary brigade was to respect native values, use native workers, promote smallpox vaccination, improve sanitation, fight typhus, and so forth. The census of 1940 indicated that this region had a ratio of one health worker per 24,000 people. The ratio in Lima was one medical professional per 350 people. Members of the brigade served as itinerant doctors, but within little more than a decade, the call for modernization replaced the idealization of traditional culture and the brigades disappeared.

## DISEASES IN THE AMERICAS

The high civilizations of the Americas provide some specific focus for analysis of the impact of the earliest European intrusions, but the effect on other native peoples is more difficult to assess because of the diffuse web of contacts and the great diversity of populations, cultures, and environments. Speculative generalizations continue to arise, as do detailed studies of particular regions and peoples. Still, even the total population and settlement patterns of pre-Contact America are matters of debate. There is essentially no debate about the fact that Native American populations collapsed after European contact; the magnitude of that impact, the severity of epidemics, the pathways by which epidemic diseases were disseminated, with and without direct European contact, and other aggravating factors, are uncertain and controversial. Although European diseases were obviously devastating to Native Americans, the impact of disease depends on complex cultural, social, economic, and institutional factors, as well as the natural history of disease.

The European conquest of the Empires of the Aztec, Incas, and Maya brought about what historians have called a catastrophic conjunction of "virgin soil epidemics" (outbreaks of diseases new to the area) and "ungulate irruptions" (the environmental degradation that follows the introduction of grazing animals into new ecosystems). The introduction of European domesticated grazing animals altered the landscape and patterns of access to natural resources. Peacefully grazing sheep, for example, devoured new pastures and reproduced beyond the carrying capacity of the land. Seeking more and more land for their animals and crops, Europeans disrupted traditional agricultural practices, ruined the land, and increasingly displaced native peoples.

In a virgin soil epidemic, no members of the affected group have immunity, because the entire population lacks prior experience with the disease. If all members of a community become ill simultaneously, mortality explodes because no healthy individuals are left to provide the simplest kinds of nursing care. When parents and grandparents are sick or dead, infants and children may die from dehydration and starvation even if they do not acquire the disease. This does not mean that those who died had defective or weak immune systems. Moreover, as a result of epidemic diseases, food supplies may be lost because no able-bodied individuals are available to manage planting or harvesting crops, or caring for domesticated animals.

Of course the New World was not a disease-free utopia, but Old World diseases like smallpox and measles were devastating to Native Americans and, therefore, served as allies in the European colonization of the Americas. A catastrophic, permanent demographic collapse might have occurred when the first devastating smallpox epidemics were followed by additional waves of disease, compounded by crop failures and food shortages. Such factors could have prevented the resurgence of population that typically occurred after pandemics struck the Old World. European diseases spread from place to place even in the absence of Europeans, leaving death and confusion and obscuring the patterns of life that had previously existed.

In response to complaints that precipitous declines in the population of Indians were causing labor shortages, King Charles I of Spain agreed to the importation of slaves directly from Africa. From the early sixteenth to the late nineteenth century, the slave trade brought some 10 million Africans to the New World. The mortality of slaves during the horrific voyage to the Americas was so high that some historians estimate that perhaps only about 25 percent of the Africans forced into slave ships survived the voyage to the Western hemisphere. Nevertheless, Europeans came to believe that African people were better adapted to laboring in the New World than Native Americans, primarily because of their alleged immunity to yellow fever and malaria. The medical consequences of the African slave trade were complex, as might be expected from this unprecedented mixing of the germ pools of Europe, Africa, and the Americas. Some diseases were especially fatal to the Indians, but seemed to spare whites and blacks; others were fatal to whites and Indians, but seemed to spare blacks.

Eighteenth-century observers noted that certain diseases—such as diarrhea and dysentery, parasitic worms, venereal diseases, pneumonia, lung abscesses, pica (dirt eating), yaws, smallpox, lockjaw (tetanus), the itch, eye diseases, fevers, and sleeping sickness—were typically associated with the slave trade. Many African diseases became permanent residents of the New World, but sleeping sickness did not because of the absence of its vector, the tsetse fly. To treat dysentery, Europeans adopted ipecac, an Indian remedy for diarrheal diseases and certain kinds of poisoning. African "remittent" and "bilious remittent" fevers might have been malaria or yellow fever. Quarantine of new African slaves would not have prevented the importation of certain diseases: those with long latent periods, diseases disseminated by healthy carriers, and those transmitted by ubiquitous insect vectors. The slave trade might, therefore, be associated with the global redistribution of amebiasis (amebic dysentery), hookworm, leprosy, filariasis, Guinea worm, yaws, syphilis, trachoma, malaria, yellow fever, and other diseases.

Epidemics probably preceded Spanish explorers, like Cabeza de Vaca (1490?–1557?) and Francisco Vásquez de Coronado (1510–1554), into the Southwest and Great Plains of North America. Explorers who followed de Vaca and Coronado saw empty land and scattered peoples. Their observations created the myth of the Great Plains as a "vast and empty hunting ground." The demographic collapse that apparently preceded European incursions into much of North America means that Europeans did not see the cultures of this region at the peak of their complexity and population density. By the 1730s, bands of hunters were engaged in trade relationships with Europeans, which led to the adoption of horses and guns and the transformation of hunting, trade, warfare, and patterns of disease.

Despite the introduction of Jennerian vaccination in the early nineteenth century, sporadic and often deadly epidemics remained a threat, especially to Native Americans, throughout the Western hemisphere. In the United States, the Vaccination Act of 1832 assigned the task of protecting Indians from smallpox to the federal government, but funding and resources were always inadequate. Even when vaccines were administered, they were often ineffective because of improper preparation or storage. During some epidemics, no vaccine was available at all, as in the case of the pandemic of 1837–1839. Epidemics among the Pueblo and Hopi Indians, in New Mexico and Arizona, from 1898 to 1899 were the last major smallpox epidemics in American Indian history.

European influence on Native American peoples eventually reached the far north, areas that are now Canada and Alaska, a vast area of diverse geographic and climatic regions where distinctive Aleut, Eskimo, and Indian cultures evolved. Before significant contact with Europeans, the major health problems seemed to be a high incidence of skin infections and intestinal disorders, as well as respiratory, rheumatic, and other diseases. Early explorers and traders, both Russian and American, introduced alcohol, tobacco, smallpox, venereal diseases, tuberculosis, and other diseases. During the 1860s, a smallpox epidemic in British Columbia killed more than half of the Indian population and devastated the Indians of the Queen Charlotte Islands. Such high mortality rates are especially appalling, because smallpox vaccination was well known by that time. According to census data from the 1880s, the Indian population was less than 20 percent of that enumerated in the 1839–1842 Hudson's Bay census.

Not all Europeans saw the decline in native population in the same way, although they generally agreed that the disappearance of the Indians was inevitable. The Spanish, who expected to extract taxes and compulsory labor from the Indians, while saving their souls, found the prospect of their disappearance deplorable. English colonists clearly recognized the devastating impact that European diseases had on the indigenous people of New England. One pious seventeenth century observer wrote: "The good hand of God favoured our beginnings in sweeping away the multitudes of the Natives by the small pox." Despite the devastating effects of Old World diseases and predictions about the inevitable disappearance of American Indians, as the prevalence of small-pox and other epidemic diseases began to decline the Native American population stabilized and began to grow again. So too did interest in native languages, religions, medicine, cultures, and ancient civilizations.

Interviews with Indian shamans, medicine men, and tribal chiefs in the nineteenth and twentieth centuries provide insights into traditional beliefs, despite the inevitable admixture of European medical concepts and practices that must have occurred over the years since European contact. For example, remedies for bullet wounds and medicines containing parts of chickens and pigs are obviously not pre-Columbian in origin. But, of course, many traditional remedies included animal parts and products, including turtle shells, bezoar stones from deer, elk, and moose, and the scent sac of a skunk.

Despite differences in culture, environment, and historical experience, theories of disease, prevention, and cure among different Native American groups have much in common. Disease was usually attributed to the hostility of the spirit prototype of some animal species; but animals also were credited with inventing cures for particular diseases. Some diseases were attributed to ghosts or witches, or violation of ceremonial regulations. Rituals, songs, and herbal remedies were all considered important components of healing. Medicinal herbs, leaves, roots, and bark were used in tonics, wound dressings, antidotes for sorcery, and so forth. An idea that might appeal to members of the modern medical community was the Seminole belief that treatment will not be effective until the doctor is well paid.

## SUGGESTED READINGS

Alarcón, Hernando Ruiz de (1984). *Treatise on the Heathen Superstitions That Today Live Among the Indians Native to This New Spain, 1629* (Trans. and ed. by J. R. Andrews and R. Hassig). Norman, OK: University of Oklahoma Press.

Alchon, S. A. (2003). *A Pest in the Land: New World Epidemics in a Global Perspective.* Albuquerque, NM: University of New Mexico Press.

Ashburn, P. M. (1980). *The Ranks of Death: A Medical History of the Conquest of America.* Philadelphia, PA: Porcupine Press. (Reprint of the 1947 ed.)

Bastien, J. W. (1998). *The Kiss of Death: Chagas' Disease in the Americas.* Salt Lake City, UT: University of Utah Press.

Betanzos, Juan de (1996). *Narrative of the Incas.* (Trans. and ed. by R. Hamilton and D. Buchanan from the Palma de Mallorca Manuscript). Austin, TX: University of Texas Press.

Blanton, R. E., ed. (1993). *Ancient Mesoamerica: A Comparison of Change in Three Regions.* New York: Cambridge University Press.

Boone, E. H., ed. (1984). *Ritual Human Sacrifice in Mesoamerica.* Washington, DC: Dumbarton Oaks Research Library and Collection.

Boone, E. H. (2000). *Stories in Red and Black: Pictorial Histories of the Aztecs and Mixtecs.* Austin, TX: University of Texas Press.

Boyd, R. (1999). *The Coming of the Spirit of Pestilence: Introduced Infectious Diseases and Population Decline among Northwest Coast Indians, 1774–1874.* Seattle, WA: University of Washington Press.

Cook, N. D. (1998). *Born to Die: Disease and New World Conquest, 1492–1650.* New York: Cambridge University Press.

Crosby, A. W., Jr. (1972). *The Columbian Exchange: Biological and Cultural Consequences of 1492.* Westport, CT: Greenwood Press.

Cruz, M. (1940). *The Badianus Manuscript; An Aztec Herbal of 1552.* Facsimile. Introduced, translated, and annotated by E. W. Emmart. Baltimore, MD: Johns Hopkins Press.

Dobyns, H. F., and Swagerty, W. R. (1983). *Their Number Became Thinned: Native American Population Dynamics in Eastern North America.* Knoxville, TN: University of Tennessee Press.

Fortuine, R. (1989). *Chills and Fever: Health and Disease in the Early History of Alaska.* Fairbanks, AS: University of Alaska Press.

Henige, D. (1998). *Numbers from Nowhere: The American Indian Contact Population Debate.* Norman, OK: University of Oklahoma Press.

Jackson, R. H. (1994). *Indian Population Decline: The Missions of Northwestern New Spain, 1687–1840.* Albuquerque, NM: University of New Mexico Press.

Jarcho, S. (1993). *Quinine's Predecessor: Francesco Torti and the Early History of Cinchona.* Baltimore, MD: Johns Hopkins University Press.

Josephy, A. M., Jr., ed. (1993). *America in 1492. The World of the Indian Peoples Before the Arrival of Columbus.* New York: Vintage Books.

Kunitz, S. J. (1994). *Disease and Social Diversity: The European Impact on the Health of Non-Europeans.* New York: Oxford University Press.

Lockhart, J., ed. and trans. (1993). *We People Here: Nahuatl Accounts of the Conquest of Mexico.* Berkeley, CA: University of California Press.

Marcus, J. (1992). *Mesoamerican Writing Systems. Propaganda, Myth, and History in Four Ancient Civilizations.* Princeton, NJ: Princeton University Press.

Melville, E. G. K. (1994). *A Plague of Sheep. Environmental Consequences of the Conquest of Mexico.* New York: Cambridge University Press.

de Montellano, B. O. (1990). *Aztec Medicine, Health, and Nutrition.* New Brunswick, NJ: Rutgers University Press.

Numbers, R. L., ed. (1987). *Medicine in the New World: New Spain, New France, and New England.* Knoxville, TN: University of Tennessee Press.

Orellana, S. L. (1987). *Indian Medicine in Highland Guatemala: The Pre-Hispanic and Colonial Periods.* Albuquerque, NM: University of New Mexico Press.

Perleth, M. (1997). *Historical Aspects of American Trypanosomiasis (Chagas' Disease).* Frankfurt am Main: Peter Lang.

Ramenofsky, A. F. (1987). *Vectors of Death. The Archaeology of European Contact.* Albuquerque, NM: University of New Mexico Press.

Restall, M. (2003). *Seven Myths of the Spanish Conquest.* New York: Oxford University Press.

Robertson, R. G. (2001). *Rotting Face: Smallpox and the American Indian.* Caldwell, Idaho: Caxon Press.

Robicsek, F. (1978). *The Smoking Gods: Tobacco in Mayan Art, History and Religion.* Norman, OK: University of Oklahoma Press.

Roys, R. L. (1976). *The Ethno-Botany of the Maya.* (With a new introduction and supplemental bibliography by S. Cosminsky). Philadelphia, PA: Institute for the Study of Human Issues.

Sahagún, Berardino de (1989). *Conquest of New Spain.* Salt Lake City, UT: University of Utah Press.

Schleiffer, H., compiler (1973). *Sacred Narcotic Plants of the New World Indians. An Anthology of Texts from the Sixteenth Century to Date.* New York: Hafner Press.

Thornton, R. (1987). *American Indian Holocaust and Survival: A Population History Since 1492.* Norman, OK: University of Oklahoma Press.

Varey, S., Chabrán, R., Weiner, D. B., eds. (2000). *Searching for the Secrets of Nature: The Life and Works of Dr. Francisco Hernández.* Stanford, CA: Stanford University Press.

Verano, J. W., and Ubelaker, D. H., eds. (1992). *Disease and Demography in the Americas.* Washington, DC: Smithsonian Institution Press.

Vogel, V. J. (1970). *American Indian Medicine.* Norman, OK: University of Oklahoma Press.

Waldram, J. B., Herring, D. A., and Young, T. K. (1995). *Aboriginal Health in Canada: Historical, Cultural, and Epidemiological Perspectives.* Toronto: University of Toronto Press.

Webster, D. L. (2002). *The Fall of the Ancient Maya: Solving the Mystery of the Maya Collapse.* New York: Thames & Hudson.

# 8

# The Americanization of Old World Medicine

The stories told by Columbus and other early explorers about the discovery of a New World may have seriously challenged European ideas about the nature of the world and its peoples, plants, and animals. But in a remarkably short time, Europeans managed to absorb and adapt reports of the exploration, conquest, and settlement of the Americas into both their biblical belief system and their universal sense of entitlement. Having heard stories of the Americas as a virtual Garden of Eden, many people coming to Britain's North American colonies early in the seventeenth century had unrealistic ideas about their prospects for economic and physical well-being in the New World.

After an exhausting voyage, even those who were not drastically debilitated by seasickness, malnutrition, and disease confronted an often hostile climate, unfamiliar foods, famines, and the difficult task of establishing new settlements with limited resources. The high mortality rates of settlers during the early colonial period reflect the effects of hardship and disease. Despite ubiquitous complaints about the unfamiliar and harsh environment, disease patterns established during the Colonial period differed from region to region. Settlers in all the British colonies reported respiratory and gastrointestinal infections, fevers, childhood diseases, and chronic conditions well known in Europe. Harsh extremes of weather were blamed for many disorders in the North, while in the South malaria, hookworm, and yellow fever became endemic. These debilitating diseases, often amplified by malnutrition, were regarded as signs of Southern backwardness and inferiority.

Nevertheless, unlike the Europeans who attempted to conquer and colonize Africa and the Indian subcontinent, those who came to the New World were originally more inconvenienced by hunger than by new diseases. Early European settlers endured many hardships, but it is likely that their major problems came from malnutrition and food shortages. Unless they were willing to seek out advice from Native

Americans, they may have failed to recognize the availability of indigenous foods and the hazards to be found in poisonous plants and animals.

Whatever privations and diseases affected settlers from Europe, the impact of their arrival had far greater consequences for Native Americans. English colonists clearly recognized the devastating impact that European diseases had on the native people of New England. One pious observer wrote: "The good hand of God favoured our beginnings in sweeping away the multitudes of the Natives by the small pox." Colonists in New England and British soldiers have been accused of deliberate attempts to transmit smallpox to the Indians through trade goods, such as contaminated blankets, but contacts between Native Americans and European sailors, fishermen, and traders might have been enough to trigger epidemics long before permanent European settlements were established.

The idea that the human body is as much a sociocultural construct as it is a physical entity came to academic prominence in the late 1980s. Historians have used this approach to analyze the manner and methods by which English colonizers came to understand the physiological differences between themselves and indigenous Americans. As the devastation caused by Old World diseases decimated Native populations, Europeans saw their successful colonization of the New World as proof that Native Americans were actually poorly adapted to the demands of the American environment. The apparent inability of Native Americans to resist European diseases and weaponry confirmed the sense of entitlement that European colonists assumed towards all the treasures, resources, and "virgin and empty lands" of the New World. By the end of the seventeenth century, English colonizers felt they had successfully established resistance to the American disease environment. Their success confirmed their belief that they—rather than the Indians—were the natural inhabitants of America.

Initially, English, French, and Spanish settlers attempted to deal with disease by employing the methods familiar to them from the Old World. In the Spanish and French colonies, the authorities attempted to establish European medical institutions and practices, although the small numbers of practitioners made it impossible to replicate the strict hierarchical patterns of the Old World. In the British colonies, relatively little was done to transplant the professional and educational institutions of the mother country. Most British colonial towns were too small to attract professional physicians. For the first half of the eighteenth century, the British colonies had no medical societies, medical schools, or permanent general hospitals.

In colonial America, physicians, lawyers, and clergymen might not have been wealthy, but they shared the distinction of membership in the class of learned men. Although their professional roles were different, as educated men they had presumably mastered a common heritage of scholarship that included standard treatises on theology, philosophy, science, and medicine. Clergymen, as the most highly educated and respected members of their community, ministered to the medical as well as the spiritual needs of their people. As Reverend Cotton Mather (1663–1728) explained, it was an "angelical conjunction" of duties and compassion that led clergymen to provide both spiritual and physical care for their followers. Moreover, clergymen did not need to compete for status in the medical marketplace, because their place in society was secured by their religious calling. Although clergymen and physicians might be respected for their theoretical knowledge and academic credentials, the medical marketplace of colonial America included apothecaries, surgeons and barber-surgeons, midwives, nurses, herbalists, folk healers, and itinerant practitioners with no special qualifications.

Preacher-physicians were presumably especially adept at dealing with the topics of illness and suffering in their sermons. Aware of the scarcity of medical practitioners in the British colonies, many seventeenth- and eighteenth-century clergymen supplemented their theological studies with courses in anatomy and physiology. Even if the most highly educated clergyman had no clinical experience when he came to the colonies, he could, at least, offer prayers and words of comfort. Perhaps the best example of a colonial clergyman-physician, John Winthrop, Jr. (1606–1676), was respected by his contemporaries as a healer and a scientist. Although he had been educated as a lawyer, Winthrop's interests included alchemy, astronomy, chemistry, medical theory, natural history, and pharmacy. His library included works by Hippocrates, Galen, Avicenna, Paracelsus, von Helmont, and so forth. Having immigrated to New England in 1631, Winthrop left Massachusetts in 1646 to found the colony of Connecticut. At the time, New England had no formal hospitals and few doctors. Well educated, respected, and financially secure, Winthrop treated local colonists and Indians, and answered queries from distant patients. Rather eclectic in his approach to healing, Winthrop prescribed remedies that included Paracelsian drugs as well as botanical preparations and animal parts or products. In general, although his medical devices included a set of cupping vessels, he avoided venesection and leeching. While in England to attain a charter for the Connecticut colony, Winthrop was elected to the Royal Society of London.

Clergymen were not alone in assuming the role of physician. Benjamin Franklin (1706–1790), for example, admitted that he had prescribed medicines and felt free to give medical advice. Yet when members of his immediate family were ill, he consulted a physician and followed his advice. Still, he insisted that it was important for those who employed a doctor to think for themselves rather than blindly follow the doctor's directions. Because of the scarcity of medical practitioners and the expenses incurred when consulting them, most colonists relied on traditional home remedies, or sought advice from almanacs and health handbooks. Popular texts included John Tennent's *Every Man His Own Doctor: Or, the Poor Planter's Physician* (1734), John Wesley's *Primitive Physic* (1747), Samuel-Auguste-André-David Tissot's *Advice to the People [on] Health* (1761), John Theobald's *Every Man His Own Physician* (1768), and William Buchan's *Domestic Medicine* (1769). Almanacs and newspapers also offered medical information. Eventually, self-taught herbalists learned the medicinal virtues of local plants and substituted them for imported remedies.

Formally educated physicians were few in number, but even in the eighteenth-century society they were demanding professional prerogatives and trying to establish restrictive medical licensing laws. Attempts to restrict the art of healing to a small class of elite physicians were, however, offensive to prevailing egalitarian principles and had little impact on the American medical marketplace. Outside major cities, in the colonies as in England, practitioners and patients ignored attempts to professionalize and control the practice of medicine. Formally educated doctors were particularly likely to complain about competition from quacks, empirics, and old women, but their potential patients generally preferred common sense to abstract theories. Colonists distrusted those arrogant enough to presume that claims of erudition should grant them status, deference, and a monopoly in the medical marketplace. The idea that proper physicians were gentlemen, who did not perform manual labor but were valued for their theoretical knowledge, was not in accord with early American reality.

In contrast to the strict hierarchy characteristic of Europe, in the British colonies men who performed the roles of apothecary, surgeon, or physician were customarily addressed as "doctor." In the colonies, most men became doctors through apprenticeship with an experienced physician and the study of standard medical texts. Wealthy families might send their sons to Europe for formal medical education and clinical experience. A few colonial era doctors had attended medical schools in Europe, but immigrated before they completed their studies or earned a formal medical degree.

Women might be recognized for their healing skills, whether they practiced as herbalists, midwives, or nurses, but they were not likely to be called "doctor." Similarly, men known locally for specialized skills, such as bone-setting or tooth-pulling, were not accorded the title. Although women could earn money by selling remedies and treating the sick, most of their healing activities involved family, friends, or neighbors. Midwifery was usually practiced informally, but some communities followed European custom in enacting regulations to control the practice of midwives. To protect the social order, the regulations issued by New York City in 1738 prohibited midwives from concealing the birth of illegitimate children, hiding the identity of the father, or letting a man participate in childbirth, except in emergencies. Nevertheless, by the 1750s male doctors were practicing midwifery in New York.

By the end of the eighteenth century, immigration from England had declined and the pattern of life in the English colonies had become more settled and secure. Although the structure of the British medical community still served as a model and ideal, colonists believed that medical practice had to be modified in response to American social and environmental conditions. Colonial cities and towns might attempt to emulate European public health measures, such as isolating the sick, establishing quarantine regulations, and eliminating sources of filth, but the enforcement of public health and sanitary regulations was generally lax and ineffectual. When colonial communities were threatened by epidemic disease, doctors and town leaders could do little more than join the clergy in urging people to pray, participate in days of fasting, and provide charitable aid for the sick poor.

Despite the low population density in colonial New England, epidemic diseases were a common, but unpredictable threat. Tracing the pathways of infectious epidemic diseases, therefore, may reveal otherwise hidden social, religious, and commercial networks. Smallpox was a familiar enemy, but colonial doctors considered a disease known as the "throat distemper" both novel and dangerous. In some towns and villages almost half the children died of the disease. Although most families in New England in the 1730s were quite isolated and self-sufficient, contagious diseases could still become epidemics. Even people living in small towns and rural areas regularly came in contact with others in churches, schools, and marketplaces, and itinerant peddlers, doctors, and clergymen visited isolated households. The traditional response to contagious epidemic diseases was to isolate the sick and impose quarantine on new arrivals, but these measures were considered useless for diseases where person-to-person transmission was not obvious. By deciding that the throat distemper was not contagious, doctors and pastor-physicians probably allowed themselves to play a significant role in disseminating the disease.

The epidemic exposed tensions between the people and physicians of Boston and those of the afflicted towns. Many Boston physicians assumed that the virulence of the disease was only a reflection of the incompetence of rural doctors. The better-trained doctors of Boston were sure that they would be able to name and cure the disease if it came to the city. Not surprisingly, when the disease was discovered in Boston, doctors there had little success in treating the sick. Epidemiologists consider Dr. William Douglass's (1691–1752) detailed description of what he called the "new epidemical eruptive miliary fever, with an angina ulcusculosa" an early American medical classic. Medical historians, however, have argued about whether the disease that occurred in New

England in 1735 and 1736 was scarlet fever or diphtheria, or whether both diseases were epidemic in New England at the time.

## THE REVOLUTIONARY WAR AND NEW REPUBLIC

By the end of the eighteenth century, the population of the British colonies had grown to over 1.6 million. Occupying and expanding into an area much larger than Britain, the colonists were well aware of their successes in establishing an economic, social, religious, and even political life quite different from that of the mother country. Rising tensions culminated in the American Revolution, a war that began in 1775 in Lexington and Concord, Massachusetts, led to the signing of the Declaration of Independence on July 4, 1776, and finally ended seven years later in 1781 with the surrender of the British at Yorktown, Virginia.

The military activities and general disruption of ordinary life associated with the Revolutionary War obviously increased the demand for the services of physicians, surgeons, drugs, and hospitals. During the war supplies of imported drugs and surgical instruments were limited by the British blockade. The lack of experience and cooperation among the colonies, as well as the chronic shortage of funds and supplies, meant that little was accomplished in terms of organizing military medicine during the Revolution. Finding competent leaders for the revolutionary medical services proved exceptionally difficult. Indeed, the first three Directors General of medical services were quickly discharged for reasons ranging from alleged treason to fraud and speculation in medical supplies. The War of 1812 revealed that the chaotic situation during the Revolutionary War had taught the new nation almost nothing about the importance of organizing a military medical service.

Having been largely isolated from the formal medical practices, educational system, licensing restrictions, and professional institutions of Great Britain, the former colonies experienced little change in medical and public health activities after the Revolution. Medical practitioners in the new republic could generally be divided into two groups: those referred to as regular, orthodox, or mainstream physicians and a diverse group of competitors, usually referred to as unorthodox or irregular practitioners.

Orthodox practitioners claimed to represent the mainstream of learned, respectable medical theory and practice going back to Hippocrates. Few American doctors had attended European universities or participated in clinical or scientific research, but they did claim that orthodox medicine represented all the scientific advances of the Renaissance and Scientific Revolution. In practice, however, most medical men followed some simplified version of one of the medical systems constructed by eminent theoreticians like Georg Stahl, Friedrich Hoffmann, Herman Boerhaave, William Cullen, and John Brown. Other than an intense opposition to orthodox practitioners, members of competing medical sects had little in common. Irregular practitioners often dismissed orthodox practitioners as members of a competing sect that they called allopathic medicine.

During the post-Revolutionary period of growth and social transformation, new civic, cultural, educational, and scientific institutions were established. As part of this rush to create indigenous institutions, American physicians established local, county, and state medical societies. Elite physicians, who had studied in Europe, believed that observation and experiment would lead to new understanding of human physiology, but most practitioners emphasized the importance of common sense and experience. Many medical societies adopted codes of professional ethics and standardized fee tables for specific medical services as a means of unifying the profession, limiting economic competition, establishing professional prerogatives, and excluding irregular practitioners. Physicians also organized scientific societies that sponsored journals and lectures. If little that was original appeared in these journals, they did, at least, provide information about scientific and medical advances in Europe.

Health and the circumstances that would promote public welfare were topics of great concern to eighteenth-century Americans. Several of the most eminent of the nation's revered Founding Fathers—Benjamin Franklin, Thomas Jefferson, and Benjamin Rush—had serious scientific interests. Five of the 56 signers of the Declaration of Independence (Josiah Bartlett, Matthew Thornton, Oliver Wolcott, Lyman Hall, and Benjamin Rush) were physicians who also shared a passionate interest in public affairs. Practical issues may have dominated discussions of American society, but Enlightenment concepts also influenced debates about the relationship between the political and social organization of the new republic and the health of the people. The writings and activities of Thomas Jefferson and Benjamin Rush (1745–1813), in particular, exemplify the ways in which leaders of the Revolution and framers of the new republic thought about these issues.

Benjamin Rush, known to history as the "Revolutionary gadfly," served as a member of the Continental Congress, a signatory of the Declaration of Independence, and Treasurer of the U.S. Mint. He was a passionate opponent of alcohol, tobacco, and slavery who described himself in the words of the prophet Jeremiah as "a man of strife and a man of contention." Although his abrasive nature earned him many enemies, John Adams eulogized him as "a man of science, letters, taste, sense, philosophy, patriotism, religion, morality, merit, and usefulness" without equal in America. Revered by his admirers, Rush was called the foremost physician of the new republic and the father of American psychiatry.

A learned man by any standard, Rush attended the College of New Jersey and served a five-year apprenticeship with Doctor John Redman (1722–1808), a disciple of Herman Boerhaave (1668–1738). Rush earned a medical degree from Edinburgh in 1768 and spent an additional year in London and Paris studying chemistry and medicine. Returning to Philadelphia, Rush accepted a series of professorial appointments in chemistry, the theory and practice of physic, physiology, pathology, and clinical medicine. He also served as physician to the Pennsylvania Hospital.

Both Jefferson and Rush believed that only an agricultural society provided an authentic foundation for health and prosperity. "Those who labor in the earth," Jefferson proclaimed, "are the chosen people of God." Urbanization and industrialization, in contrast, led to poverty, disease, political inequality, and social injustice. Industries that restricted men to indoor, sedentary work were unhealthy. Unless men enjoyed the benefits of fresh air and exercise they were susceptible to rickets and other debilitating conditions. Women and children, however, were suited to sedentary, indoor work. Urban epidemics, though tragic in many ways, offered confirmation and consolation to these Founding Fathers, because, as Jefferson said in a letter to Rush, such epidemics would "discourage the growth of great cities as pestilential to the morals, the health and the liberties of man." Rush agreed with Jefferson that cities were like "abscesses on the human body," but he lived and worked among the approximately 40,000 residents of Philadelphia.

Because political liberty was associated with individual and social health, Rush asserted that patriots enjoyed good health, cheerful dispositions, and fruitful marriages. Enemies of the Revolution, in contrast, were subject to both mental and physical decay. Good political principles encouraged good health, but, Rush warned, an excess of liberty, leading to social instability and anarchy, could cause illness and insanity. Even though liberty, freedom, and good government promoted the physical, moral, and political well-being of the American people, they could not completely eradicate all forms of disease and disability. Physicians, therefore, had to develop therapies for physical and mental disorders that were appropriate to the American environment. Rush's *Medical Inquiries and Observations upon the Diseases of the Mind* (1812), the first general treatise on psychiatry written in America, served as a guide for the management of America's early institutions for the care of the insane. In addition to advice about immobilizing patients with mental illness when necessary, Rush generally prescribed the usual therapeutic approach, that is, bleeding and purging.

According to Rush, all diseases were due to the accumulation of putrid materials that caused a nervous constriction of the blood vessels. Symptoms seemingly associated with different diseases were actually modifications of the same primary disorder, which could be explained as an "irregular convulsive or wrong action" in the affected system, or a "morbid excitement" of the vascular system. Effective therapeutic measures should, therefore, rid the body of morbid materials and bring about relaxation of nervous excitement. In practice, this invariably meant depleting the body of harmful materials by bleeding, cupping, vomiting, purging, sweating, and salivation. Nevertheless, Rush insisted that treatment had to be modified according to local conditions and the specific characteristics of the patient. In an age where diseases were ubiquitous, unpredictable, and often fatal, doctors generally assumed that in the absence of active intervention the natural result of illness was death. Since few diseases were recognized as specific entities, and the early stages of many illnesses are quite similar, doctors could easily convince themselves and their patients that medical treatment of what might have been a minor illness had warded off death.

Although all diseases were attributed to the same primary disorder within the body, Rush was very interested in the environmental conditions associated with epidemic diseases. His first contribution to epidemiology was an essay published in 1787, "An Enquiry into the Causes of the Increase of Bilious and Remitting Fevers in Pennsylvania with Hints for Preventing Them." But the city remained notoriously unsuccessful in preventing epidemic fevers, as indicated in Rush's account of "The Bilious Remitting Yellow Fever as it appeared in the City of Philadelphia in the Year 1793."

The origin of yellow fever is almost as mysterious as that of syphilis and concerns the same problem of Old versus New World distribution of disease in pre-Columbian times. Claims that Mayan civilization was destroyed by yellow fever or that epidemics of this disease occurred in Vera Cruz and San Domingo between 1493 and 1496 remain doubtful. By the eighteenth century, yellow fever was one of the most feared diseases in the Americas. An attack of yellow fever begins with fever, chills, headache, severe pains in the back and limbs, sore throat, nausea and vomiting. Experienced physicians might detect diagnostic clues during the early stages of the disease, but mild cases are easily misdiagnosed as influenza, malaria, or other fevers. Characteristic symptoms in severe cases include jaundice, fever, delirium, and the terrifying "black vomit" (caused by hemorrhaging into the stomach). Damage to the heart, kidneys, and liver can lead to death.

Although outbreaks of the disease occurred in many American cities, the situation in Philadelphia was particularly striking. Eighteenth-century Philadelphia was America's cultural, social, and political center and an active trading partner with the West Indies. The 1798 yellow fever outbreaks in Philadelphia, New York, Boston, and other American cities proved that very little had been learned during the 1793 epidemic in terms of prevention and treatment. For his conduct during the 1793 yellow fever epidemic in Philadelphia, Benjamin Rush is often cited as the very model of the American practitioner of "heroic medicine." Certainly, he was very enthusiastic about the value of therapeutic bloodletting and vigorous purgation, and he aggressively attacked the arguments of his opponents and their therapeutic timidity. He did not, however, claim that he had invented a new therapeutic system, nor did he call his methods "heroic." Instead, he spoke about the value of "copious depletion" achieved by means of large doses of jalap and calomel, bloodletting, cold drinks, low diet, and the applications of cold water to the body. After the epidemic of 1793, Rush extended his yellow fever therapies to other diseases, and began to consolidate his medical ideas and experiences into a new system of medicine.

In general, the term heroic medicine refers to the treatment of disease by means of copious bloodletting and the aggressive use of harsh drugs or techniques that cause purging, vomiting, and sweating. Some historians have questioned the use of the term, but Oliver Wendell Holmes (1809–1894), physician and poet, had no problem using it when reflecting on the history of American therapeutics. In his most rhetorical manner, Holmes asked how it could have been possible for the people of the Revolution to adopt any system of medicine other than "heroic" practice. That brave generation, he explained, was accustomed to consuming "ninety grains of sulfate of quinine" and "three drachms of calomel." In any case, the term heroic medicine had already been popularized in the 1830s by doctors, both orthodox and sectarian, who were adopting more moderate approaches than the aggressive bleeding, purging, and puking of their predecessors.

Given prevailing concepts of the vital functions of the body in health and disease, extreme measures of depletion were considered rational and necessary. Physicians and patients generally thought about health and disease in terms of humoral balance and the movement of the blood. If blood could not move freely it could become thick, weak, and putrid. Just as a healthy society demanded the free movement of people and goods, a healthy body required the free movement of blood through the vessels and the therapeutic or prophylactic removal of putrid blood. In theory, toxins and impurities could also be removed from the body through other fluids, such as sweat, urine, stools, pus, and vomit.

The term "heroic" seems especially appropriate for Rush's actions during the 1793 epidemic in Philadelphia. With hardly time to rest, sleep, or eat, Rush visited hundreds of patients throughout the city and responded to dozens of others who came to his house. Critics of the good doctor might say that those who were unable to obtain his services were actually better off than those subjected to his routine of bleeding and purging. In a direct assault on raging fevers, Rush wrapped his patients in cold, wet sheets and dosed them with buckets of cold water and cold enemas. Daily bleeding and purging continued until the patient either recovered or died. Rush knew that his critics thought his purges were too drastic and his bloodletting was "unnecessarily copious," but he believed that disease yielded to such treatment and insisted that the only danger in treatment was excessive timidity.

Physicians in Europe might have prescribed different treatments for yellow fever, but their recommendations were not necessarily milder. In an autopsy report on a soldier who died of yellow fever, P. C. A. Louis (1787–1872), the great French clinician, provided details of the treatment prescribed by a French army doctor. On the first day the patient was given a large dose of castor oil, an enema, and several doses of calomel, while leeches were applied to his temples. On the second day, in addition to a large dose of calomel, the patient was bled by leech and lancet. On the third day, the patient was given several enemas and 25 drops of laudanum before he died.

William Cobbett (1763–1835), a British journalist and social reformer, made Rush the special target of the wit and sarcasm that enlivened his polemical writings. While living in Philadelphia, Cobbett (also known as Peter Porcupine) established a newspaper called *Porcupine's Gazette*. Like Rush and Jefferson, Cobbett glorified traditional rural life and deplored the impoverishment and deterioration brought about by the Industrial Revolution. But where medical practice was concerned, Cobbett and Rush were implacable enemies. Based on studies of the Philadelphia yellow fever epidemic, Cobbett asserted that Rush had an unnatural passion for taking human blood and that many of his patients actually died of exsanguination. According to Cobbett, Rush's method was "one of those great discoveries which have contributed to the depopulation of the earth." In response, Rush sued Cobbett for libel. Not surprisingly, the American jury favored the Revolutionary hero and granted Rush a $5,000 judgment against Cobbett.

Losing the libel suit did not silence Cobbett, who proclaimed that the death of George Washington (1732–1799) on the very same day that Rush enjoyed his legal victory was the perfect example of death by exsanguination "in precise conformity to the practice of Rush." After the trial Cobbett launched a new periodical for the express purpose of attacking Rush's methods, but he later returned to England to publish a journal dedicated to social and parliamentary reform. Prevailing methods of education also attracted Cobbett's blistering contempt. Many of the best years of a young man's life, he complained, were "devoted to the learning of what can never be of any real use to any human being."

Although it is impossible to diagnose George Washington's final illness with certainty, it probably involved inflammation of the throat caused by infection with streptococci, staphylococci, or pneumococci. In order to show that everything medically possible had been done, Washington's physicians published an account of his death in the newspapers. Doctors James Craik and Elisha C. Dick blamed Washington's illness on exposure to rain while riding about Mount Vernon on horseback. Suffering from a violent ague, sore throat, and fever caused by what the doctors called *cynanche trachealis*, Washington realized that bloodletting was necessary. A local bleeder took 12 or 14 ounces of blood from his arm. The next day the attending physician, worried by the "fatal tendency of the disease," performed two "copious bleedings," blistered the throat, dosed the patient with calomel, and administered an enema before the arrival of two consulting physicians. Seeing no improvement, the physicians carried out another bleeding of about 32 ounces of blood, and dosed the patient with more calomel, emetic tartar, and fumes of vinegar and water. Despite further treatments, including blisters applied to the extremities and a cataplasm of bran and vinegar for the throat, the patient "expired without a struggle."

During the summer of 1793, Philadelphia was plagued by great swarms of mosquitoes, as well as unusually large accumulations of filth and putrefaction in the streets, alleys, and wharves. Doctors anticipated an increase in the usual "autumnal fevers." Observing the great numbers of "moschetoes" in the city, Rush noted this as another sign of unhealthy atmospheric conditions. [The role of mosquitoes in the dissemination of yellow fever was not demonstrated until the early twentieth century by Walter Reed (1851–1902) and his colleagues on the U.S. Army Yellow Fever Commission.] As soon as a few suspicious cases appeared, Rush warned the authorities that yellow fever had returned to Philadelphia for the first time since 1762. As the number of deaths climbed, thousands of residents fled from the city. Within months, more than 10 percent of Philadelphia's 40,000 inhabitants had died of yellow fever. Mayor Matthew Clarkson convened a committee of citizen volunteers to establish a hospital and orphanage, supervise the collection and burial of abandoned corpses, organize efforts to clean the streets, distribute supplies to the poor, and fight the panic that gripped the city.

Blaming the epidemic on the morbid vapors emanating from coffee putrefying on the wharf, Rush warned that the exhalations of other rotting materials would eventually produce fevers miles away from the original outbreak. Other physicians ridiculed this theory and argued that the disease had been imported by ships coming from the West Indies. Despite the controversy among the physicians, the mayor did order the removal of rotten materials along the wharf. Fear of epidemic disease generally inspired sanitary reforms in cities that otherwise tolerated offensive odors and mountains of garbage. For example, in 1797, when landfills along the waterfront on Manhattan became unbearably putrid, public health authorities blamed these "filthy nuisances" for an outbreak of yellow fever. To fight filth, stench, and disease, the mayor had the area covered with "wholesome earth and gravel." South Street was built on top of the fill. Such sanitary campaigns might not affect yellow fever directly, but they did improve the atmosphere in a general way.

Debates about the proper response to yellow fever became entangled in the political conflicts that wracked Philadelphia in the 1790s. Generally following partisan divisions, some Philadelphians blamed the epidemic on the influx of foreigners coming by ship from Haiti, while others insisted that the epidemic was caused by unsanitary local conditions. For the most part, Republican (Jeffersonian) doctors and politicians said the fever was caused by local conditions. Republicans opposed contagionist theories, quarantine regulations, and restrictions on trade with the West Indies.

The strength of anticontagion sentiment was demonstrated by physicians who attempted to prove that the fever was not contagious by inoculating themselves with the vomit, blood, or saliva of yellow fever patients. Even a strict anticontagionist needed great dedication and bravery to care for the sick, because most doctors believed that even if an epidemic were generated first by noxious vapors, the exhalations of the sick might also generate a dangerous miasmatic condition. Contagionists, of course, greatly feared the sick and demanded their isolation, which often meant that the sick died of neglect. Arguing that his method was democratic and egalitarian because it could be used by virtually anyone, Rush claimed that attacks on his therapeutics were politically motivated and dangerous. Perhaps his decision to publish directions for treatment in the newspapers so that any reader could treat the disease alienated many doctors.

Physicians of the eighteenth century had good and cogent reasons for rejecting the idea that yellow fever was transmitted by a contagion, which was defined as "a force operating within a distance of ten paces." Many people contracted the disease even though they had no contact with the sick, people who cared for the sick did not necessarily contract the illness, epidemics ended with the onset of cold weather, and people who fled from affected cities did not carry the disease with them. All these observations suggested that yellow fever epidemics were generated and sustained by specific local conditions. These ideas about yellow fever were collected by Noah Webster (1758–1843), American lexicographer, from questionnaires he sent to physicians in Philadelphia, New York, Baltimore, Norfolk, and New Haven. In 1796, he published this information along with his own comments and conclusions as *A Collection of Papers on the Subject of Bilious Fever, prevalent in the United States for a Few Years Past.*

Federalist physicians and politicians generally accepted contagionist doctrines and favored quarantine and limitations on foreign trade. Blaming an epidemic on local conditions, they believed, was unpatriotic and detrimental to the economic well-being of American cities. Therefore, Hamiltonians insisted that yellow fever had been imported from Haiti, along with French refugees. In the West Indies, stimulants such as quinine and wine were traditionally prescribed for yellow fever. In the Philadelphia epidemic, this approach became known as the "Federalist cure." At the beginning of the epidemic, Rush used relatively gentle purges and experimented with remedies used in the West Indies, but he soon decided that only strong purges and vigorous bleedings were effective.

Some physicians resorted to chemical theories and tried to analyze the hypothetical vapors associated with putrefaction, as well as the much-feared black vomit that seemed to characterize the most lethal cases of the disease. Lacking specialized chemical tests, but not lacking in bravado, some doctors tasted the black vomit and survived. This did not provide significant chemical information, but it did show that even the most revolting product of the disease did not transmit the fever.

Since yellow fever is caused by a virus, careful nursing, relief of symptoms, and rest might do the most good or the least damage to the patient. But eighteenth-century physicians were unlikely to meet a challenge like yellow fever with such timid measures as rest and fluids. Innovative physicians prescribed everything from rattlesnake venom to castor oil and laudanum. Sir William Osler (1849–1919), author of the widely used textbook *Principles and Practices of Medicine* (1892), advised a course of therapy that included generous doses of cold carbonated alkaline water, moderate doses of calomel, saline purges or enemas, cool baths for the fever, and perchloride of iron or oil of turpentine for the gastric hemorrhages. To relieve uremic symptoms, Osler suggested hot baths, hot packs, and hot enemas. Stimulants, such as strychnine, were prescribed to counter feeble heartbeat.

After the epidemic ended and those who had fled returned to the city, Philadelphia observed a day of thanksgiving and remembrance: over four thousand had died out of a population of approximately forty thousand. Rush was overcome with "sublime joy" that his methods had finally conquered this formidable disease. Even the fact that the disease had killed three of his apprentices and his beloved sister did little to shake his faith in his therapeutics. The compulsion to ascribe success to medical treatment when recovery actually occurred in spite of the best efforts that medicine had to offer was certainly not unique to Benjamin Rush.

A famous eyewitness account of the epidemic by Mathew Carey (1760–1839), *A Short Account of the Malignant Fever, Lately Prevalent in Philadelphia*, contains a vivid description of the symptoms of the disease, comments on the "astonishing" quantity of blood taken by medical practitioners, and gives a list of those who died. In particular, Carey noted, the disease was "dreadfully destructive among the poor." When the epidemic began, many physicians believed that blacks were less susceptible to the disease than whites, but the list of the dead proved that this was not true. Nevertheless, Carey noted that during the early phase of the epidemic, when no white nurses would care for the sick, members of the African church offered to serve as nurses and to assist in burying the dead. Nurses were very important, Carey wrote, because many died from lack of care rather than the virulence of the disease itself.

Determining the case fatality rate for yellow fever is difficult because mild cases might be ignored or misdiagnosed. During the 1878 epidemic in New Orleans, the mortality rate in hospitals was over 50 percent among whites and 21 percent among blacks. However, physicians estimated the mortality rate among their private white patients at less than 10 percent. Presumably, these differences reflect the different health status of wealthy versus poor patients. Only the most impoverished whites were likely to be taken to hospitals.

Benjamin Henry Latrobe (1764–1820), an engineer who helped plan Washington, DC, believed that safe water systems would limit the threat of epidemic disease. In 1798, Latrobe visited Philadelphia and concluded that pollution of wells with "noxious matter" from the city's privies was the cause of epidemic disease. In 1801, after following Latrobe's plans, Philadelphia had a citywide safe water system, with streetside pumps that provided free water to all, and private lines connected to the homes of the wealthy. A few other large cities, most notably New York and Boston, also invested in municipal water systems in the first half of the nineteenth century, but water, sewage and garbage disposal problems plagued many cities into the twentieth century. Although drinking contaminated water does not cause yellow fever, improved water supplies played a role in decreasing the danger of epidemic diseases, both directly and indirectly. Moreover, the elimination of swamps, ditches, wells, and cisterns as cities grew and modernized decreased the areas available as mosquito breeding grounds.

## THE MEDICAL PROFESSION

During the colonial period, there were few legal or social obstacles to the practice of medicine. Individuals with or without special education or training could present themselves as healers. Eventually, physicians established a legally protected professional identity by banding together in professional societies that lobbied for medical licensing laws that would exclude sectarian practitioners. But claims for professional expertise and legal restraints on medical practice did not accord with the cultural climate of the developing nation. By 1845, several states had repealed their medical licensing laws. Aware that licensing laws were increasingly unpopular and that state societies were unable to achieve their goals, regular physicians established the American Medical Association in 1847 in order to provide a national platform to promote the interests of the profession. By the end of the nineteenth century, despite the efforts of competing medical sects, physicians had essentially achieved an effective monopoly on state sanctioned medical licensing.

In pursuit of professional recognition, orthodox practitioners also attempted to gain control over medical education. Most aspiring doctors could not afford to study abroad, but attendance at a formal medical school became increasingly more respectable than training through apprenticeship alone. By the 1820s, proprietary medical schools began to compete with the few medical schools that had been established in connection with medical societies or colleges. Usually founded by one or more doctors as a for-profit enterprise, these independent schools were supported by students' fees. Thus, the ability to pay tuition was usually the only qualification students needed to meet.

As the proprietary schools continued to multiply, physicians realized that they had transformed the medical marketplace from a venue with a chronic shortage of regular doctors to one with an excess. Between 1765 and 1800, less than 250 doctors had graduated from American medical schools. During the 1830s, American medical schools produced almost 7,000 graduates; during the 1850s the number of graduates was approaching 18,000. Although graduates of the proprietary medical schools might have mastered very little of medical theory or clinical practice, they were formally qualified and could join the battle against sectarians and quacks. Regular physicians like Dr. William Currie (1754–1828), author of *An Historical Account of the Climates and Diseases of the United States of America* (1792), warned against the unorthodox practitioner: "though he may kill by license, he can only cure by chance." The bills of mortality, Currie argued, would show that "more lives have been destroyed by the villainy of quacks ... than by disease." He expressed surprise that "our enlightened legislatures" had not prevented the activity of quacks.

In addition to denouncing the "villainy of quacks," regular physicians argued that medical practices that had been developed in other countries were not directly applicable to the needs of American patients. Because epidemic diseases varied with specific environmental, climatic, social, and occupational conditions, only physicians with extensive experience and training appropriate to the American environment should practice in America. Like Jefferson and Rush, nineteenth-century American doctors assumed that residents of the countryside would be healthier than those who lived in towns and cities. Only experienced doctors would understand that the kinds of treatment tolerated by active farmers were quite different from those appropriate to sedentary city people. A farmer with acute rheumatism might easily lose 60 to 70 ounces of blood in treatment, but a sedentary resident of the city could hardly tolerate the loss of half that quantity.

In contrast to Europe, most doctors in early America had to serve as physicians, surgeons, and pharmacists. By the mid-nineteenth century, however, as urban populations expanded, some doctors found it possible to focus on the treatment of disorders of the nerves, lungs, eyes, ears, and so forth, while others were able to confine their practice to surgery or even the traditionally female field of midwifery. This was a great departure from the past, when "specialists"—such as those who set broken bones or removed decayed teeth—were dismissed as quacks. Dentistry and pharmacy actually established a separate professional identity in America before the Civil War. The first American dental text and journal were published in 1839, just a year before the Baltimore College of Dental Surgery and the American Society of Dental Surgeons were founded. Pharmaceutical journals, professional societies, and schools of pharmacy were established in the 1820s, but national and state professional societies were not founded until the 1850s.

Medical societies in the nineteenth century provided a forum in which orthodox physicians could claim membership in the international scientific community. Knowledge of recent developments in European medicine allowed some physicians to look at patients in hospitals and asylums, and even private practice, as clinical material for research, or at least focused observation. Admirers of the work of the great French physician P. C. A. Louis, such as Henry I. Bowditch and George C. Shattuck, attempted to apply his "numerical method" in American hospitals. Bowditch established the first physiological laboratory in America at the Harvard Medical School in 1871. Physicians who had studied abroad were eager to import and translate new scientific and medical texts and adapt European research for American practitioners. As the numbers of medical schools increased, so did the market for textbooks.

Despite the well-known deficiencies of most American medical schools, before the Civil War they served as a key source of science education for American students. Even the medical schools with the lowest admission standards and the worst facilities accepted the concept that medical education required lectures in anatomy and pathology, or morbid anatomy supplemented by the dissection of human bodies. Although postmortems were historically important to coroners and in criminal proceedings, few families were receptive to the use of the autopsy as a way of achieving diagnostic specificity or for the advancement of medical science. In America, as in Europe, cadavers for anatomical demonstrations were always in short supply. Because the practice of human dissection was generally regarded with horror and legal means of providing cadavers for medical education were rare, rumors of grave-robbing led to fear, hostility, and even violence, such as New York's "Doctors' Riot" in 1788.

When American doctors were involved in scientific studies, they tended to follow a practical path that could expand botanical knowledge and lead to new remedies. By collecting geological and meteorological observations, and keeping careful case records, they tried to corroborate ideas about the relationship between local environmental factors—soil conditions, temperature, humidity, rainfall, and so forth—and health. In addition, they searched for correlations between what might be called sociological data and patterns of disease. By comparing patterns of morbidity and mortality in the new nation with those of the Old World, American doctors expected to provide scientific proof that the American environment and the institutions of the new nation promoted physical and mental health.

The life and work of William Beaumont (1785–1853) demonstrates that when presented with the opportunity to carry out physiological research, even a doctor with little formal training could plan and execute ingenious experiments. Indeed, Sir William Osler called Beaumont "the first great American physiologist." Beaumont's reputation is based on the remarkable series of observations and experiments described in his *Experiments and Observations on the Gastric Juice and the Physiology of Digestion* (1833). Beaumont's work was important not only in terms of his scientific observations, but as a landmark in the history of human experimentation and biomedical ethics.

Except for his apprenticeship with Dr. Benjamin Chandler, in St. Albans, Vermont, Beaumont was a self-educated man, without benefit of university or college. Beaumont grew up on a farm in Connecticut and became a schoolteacher in order to escape from farming. Compensating for the lack of formal education, Beaumont, like many of his contemporaries, pursued an extensive program of reading that included important medical authorities, as well as the writings of Shakespeare and Benjamin Franklin. His notebooks from 1811 to 1812 describe his training, reading program, and early medical practice.

In 1812, just before the United States' declaration of war with England, Beaumont was able to secure a position as surgeon's mate. His experiences in dealing with diseases and wounds support the adage "war is the best medical school." After the war, Beaumont's attempts to establish a private practice were unsuccessful and he reenlisted in the Medical Department of the Army. He was sent to Fort Mackinac, which was then a remote army post on the Western frontier. Mackinac Island, in the straits of the Great Lakes, was an outpost of the American Fur Company. Here, Beaumont frequently encountered patients with intermittent fevers, typhus, dysenteries, and rheumatism. Gunshot wounds were not uncommon, but the accidental shot that struck

Alexis St. Martin, a young French Canadian, in the abdomen in 1822 had unique results. The shot created a wound bigger than the size of a man's hand, fractured the lower ribs, ruptured the lower portion of the left lobe of the lungs, and punctured the stomach. Beaumont thought the wound would be fatal, but he cared for St. Martin to the best of his ability with poultices of flour, charcoal, yeast, and hot water. He changed the dressings frequently, cleaned the wound, removed debris, and bled the patient to fight against fever. Surprisingly, St. Martin survived, but all attempts to close the wound were unsuccessful. Beaumont soon realized that St. Martin's permanent gastrostomy (new opening into the stomach) provided a unique opportunity to study digestion in a healthy human being. Various kinds of foods and drugs could be inserted directly into St. Martin's stomach and samples of the gastric juices could be removed. Beaumont planned to conduct lecture tours to demonstrate his experiments, but St. Martin frequently ran away. In 1832, Beaumont and St. Martin signed a contract that gave Beaumont the exclusive right to perform experiments on St. Martin. This document was the first such contract in the history of human scientific experimentation. Despite St. Martin's later complaints about the discomforts of being a human guinea pig, Beaumont's physiological experiments did not seem to harm him. St. Martin and his wife Marie had seventeen children, but only five were alive when he died in 1880.

In addition to Beaumont's famous contributions to the physiology of digestion, his career provides insights into the evolution of medical education, professionalism, and even medical malpractice law in the first half of the nineteenth century. Although malpractice suits were rare in the 1840s, Beaumont was involved in two such battles. The first was the result of Beaumont's unsuccessful attempt to save the life of a man who had been struck on the head with an iron cane by a carpenter named Darnes Davis. Beaumont attempted to relieve cranial pressure by performing a trephination. When the case came to trial in 1840, Davis's lawyers argued that Beaumont had caused the death by drilling a hole into the victim's skull in order to perform experiments on the brain, just as he had left a hole in St. Martin's stomach in order to do experiments on digestion.

Four years later, Beaumont and Dr. Stephen Adreon were sued for medical malpractice by an indigent patient named Mary Dugan. In the 1840s, the regular physicians in the St. Louis area were battling for strict licensing laws that would give them control over medical practice and inhibit the activities of irregular practitioners and quacks. Thus, the trial threatened to become a major landmark in establishing the limits of malpractice jurisprudence. Despite the efforts of the regular physicians to distinguish themselves from their irregular rivals, prevailing popular sentiment at the time favored the repeal of whatever state and local regulations of medical licensure still existed. This malpractice suit revealed a great deal about tensions within the medical community and the fact that the regulars were not only battling irregulars and quacks; they were also diverting much of their energy into internal rivalries.

Adreon had examined Dugan before asking Beaumont and his partner Dr. James Sykes to act as consultants. After all three physicians agreed on a diagnosis, Adreon lanced the patient's abscess, drained it, and applied poultices. But Dugan later complained of complications that the doctors diagnosed as "typhlo-enteritis" (purulent inflammation in the intestinal tract) unrelated to the surgical procedure. Dr. Thomas J. White, who was extremely hostile to Beaumont and Adreon, persuaded Dugan to file a malpractice suit for $10,000 in damages. White argued that that Adreon punctured a hernia and cut the intestines through negligence and lack of skill. The jury sat through a two-week trial before acquitting Adreon and Beaumont. When Dugan died in 1848, White performed the autopsy. The autopsy results, which were published in the *St. Louis Medical and Surgical Journal* (1848), seemed to refute the original diagnosis of Adreon and Beaumont. Being acquitted was little consolation to Beaumont in the face of such hostility from rivals within the medical community. In response, Beaumont refused to deal with the Medical Society of St. Louis or participate in the establishment of the American Medical Association.

## REGIONAL DISTINCTIVENESS

Many Americans shared the belief that there were "differences in salubrity" from one region of their vast nation to another. Physicians argued that regional differences in therapeutics were, therefore, necessary. Southern physicians were especially supportive of the concept of a distinctive medical environment, but physicians in other regions shared an interest in the study of race and possible racial differences in disease patterns. Southern medical societies, journals, and medical schools served as forums in which physicians could express and promote their doctrine of intrinsic racial differences in physiological and mental faculties. Studies of craniometry and phrenology were invoked as if they could supply scientifically valid answers to questions about race. In attempts to support their racial hypotheses, some Southern physicians assembled major collections of human skulls. Slave owners used these racial hypotheses of physiological and medical differences as a rationalization for slavery. Being medically different from whites and allegedly immune to certain diseases, black slaves should be capable of working in the fields in all seasons and weathers. Some doctors believed that blacks were more susceptible to cold and frostbite than whites, more tolerant of heat, and less tolerant of blood loss through venesection.

Although black women were expected to work throughout their pregnancy, doctors warned that they were more likely to develop prolapsed uterus than white women. Southern doctors concluded that blacks were very susceptible to tuberculosis, particularly a very severe condition known as "Negro consumption," or "struma africana," which was probably miliary tuberculosis.

From the Revolution to the Civil War, the medical problems of the South included malaria, parasitic worms, dysentery, and, in major port cities, yellow fever. Blacks in particular suffered from a heavy burden of parasitic infections, respiratory diseases, malnutrition, and high rates of infant and maternal mortality. The black infant mortality rate appeared to be twice as high as that of white infants. Environmental factors, primarily lack of proper sanitation and clean water, probably account for the perception that blacks were particularly susceptibility to typhoid fever, parasitic worms, fungal infections, and dysentery. The habit of clay eating (pica or geophagy) was another way to acquire parasites.

Harvest times for many crops, late summer and early fall, coincide with the peak season for malaria. Blacks were allegedly less susceptible to malaria than whites, but "resistance" was very unpredictable. In modern terms, differences in the severity of malarial fevers and susceptibility to the disease might be explained in terms of more or less virulent strains of the malaria parasites found at different locations and human genetic variations. The genes for sickle cell anemia and thalassemia, for example, apparently enhance resistance to malaria (in heterozygotes; i.e., carriers). Sickle cell anemia might also explain joint pain, lung infections, chronic leg ulcers, and the deaths of children with this genetic variant.

Importing slaves from Africa meant importing infectious diseases, such as malaria, smallpox, yaws, leprosy, guinea worm, filariasis, ascariasis, tapeworm, hookworm, and trypanosomiasis. When the direct importation of slaves from Africa ended, those African diseases that could not survive in the Americas essentially disappeared. Some imported diseases, however, became permanently established. For example, the parasite for sleeping sickness (*Trypanosoma gambiense*) arrived in the Americas, but without the tsetse fly, the disease could not become endemic. In contrast, the filarial roundworm, *Wuchereria bancrofti*, which causes elephantiasis, became endemic in parts of the South. Adult worms invade the human lymphatic vessels and lymph nodes, causing an inflammatory response that may result in gross swelling of affected areas. The parasite can be transmitted by the American mosquito *Culex quinquefasciatus*. An endemic focus of filariasis existed in Charleston, South Carolina, until the 1920s, but elephantiasis made incursions into other parts of the South and even the North. Elephantiasis was so prevalent in Barbados in the West Indies that the disease was called "Barbados-leg." The disease was also common in Charleston, apparently because both Charleston and Barbados were primary ports of entry for slaves. Recognition of the relationship between the disease and the mosquito vector led to an intensive mosquito control campaign in the 1920s in the city. By the 1940s, Charleston was considered "filaria-free."

Fragmentary evidence in plantation records, diaries, slave narratives, interviews with former slaves, and folklore collections suggest that slaves used their own healing methods, perhaps derived from traditional African herbal medicine, in order to avoid the imposition of remedies prescribed by white doctors. Wherever possible, slaves apparently consulted black midwives, nurses, herbalists, root doctors, and magicians. In addition to diagnosing and treating illness, some black healers and magicians claimed the ability to protect slaves from whites and from other slaves. Some African healing traditions, especially those linked to spirituality and religion, as well as medicinal teas, herbs, poultices, prayers, songs, and sickbed gatherings, presumably survived in black families and communities after the Civil War.

## THE CIVIL WAR

Southern distinctiveness, especially as manifested in its commitment to slavery, its "peculiar institution," was only one of the complex causes of the conflicts that resulted in the Civil War, but there is little doubt that slavery was—as Lincoln said—"somehow" at the heart of the conflict. Decades before the outbreak of the war, with the Confederate bombardment of Fort Sumter on April 12, 1861, the gap between North and South in terms of social, economic, and cultural experiences had become unbridgeable. Nevertheless, neither side was prepared for the awesome bloodbath of a war that did not end until April 9, 1865, when Robert E. Lee surrendered to Ulysses S. Grant at Appomattox Court House in Virginia.

Neither the Union nor the Confederacy expected the War Between the States to last very long; thus, neither side made suitable provisions for sanitation or care of the sick and wounded. Many volunteer fighting units joined the war effort without hospital tents, supplies, surgeons, or record keepers. Temporary, overcrowded, unsanitary facilities, such as old barns, tobacco warehouses, and private homes, served as makeshift hospitals. Medical staff and facilities were immediately overwhelmed by the troops suffering from fevers and fluxes. In the first six months of the war, 30 percent of the soldiers contracted malaria, typhoid fever, smallpox, and dysentery. Other debilitating conditions included asthma, tuberculosis, epilepsy, sunstroke, venereal diseases, rheumatism, dyspepsia, and boils at sites that made mounting a horse very difficult. Surgical services were more primitive than necessary, considering the state of the art in the

1860s, because of the lack of supplies, equipment, and facilities, and the poor training of many surgeons. But war wounds and diseases provided a grisly proving ground for inexperienced surgeons and physicians. Although anesthesia had been in use since the 1840s, many military surgeons thought it unnecessary in amputations and claimed that anesthetics prolonged shock and bleeding and inhibited healing.

The medical situation of the South was even worse than that of the North. Because of the naval blockade of the South, medical supplies, such as chloroform, quinine, belladonna, digitalis, and opium, were almost impossible to obtain. Robert E. Lee admitted that his army did not have proper medical and sanitary support. Indeed, it had no Sanitary Commission and its Medical Department was not properly equipped.

As the war dragged on, military activities consumed more and more medical resources, medical school enrollments declined, and civilian asylums and hospitals lost critical staff members. Even plans for urban sanitary improvements and the collection of vital statistics were suspended as resources were increasingly consumed by war-related activities.

The struggles of nurses and doctors during the war and the suffering of their patients make painfully evident the disproportion between advances in the techniques of healing and those of killing. Almost three million men served in the war; about six hundred thousand died. Of this total mortality, the Union loss was about 360,000; the Confederate army lost about 260,000 men. As in all wars up to the twentieth century, more soldiers died of disease than in battle. Union medical officers reported more than six million cases of sickness. There were more than a million cases of malaria among white Union troops, about 140,000 cases of typhoid fever, 70,000 cases of measles, 60,000 cases of pneumonia, 70,000 cases of syphilis, and 110,000 cases of gonorrhea between May 1, 1861, and June 30, 1866. The huge assemblies of men and animals that had previous lived in rural isolation and their movement through unfamiliar regions provided the perfect environment for the dissemination of previously localized diseases. Many thousands of soldiers who had been weakened by diseases, injuries, and wounds during the war died at home; their deaths and those of others they infected were not part of the Army's mortality figures. Many others suffered chronic illnesses and disabilities because of their injuries or loss of limbs.

Scurvy, sunstroke, colic, diarrhea, dysentery, and typhoid fever were common, which was not surprising considering the lack of nutritious food and safe drinking water. Military doctors warned their "superiors" that scurvy undermined the "fighting powers of the army" even if soldiers did not realize that they were sick, but it was a battle to secure well-known antiscorbutics, such as potatoes, onions, cabbage, tomatoes, squash, beets, and fresh lemons. One surgeon described using water from the Chickahominy swamp, which was full of the bodies of dead horses and soldiers. Perhaps attempts to disguise the noxious quality of drinking water by adding a "gill of whisky" per canteen helped disinfect the water. The stench of the army camp and hospital, he reported, was enough to "cause a turkey buzzard to contract typhoid fever." Many soldiers were tormented by hordes of lice, which they referred to as "bodyguards." Doctors also complained about soldiers who had been recruited despite constitutional defects that made them unfit for army life. Cursory medical exams failed to detect recruits who were too young, others who were too old, and a few who were actually female.

In addition to the many soldiers who survived physical wounds and surgical amputations, some returned to their homes with severe psychological trauma caused by the stress of the war. Having analyzed pension records and case studies of Civil War veterans who were committed to insane asylums, historians have suggested that their symptoms would now be diagnosed as post-traumatic stress disorder. Civil War diagnostic categories that might now come under this heading include sunstroke, homesickness, and irritable heart. The symptoms of a condition diagnosed as irritable heart, soldier's heart, or neurocirculatory asthenia included chest pains, palpitations, breathlessness, fatigue, syncope, and exercise intolerance. Irritable heart was first recognized as an important issue during the Civil War because it incapacitated thousands of soldiers.

All areas of the country were affected, directly or indirectly, by the war. Years of turmoil left a legacy of malnutrition, hookworm infestation, and malarial fevers that affected the health of returning troops, their families, and communities for many years. In the South, the war caused the destruction of many libraries, medical schools, and other educational institutions. Medical societies and journals vanished and many Southern physicians emigrated to the North. Many farmers returned home to discover that their homes, barns, crops, and livestock had been destroyed.

The Civil War triggered major epidemics among horses, mules, cattle, and hogs. Hog cholera, which was first reported in Ohio in the 1830s, spread to at least twenty states by 1860. One probable mode of transmission foreshadows the Mad Cow story: meat scraps from diseased carcasses were fed to healthy animals, which then became infected. Bovine pleuropneumonia, or lung fever, caused by *Mycoplasma mycoides* and transmitted via droplet infection, was a localized problem before the Civil War. Imported animals from Europe during the 1840s exacerbated the problem. The disease kills about half of the infected animals, but many of the survivors became carriers. After the war, cattle fever, pleuropneumonia, bovine tuberculosis, and hog cholera remained as major problems for agriculture. Cattle and horses were attacked by brucellosis, equine influenza, vesicular stomatitis, Eastern equine encephalomyelitis, Potomac fever, and glanders. Advances in transportation and increased commerce after the war exacerbated the dissemination of the diseases of livestock.

Although the development of nursing in America is a complex story, the Civil War was a transforming event for the thousands of women who participated in nursing and other philanthropic activities during the war. Memorable descriptions of military hospitals, the suffering of the sick and wounded, and the tasks undertaken by male and female nurses were written by celebrated authors, like Louisa May Alcott and Walt Whitman, and little known figures, such as Jane Stuart Woolsey, who wrote *Hospital Days: Reminiscence of a Civil War Nurse* (1868) to describe her work as the superintendent of nursing at a Union barrack hospital near Alexandria, Virginia. Alcott worked as a nurse's aide in a 40-bed ward in a hotel turned into a hospital after the first battle of Bull Run. Stories of the staff's struggles to care for wounded soldiers, as well as those stricken by diphtheria, pneumonia, typhoid, and other diseases, were published in a Boston newspaper as "Hospital Sketches."

Dr. Elizabeth Blackwell and other medical women founded the Women's Central Association for Relief and organized programs in several New York City hospitals to train women to serve as nurses. Most nurses had little or no training, but the tasks assigned to them were simple: bathing patients, dressing wounds, providing clean linens, preparing and serving nourishing meals, administering medications, and writing and reading letters for their patients. Civil War nurses were expected to provide care and comfort, rather than medical support, but were burdened by the disparity between the availability of humanitarian aid and the enormity of the suffering and loss of life caused by the war.

Dorothea Lynde Dix (1802–1887), who had devoted her life to improving the treatment of the insane, was appointed Superintendent of Female Nurses in 1861. The responsibilities assigned to Dix by the Secretary of War included recruitment of female army nurses, hospital visitation, distribution of supplies, management of ambulances, and so forth. Despite her official position, Dix had no real authority or means of enforcing her rules and directives. Famous for her demand that war nurses should be middle-aged women, plain in appearance, Dix was not popular with Army doctors, hospital surgeons, volunteer nurses, and the leaders of the U.S. Sanitary Commission. Because of disputes between Dix and the Sanitary Commission about their overlapping areas of authority, leaders of the Commission portrayed her as a "philanthropic lunatic" and an obstacle to the war effort. Louisa May Alcott said that, although Dix was regarded as a "kind old soul," nurses considered her "very queer, fussy, and arbitrary." Displaced from her old position as noble role model for American girls, Dix has been analyzed by modern historians and pronounced a "disastrous failure" and a rival, rather than a supporter, of Clara Barton, another former female icon.

Clara Barton (1821–1912), founder of the American branch of the Red Cross, was also involved in nursing during the war, but she was primarily associated with the monumental task of obtaining supplies, including medicines, and identifying the dead and wounded. When the war ended, Barton helped organize the exchange of prisoners of war and a bureau of records to search for missing men. She went to Andersonville, the notorious Confederate prison camp in Georgia, to lead the effort to identify and mark the graves of Union soldiers. During the war about 13,000 of some 32,000 prisoners died at the camp, from scurvy, dysentery, typhoid, gangrene, and other conditions caused by malnutrition, filth, and neglect. As President of the American Red Cross, Barton attempted to expand the role of the organization beyond war relief to the provision of aid for other forms of disaster.

In support of the Union Army, representatives of the Women's Central Association of Relief and other religious, medical, and reform organizations, including the Lint and Bandage Association, and the Physicians and Surgeons of the Hospitals of New York, went to Washington to formally request the establishment of a sanitary commission. Despite some resistance from military leaders, the Secretary of War authorized the U.S. Sanitary Commission in June 1861. Operating as a voluntary organization, the Sanitary Commission attempted to provide food, medical supplies, and other forms of humanitarian assistance to soldiers, investigate and improve sanitary conditions at military camps and hospitals, and implement a comprehensive system of record keeping. The Sanitary Commission actively solicited donations in order to purchase and distribute supplies, organize transportation to hospitals, and provide support for soldiers' aid societies.

Under the auspices of the Commission, volunteers provided humanitarian services for sick and wounded soldiers, distributed soap and other toiletries, and established kitchens for the preparation of special diets for invalids, hospital libraries, and rest facilities for soldiers. Historians suggest that participation in the work of the Sanitary Commission prepared many women for the roles they created in post-war reform movements at the local and national level. Many Sanitary Commission branches refused to allow blacks to participate in volunteer work, forcing many African-American men and women to participate in other war relief societies. In order to reach a general audience, especially the families of Union soldiers, the Commission published a newspaper called the *Sanitary Reporter* and created a hospital directory to help relatives locate wounded and missing soldiers. The lists compiled by 1864 contained the names of close to six hundred thousand sick, wounded, and dead soldiers. Publication of statistical data about the

Army's incompetence in the distribution of food, clothing, bedding, and medical supplies, camp sanitary conditions, and hospital management was an obvious source of embarrassment to military bureaucrats.

Memoirs and letters of Civil War surgeons provide intimate portraits of camp life, army politics, and their often frustrating attempts to care for sick and wounded soldiers. Doctors complained that it was almost impossible to get medical supplies from "drunken and incompetent quartermasters." Supplies of food were often inadequate, but whisky was freely available—perhaps as "medicinal whiskey." Doctors suspected that whisky was always transported even if medical supplies were left behind. Daniel M. Holt, for example, assistant surgeon in the 121st New York Volunteers, quickly discovered that the demands on a military doctor were quite different from those of a country doctor. During his two years of army life, Holt lost 21 pounds, suffered from gastrointestinal problems, and contracted tuberculosis. Sick, discouraged, and worried about re-establishing his practice, Holt left the army in 1864. He died in 1868, only 47 years of age.

John Vance Lauderdale, another doctor from New York, served as a contract surgeon on a hospital ship that brought the sick and wounded from southern battlefields to northern hospitals. His brother told him that all doctors agreed that he would "learn more of surgery in one year in the Army than in a life time of private practice or in the hospitals of New York." But Lauderdale felt he learned little at all except about his own therapeutic inefficacy. Patients died from dysentery, malaria, hospital gangrene, and typhoid fever, but he had nothing better to dose them with than whisky. After surgical operations, soldiers might die of shock, bleeding, or infection, or they might succumb to the diarrheas, dysenteries, and fevers so common at camps and hospitals. Many doctors confessed that they had learned a great deal about the horrors of war, the futility of contemporary medicine, and their own deficiencies.

Perhaps surgeons also returned home with folklore about wounds and healing. Maggot therapy, for example, was based on the observation that certain "worms" seemed to cleanse a wound of pus, while ignoring healthy flesh. This technique had already been described by military surgeons during the Napoleonic wars. Bacteria that can make insects sick may have been responsible for the exceptional healing of Civil War soldiers' wounds that glowed in the dark. According to Civil War folklore, soldiers with wounds that glowed in the dark had better survival rates than soldiers with nonglowing wounds. Microbiologists think this might have some basis in fact. The luminescent bacterium *Photorhabdus luminescens*, an insect pathogen, has been investigated as a potential biocontrol agent. Some *Photorhabdus* strains produce antibiotics that inhibit the growth of bacteria that could cause infections in open wounds.

Nevertheless, military medicine gave many doctors an unprecedented opportunity to gain surgical experience, if not competence,
and some appreciation for the importance of sanitation and hygiene.
Doctors also learned about pathology and neurology by carrying out
autopsies and by attempting to rehabilitate soldiers who had survived
amputations. Civil War surgeons became notorious for amputating legs
and arms that might have been saved under different circumstances. On
the other hand, soldiers with fractures and wounds that might have been
treated conservatively in private practice were probably saved by the
amputation of limbs that were already hopelessly mangled and infected
by the time they received medical care. When civilian surgeons blamed
army doctors for being too eager to cut off limbs, Jonathan Letterman
(1824–1872), Medical Director of the Army of the Potomac, argued that
amputations done as soon as possible after injury were essential to saving lives. "If any objection could be urged against the surgery of those
fields," Letterman wrote, "it would be the efforts... of surgeons to
practice 'conservative surgery' to too great an extent."

Caricatures showed the beleaguered field surgeon holding a knife
between his teeth between amputations, throwing amputated limbs onto
an ever-growing pile. Even during the war, reporters and commentators
were especially harsh in their judgments of military surgeons, despite the
fact that the mistakes of commanders and generals were the true causes
of so much suffering and death. In response to critics, Letterman did not
claim that there were no incompetent surgeons in the army, but he urged
them to remember the medical officers who "lost their lives in their
devotion to duty... and others sickened from excessive labor which they
conscientiously and skillfully performed." Of course military doctors
lost many patients to disease and wounds, but even the best doctors,
under optimum conditions in the 1860s could do little to cure or prevent
most diseases; nor could they cure post-surgical infections. The work of
the field surgeon was brutal, rushed, and stressful, but Civil War surgeons were not necessarily careless, heartless, and incompetent. Most
began military service with about the same training as any of their typical contemporaries, but they were often worn down by the stresses and
deficiencies of military medicine. Civil War doctors were expected to
function as public health officer, dietician, dentist, nurse, and psychologist, with only minimal resources or help. Many doctors contracted
camp illnesses or became disabled by accidents or enemy fire, and many
died. Turning the tables on civilian doctors, Letterman said that in his
experience it was impossible to rely on civilian surgeons "during or after
a battle. They cannot or will not submit to the privations and discomforts which are necessary, and the great majority think more of their
own personal comfort than they do of the wounded."

Civil War surgeons established some improvements in the management of external wounds, but mortality rates for chest, head, and

abdominal wounds were very high. Amputations, which constituted about 75 percent of all Civil War operations, saved many lives, despite the crudity of surgical procedures and facilities. Many amputees recovered and returned to active duty, sometimes with a prosthetic limb. Anecdotes about amputees who continued to fight led to the saying that if all the soldiers and officers who had lost limbs in battle were brought together they could form their own brigade. In a grim version of recycling, new amputees sometimes appropriated the prosthetic limbs of soldiers who had died in battle. In Jules Verne's 1864 novel *From the Earth to the Moon*, the members of the Baltimore Gun Club, veterans of the Civil War, were notable for their "crutches, wooden legs, artificial arms with iron hooks at the wrist, rubber jaws, silver skulls, platinum noses." Mutilated in the war, these men were the ingenious inventors who designed a gigantic cannon for their voyage to the moon. Thus, although accounts of Civil War amputations focus on the brutality of the procedure, the thousands of veterans who returned home with missing limbs could be regarded as success stories.

Prior to the war, when faced with the prospect of performing surgery, most doctors subscribed to the principle of "conservative therapeutics," that is, doctors tried to avoid surgical interventions and surgical mutilations. Civil War surgeons, however, had to make decisions about treatment under very different conditions. Unless surgeons acted quickly and without pity, many of the wounded would probably have died of their injuries. When treating men whose arms and legs had already been fractured and torn open by bullets, amputation was the course of action most likely to save the patient from gangrene, tetanus, pyemia, and other deadly infections almost invariably acquired on the battlefield or in the hospital. Army surgeons believed that: "Life is better than a limb; and too often mutilation is the only alternative to a rapid and painful death." The U.S. Sanitary Commission recommended amputation for patients whose limbs had been badly lacerated and for those with compound fractures. The *Manual of Military Surgery* used by Confederate surgeons also suggested amputation when the limb had been badly injured.

An estimated 60,000 amputations were performed during the war; about 35,000 men survived such operations, but mortality statistics were imprecise and unreliable. Anesthesia made it possible to perform amputations that would have been impossible or invariably fatal previously. The outcome of surgery depended on many variables: the time since injury, part of the body, and type of surgical procedure. Official Union records suggest that amputation at the hip performed more than 24 hours after the wound was incurred were almost invariable fatal, but the mortality rate for amputation at the ankle was about 25 percent. Physicians discovered also that artificial limbs might make mobility possible again, but prosthetic devices did not trick the body into forgetting its lost parts. Silas Weir Mitchell (1829–1914), one of the founders of American neurology, carried out studies of causalgia and a problem he labeled "phantom limb pain" at the hospital for "stumps and nervous diseases" established by Surgeon General John Hammond to care for amputees suffering from chronic pain and disability. Mitchell's research provided fundamental insights into the workings of mind and body. Previously, the phantom limb phenomenon had been dismissed as a hallucination or neurosis. But, based on his observations and his knowledge of the physiology of the nervous system, Mitchell attributed the phenomenon to an ascending neuritis associated with some change in the central nervous system.

Oliver Wendell Holmes noted the relationship between the war and the American prosthetics industry. "War unmakes legs," Holmes wrote, and "human skill must supply their places." Those who lost a limb provided an unprecedented market for prosthetic devices; tens of thousands of men returned from the war without arms and legs. The war stimulated the pharmaceutical industry, along with the business of supplying prosthetic devices. Civil War pensions involved compensation related to the loss of body parts and funding for the purchase of artificial limbs. Between 1861 and 1873, the United States Patent Office granted 150 patents for artificial limbs and related devices. After the war the flourishing prosthetic device industry remained profitable by providing artificial limbs for those wounded while working in factories and mines and the accidents associated with the railroads and other forms of mass transportation.

In many ways, the role of the Federal government in policies and practices related to agriculture, education, medicine, and science was transformed by the Civil War. During the long and bloody war, both the Union and the Confederate governments had to create and expand military medical establishments to supervise camp sanitation and cope with the management of the sick and wounded. Medical officers had to carry out medical inspections of recruits, establish ambulance corps, obtain and distribute medical supplies, and oversee hospital trains and hospitals. When the war began, the number of regularly appointed army surgeons and assistant surgeons in the Union Medical Department was totally inadequate to the unprecedented medical demands. Contract surgeons were hired for three to six months with the nominal rank of acting assistant surgeon. Medical duties for surgeons and assistant surgeons were essentially the same, but the surgeon did more administrative work and was better paid. Other personnel in the Medical Department were brigade surgeons, regimental and assistant surgeons, contract surgeons, nurses, and hospital stewards who worked as apothecaries and wound dressers.

William A. Hammond (1828–1900), who served as Surgeon General from 1862 to 1864, improved the efficiency of the Army's

Medical Department, built large general hospitals, instituted an ambulance service, and won the admiration of the Sanitary Commission. In modern bureaucratic organizational charts, the U.S. Army Surgeon General and the Public Health Service Surgeon General are quite separate and distinct officials. Before the Civil War, the term "Surgeon General" was the title of the senior officer in the United State Army Medical Department. After the war, the Navy adopted the title for the Chief of its Bureau of Medicine and Surgery. When the Marine Hospital system evolved into the Marine Hospital Service, the title Supervising Surgeon was given to the newly created senior government doctor directing the MHS. Further reforms transformed the Marine Hospital Service into the United States Public Health Service. The director of the United States Public Health Service was called the Surgeon General, or more specifically the Surgeon General of the United States, or the Surgeon General of the United States Public Health Service. Today the Surgeon General is a political appointee, with direct command of a rather small staff, but the title traditionally confers a great deal of moral authority and the individual holding the office often acts as the chief spokesperson for the government on health issues. The Army, Navy, and Air Force still award the title of Surgeon General to their chief medical advisors. These officials are also involved in providing advice to the Defense Department on medical policy and health issues.

Surgeon General Hammond, an energetic and imposing figure at 6 feet 2 inches, and 250 pounds, was quite a change from his dogmatic 64-year-old predecessor, C. A. Finley, who had become Surgeon General in 1861. Hammond graduated from New York University's Medical College in 1848 and entered the U.S. Army as an assistant surgeon. In 1860, Hammond resigned from the army and accepted a position as Professor of Anatomy and Physiology at the University of Maryland Medical School. He re-enlisted at the start of the Civil War and served as inspector of hospitals and army camps. Members of the U.S. Sanitary Commission were impressed by his work and exerted considerable pressure to have him appointed Surgeon General of the Medical Department with the rank of brigadier general.

Hammond created the general hospital service, oversaw the establishment of an efficient ambulance corps, and created two large government-operated drug laboratories to produce high-quality medicines for the army. He also alienated many conservative regular and volunteer medical officers when he removed popular drugs like calomel and tartar emetic from the Army's official list of medical supplies. The American Medical Association passed a resolution condemning Hammond's decision. Inevitably Hammond's rapid promotion and obvious contempt for incompetents created powerful enemies, including Secretary of War Edwin M. Stanton, who charged him with graft, fraud, and exceeding his authority. After a trial that lasted from January to August 1864,

Hammond was court-martialed and dismissed from the Army. George Strong, head of the Sanitary Commission, said that Hammond, who tended to avoid bureaucratic rules in pursuit of efficiency, had been guilty of "little more than the technical sin of purchasing supplies too freely." Returning to New York, Hammond became Professor of the Diseases of the Mind and Nervous System at Bellevue Hospital Medical College. Widely recognized for his work in neurology, Hammond was a leader in the establishment of the American Neurological Association. Hammond's court-martial was overturned in 1879, and he was restored to the rank of brigadier general.

Many of the improvements in Civil War medical services were the work of Jonathan Letterman (1824–1872), Medical Director of the Army of the Potomac. Often called the father of modern battlefield medicine, Letterman acknowledged his debt to the work of the French military surgeon Dominique-Jean Larrey (1766–1842). During the Napoleonic wars, Larrey introduced *ambulances volantes* to expedite the removal of injured soldiers from the battlefield. Working closely with Hammond, Letterman established an ambulance corps, raised standards for army surgeons and medical inspections, standardized triage and treatment, improved hospital and camp sanitation, simplified the collection and processing of medical data, and created a system of mobile field hospitals using large tents. The "Letterman system" remains the basis of the modern organization and operation of military medical systems in all armies.

The importance of the ambulance corps is apparent in a comparison of the time taken to remove the injured after the battle of Manassas and the battle of Antietam, the bloodiest one-day battle of the war. It took one week to remove the wounded at Manassas, but with Letterman's transportation system in operation at the battle of Antietam, the ambulance corps was able to remove all the wounded from the battlefield within 24 hours. Letterman also developed the three-tiered evacuation system that is still used today. Medical officers at Field Dressing (Aid) Stations located next to the battlefield applied dressings and tourniquets. The wounded were then brought to the Field Hospital (now MASH units) closest to the battlefield for emergency surgery and treatment. Large hospitals at some distance from the battlefield provided long-term care.

Although much of the medical organization of the war was soon dismantled, the Surgeon General's office did retain significant responsibilities and created institutions that provided materials for research and teaching. In 1862, Hammond established the Army Medical Museum in Washington to collect and study unusual anatomical and pathological specimens, projectiles, and other foreign objects found during surgical operations in military hospitals. The museum eventually became the Armed Forces Institute of Pathology. Hammond also was responsible for initiating the compilation of a comprehensive medical and surgical history of the war. Using the pathological specimens collected during the war and mountains of wartime records, Joseph J. Woodward, George Alexander Otis, and others organized the six thousand page, six volume *Medical and Surgical History of the War of the Rebellion (1861–1865)*. Woodward and Otis, medical officers in the Surgeon General's Office, were the major editors of the *History*. Otis was curator of the Army Medical Museum from 1864 to 1881. The Civil War also left a unique, unprecedented legacy in photographs, especially photographic studies of medical and surgical cases related to injuries sustained during the war.

Another distinguished member of the Surgeon General's Office, John Shaw Billings (1838–1913), established the Army Medical Library, which became the National Library of Medicine. In addition to creating the *Index Catalogue* for the collection in the Library of the Surgeon General, Billings also established the *Index Medicus*, so that information in the rapidly growing medical and scientific literature would be accessible to researchers. In 1883, Billings became director of the newly combined Library of the Surgeon General's Office and the Army Medical Museum, which became the Army Medical Library and Museum. Through a law passed in 1976, the Armed Forces Institute of Pathology became the nation's official medical repository. Specimens submitted to the Armed Forces Institute of Pathology for diagnosis, either by military or civilian doctors, are kept as part of the repository. Specimens in the repository have been invaluable for research on the history of disease. For example, lung tissue preserved in paraffin wax from the World War I period was used to identify the virus that caused the 1918–1919 influenza pandemic. The National Museum of Health and Medicine, which is now a division of the Army Medical Museum, has pathological specimens on display in exhibits on the Civil War, the Korean Conflict, and the human body.

## SUGGESTED READINGS

Adams, G. W. (1996). *Doctors in Blue: The Medical History of the Union Army in the Civil War.* Baton Rouge, LA: Louisiana State University Press.

Bankole, K. (1998). *Slavery and Medicine: Enslavement and Medical Practices in Antebellum Louisiana.* New York: Garland Publishing.

Beaumont, W. (1959). *Experiments and Observations on the Gastric Juice and the Physiology of Digestion.* New York: Dover.

Benes, P., ed. (1992). *Medicine and Healing, The Dublin Seminar for New England Folklife, Annual Proceedings, 1990*. Boston, MA: Boston University Press.

Bengston, B. P., and Kuz, J. E. (1996). *Photographic Atlas of Civil War Injuries: Photographs of Surgical Cases and Specimens of Orthopaedic Injuries and Treatments during the Civil War*. Otis Historical Archives. Grand Rapids, MI: Medical Staff Press.

Bollet, A. J. (2002). *Civil War Medicine: Challenges and Triumphs*. Tucson, AZ: Galen Press.

Brown, T. J. (1998). *Dorothea Dix. New England Reformer*. Cambridge, MA: Harvard University Press.

Burbick, J. (1994). *Healing the Republic: The Language of Health and the Culture of Nationalism in Nineteenth-Century America*. Cambridge: Cambridge University Press.

Byrd, W. M., and Clayton, L. A. (2000). *An American Health Dilemma: A Medical History of African Americans and the Problem of Race*. 2 vols. New York: Routledge.

Cash, P., ed. (1980). *Medicine in Colonial Massachusetts*. Boston, MA: Colonial Society of Massachusetts.

Cassedy, J. H. (1986). *Medicine and American Growth, 1800–1860*. Madison, WI: University of Wisconsin Press.

Craighill, E. A. (1989). *Confederate Surgeon: The Personal Recollections of E. A. Craighill*. Edited by P. W. Houck. Lynchburg, VA: H. E. Howard.

Cunningham, H. H. (1958). *Doctors in Gray: The Confederate Medical Service*. Baton Rouge, LA: Louisiana State University Press.

Currie, W. (1972). *An Historical Account of the Climates and Diseases of the United States of America; and of the Remedies and Methods of Treatment, Which Have Been Found Most Useful and Efficacious, Particularly in Those Diseases Which Depend Upon Climate and Situation. Collected Principally from Personal Observation, and the Communications of Physicians of Talents and Experience, Residing in the Several States*. New York: Arno Press Inc. Reprint of 1792 edition.

Dean, E. T., Jr. (1997). *Shook Over Hell. Post-Traumatic Stress, Vietnam, and the Civil War*. Cambridge, MA: Harvard University Press.

Estes, J. W., and Smith, B. G., eds. (1997). *A Melancholy Scene of Devastation: The Public Response to the 1793 Philadelphia Yellow Fever Epidemic*. Canton, MA: Science History Publications.

Fatout, P., ed. (1996). *Letters of a Civil War Surgeon*. West Lafayette, IN: Purdue University Press.

Fett, S. M. (2002). *Working Cures: Healing, Health, and Power on Southern Slave Plantations*. Chapel Hill, NC: University of North Carolina Press.

Fox, C. G., Miller, G. L., and Miller, J. C., comps. (1996). *Benjamin Rush, M.D.: A Bibliographic Guide*. Westport, CT: Greenwood Press.

Freemon, F. R. (1993). *Microbes and Minnie Balls: An Annotated Bibliography of Civil War Medicine.* Rutherford, NJ: Fairleigh Dickinson University Press.

Freemon, F. R. (1998). *Gangrene and Glory: Medical Care During the American Civil War.* Madison, NJ: Fairleigh Dickinson University Press.

Friendenberg, Z. B. (1998). *The Doctor in Colonial America.* Danbury, CT: Rutledge Books.

Giesberg, J. A. (2000). *Civil War Sisterhood: The U.S. Sanitary Commission and Women's Politics in Transition.* Boston, MA: Northeastern University Press.

Gillett, M. C. (1987). *The Army Medical Department, 1818–1865.* Washington, DC: Center of Military History, United States Army.

Greiner, J. M., Coryell, J. L., and Smither, J. R., eds. (1994). *A Surgeon's Civil War. The Letters and Diary of Daniel M. Holt, M.D.* Kent, OH: Ohio State Press.

Harris, B., and Ernst, W., eds. (1999). *Race, Science and Medicine, 1700–1960.* London: Routledge.

Horsman, R. (1996). *Frontier Doctor: William Beaumont, America's First Great Medical Scientist.* Columbia, MO: University of Missouri Press.

Josyph, P., ed. (1993). *The Civil War Letters of John Vance Lauderdale, M.D.* East Lansing, MI: Michigan State University Press.

King, L. S. (1990). *Transformations in American Medicine: From Benjamin Rush to William Osler.* Baltimore, MD: Johns Hopkins University Press.

Kiple, K. F., ed. (1987). *The African Exchange: Toward a Biological History of Black People.* Durham, NC: Duke University Press.

Kuz, J. E., and Bengston, B. P. (1996). *Orthopaedic Injuries of the Civil War: An Atlas of Orthopaedic Injuries and Treatments during the Civil War.* Kennesaw, GA: Kennesaw Mountain Press.

Melosi, M. V. (2000). *The Sanitary City: Urban Infrastructure in America from Colonial Times to the Present.* Baltimore, MD: Johns Hopkins University Press.

Oates, S. B. (1994). *A Woman of Valor. Clara Barton and the Civil War.* New York: The Free Press.

Pryor, E. B. (1987). *Clara Barton. Profession Angel.* Philadelphia, PA: University of Pennsylvania Press.

Robertson, J., Jr. ed. (1992). *The Medical and Surgical History of the Civil War.* (Formerly entitled *Medical and Surgical History of the War of the Rebellion.*) Wilmington, NC: Broadfoot Publishing Co. Reprint of 1883 edition.

Rush, B. (1972). *Medical Inquiries and Observations.* New York: Arno Press. Reprint of 1815 edition.

Savitt, T. L. (2002). *Medicine and Slavery: Diseases and Health Care of Blacks in Antebellum Virginia.* Chicago, IL: University of Chicago Press.

Savitt, T. L., and Young, J. H., eds. (1988). *Disease and Distinctiveness in the American South*. Knoxville, TN: University of Tennessee Press.

Smith, G. W. (2001). *Medicine for the Union Army: The United States Army Laboratories During the Civil War*. Binghamton, NY: Pharmaceutical Products Press.

Snow, L. F. (1993). *Walkin' over Medicine: Traditional Health Practices in African-American Life*. Boulder, CO: Westview Press.

Steiner, P. E. (1968). *Disease in the Civil War: Natural Biological Warfare in 1861–1865*. Springfield, IL: Charles C. Thomas Publisher.

Tripler, C. S., and Blackman, G. C. (1989). *Hand-Book for the Military Surgeon*. American Civil War Surgery Series. San Francisco, CA: Norman Publishing.

Valencius, C. B. (2002). *The Health of the Country: How American Settlers Understood Themselves and Their Land*. New York: Basic Books.

Watson, P. A. (1991). *The Angelical Conjunction: The Preacher-Physicians of Colonial New England*. Knoxville, TN: University of Tennessee Press.

Wooley, C. F. (2002). *The Irritable Heart of Soldiers: The US Civil War to Soldier's Heart: World War I*. Burlington, VT: Ashgate.

Woolsey, J. S. (1996). *Hospital Days: Reminiscence of a Civil War Nurse*. Roseville, MN: Edinborough Press.

# 9

# Clinical and Preventive Medicine

Throughout Europe, the seventeenth century was a period of political, social, and spiritual unrest, manifested by warfare and revolution, Reformation, and Counter-Reformation. Bitter controversies were as characteristic of medicine and science as they were of religion and politics. An increasingly literate public was becoming skeptical of ancient medical dogma; chemical remedies were challenging traditional Galenicals, and instruments like the telescope, microscope, barometer, pulse clock, and thermometer were providing new means of investigating the natural world.

England's own philosopher of science and Lord High Chancellor, Francis Bacon (1561–1626), called for a more pragmatic approach to medicine and nature. If physicians collected data empirically, without regard to ancient doctrines, Bacon predicted that they would be able to form new theories, make new discoveries, prolong life, and understand the workings of the body in health and disease. Bacon's vision of the "Grand Instauration" that would transform the sciences and improve the human condition helped inspire the establishment of new scientific societies and novel medical philosophies.

Changes in medical philosophy and practice probably affected few patients directly. Learned physicians served only the rich; most people lived and died without the assistance of physicians or surgeons. Seeking medical attention was impossible for impoverished peasants and workers, who could afford neither the physician's fees nor the elaborate remedies he prescribed. It was not the physician who dealt with the afflictions of the common people, but the great army of "irregular practitioners"—barber-surgeons, apothecaries, midwives, empirics, and peripatetic quacks.

Pretentious physicians, more interested in their purses than their patients, provided a favorite target for satirists. Jean Baptiste Molière (1622–1673), the witty French playwright, aimed some of his sharpest barbs at the affectations of the fashionable physician, in his fancy wig, ornate velvet coat, and gold-handled cane. At least the hollow handle of the cane had a practical purpose; stuffed with smelling salts and perfumes it provided an antidote to the aroma of the sickroom. Perhaps all too many physicians resembled Molière's caricature of the physician, whose prescription for any illness was always "clyster, bleed, purge," or "purge, bleed, clyster." (Clyster is an archaic term for enema.) In Molière's play *Love's the Best Doctor*, we learn that "we should never say, such a one is dead of a fever," because, to tell the truth, the patient died of "four doctors and two apothecaries."

Nevertheless, physicians were mastering the art of using new drugs, such as quinine and ipecac, while the introduction of New World foods, especially potatoes and corn, had a remarkable effect on health and population growth. The potato became the staple food of the poor in northern Europe, the British Isles, and Ireland. A one-acre plot of potatoes could feed a family of six all year. Over-dependence on a single crop has always been one of the risks of agricultural societies, as demonstrated by the Irish potato famine of 1845. (In 2001, scientists were able to use PCR amplification of samples taken from historic specimens to identify the specific strain of the plant pathogen, *Phytophthora infestans*, that was responsible for the devastating potato blight.) Corn, which was usually called maize, or Turkish wheat, provided much needed calories, but also made pellagra (a nutritional disease caused by insufficient niacin and protein in the diet) an endemic disease in many areas. Some New World plants, such as tobacco, were simultaneously credited with medicinal virtues and condemned as poisons.

Although mortality rates for this period are generally crude estimates, interest in the accurate measurement of births and deaths was growing. John Graunt (1620–1674), author of *Observations upon the Bills of Mortality* (1662), the first book on vital statistics, attempted to derive general trends from the local Bills of Mortality (weekly lists of burials) and the records of marriages and baptisms kept by parish clerks. Graunt called attention to the fact that the urban death rate was greater than that of rural areas. Infant mortality, a good index of general health and sanitation, was very high: probably 40 percent of all infants died before reaching their second birthday. Renowned astronomer Edmond Halley (1656–1742), who was interested in the theory of annuities and mortality rates, noted that those who reached maturity should not complain about the shortness of their lives, because half of all those born were dead within 17 years. Nevertheless, the physical sciences had been transformed and it seemed reasonable to expect a similar revolution in medicine. To this end, physicians devoted to scientific research developed elaborate theories, which had little to do with the practical details of patient care. Thomas Sydenham, who has been honored as the English champion of clinical, or bedside medicine, provides an instructive example of a physician who recognized the growing tension between medicine as science and medicine as the care of the sick.

## THOMAS SYDENHAM, THE "ENGLISH HIPPOCRATES"

Thomas Sydenham (1624–1689) epitomized the reaction of the clinician to abstract and speculative medicine and the pretensions of physicians who behaved as if their scientific research was more significant than medicine practiced at the bedside of the patient. When scientific medicine was generally carried out in the autopsy room, patients with long, lingering illnesses might well frustrate a physician who was overly devoted to his research.

Like Hippocrates, Sydenham believed that it was the task of the physician to assist the body's natural healing processes, while finding patterns in symptoms and searching for the cause of disease. Since clinical medicine was an art that demanded acute observation, experience, and balanced judgment, the true physician should dedicate himself to useful techniques, common sense, and the principles of Hippocrates. Revered as the English Hippocrates, Sydenham was eulogized as "the great representative of the practical medicine of practical England" and the man who recognized "the priority of direct observation, and its paramount supremacy to everything else."

Politically, as well as professionally, Sydenham might be regarded as the antithesis of William Harvey. Indeed, Sydenham's goals and achievements have been ascribed to the events that made him a highly politicized person; that is, his attempts to reform medicine were apparently inseparable from his political stance. Sydenham and his brothers fought as soldiers in the Parliamentary Army; their mother was killed in a Royalist raid. Several close encounters with death during the war convinced Sydenham that a special providence had spared his life.

After the Royalists were defeated, Sydenham resumed his studies at Oxford and, in less than two years, he was granted a bachelor's degree in medicine. When hostilities began again, Sydenham rejoined the army. In 1655, Sydenham resigned his Oxford fellowship and established a private practice in an aristocratic London neighborhood close to the malarial marshes that generated a steady supply of fever patients. He also attended the sick poor at various London hospitals. Although Sydenham became a Licentiate of the Royal College of Physicians in 1663, he was never granted the honor of becoming a Fellow of that prestigious association. His enemies even tried to rescind his license and banish him from the College of Physicians for medical heresy and irregular practice. In an age where personal abuse was a common form of professional discourse, Sydenham was always ready to return real or imagined insults. Defensive about the deficiencies in his formal education, Sydenham boasted of his ability to "think where others read."

Puritan principles, especially the idea that increasing useful knowledge was a paramount religious duty, guided Sydenham's approach to medicine. Studying cadavers was useless, because death was an admission of defeat, or proof of inadequate care. Medical education, according to Sydenham, could take place only at the bedside of the sick, not in the classroom, library, or anatomy theater. Despite his admiration for Hippocrates, Sydenham insisted that experience had been his only teacher. Many of the anecdotes treasured by Sydenham's followers reflect this attitude. For example, when Dr. Richard Blackmore asked Sydenham to recommend the best books for learning medicine, he replied: "Read 'Don Quixote'; it is a very good book; I read it myself still." Perhaps this retort reflected his opinion of both young doctor Blackmore and the medical literature of his time, along with microscopy and pathological anatomy, which he dismissed as frivolous and irrelevant.

Although Sydenham ridiculed attempts to study the ravages of disease through postmortems, he considered close study of the natural history of disease among hospital patients valuable training. According to Dr. Robert Pitt, by carefully studying the course of disease in a hospital for the "meaner class" of patients, Sydenham was able to determine whether a fever could be cured by "Natural Power," or whether it required "Bleeding, Vomiting, Purgatives... before risking the lives of people of quality." When accused of diminishing the dignity of the healing art by recommending plain and simple medicines, Sydenham countered that wise men understood that "whatever is useful is good." Not only were simple remedies useful, they were safer than "superfluous and over-learned medicines" that were likely to aggravate the disease until the tormented patient "dies of his doctor." Recommending moderation in all things, Sydenham prescribed appropriate diets, drugs, exercise, and opium, the drug God had created for the relief of pain. Even a simple remedy, like a rag dipped in rosewater and applied to the forehead, often did more good than any narcotic.

In 1665, the year of the Great Plague, Sydenham and his family fled from London. While living in the countryside, he found the time to complete his *Medical Observations Concerning the History and Cure of Acute Diseases*. As an admirer of the rapidly developing science of taxonomy, Sydenham prescribed analogous methods for the study of the natural history of disease. Because Nature produced uniform and consistent species of diseases, Sydenham assumed that close attention to a small number of cases would produce information that applied to all similar cases. Combining direct observations and Robert Boyle's chemical theories, Sydenham suggested that subterranean effluvia generated disease-causing miasmata when they came in contact with certain corpuscles in the air. As the atmosphere became "stuffed full of particles which are hostile to the economy of the human body," each breath became saturated with "noxious and unnatural miasmata" that mixed with the blood and engendered acute epidemic diseases.

In his attempt to extend scientific taxonomy to medicine, Sydenham envisioned disease as an entity existing independently of the person who might become its victim. Acute diseases caused by changes in the atmosphere that affected great numbers of people at the same time were called epidemics; other acute diseases attacked only a few people at a time and could be called intercurrent or sporadic. Physicians had long been content with vague designations of diseases in terms of major symptoms, but Sydenham believed that the physician must learn to distinguish between different diseases with similar symptoms. For example, fevers were vaguely classified as continued, intermittent, and eruptive. Typhus was the most common of the continued fevers, malaria was the prime example of an intermittent fever, and smallpox was the most dreaded eruptive fever.

Smallpox, which Sydenham carefully distinguished from scarlet fever and measles, was so common in the seventeenth century that, like Rhazes, Sydenham regarded it as essentially part of the normal maturation process. Physicians generally kept smallpox patients confined to bed under a great weight of blankets and prescribed heating cordials to drive out diseased matter. Sydenham contended that the orthodox "heating regimen" caused excessive ebullition of the blood, which led to improper fermentation, confluent pustules, brain fever, and death. To assist nature, Sydenham prescribed a simple and moderate "cooling regimen" featuring light covers, moderate bleeding, and a liberal allowance of fluids.

Sydenham's short treatise on mental illness has been called the most important seventeenth-century work on psychological disorders and their treatment. According to Sydenham, psychological disorders were as common as physical complaints. Moreover, hysteria, a disorder the ancients attributed to the wanderings of the uterus, seemed to be the most common of all chronic diseases. Perhaps it was no surprise that hardly any women were wholly free of this disorder, but it was certainly remarkable to learn that men were also subject to hysterical complaints. Faced with the challenge of determining a new etiology, Sydenham ascribed hysteria to disordered animal spirits. Time, the prince of physicians, healed many of these patients, but Sydenham also recommended "steel syrup" (iron filings steeped in wine) and horseback riding. For both mental and physical complaints, Sydenham was as enthusiastic about horseback riding as modern health activists are about jogging. Some patients had to be tricked into health-restoring exercise. Frustrated by one patient who stubbornly refused to get well, Sydenham suggested a consultation with the wonder-working Dr. Robinson at Inverness. The patient made the long trip on horseback only to find that there was no such doctor, but, as Sydenham expected, anticipation, exercise, and anger effected a cure.

## ON THE MISERIES OF GOUT AND THE VIRTUES
## OF COLCHICINE

Some of Sydenham's most vivid writings are those describing the onset, pain, and progress of gout, a disease also known as podagra. Sydenham confessed that he had endured the agonies of gout for 34 years without discovering anything useful about its nature or treatment. Many physicians, especially those who suffered from gout, considered the condition incurable. In its typical form, the disease announced itself by intense pain in the big toe. Victims were told that it was better for their "bad humors" to accumulate in a peripheral joint rather than in vital interior parts of the body. For the miseries of gout, stone, and chronic hematuria (which Sydenham bluntly referred to as "a great pissing of blood"), his only antidote was opium and more opium.

Until the twentieth century, little could be added to Hippocrates' observations that gout generally attacked young adult males, while sparing women and eunuchs. Victims of the disease were thought to be wealthy men who indulged themselves in heavy wines, rich foods, excessive sexual activity, and those with an "unhappy hereditary tendency." Seneca said the disease had "Bacchus for its father and Venus for its mother." Today, primary gout is described as an inherited disorder of purine metabolism, which results in the accumulation of uric acid. Secondary gout is a condition apparently caused by noxious chemicals, such as lead and various drugs. Seventeenth-century microscopists depicted crystals teased from a gouty joint: these crystals were eventually identified as uric acid. In 1847, Sir Alfred Baring Garrod (1819–1907), an eminent London physician and professor of medicine, noted an elevated level of uric acid in the blood of victims of gout; uric acid levels were not elevated in patients with other forms of arthritis or rheumatism. In addition to developing tests for gout, Garrod correctly suggested that gout might be caused by the inability of the kidney to excrete uric acid or an increase in the formation of this chemical, and that acute attacks of gout might be the result of the precipitation of sodium urate in the affected joints.

Gout attacks are not fatal, but they are so painful that some victims have been driven to suicide. An attack usually begins with intense pain in the great toe, chills, shivers, restlessness, and fever. Eventually, gout cripples the major joints and results in the chronic torment of kidney stones. Sometimes, Sydenham observed, the stones killed the patient "without waiting for the gout." Living with fear, anxiety, and pain, the victim's mind "suffers with the body; and which suffers most" even the long-suffering Sydenham could not say.

The only comfort Sydenham had to offer his fellow victims was the thought that gout "kills more rich men than poor, more wise men than simple." Nature, Sydenham believed, balanced her accounts by giving those she had favored an appropriate affliction in order to produce a mixture of good and evil. Gout was the disease of kings, emperors, admirals, and philosophers. Despite Sydenham's belief that gout reflected divine justice, the alleged relationship between gout and wealth and wisdom is simply an artifact of historical interest in the medical problems of the rich and famous and general indifference to the anonymous victims of disease who suffered the torments of gout without benefit of medical or biographical attention. Still, the list of distinguished victims of gout is so impressive that the British psychologist Henry Havelock Ellis (1859–1939) thought the disease was associated with genius. The victims of gout included Erasmus, Francis Bacon, William Harvey, Benjamin Franklin, Joseph Banks, Tobias Smollett, Edward Gibbon, Benjamin Disraeli, and Joseph Conrad. Lord Chesterfield said that "gout is the distemper of a gentleman, rheumatism... of a hackney coachman." Franklin, who wrote a witty "Dialogue" between himself and the gout, also suffered from kidney stones. He concluded that "the Gout is bad, and... the Stone is worse." Comforting himself with the idea that those who lived long and well must expect to encounter some diseases, Franklin reflected that there were maladies far worse than kidney stones and gout. Still, the torments of gout and stone drove him to seek out dubious remedies, including a good dose of "Jelly of Blackberries."

Physicians traditionally attacked the gout with bleeding, sweating, purges, cathartics, emetics, diuretics, blisters, massage, and cauterization. From his own experience, Sydenham could testify that none of these methods worked any better than ancient Roman charms and incantations. Abstinence in diet and drink was advisable, but in Sydenham's experience: "If you drink wine you get gout—if you do not, gout gets you!" In 2004, scientists actually corroborated the traditional belief that alcohol consumption increases the risk of developing gout. Sydenham would be surprised to learn, however, that beer is more likely to lead to gout than liquor, or wine.

Unfortunately, Sydenham failed to appreciate the value of colchicum, the one remedy that could have mitigated his sufferings. Colchicum, a crude extract of the autumn crocus, was used in many traditional purges. The Doctrine of Signatures provided a tenuous link between colchicum and gouty arthritis by associating the shape of the flower with that of the crippled arthritic hand. Although colchicum was reputed to have aphrodisiac properties, it also caused unpleasant side effects, including stomach irritation, nausea, and death. Colchicum generally produced dramatic relief from the pain of gout, as demonstrated by the success of the secret remedies of various quacks and empirics. By the eighteenth century, physicians had joined the quacks in recommending colchicum for the relief of gout. The mechanism by which colchicine, the active ingredient in colchicum, relieves gout attacks is still obscure. Colchicine was first isolated in 1820 by Joseph Pelletier (1788–1842) and Joseph Bienaimé Caventou (1795–1877), who are considered the founders of alkaloid chemistry. In addition to its therapeutic virtues, colchicine is invaluable to cell biologists and horticulturists, because it arrests mitosis (cell division) at metaphase. In plants this can cause polyploidy (increase in chromosome number), leading to the production of new varieties.

## QUININE AND MALARIA

Misjudging the value of colchicine for gout caused Sydenham much personal discomfort, but his studies of quinine for malaria offered relief from the debilitating intermittent fever that is still worthy of the title "million-murdering Death." Symptoms of malaria include raging thirst, headache, fatigue, and delirium. Patients suffer from bouts of fever and chills that alternate with periods of apparent remission. If we consider the impact of diseases on populations over time, as measured by the greatest harm to the greatest number, malaria has been the most devastating disease in history. Scientists and historians generally agree that malaria has been a significant force in human evolution and in determining the success or failure of settlement patterns and colonial ventures throughout the world. Malaria seems to have achieved its widest distribution in Europe during the seventeenth century, but it was not uncommon there even in the nineteenth century. According to the World Health Organization, malaria attacks about 300 million people a year, and causes more than 1 million deaths, about 90 percent of them in Africa. Some authorities say that deaths from malaria may actually number about 2.7 million a year. Malaria was Africa's leading killer until 1999, when it was displaced by AIDS.

One of the great accomplishments of seventeenth-century medical science was the discovery that quinine could be used as a specific remedy for malaria. Quinine is the active ingredient in cinchona (also known as Peruvian bark, Jesuits' powder, or Devil's bark), a traditional Peruvian remedy supposedly named after the Countess of Chinchón, wife of the Governor of Peru. The story of the feverish Countess appears to be pure fiction, but, with or without her blessings, the New World remedy spread quickly throughout Europe. As demand for the wonder-working bark drove its price higher and higher, charlatans amassed great fortunes selling secret remedies containing Peruvian bark or useless imitations that mimicked quinine's bitter taste. By the end of the 1660s, confidence in Peruvian bark had dropped precipitously because many physicians claimed that the drug was responsible for dangerous relapses and sudden deaths. Careful study convinced Sydenham that the bark was safe and effective; adverse reactions were due to improper use rather than to any evil in the drug itself.

Peruvian bark was important not only as a remedy for malaria, but also for its symbolic value in challenging the ancient foundations of pharmacology. Medical dogma called for remedies that were complex and purgative, but Peruvian bark cured malaria without purgation. Orthodox medical theory condemned the new remedy as "irrational" because it was theoretically impossible for healing to occur without the expulsion of morbid matter. Therefore, while the bark seemed to interrupt cycles of intermittent fevers, opponents of Peruvian bark assumed that its use led to the accumulation of dangerous materials within the body. Sydenham argued that experience was more compelling than theory; the drug was safe and effective if dosage, timing, and duration of treatment were carefully regulated. In terms of medical practice and theory, therefore, quinine was as revolutionary as gunpowder had been to the art of warfare.

Despite Sydenham's conviction that the bark was harmless, the use of quinine can cause some very unpleasant side effects, including headaches, vomiting, rashes, and deafness. Indeed, some physicians used complaints about ringing in the ears to determine the optimum dosage for each patient. Because few practitioners, or patients, could accept the concept of specificity in diseases and remedies, Peruvian bark was freely prescribed for fevers, colds, flu, seasickness, headache, and hangovers. But quinine is a specific remedy for the specific intermittent fever known as malaria. Its use as a general febrifuge and tonic exposed many people to risks without benefits.

Peruvian bark prepared Europe for a new relationship with malaria. For hundreds of years, malaria and other murderous diseases kept Europeans from penetrating the vast African continent. Thus, quinine became one of the tools that made European exploitation of Africa, and much of Asia, possible. In areas where malaria is highly endemic, slight genetic variations that enhance resistance to the disease may provide a powerful evolutionary advantage. The prevalence of genes for disorders known as sickle cell anemia and thalassemia suggests such an evolutionary pattern. Biologists as well as anthropologists, therefore, have been intrigued by the relationship between genes for abnormal hemoglobins and resistance to malaria.

Quinine, the compound responsible for cinchona's effectiveness against malaria, was isolated in 1820. Within 10 years, the purified drug was being produced in large quantities. Until the 1850s, the forests of Peru, Bolivia, and Colombia were the only sources of the bark, but the Dutch and British established cinchona plantations in Indonesia and India. Intensive experimentation led to significant increases in the yield of active alkaloids. By the turn of the century, the Dutch had captured more than 90 percent of the world market. The Dutch monopoly on this vital drug was not broken until the 1940s, with the Japanese conquest of Indonesia and the European development of synthetic antimalarial drugs.

A type of protozoan belonging to the genus *Plasmodium* causes malaria. The minute parasite has a complex life cycle that includes forms that grow and multiply in blood-sucking mosquitoes and other forms that live in the liver and red blood cells of vertebrate hosts. The female *Anopheles* mosquito transmits the parasite from infected individuals to new victims. Four species of the protozoan parasites cause human malaria: *Plasmodium vivax*, *Plasmodium falciparum*, *Plasmodium malariae*, and *Plasmodium ovale*. All forms of malaria may have serious consequences, but *P. falciparum* (malignant tertian malaria) is particularly dangerous. Other members of the genus *Plasmodium* are parasites of various species of birds, reptiles, amphibians, and mammals.

Because anopheline mosquitoes prefer to lay their eggs in stagnant waters, malaria typically becomes endemic in marshy areas. The ancient Greeks and Romans noted the connection between malaria and marshes, but the basis of this relationship was not discovered until the end of the nineteenth century. During the first half of the twentiethth century, the conquest of malaria seemed to be a real possibility, but the optimism raised by the anti-malaria campaigns of the 1950s and 1960s ended in the 1970s as the resurgence of malaria became obvious. By the 1980s, the hope that malaria could be eradicated by pesticides and drugs had been abandoned. The increasing prevalence of pesticide-resistant mosquitoes and drug-resistant malarial parasites was only part of the problem; socioeconomic and geopolitical issues were even more significant. Although the global campaign to eradicate malaria that was launched in 1955 has been called a misguided failure, it did provide valuable lessons. Public health workers realized that even though global eradication of malaria was not a realistic goal, sustained control was essential to economic development in areas where the disease remained endemic.

Malaria has continued to flourish because global recessions, large-scale population migrations, political upheavals, and warfare militated against the high levels of financial and administrative support, sophisticated organizational infrastructure, and international cooperation needed to sustain anti-malarial campaigns. To reverse this dismal trend, the World Health Organization established special programs to support research on malaria, schistosomiasis, trypanosomiasis, leishmaniasis, filariasis, and leprosy in areas where these diseases were still endemic. Many anti-malaria initiatives were launched in the 1990s, including Roll Back Malaria (RBM), funded by a consortium of the WHO, World Bank, United Nations Development Program, and United Nations Children's Fund.

Because of advances in molecular biology culminating at the end of the twentiethth century, parasitology—once known as tropical medicine—became an attractive and challenging area of biomedical research. Basic research on the biology and immunology of malaria raised hopes for the development of anti-malaria vaccines. Certainly, Sydenham would pronounce such "mission oriented" therapeutic research both good and useful, but he might disparage the hyperbole surrounding the sequencing of the genome of the parasite and the mosquito as too far removed from the needs of patients. Many public health experts would agree with him and object to diverting funds from practical efforts to control malaria into projects that have been called the Star Wars approach to infectious disease. Decoding the genome of *Plasmodium falciparum*, the most dangerous of the four strains of malaria parasites, took six years. The genome of *Anopheles gambiae*, the primary vector of the parasite, took about 15 months. In 2002, the genome sequence of *A. gambiae* was published in *Science*; the genome sequence of *P. falciparum* was published in *Nature*. Understanding the genetic make-up of both the mosquito and the plasmodium might, however, facilitate the development of new drugs, insect repellents, and mosquito traps.

Advances in the techniques of molecular biology provided sophisticated insights into the machinations of the malaria plasmodium, but the most intractable obstacles to the development of a malaria vaccine have generally been economic and geopolitical factors. Disputes between the WHO and the biotechnology companies that have the technical competence to manufacture novel vaccines reflect the central problem in tropical medicine: the tension between the poorest nations, which need remedies and vaccines for malaria and other infectious diseases, but lack the resources to produce them, and the developed nations, which could develop such medicines, but do not need them. Given the role malaria has played in history, it would be ironic indeed if the question of whether or not it is possible to develop a malaria vaccine is subverted by the problem of whether it is politically or economically expedient to do so.

## THE EIGHTEENTH-CENTURY FOUNDATIONS OF MODERN MEDICINE

The eighteenth century has been aptly described as the adolescence of modern medicine, the era in which the foundations of scientific medicine were first established. During this period, the ideas of the philosophical movement known as the Enlightenment inspired the search for rational systems of medicine, practical means of preventing disease, improving the human condition, and disseminating the new learning to the greatest number of people possible. Although historians continue to argue about the definition, meaning, and even the existence of a specific era popularly known as the Enlightenment, there is general agreement that Enlightenment thought may be interpreted as the optimistic belief that human beings have the capacity to subject all inherited beliefs to rational analysis and open debate. The eighteenth century boasts a prodigious who's who of physicians and scientists, easy to list, but impossible to discuss in the detail they deserve. A few of the leading lights of clinical medicine will have to serve as exemplars of this era.

Just as Thomas Sydenham is honored for following Hippocrates in his emphasis on patient care and epidemiological observations, Hermann Boerhaave (1668–1738) is remembered for his role in revitalizing the teaching of clinical medicine. Teacher, writer, and chemist, Boerhaave was probably the most influential physician of the eighteenth century. His contemporaries thought of him as the "Newton of Medicine." Speaking of his own sources of inspiration, Boerhaave emphasized the work of Hippocrates, Francis Bacon, and Thomas Sydenham. It was said that, in deference to the "English Hippocrates," Boerhaave tipped his hat every time Sydenham's name was mentioned. As a student, Boerhaave immersed himself in botany, chemistry, philosophy, and languages. Although, like Sydenham, he suffered the torments of gout, Boerhaave possessed boundless energy as well as erudition, as demonstrated by his simultaneous commitment to professorships in botany, chemistry, medical theory, and clinical medicine at Leiden.

By establishing a hospital especially for teaching purposes, Boerhaave was able to combine theoretical and practical instruction at the patient's bedside. Bedside instruction, which remedied one of the greatest deficiencies of academic medicine, made Leiden a major center of medical education—at least until Boerhaave's disciples succeeded in bringing clinical instruction to other schools. Bedside medicine prepared the way for hospital medicine, which developed during the last years of the eighteenth century and flourished in the nineteenth century.

No major biomedical discovery can be attributed to Boerhaave, but medical students were taught to think of his system as "perfect, complete, and sufficient," and powerful enough to fill the void created by the demise of Galenism. Those who dared to differ from the great Boerhaave were denounced as medical heretics. Through lectures faithfully recorded by his disciples, Boerhaave became teacher to the world. The books that expressed Boerhaave's ideas, *Institutiones medicae* (1708), *Book of Aphorisms* (1709), *Index plantarum* (1710), and *Elementia chemiae* (1732), remained in use for almost one hundred years. Boerhaave taught his followers that the study of human health and disease must be based on anatomy and physiology, chemistry and physics. Unfortunately, like Galenism, Boerhaave's beautifully crafted system so thoroughly satisfied his contemporaries that it tended to stifle curiosity and innovation.

The great virtue, and ultimately the equally great flaw, of Boerhaave's system was the way he integrated classification and natural science with considerations of the nature, causes, and treatment of disease. For example, eighteenth-century physiologists regarded the study of the chemistry of digestion as part of a deep philosophical argument about life. If one could understand how the dead matter of plant and animal foods could nourish living tissue, one would discover the secret of life. According to Boerhaave, if the digestive processes were inadequate, various foods gave rise to acids. Since acids were supposedly foreign to bodily humors, the resultant state of *acid acrimony* would produce disorders of the intestinal tract, which then affected the blood, milk, skin, and brain. Obviously, such disorders should be treated with *anti-acids* such as meat, fish, leafy vegetables, and alkaline powders.

The chemistry of Boerhaave's medical system is intriguing, but often confusing, because terms that seem familiar to modern chemists meant something quite different within an eighteenth century context. For example, *earth* signified an inert material that could not be liquefied by fire or dissolved in water. A *salt* was a substance that dissolved in water and was liquefied by fire. *Sulfur* and *oil* were substances that melted and burned, but did not mix with water. Eventually, the deficiencies and failures of eighteenth-century medical systems became all too apparent. New discoveries and unlovely facts forced nineteenth-century physicians to confine themselves to formulating more modest and limited explanatory frameworks.

The eighteenth century is also notable for the work of Giovanni Battista Morgagni (1682–1771), author of *De sedibus et causis morborum* (*On the Seat and Cause of Disease*, 1761) a five-volume landmark in the evolution of pathological anatomy. After studying medicine in Bologna, Morgagni became Professor of Theoretical Medicine and Anatomy at the University of Padua. Like his predecessor, Andreas Vesalius, Morgagni brought great glory to the University through his anatomical research. Morgagni's attempt to find correlations between clinical symptoms and postmortem findings was based on over six hundred dissections. Careful observations of the appearance and course of various diseases were essential to Morgagni's research program, as were dissections and experiments on various animals as a means of understanding clinical patterns of disease in humans.

Convinced that normal human anatomy had been well established, Morgagni focused his considerable energies on exploring the origin and seat of diseases that caused pathological changes demonstrable in the cadaver. His meticulous observations and case histories were carefully arranged and published when he was 80 years old. After summarizing each case history, Morgagni attempted to correlate observations of the course of illness with his findings at autopsy. Autopsies sometimes revealed errors in diagnosis and treatment that contributed to, or caused, the death of the patient. In one case, the attending physician had diagnosed a stomach complaint, but the postmortem revealed that the patient had a normal stomach and diseased kidneys.

Autopsies sometimes revealed sad and bizarre behaviors. For example, in discussing findings related to the suppression of urine, Morgagni noted several cases where girls had damaged the bladder by introducing needles or pins into the urethra. Some girls claimed to have swallowed these items, but others tried to conceal their injuries, even if it meant death. Similarly, at autopsy Morgagni discovered that some males had died with needles in their urinary organs. Morgagni boasted that he had dissected more male urethras than any other anatomist, but he complained that he had not found as many cases of damage to the urethra due to gonorrhea as he had expected. He was unsuccessful in discovering the seat of gonorrhea in males and females, but dissections did prove that over the course of many years the disease insidiously made its way throughout the body.

In compiling case studies, the morbid anatomist needed a healthy dose of skepticism. Colleagues offered Morgagni reports of bizarre hungers brought on by lice growing in the stomach and worms in the appendix. He was quite suspicious of the first report, but thought that the second seemed plausible. In discussing various kinds of fluxes (diarrheas) he urged his readers to be suspicious when evaluating reports of the ingestion or excretion of frogs, toads, lizards, and so forth. The anatomist should examine the physical evidence and determine what kind of bodily parts and products were actually involved.

Morgagni is regarded as a pioneer of morbid anatomy and a guide to a new epoch in medical science. Even though Morgagni remained essentially a humoralist, his work may be seen as part of the transition from general humoral pathology towards the study of localized lesions and diseased organs. By encouraging physicians to think of disease in terms of localized pathological changes rather than disorders of the humors, Morgagni's work brought about a new attitude towards specific diagnostic and surgical interventions. He was the first person to attempt a systematic examination of the connection between the symptoms of disease in the living body and post-mortem results revealed only to the dedicated investigator. His work helped to establish an anatomical orientation in pathology and the recognition that unseen anatomical changes within the body were reflected in the clinical picture. Confirmation could be found only in the autopsy room, but recognition of the relationship encouraged interest in finding ways of *anatomizing* the living—that is, detecting hidden anatomical lesions in living patients. This goal would be realized in Leopold Auenbrugger's (1722–1809) studies of chest percussion, René Théophile Hyacinthe Laënnec's (1781–1826) invention of the stethoscope, and the remarkable rise of medical instrumentation that followed.

## ENLIGHTENMENT PHILOSOPHY AND MEDICAL REFORM

Although elaborate systems fascinated many eighteenth-century physicians, this period also produced pragmatic reformers who realized that one could not heal sailors and soldiers or peasants and workers with learned speculations. Social and medical reformers, inspired by the Enlightenment belief that it was possible to improve the human condition through the application of reason to social problems, turned their attention to public health and preventive medicine. In the eighteenth century, to an unprecedented extent, the ship, the army barrack, the factory, the prison, the hospital, and the boarding school were closed worlds in which unrelated people were confined, sharing unhygienic conditions, unhealthy diets, polluted air, and communicable diseases.

Reformers and philanthropists argued that scientific investigations of the abominable conditions of cities, navies, armies, prisons, lunatic asylums, and hospitals could improve the health and prosperity of society as a whole. Sometimes this battle was led by medical men familiar with specific constituencies, such as Sir John Pringle, surgeon general of the British armies, or James Lind, Charles Blane, and Thomas Trotter, pioneers of naval medicine and hygiene. The English philanthropist John Howard called for the reform of prisons, while French physician Philippe Pinel attempted to reform the abysmal conditions in mental asylums.

The goals and ideals, as well as the sometimes authoritarian methods that characterized the developing field of public health medicine, are reflected in the work of Johann Peter Frank (1745–1821), a pioneer of what is now called social medicine. His philosophy was encapsulated in his 1790 oration, "The People's Misery—Mother of Diseases," and expounded in great detail in the six volumes of his *System of Complete Medical Police* (1777–1817). This monumental work was a widely known and influential exposition of the social relations between health and disease. Weaving together the noblest ideals of Enlightenment thought, enlightened absolutism, and pragmatic public health goals, Frank devoted his life to teaching Europe's monarchs that the people constitute the state's greatest wealth and that it was in the state's best interest to see that its subjects should be "as numerous, healthy, and productive as possible." Human resources could best be maintained through "rational hygienic measures" by combining the power of the state with the knowledge of the physician. For the welfare of the people, the physician must be responsible for the two branches of state medicine: forensic medicine and the medical police who enforced the dictates of the state.

Even as a student, Frank felt himself driven by a profound inner restlessness. He attended various universities in France and Germany before he obtained his medical degree from Heidelberg in 1766. When Frank became personal physician to the Prince-Bishop of Speyer, he began to test his ideas about a new social medicine by studying the conditions of the serfs and determining how the government could affect the health of its subjects. Among other things, Frank established a school to train midwives, hospitals to serve the poor, and a school for surgeons.

In 1779, Frank published the first volume of his *Medical Police*. Subjects covered included marriage, fertility, and childbearing. The next two volumes dealt with sexual intercourse, prostitution, venereal diseases, abortion, foundling hospitals, nutrition, clothing, and housing. Although these books made Frank famous, they did not please the Prince-Bishop. A position in the service of Emperor Joseph II provided better conditions for Frank's studies of medical practitioners and institutions, public health measures, and the condition of working people and peasants.

By the second half of the twentiethth century, the population explosion was generally recognized as a major threat to global economic and social welfare, but Frank was most concerned with the opposite problem. *Medical Police* reflects the economic and political concerns of the rulers of Austria, Prussia, France, and Spain, who were convinced that they needed more people for their armies, industries, and farms. The so-called enlightened despot and his physicians understood that people could only be productive if they were healthy and able-bodied; in other words, the welfare of the people was the welfare of the state. No detail was, therefore, too small to escape Frank's attention if it might conceivably affect the future fertility of the people.

Medical police would be authorized to supervise parties, outlaw unhealthy dances like the waltz, enforce periods of rest, and forbid the use of corsets or other fashionable articles of clothing that might constrict or distort the bodies of young women and jeopardize childbearing. If Frank's concept of medical police seems harsh, his definition of the qualities of the true physician reflects his heartfelt belief that the most important qualities of the physician were the love of humanity and the desire to alleviate suffering and provide consolation where there was no cure. Concerned that people might make mistakes in determining when death had occurred, Frank provided advice about resuscitation and rescue, dealing with accidents, and the appointment of specialized rescue workers.

By studying the lives of peasants and workers, Frank hoped to make physicians and philosophers see how diseases were generated by a social system that kept whole classes of people in conditions of permanent misery. Eighteenth-century social classes, as Frank knew them, consisted of the nobility, bourgeoisie, and paupers. The great majority of all people fell into the last category. Convinced that one of the worst aspects of the feudal system was the harsh conditions imposed upon peasant women and children, Frank argued that all pregnant women needed care and kindness in order to successfully carry out their duty to the state, which was to produce healthy new workers. Reports of the accidents that maimed and killed children left alone while their mothers worked in the fields prove that the past was not a golden age of prefeminist family life. Babies cried themselves almost to death with fear, hunger, thirst, and filth. Sometimes pigs or dogs got into the house and attacked infants; sometimes small children wandered away from home and died by falling into wells, dung pits, or puddles of liquid manure.

Other aspects of medicine and its place in eighteenth-century society are reflected in the changing pattern of medical professionalization in Europe. France, for example, entered the eighteenth century with a medical system dominated by learned physicians steeped in traditional Hippocratic doctrines. Endless academic debates about abstract medical philosophies obscured a broad range of therapeutic practices, as well as the work of unorthodox and unlicensed healers. By the end of the century, however, French medicine had been transformed by two very powerful catalysts: revolution and war. Ignorant of medical philosophy, military men were known to say that many lives could be saved by hanging the first doctor found bleeding the wounded with his right hand and purging them with the left. Promoting the ideology of equality, revolutionary leaders denounced academic medicine as the embodiment of all the worst aspects of the Old Regime, from favoritism and monopoly to neglect and ignorance. Ironically, the revolutionary movement that intended to eradicate doctors, hospitals, and medical institutions generated a new public health policy, better trained doctors, new medical schools, and hospitals that offered unprecedented opportunities for clinical experimentation, autopsies, and statistical studies. Hospital reform was especially difficult, costly, and painful, but the revolutionary era established the hospital as the primary locus of sophisticated medical treatment, teaching, and research.

## NUTRITION, MALNUTRITION, HEALTH, AND DISEASE

Although nutrition is generally regarded as a twentieth-century science, the belief that health and longevity depend on regulating the consumption of food and drink is one of the most ancient and universal principles of medical theory. Foods were generally classified in terms of opposing qualities such as hot or cold, moist or dry, which determined whether particular foods would be strengthening, weakening, purgative, or constipating. These concepts were not seriously challenged until well into the eighteenth century, when new chemical theories sparked an interest in the *acidity* or *alkalinity* of foods. By the end of the nineteenth century, these chemical distinctions were giving way to a new physiological concept of the role of food substances in the animal economy. Since that time, nutrition scientists have lamented that the development of their field has been hampered, not by neglect, but by enormous amounts of misinformation, generated, at least in part, by its uniquely popular appeal. Critics of the modern food industry see diet as a political issue, especially in societies where food deficiencies have been replaced with the problems of excess and confusion about rational dietary guidelines.

The modern science of nutrition grew out of efforts to understand and isolate the dietary factors promoting health and preventing disease. Finding the causes of vitamin deficiency diseases was no simpler than unraveling the etiology of infectious diseases. Indeed, both kinds of disorders often seemed to occur in the form of devastating plagues and pestilences. Despite the accumulation of empirical evidence about the relationship between diet and disease, scientists could not unequivocally establish the existence of putative micronutrients without substantial progress in chemistry. Nevertheless, naval surgeon James Lind (1716–1794) and other pioneers of nutritional science proved it was possible to prevent certain diseases by specific changes in diet. Although there are many vitamin deficiency diseases, scurvy is of special interest because the experimental foundations of our understanding of this disease are part of the abiding legacy of the eighteenth century.

Scurvy may be among the most ancient and ubiquitous pestilences, tormenting its victims with rotting of the gums and teeth, deep aches and pains, blackening of the skin, and an overwhelming lassitude. Seeing whole families, monasteries, or armies afflicted with scurvy, ancient writers variously concluded that the disease was contagious, congenital, inherited, transmitted by scorbutic nurses, or generated by malign combinations of diet and atmosphere. Hermann Boerhaave, for example, considered scurvy a very infectious poison.

As sailing ships replaced oared galleys and long ocean voyages became possible, the old army sickness became known as the sailors' disease. Nostalgic visions of graceful tall ships notwithstanding, these sailing vessels were more accurately called floating hells. The common sailor could expect accommodations that were dirty, damp, vermin-infested, and a moldy, monotonous diet of salt pork, indigestible oatmeal, and ship's biscuits. Lord George Anson, to whom James Lind dedicated his *Treatise on Scurvy*, lost more than half of his men to scurvy during his voyage of circumnavigation in 1741. Deaths of sailors were so common that they were hardly worth noting. As long as one in five ships returned with a cargo of spices, the sponsors of an expedition could make a good profit. Between 1500 and 1800, scurvy killed more sailors than all other diseases and disasters combined. Thus, it is not surprising that naval surgeons were among the first to provide good clinical descriptions of the disease and remedies to prevent and cure it.

Before obtaining his M.D. at the University of Edinburgh in 1748, James Lind served as ship's surgeon on voyages to the West Indies, Guinea, and the Mediterranean. In 1758, Lind was appointed Senior Physician to Haslar Hospital, where he saw hundreds of scorbutic patients. Lind's lesser known contributions to medicine include observations on tropical medicine, a distillation apparatus for making safe drinking water, and a remedy composed of quinine, spirits, and citrus peel that sounds like the quintessential summer restorative, the gin and tonic. A practical man, proud of his experience, but well read and thoughtful, Lind was ready to take exception to the most learned physicians of his day. While his contemporaries deferred to scholars like Hermann Boerhaave, Lind was not equally impressed. After reviewing scholarly writings on scurvy, Lind insisted that theories must stand or fall according to the test of experience.

Clearly, Lind saw himself as more original and less gullible than Boerhaave and his disciples, including one who published a book in which scurvy was attributed to sin and the Devil. Scholars who attributed scurvy to a "very infectious poison" could not explain why no officers contracted the disease when it raged with remarkable virulence among common soldiers. Learned physicians felt obliged to ground their ideas about scurvy in theoretical rationalizations derived from classical authors. For the scholar, remedies were only of interest if theory rationalized their action. Similarly, if an idea was theoretically sound, no empirical tests were necessary. For example, according to Boerhaave, the blood serum of patients with scurvy was too thin and acrid, while the material that made up the portion that clotted was too thick and viscid. It was, therefore, the physician's delicate task to thicken and neutralize the acridity of the serum while simultaneously thinning the clot-forming portion of the blood.

Although scurvy took many forms, its characteristic signs were putrid, bleeding gums and blue-black spots on the body. Generally, the first signs of the disease were pale and bloated complexion, listlessness, and fatigue. Eventually, internal hemorrhages caused weakness, lethargy, stiffness and weakness of the knees, swelling of the ankles and legs, chronic sores, putrid ulcers, and breathlessness following any exertion. Advanced cases were marked by coughing and pains in the bones, joints, and chest. Profuse hemorrhages and violent dysenteries reduced the patient to extreme weakness. Sudden death might occur in patients suffering from the breakdown of previously healed ulcers, chest pains, and difficult respiration.

During two cruises of 10 and 11 weeks in 1746 and 1747, scurvy attacked the British frigate *Salisbury* with great virulence after only 4 weeks at sea. Although the captain generously provided the sick with fresh provisions, including mutton broth and meat from his own table, 80 of the 350 crewmen suffered from scurvy. Generally, the sailor's diet consisted of putrid beef, rancid pork, moldy biscuits, and bad water. Probably only a liberal allowance of beer, brandy, and rum could make such food palatable. While greens, fresh vegetables, and ripe fruits were regarded as preservatives against scurvy, Lind could not tell whether these foods were needed to counteract the bad effects of the moist sea air, or to correct the quality of hard, dry ship's rations. One hundred years previously, John Woodall (1570–1643), author of *The Surgeon's Mate, or Military and Domestic Medicine* (1636), had called attention to the antiscorbutic virtues of lemon juice. Woodall's observations were interesting, but essentially anecdotal. It was Lind's special genius to test possible antiscorbutics with a controlled dietary experiment.

A group of scorbutic sailors were put on a diet of gruel, mutton broth, puddings, boiled biscuits, barley, raisins, rice, currants, and wine. In addition to this basic diet, two of the men were given a quart of cider a day; two were given *elixir vitriol* (sulfuric acid diluted with water and alcohol); two received rations of vinegar; two were given sea water; two received a combination of garlic, mustard seed, balsam of Peru, gum myrrh, and barley water, well acidulated with tamarinds and cream of tartar; two others were given two oranges and one lemon per day. Within six days one of the sailors given oranges and lemons was fit for duty and the other was strong enough to serve as a nurse. Lind's experiment not only demonstrated that oranges and lemons cured scurvy, it also showed that it was possible to test and compare alleged remedies.

Proving that lemons and oranges cured scurvy was easier than convincing the authorities to utilize the information. There was no scientific obstacle to the eradication of sea scurvy, but it was essentially impossible for a naval surgeon to force his so-called superiors to abandon entrenched opinions, sanctioned by "time, custom, and great authorities." The British Admiralty did not adopt Lind's remedy until 1795, when it proposed that lemon juice should be provided *after* six weeks on standard rations. The British Board of Trade did not require rations of lime juice in the merchant marine until 1865. Lemons did not become part of standard rations in the American Navy until 1812. Even without official blessings, some naval surgeons included a form of lemonade in their medical kit, but supplies of antiscorbutics were generally inadequate and unreliable. Army doctors ignored or rejected Lind's work and argued that a great many factors, especially a history of "evil habits," along with fatigue, depression, and bad food, could cause scurvy.

Apathy and ignorance only partially explain the failure of the medical community to call for the universal adoption of Lind's remedy. Although naval surgeons and sailors were well acquainted with the natural history of scurvy, confusion about the nature of the disease persisted into the twentieth century. Moreover, experience seemed to prove that scurvy had no single cause or cure. One argument against the dietary deprivation theory of scurvy was the observation that cooks were often the first to die of the disease. A certain degree of skepticism is certainly valid in the face of any claim for a cure too wonderful and too simple to be true. Indeed, marvelous health-giving fruits seemed more at home in a utopian fantasy such as Francis Bacon's (1561–1626) *New Atlantis*, than in a medical treatise. In Bacon's allegory, a wonderful fruit that resembled an orange cured the sickly crew members of a lost British ship that landed in the mythical New Atlantis.

Physicians had heard of many equally miraculous antiscorbutics touted by sailors and explorers. For example, when Jacques Cartier's expedition in search of a northern route through North America was trapped by the ice during the winter in 1536, his crew was attacked by scurvy. Native Americans showed the French how to make a remedy from the bark and leaves of a certain tree. At first, most of the sick refused to try the Indian remedy, but when those who tried it recovered it was soon in great demand. The French had to admit that all the learned doctors of France could not have restored their health and strength as successfully and rapidly as the Indian remedy. Other sailors and doctors ascribed antiscorbutic virtues to high morale, good food, water distilled over powdered scurvy grass, cleanliness, dry clothing, wholesome exercise, sour oranges and lemons, oil of vitriol, and periodic access to fresh country air. Many sailors believed that all complex medical approaches were useless. Instead of medicines, they insisted that being buried in the earth up to the neck cured scurvy.

One of the most distinguished and influential of all naval physicians, Sir Gilbert Blane (1749–1834), Physician of the Fleet, and personal physician to Lord Rodney, Commander-in-Chief, was able to implement reforms that naval surgeons had long desired. Sir Gilbert earned the nickname "Chilblain" because his concern for the welfare of the common sailor was so well hidden by his icy demeanor. Throughout history, it had been taken for granted that armies would lose more men by sickness than by the sword, but in the eighteenth century new approaches to vital statistics provided disconcerting evidence of the human and economic toll. As physician to the Fleet, Blane received a monthly report of the prevalence of diseases, mortality, and other matters related to health from every naval surgeon. In order to improve the condition of Britain's sailors, Blane used these reports to prepare his first treatise on naval hygiene. Later, in his *Observations on the Diseases of Seamen*, Blane advised the authorities that preserving the health of seamen was not only a matter of basic humanity, but also a form of enlightened self-interest spurred by economic and political necessity. As warfare and economic ventures required ever-greater numbers of sailors and soldiers, statistical methods proved that the state could not afford to waste its valuable stock of able-bodied men. These common sailors, "the true sinews of war," were essential to the public defense (and offense). As a nation dependent on her navy, Britain had to realize that, even if her officials thought of sailors as a "commodity," economic and political necessities indicated that it was less expensive to maintain life and health than to support invalids and replace the dead.

In 1795, Blane became Commissioner of the Board of the Sick and Wounded Sailors, a position that he used to sponsor many much needed reforms. After 1796, the incidence of sea scurvy declined dramatically. The inexorable logic of numbers demonstrated that, in the years before Blane's reforms were instituted, about 1 of every 7 British sailors died, while many others were permanently disabled. At the beginning of the war in America, 1 in 2.4 men became ill and 1 in 42 died. By the end of the Napoleonic wars, these rates had been reduced to 1 in 10.7 sick and 1 in 143 dead. Blane calculated that if the 1779 mortality rate had not been reduced, Britain's entire stock of seamen would have disappeared long before the defeat of Napoleon.

By 1815, although fevers, pulmonary inflammation, and dysentery continued to plague British sailors, sea scurvy had been nearly eradicated. Whatever expenses had been incurred in provisioning ships with citrus fruits were clearly offset by lower manpower costs. Thomas Trotter (1760–1832), another Physician to the Fleet, continued the battle for the health of sailors. In addition to dietary reform, Trotter recognized the value of inoculation against smallpox and became an early champion of vaccination. Indifferent to scholarly theories about scurvy, Trotter simply argued that fresh citrus fruits provided "*something* to the body" that fortified it against the disease and warned his readers to resist "imaginary facts and fallacious conclusions."

Despite lime rations, sporadic outbreaks of scurvy continued to occur at sea, while army surgeons fatalistically accepted scurvy as one of the pestilences of war, along with typhus, typhoid, and dysentery. Nevertheless, when a British naval expedition returned from the arctic in 1876 with the news that half the 120 men had suffered from scurvy, and 4 had died, the House of Commons called for an inquiry. Similar scandals caused doubt and confusion among scientists as to the nature of scurvy and antiscorbutics.

In the 1870s, physicians were surprised to find scurvy appearing among the children of middle-class families in London's suburbs. Unlike the poor, who relied on potatoes, well-to-do people were likely to feed their children bread and butter and tinned milk (canned, sterilized milk). In this situation we can see how some medical and hygienic advances help solve one problem, but create unforeseen difficulties. Although sterilization of milk helped reduce the problem of infantile diarrheas, as more families switched to tinned milk, infantile scurvy appeared in both rich and poor families. Even today, problems associated with artificial feeding continue to arise and spread throughout the world because the manufacturers of infant formulas promote their products as the modern way to feed the baby. A new class of adult scorbutics was created in the 1960s as Zen macrobiotic diets became more fashionable and more extreme. Some followers of such dietary regimens consumed nothing but brown rice sprinkled with sesame seeds.

Many people living in climates more inhospitable than Europe avoided scurvy through the ingenious use of plant and animal resources. For example, American Indians made teas and tonics from the needles, sap, or bark of appropriate trees, and the indigenous people of Australia used a green plum for medicinal purposes. Cereals, peas, and beans lack antiscorbutic properties in their dry, dormant state, but during their sprouting stage they are good sources of vitamin C. The nutritional value of bean sprouts has long been appreciated in Asia. Although some groups of Eskimos were able to gather berries and others ate the vegetable material found in the rumen of caribou, for the most part, the Eskimo menu was limited to meat and fish. Since vitamin C is present at low levels in animal tissues, it is possible to avoid scurvy by consuming fresh meat and whole fish without the niceties of cleaning and cooking.

Even though physicians generally agreed that the prevalence and severity of scurvy were related to diet, other factors, such as contagion, climate, and physical condition, were considered equally important. For example, Jean Antoine Villemin (1827–1892) attributed scurvy to a contagious miasma, similar to that which caused epidemic typhus. Fresh vegetables and lemons might have some therapeutic value, but, Villemin argued, that did not mean a deficiency of lemons caused scurvy any more than a deficiency of quinine caused malaria. Russian physicians expressed a similar belief as late as World War I, when they suggested that scurvy was an infectious disease spread by lice. A chemical theory of scurvy reminiscent of Boerhaave's was proposed by Sir Almroth Wright (1861–1947), who argued that scurvy was caused by acid intoxication of the blood. Wright insisted that the direct administration of antiscorbutic chemicals, such as sodium lactate, would restore normal alkalinity to blood more efficiently than lime juice.

As scientists attempted to determine the antiscorbutic value of various foods, they found that animal experiments often added to the confusion, because different animal species vary in their vitamin requirements. In 1907, Axel Holst (1860–1931) and Theodor Frölich (1870–1947) discovered an appropriate animal model for the systematic evaluation of antiscorbutics. Holst, Professor of Hygiene and Bacteriology at the University of Christiana, Oslo, had studied bacteriology in France and Germany. He had also visited the laboratory of the Dutch physician and bacteriologist Christiaan Eijkman (1858–1930) in Indonesia to learn about a disease known as beriberi. Searching for a mammalian model for beriberi, Holst tested the guinea pig. When he noted signs of scurvy, he enlisted the assistance of Frölich, a pediatrician concerned with infantile scurvy. Holst and Frölich demonstrated that scurvy in the guinea pig was induced by diet and cured by diet. If Holst had used the rat as his experimental animal, the story would have been quite different. Although some scientists considered the rat the ideal and universal model for deficiency diseases, unlike guinea pigs and primates, rats are not readily susceptible to scurvy.

Beriberi is now known as a nutritional disorder caused by a deficiency of thiamine (vitamin B1). Its symptoms and severity, however, may vary from swelling of the legs, arms, and face, to a gradual loss of sensation that may culminate in paralysis. Eventually, damage to the cardiovascular system and the nerves may lead to severe debility and even death. Although beriberi occurred throughout the world, it was particularly prevalent in Asia. In some Asian nations, beriberi was one of the leading causes of death. The best-known example of the relationship between food preparation methods and beriberi is the milling of rice, which removes the thiamine-containing bran and germ layers. While working in Indonesia, Eijkman realized that chickens could be used as a model experimental system to study this ancient disease. In 1929, Eijkman was awarded the Nobel Prize in Physiology or Medicine for his contributions to the study of vitamin deficiency diseases. Thiamine was chemically characterized and synthesized in the 1930s by Robert R. Williams (1886–1965). His brother, Roger John Williams (1893–1988) isolated two other important B vitamins, pantothenic acid and folic acid. At the University of Texas, Roger Williams founded and directed the Clayton Foundation Biochemical Institute, where many other vitamins were discovered. Williams thought that pantothenic acid might be helpful in the management of rheumatoid arthritis and other diseases.

As early as the eighteenth century, experiments deliberately conducted on human guinea pigs had provided support for Lind's hypothesis. William Stark (1740–1770), who served as his own guinea pig, was probably the first physician to attempt a systematic series of dietary deprivation experiments. Weakened by a diet of bread and water, to which he had added tiny amounts of various oils, bits of cooked meat, and honey, Stark, with gums swollen and purple, consulted the great Sir John Pringle (1707–1782), founder of modern military medicine. Although Pringle had considerable experience with scurvy, instead of recommending fruits or vegetables, he suggested that Stark reduce his salt intake. Less than nine months after beginning his experiments, Stark was dead. Had his eminent colleagues suggested oranges and lemons instead of venesection, Stark might have recovered and demonstrated the value of Lind's dietary experiments.

In 1940, John Crandon, a young American surgeon, served as his own guinea pig in a study of the relationship between vitamin C deficiency and wound healing. Perhaps the most surprising finding in Crandon's experiment was that signs of scurvy did not appear until he had endured about 19 weeks on a restricted diet. In similar experiments conducted in England during World War II, it took several months to provoke signs of scurvy. Presumably, the nutritional status of twentieth-century volunteers was very different from that of the wretched sailors Lind had described. Moreover, Lind believed that exhaustion, hunger, and desperation—factors now subsumed by the term *stress*—predisposed sailors to scurvy.

Although progress in bacteriology and surgery helped reduce the death toll from battlefield injuries during World War I, dysentery and deficiency diseases rendered some military units totally unfit for any kind of action. Indeed, even after the First World War, doctors still considered it possible that certain foods produced scurvy and that others functioned as antidotes. Laboratory experiments and historical research on the antiscorbutics that had been used by the British navy helped explain many paradoxical reports. While it may be true that "a rose is a rose is a rose," we cannot assume that "a lime is a lime is a lime." During the first half of the nineteenth century, the lime juice used by the British navy usually came from Mediterranean sweet limes or Malta lemons. In the 1860s, the Navy began using West Indian sour limes. Scientists eventually discovered that the antiscorbutic potential of this lime was negligible. Using guinea pigs to test antiscorbutic diets, Harriette Chick (1875–1977) and associates at the Lister Institute carefully measured the antiscorbutic quality of various foods. Researchers proved that not all species of lemons and limes were effective as antiscorbutics; moreover, preserved citrus juices were often totally useless. As a result of such studies, during World War II discussions about provisions for the armed forces focused on how to allow a safety margin against scurvy rather than emergency measures to combat epidemic scurvy.

Many researchers were actively pursuing the antiscorbutic factor, but it was the biochemist Albert Szent-Györgyi (1893–1986), who was not actually looking for dietary factors, who discovered it. Although Szent-Györgyi began his career as a doctor, he was more interested in chemistry, histology, physiology, the biochemical mechanism of respiration, and the biological oxidation of carbohydrates. The path that led to Szent-Györgyi's discovery of vitamin C was extremely circuitous. It began with studies of Addison's disease (chronic adrenocortical insufficiency).

In his classic monograph, *The Constitutional and Local Effects of Disease of the Suprarenal Capsules* (1855), Thomas Addison (1793–1860) described the symptoms of this disorder as "anemia, general languor or debility, remarkable feebleness of the heart's action, irritability of the stomach, and a peculiar change of color in the skin." Weakness, nausea, vomiting, anorexia, and abdominal pains usually preceded changes in pigmentation, but bronzing of the skin was often the first symptom to attract attention. Szent-Györgyi associated the darkening of the skin in Addison's disease with the browning of fruits and vegetables like apples and potatoes. Using this rather tenuous connection, he attempted to isolate the mysterious anti-bronzing factor from fruits that did not undergo browning on withering, such as lemons and oranges. In 1927, Szent-Györgyi isolated a novel substance that he planned to call "ignose," meaning, "I don't know," because it could not be chemically identified. When editors refused to publish a paper about ignose, Szent-Györgyi suggested "godnose," but he finally had to settle for "hexuronic acid." Nutritional experiments conducted in collaboration with the American biochemist Joseph L. Svirbely in 1931 demonstrated that hexuronic acid was vitamin C. In keeping with its nutritional role in the prevention of scurvy, hexuronic acid was renamed ascorbic acid. Szent-Györgyi was awarded the 1937 Nobel Prize in Medicine or Physiology for his work on biological oxidation reactions and vitamin C.

Ascorbic acid plays an essential role in the final stages of the synthesis of collagen, a protein that serves as a kind of intercellular cement and plays a major structural role in connective tissue. The role of vitamin C in preventing scurvy was, therefore, clearly established, but the activities ascribed to this vitamin and the appropriate daily dosage for human beings remain controversial. The mystique of vitamin C has continued to evolve since the 1960s, when Irwin Stone, an industrial chemist, made the claim that primates suffer from an inborn error of metabolism that could be corrected by consuming large amounts of vitamin C. Megavitamin therapy, also known as orthomolecular medicine, acquired some eminent spokesmen, such as Roger Williams, the discoverer of pantothenic acid, and the ingenious chemist and two-time Nobel Laureate, Linus Pauling. Vitamin C enthusiasts claimed that the vitamin has antiviral and antibacterial activity, lowers blood cholesterol, cures the common cold, and increases mental alertness, intelligence, and general well being. Predictably, as AIDS hysteria mounted, reports appeared in newspapers and magazines about victims of AIDS who had been cured by megadoses of vitamin C. Expensive vitamin preparations called HIM (Health and Immunity for Men) were marketed to the "sexually active male" as a means of maximizing the ability of the immune system to fight infections, while allowing the body to maintain "sexual vitality and potency."

With so many self-proclaimed authorities promoting megadose vitamin products for mental and physical illness, a hearty dose of skepticism and caution is absolutely necessary. The idea that if a little bit is good, a lot must be better does not fit the facts about vitamins. In large doses, some vitamins may be toxic or teratogenic (causing deformity in the fetus). For example, a report released by the Institute of Medicine in 2001 warned that megadoses of vitamin A, such as those sold in health food stores, can cause severe liver disease, as well as birth defects when they are taken by pregnant women, and excessive doses of vitamin E can cause uncontrolled bleeding. Vitamin A is, of course, essential for good vision, immune function, and so forth. In poor countries, vitamin A deficiency is a major cause of blindness. The vitamin is found in meat, fish, eggs, fruits and vegetables (oranges, carrots, spinach), and in vitamin-fortified breakfast cereals. People who believe that raw foods are better sources of vitamins might be surprised to learn that cooking doubles the body's absorption of vitamin A.

In an era of food abundance, dietary and nutritional standards may be more powerfully influenced by political and economic forces than by scientific research. Scientists, nutritionists, and public health experts argue that the food industry has effectively campaigned to confuse the American public and block efforts to provide rational nutritional guidelines. The industry won a major victory in 1994 with the passage of the Dietary Supplement Health and Education Act, which deregulated dietary supplements and exempted such products from FDA oversight. Based largely on economic factors clad in the rhetoric of freedom of choice, the Dietary Supplement Act broadened the definition of supplements to include herbs, diet products, and essentially any product that could be called a dietary supplement. Manufacturers of dietary supplements, "Techno Foods," or nutraceuticals do not have to prove that their products are essential or specifically beneficial to the body. With the completion of the Human Genome Project, some food supplement producers claimed that the new science of nutritional genomics, or nutrigenomics, could provide diets specifically calibrated to an individual's genetic makeup. Potential customers were given kits for the collection of DNA in order to obtain dietary advice and purchase very expensive customized vitamins and supplements. Many scientists expressed skepticism about such claims.

Despite the increased emphasis on nutrition and dietary supplements, specific vitamin deficiency diseases still occur even in wealthy nations. In 2000, physicians were surprised to see an apparent resurgence of nutritional rickets, a disease of infants caused by a deficiency of vitamin D. Without vitamin D, the cartilage of developing bones cannot properly mineralize, but the symptoms of rickets include enlarged heart and organ failure, as well as soft bones and deformed limbs. Physicians and nutritionists generally assumed that rickets had been eradicated, because vitamin D has been added to milk since the 1930s. Moreover, people make their own vitamin D when a precursor molecule in the skin is activated by sunlight. Rickets can, however, occur in infants who have been breastfed and carefully protected from sunlight, in order to prevent skin cancers. Vitamin D deficiency in adults, especially the elderly, can lead to osteomalacia (adult rickets), bone fractures, seizures, or heart failure due to very low blood levels of calcium.

Whether nutritional guidelines are based on clinical observations or laboratory research, the history of scurvy indicates that the well-being of populations is more likely to be affected by the *politics* than the *science* of nutrition. The economic and political aspects of nutrition are most apparent in the frequent rediscovery of the trinity of malnutrition, poverty, and disease. Obviously, in the case of vitamin deficiency diseases, preventive measures were available long before any specific dietary factors were discovered. Advances in the science of nutrition proved that certain diseases, such as scurvy, beriberi, and pellagra, were not due to infectious microbial agents and were not, therefore, a direct threat to those with adequate diets.

During the late nineteenth century, the threat of infectious diseases and the development of germ theory diverted attention from other kinds of diseases. But today, in wealthy, industrialized nations, the growing burden of chronic disorders has overshadowed the threat of infectious disease. By the 1970s, the United States Congressional Office of Technology Assessment was chastising researchers for neglecting dietary links to cancer, stroke, hypertension, diabetes, and dental disorders. Although there is general agreement about the importance of nutrition for good health, physicians and researchers remain cautious when confronted with claims that the diet–disease connection provides an immediate panacea for the heavy burden generated by chronic degenerative diseases in the wealthy industrialized nations.

## SMALLPOX: INOCULATION, VACCINATION, AND ERADICATION

In the case of vitamin deficiency diseases, preventive measures were available long before effective means of control were adopted. A similar case can be made for the prevention of smallpox, a viral disease. At least in theory, smallpox could have been eradicated by the methods available at the beginning of the nineteenth century. But smallpox was not attacked on a global scale until the second half of the twentieth century, when the costs of protecting wealthy nations from the disease exceeded the costs of eliminating the disease from the world's poorest countries.

Variola, the smallpox virus, is a member of the orthopoxvirus family, which includes cowpox, buffalopox, camelpox, swinepox, gerbilpox, and monkeypox. The origin of smallpox is unknown, but epidemiologists suggest that it might have evolved from one of the poxviruses of wild or domesticated animals. Based on the characteristics of the poxviruses and genomic sequencing, virologists have suggested that smallpox and the other poxviruses might have evolved from a common ancestral virus whose natural host was a rodent. Several forms of variola, which differ in virulence, have been characterized. The complete genome of vaccinia, the virus used in vaccines that provide protection against smallpox, was decoded in 1990. Four years later, scientists established the complete genetic code of one of the more virulent strains of variola. Despite the marked differences in virulence of the two viruses, vaccinia and variola are remarkably similar in terms of their DNA sequences.

Unlike most viruses, the smallpox virus is quite stable outside its host and can retain its powers of infectivity over fairly long periods of time. Typically, the disease spreads from person to person by droplet infection; however, the virus may also be transmitted by clothing, blankets, or shrouds contaminated with pus or scabs. After a person is exposed, the virus multiplies rapidly and spreads throughout the body. Following an incubation period of about 14 days, there is a sudden onset of flu-like symptoms, including fever, aches and pains, coughing, sneezing, and fatigue. At this stage an accurate diagnosis is almost impossible, because many illnesses begin with fever, aches, sneezing, nausea, and fatigue. A few days later flat, red vesicles appear, first in the mouth and throat, then on the face, and finally on the arms, legs, palms, and soles. The vesicles turn into pus-filled blisters, which eventually dry out as scabs form, but in some cases the whole body is covered with a bloody rash. Other patients might, according to Sir William Osler, become a "dripping unrecognizable mass of pus," suffering from delirium due to high fever and giving off a putrid, stifling odor. Septic poisoning, broncho-pneumonia, cardiovascular collapse, scars, blindness, and deafness were not uncommon complications, but the worst form of the disease, known as black or hemorrhagic smallpox, was almost always fatal.

Presumably, smallpox smoldered in obscurity for centuries among the innumerable local fevers of Africa or Asia until changing patterns of human migration, warfare, and commerce carried the disease to Persia and Europe, Central Asia, and China. Characteristic scars on the mummy of Ramses V (d. 1157 B.C.E) and the existence of Indian and African deities devoted to smallpox suggest the antiquity of the disease. By the seventeenth century, smallpox was greatly feared in Europe as "the most terrible of all the ministers of death." In his *Essay on Fevers* (1750), John Huxham (1692–1768) noted the great variability in the form and severity of smallpox, even within the same village, household, and family. In some cases the pocks were mild and distinct; in others they were highly malignant and nearly confluent. Moreover, Huxham noted that some people visited the sick in order to acquire the disease at a propitious time, but remained well; then, after congratulating themselves on escaping infection, they contracted the disease from an unknown source months or years later. Even though smallpox is considered highly contagious, it is still all but impossible to predict how many of the people who have been exposed to a person with smallpox—in the sickroom or "downwind" in an airport terminal—will actually become infected.

While mortality rates for smallpox were usually about 15 to 25 percent, during some epidemics 40 percent of those who contracted the disease died. Smallpox, along with diarrhea, worms, and teething, was one of the inevitable crises of childhood; about 30 percent of all English children died of smallpox before reaching their third birthday. No medicine can cure smallpox once the infection is established, but ever since the ninth century, when Rhazes separated smallpox and measles from other eruptive fevers, physicians have added to his ingenious prescriptions. Some physicians recommended opening the vesicles with a golden needle, while others prescribed a dressing of horse or sheep dung for smallpox and goat manure for measles. A few skeptics warned that the physician's ministrations might be more dangerous than the disease.

Unable to afford the services of a physician, peasants in many parts of Europe attempted to protect their children by deliberately exposing them to a person with a mild case in order to "buy the pox" under favorable conditions. (Members of those antediluvian generations that grew up before routine immunization against measles, mumps, and rubella may remember similar attempts to get children to catch these inevitable childhood diseases at a favorable time.) Some folk practices, however, involved methods more daring than passive exposure. Ingrafting or variolation, for example, required taking fresh material from smallpox pustules and inserting it into a cut or scratch on the skin of a healthy person. In China, children were exposed to the "flower-blossom disease" by making them inhale a powder made from the crusts of smallpox scabs. Experience taught folk practitioners in Africa, Asia, India, and Turkey that deliberately exposing patients to a significant risk at a propitious time provided long-term benefits. Learned physicians, in contrast, generally dismissed these practices as barbaric and superstitious. During the eighteenth century, increasing interest in natural curiosities led to closer scrutiny of many ancient folk practices, including inoculation or variolation. (The term inoculation comes from the Latin *inoculare*, to graft; variolation comes from *variola*, the scholarly name for smallpox.)

Credit for transforming the so-called Turkish method of variolation from a curious "heathen custom" into a fashionable practice among the English elite is traditionally ascribed to Lady Mary Wortley Montagu (1689–1762), but some historians argue that the tribute to Lady Mary is more romance than history. Appropriately enough, the story begins with the elopement of Mary Pierrepont and Edward Wortley Montagu. In 1718, Lady Mary accompanied her husband to the Turkish Court at Constantinople, where he served as Ambassador Extraordinary. Among all the curious customs the inquisitive Lady Mary observed in Turkey, the practice of variolation was especially intriguing. In letters to friends in England, Lady Mary described how people wishing to "take the smallpox" arranged to share a house during the cool days of autumn. An inoculator brought a nutshell full of matter from the very best sort of smallpox and inserted some of it into scratches made at appropriate sites. About eight days after the operation, the patients took the fever and stayed in bed for a few days. To demonstrate her faith in the procedure, Lady Mary arranged to have the operation performed on her six-year-old son. Charles Maitland, the ambassador's physician, and Emanuel Timoni (d. 1718), the Embassy surgeon, were present when young Edward was variolated by an old woman with a rather blunt and rusty needle. Timoni had already published an account of the Turkish method of procuring the smallpox in the *Philosophical Transactions of the Royal Society* (1714). A similar report by Giacomo Pylarini (1659–1718) appeared in the same volume of the journal. These descriptions of the practice, published in Latin, were written for physicians, whereas Lady Mary wrote in English for a general audience.

During the smallpox epidemic of 1721, Lady Mary was back in London. When she insisted on inoculating her four-year-old daughter, Maitland demanded that several physicians be present as witnesses. According to Lady Mary, the physicians observing the inoculation were so hostile she was afraid to leave her child alone with them. Nevertheless, after the pox erupted, one of the physicians was so impressed he had Maitland inoculate his only surviving child (all the others had died of smallpox). Clergymen and physicians immediately launched an avalanche of pamphlets and sermons condemning the Turkish method. In a particularly vicious attack, the Reverend Edmund Massey denounced inoculation as a dangerous, atheistic, malicious, and sinful practice invented by the Devil. According to Reverend Massey, diseases were a form of "happy restraint" sent into the world by God to test our faith and punish our sins. God might sometimes give man the power to treat diseases, but the power to inflict them was His own. Reverend Massey feared that members of his flock might be less righteous if they were more healthy and less afraid of smallpox. In response to attacks on ingrafting, Lady Mary published "A Plain Account of the Inoculating of the Small Pox" so that ordinary people who were being "abused and deluded by the knavery and ignorance of physicians" could learn about the methods practiced in Constantinople. Emphasizing the loss of fees that physicians would suffer if smallpox were eliminated, she argued that physicians considered the Turkish method a terrible plot to reduce their income. A funeral monument for Lady Mary in Lichfield Cathedral, erected in 1789, praised her for introducing her country to the beneficial art of smallpox inoculation.

Another advocate of inoculation, the Reverend Cotton Mather (1663–1728), minister to the Second Church of Boston, also became interested in inoculation on learning of its use among "primitive, heathen" people. The indefatigable New England clergyman was the author of about 450 pamphlets and books, a corresponding Fellow of the Royal Society of London, and the victim of a series of personal tragedies, including the deaths of two wives, the insanity of a third wife, and the loss of 13 of his 15 children. John Cotton and Richard Mather, Cotton Mather's grandfathers, and his father, Increase Mather (1639–1723), were prominent spiritual leaders. Increase Mather was also president of Harvard College, from which Cotton earned his baccalaureate when he was 15 and his master's degree three years later. Insatiable curiosity, as well as an obsession with "doing good," drove Mather to seek knowledge of medicine and explanations for the "operations of the invisible world" from unorthodox sources, including Africans, Turks, dreams, and apparitions. In *The Angel of Bethesda*, a medical treatise that was not published until 1972, Mather suggested that the "animated particles" revealed by the microscope might be the cause of smallpox. To maintain a sense of balance, we must also recall Mather's ambiguous role in the Salem witchcraft troubles, and his conviction that while sheep "purles" were medicinal, human excrement was an unparalleled remedy.

By the time John Winthrop's fleet of 17 ships set out for New England in 1630, smallpox had already exerted a profound effect on the peoples of the New World. The Spanish conquistadors had found smallpox a more powerful antipersonnel weapon than gunpowder. Colonists in North America discovered that the impact of smallpox on Europeans was modest in comparison to the devastation it caused among Native Americans. Seventeenth-century settlers referred to the terrible toll smallpox took among the Indians as another example of the "wonder-working providences" by which God made room for His people in the New World.

Of course even Old World stock was not exempt from the threat of smallpox. When the disease struck Boston, a city of about 12,000 inhabitants, in 1721, prayers, fast days, quarantines, and travel bans failed to halt the epidemic. Almost half the people of Boston contracted smallpox; of those who were infected about one in seven died. During this outbreak, Mather initiated the test of inoculation he had been planning since he had learned of the practice. Reverend Mather first heard about inoculation from a young African slave given to him by members of his congregation; Mather named the young man Onesimus. When Mather asked Onesimus if he had ever had smallpox, the young man showed him a scar on his arm and explained that in Africa people deliberately exposed themselves to a mild form of smallpox in order to avoid the more dangerous natural form. Therefore, when Mather read Timoni's account of inoculation in the *Philosophical Transactions of the Royal Society*, he immediately accepted it as confirmation of what he had previously learned from Onesimus. Mather was convinced that he could rid the New World colonies of smallpox if only he could secure the cooperation of the doctors. When smallpox appeared in 1721, Mather sent out letters to Boston's doctors asking them to hold a consultation concerning inoculation.

Imbued with a firm sense of ministerial privilege, duty, and authority, Mather saw no impropriety in offering advice to townspeople and medical men, but many New Englanders resented his interference. The most dramatic statement of displeasure consisted of a granado (fire bomb) thrown through the pastor's window. By the Providence of God the device failed to explode, allowing Mather to read the attached note: "COTTON MATHER, You Dog, Dam you, I'll inoculate you with this, with a Pox to you." Many proper Bostonians agreed with the sentiments expressed by the mad bomber and rejected Mather's bizarre ideas about smallpox, whether they came from African slaves, heathen Turks, or the Royal Society.

Of all the physicians Mather appealed to, only Zabdiel Boylston (1680–1766), a practitioner whose medical training consisted of a local apprenticeship, was willing to test the efficacy of inoculation. On June 26, 1721, Boylston tried the experiment on his own 6-year-old son, a 2-year-old boy, and a 36-year-old slave. The operation was successful. After performing more than two hundred inoculations, Boylston concluded that variolation was the most beneficial and effective medical innovation ever discovered. Nevertheless, as word of these experiments spread, Boston became a true "hell on earth" for Mather and Boylston. Bostonians were shocked and alarmed by these unprecedented experiments; physicians denounced Mather and Boylston for imposing a dangerous and untried procedure on the community. Boston officials prohibited further inoculations.

Some ministers denounced inoculation as a challenge to God's plan, an invitation to vice and immorality, and an attempt to substitute human inventions for Divine guidance. But other ministers agreed with Mather and became truly zealous advocates of inoculation. The Reverend Benjamin Colman called inoculation "an astonishing mercy." In response to Massey's attack on inoculation, the Reverend William Cooper said: "Let us use the light God has given us and thank him for it." In contrast, William Douglass (1691–1752), one of Boston's most prominent and best-educated physicians, denounced inoculators for promoting "abuses and scandals." Douglass was the only university-trained physician in Boston, a graduate of Edinburgh's medical school. Sounding more like a theologian than a physician, Douglass proclaimed it a sin to deliberately infect healthy people with a dangerous disease, which they might not have contracted otherwise. How was it possible, Douglass asked, for clergymen to reconcile inoculation with their doctrine of predestination? Nevertheless, by 1730 Douglass reconsidered this "strange and suspect practice" and became an advocate of inoculation.

Reflecting on the turmoil caused by inoculation, Mather asked the people of New England to think about the many lives that might have been saved if physicians had not "poisoned and bewitched" them against the procedure. Although Mather admitted that some people died after inoculation, he reminded his critics that some people died after having a tooth pulled, while others casually risked their lives by dosing themselves with emetics and cathartics, or by smoking tobacco. As the epidemic died down, the fear and hostility aroused by the inoculation experiments also ebbed away. People began to ask whether inoculation really worked and whether it was less dangerous than smallpox contracted in the natural way.

Boylston's meticulous records, published in 1726 under the title *An Historical Account of the Small-Pox Inoculated in New England*, provided statistical evidence of the relative safety of inoculation. During the epidemic of 1721, 844 people died of smallpox. Based on the population of Boston at the time, the mortality rate for naturally acquired smallpox during this epidemic was about 14 percent. Out of 274 inoculated individuals, only 6 died of smallpox. The case fatality rate of 2.2 percent for the inoculated group was substantially lower than the case fatality rate in the general population of Boston. Of course, such crude calculations do not take into account many important complications, such as the problem of assessing the risk of acquiring smallpox naturally, or the possibility that some of those who were inoculated might have already contracted the disease. Today a vaccine with a two percent fatality rate would be unacceptable, but when compared to naturally acquired smallpox, the benefits of inoculation clearly exceeded the risk.

Inoculation had important ramifications for medical practitioners and public health officials willing to accept the responsibilities inherent in this unprecedented promise of control over epidemic disease. As Benjamin Franklin so poignantly explained, weighing the risks and benefits of inoculation became an awesome responsibility for parents. In 1736, Franklin printed a notice in the *Pennsylvania Gazette* denying rumors that his four-year-old son Francis had recently died of inoculated smallpox. Franklin was afraid that the false reports would keep other parents from protecting their children. The child acquired natural smallpox while suffering from a "flux" that had forced Franklin to postpone the operation. In his *Autobiography*, Franklin reflected on the bitter regrets he still harbored about failing to protect Francis from smallpox. Knowing that some parents refused to inoculate their children because of fear that they would never forgive themselves if a child died after the operation, he urged them to consider that uninoculated children faced the greater risk of naturally acquired smallpox.

As epidemics of smallpox continued to plague New England communities, the isolation and recovery period required for safe inoculation tended to limit the practice to wealthy families. An inoculated person with a mild case of smallpox was obviously a danger to others; inoculated smallpox was contagious. Indeed, during the Revolutionary War, the British were accused of conducting "germ warfare" by inoculating agents and sending them about the country to spread the infection. Washington initially hoped that isolation and quarantine would prevent the dissemination of smallpox among his troops, but he knew that members of the British army were routinely protected against the disease by inoculation. With smallpox a constant threat to the army, General George Washington ordered secret mass inoculations of American soldiers in order to maintain an effective military force. Through such measures, smallpox gradually ceased to be "the terror of America."

Perhaps the greatest medical accomplishment of the Age of Enlightenment was recognition of the possibility of preventing epidemic smallpox. In England, members of the Royal Society shared an interest in curious folk customs from around the world and their journal provided a vehicle for the dissemination of much curious information. Emanuel Timoni's "Account, or history, of the procuring of the smallpox by incision, or inoculation, as it has for some time been practised at Constantinople," published in the Society's *Philosophical Transactions* in 1714, provides a perfect example of an inquiry into strange and exotic folk customs. Another description of inoculation was submitted to the Royal Society by Giacomo Pylarini.

According to Timoni and Pylarini, the inoculator took pus from a favorable smallpox case by opening a pustule with a needle. The needle was placed in a clean glass vessel that was carried about in the inoculator's armpit or bosom to keep it warm. Several small wounds were made in a healthy subject's skin and a little blood was allowed to flow. The smallpox matter was mixed with the blood and the incision was covered with half a walnut shell. A magical or religious touch could be added by inoculating at several sites to form a cross.

Seven years after the appearance of these papers, a series of experimental trials was conducted under royal sponsorship and with the cooperation of the Royal Society and College of Physicians, to evaluate the safety of inoculation. Six felons, who had volunteered to participate in an experiment in exchange for pardons (if they survived), were inoculated by Maitland on August 9, 1721, in the presence of at least 25 witnesses. On September 6, the experiment was judged a success and the prisoners were released, happily free from prison and fear of smallpox. As a further test, the orphans of St. James's parish were inoculated. These experiments were closely studied by the Prince and Princess of Wales (later King George II and Queen Caroline). Based on highly favorable reports, the Princess decided to inoculate two of her daughters. Inevitably, there were some highly publicized failures, which were exploited in the war of sermons and pamphlets disputing the religious, social, and medical implications of inoculation.

Advocates of inoculation believed that protecting individuals from smallpox was only the beginning. Matthieu Maty (1718–1776), who championed inoculation in England, France, and Holland, predicted that within one hundred years people might totally forget smallpox and all its dangers. By the second half of the eighteenth century, inoculation was a generally accepted medical practice. Based on information reported by inoculators for the years 1723 to 1727, James Jurin (1684–1750), a prominent physician and advocate of inoculation, calculated a death rate from inoculated smallpox of about 1 in 48 to 60 cases, in contrast to 1 death per every 6 cases of natural smallpox. Individual inoculators reported morality rates ranging from 1 in 30 to 1 in 8,000. In general, the mortality rate for inoculated smallpox probably averaged about 1 in 200. Because inoculation was most commonly demanded during epidemic years, some of the deaths attributed to inoculation might have been the result of naturally acquired smallpox. Although inoculation probably had a limited impact on the overall incidence of smallpox, it paved the way for the rapid acceptance of Edward Jenner's cowpox vaccine and the hope that other epidemic diseases might also be brought under control.

## EDWARD JENNER, COWPOX, AND VACCINATION

Edward Jenner (1749–1823) was 13 years old when he was apprenticed to a physician. He obtained a respectable medical degree from St. Andrews, but preferred the life of country doctor to a fashionable London practice. Although he was often described as modest in both professional ambitions and intelligence, his mind was lively enough to maintain a lifelong friendship with the distinguished anatomist John Hunter (1728–1793). Thanks to a study of the rather nasty reproductive strategy of the cuckoo and Hunter's sponsorship, Jenner became a member of the Royal Society. In their correspondence, Hunter and Jenner exchanged ideas about natural history and medicine. Thus, when Jenner became intrigued by local folk beliefs about smallpox and cowpox, he asked Hunter for his opinion of the hypothesis that inoculation with cowpox might eliminate the danger of smallpox. Hunter offered the advice that guided his own work: do not speculate, do the experiment.

In 1793, the Royal Society rejected Jenner's paper "Inquiry into the Natural History of a Disease known in Gloucestershire by the name of the 'Cowpox.'" Five years later, Jenner published *An Inquiry into the Causes and Effects of the Variolae Vaccinae, a Disease Discovered in Some of the Western Counties of England, particularly Gloucestershire, and Known by the Name of the Cow Pox*. Jenner named the infective cowpox agent *Variola vaccinae* (Latin, *vacca,* meaning cow, and *variola,* the Latin name of smallpox). In view of the medical profession's tendency to resist new ideas and methods, the fact that Jennerian vaccination spread throughout Europe and the Americas by 1800 is as remarkable as the rewards and honors heaped upon the modest country doctor who championed the new technique. The Royal Jennerian Society was established in 1803 in order to provide free vaccinations for the impoverished children of London.

In the *Inquiry*, Jenner suggested that a disease of horses' hooves, called "the grease," was modified by passage through the cow and caused a disease in humans that was so similar to smallpox that it might be the primordial source of the disease. Because both men and women in Gloucestershire milked dairy cows, a man who had applied ointments to the hooves of horses suffering from the grease could transfer the infection to the udders of cows, where it appeared as an eruptive disease called cowpox. Infected milkmaids noted lesions on their hands, along with mild symptoms of generalized illness. While the cowpox was a minor inconvenience, people who contracted the infection seemed to be immune to natural and inoculated smallpox.

Eighteenth century standards of proof, medical ethics, informed consent, and clinical trials were very different from those proclaimed by modern medicine. Jenner's evidence would probably intrigue, but certainly not convince, a modern research review board. In addition to compiling case histories, Jenner performed experiments on the transmission and effect of cowpox. For example, in May of 1796, Jenner inoculated eight-year-old James Phipps with fluid taken from a cowpox lesion on the hand of a milkmaid named Sara Nelmes. About a week later, the boy complained of mild generalized discomfort, but within a few days he had completely recovered. When Jenner performed a test inoculation, using pus taken from a patient with smallpox, Phipps appeared to be immune to inoculated smallpox. After a number of successful trials, Jenner concluded that a person previously affected by cowpox virus "is forever after secure from the infection of the small pox." Jenner even inoculated his own son with cowpox fluid and later tested his immunity against smallpox pus.

To distinguish between the old practice of *inoculation* with smallpox matter and his new method, Jenner coined the term *vaccination* (Latin *vaccinus*, relating to the cow). For the sake of convenience, and to distance his procedure from unwelcome associations with "brute animals," Jenner proved that immunity could be transmitted directly from person to person. Nevertheless, some of Jenner's contemporaries denounced him as a fraud and a quack and raged against the use of vile animal matter in human beings, while others called vaccination the greatest discovery in the history of medicine. Physicians, surgeons, apothecaries, clergymen, and assorted opportunists vied for control of vaccination. But maintaining control was impossible because recipients of the vaccine could use their own vesicles to vaccinate family and friends.

Critics of Jennerian vaccination warned that deliberately transmitting disease from animals to human beings was a loathsome, immoral, and dangerous act. Experience, however, substantiated Jenner's major contention: vaccination was simple, safe, inexpensive, and effective. Vaccination, therefore, rapidly displaced inoculation despite inevitable religious, social, scientific, and pseudoscientific objections. Within one brief decade, enterprising practitioners had carried vaccination all around the world. Threads impregnated with cowpox lymph were generally the medium of transmission, but on long voyages vaccine could be kept alive by a series of person-to-person transfers. A major difficulty in assuring the continuity of the chain of vaccination was finding individuals who had not previously contracted smallpox or cowpox.

In 1802, Charles IV ordered the Council of the Indies to study ways of bringing vaccination to Spanish America. An expedition was quickly organized and Francisco Xavier de Balmis (1753–1819) was appointed director. As the Spanish ship sailed around the world, de Balmis established vaccination boards in South America, the Philippines, and China. To maintain active vaccine on these long voyages, de Balmis selected about two dozen orphans and performed arm-to-arm passage every 9 or 10 days. When necessary, he replenished his supply of unvaccinated boys and continued with his mission. Because of the remarkable dispersal of Jennerian vaccine, de Balmis sometimes found that vaccine had gotten to some parts of the world before he did.

The first vaccination in North America was probably performed by John Clinch, a physician and clergyman who had settled in the Newfoundland area. Clinch and Jenner became friends while they were students in England. In 1800, Jenner's nephew, the Reverend Dr. George Jenner, sent "pox threads" to Clinch. Physicians in Cincinnati, Lexington, St. Louis, and other communities apparently obtained samples of cowpox vaccine during the first decade of the nineteenth century. Dr. Antoine François Saugrain de Vigny (1763–1820), for example, introduced the vaccine to St. Louis in 1809, just eight years after a smallpox outbreak in the city. As early as 1800, Saugrain's relatives in France had relayed reports about the vaccine and urged him to vaccinate his children. In June 1809, Saugrain put a notice in the Missouri *Gazette* to inform readers that he had obtained "the genuine vaccine infection." Having successfully vaccinated his family and others, he felt compelled to "disseminate this blessing" and inform physicians and others about the availability of vaccine. He also offered free vaccinations for poor people and Indians.

The best-known advocate of vaccination in America during the first part of the nineteenth century was Benjamin Waterhouse (1754–1846). Born in Newport, Rhode Island, Waterhouse completed a medical apprenticeship with Newport's leading physician, John Halliburton. Like many ambitious American doctors, Waterhouse pursued medical studies in London, Edinburgh, and Leiden. Having earned his medical degree, Waterhouse returned to Newport, where he established a private practice. He also taught natural history and applied botany at the College of Rhode Island (later Brown University). Waterhouse later became the first professor of the Theory and Practice of Medicine at the newly established Harvard Medical School. In addition to his work on the cowpox, Waterhouse presented lectures in natural history, helped establish the Botanical Gardens in Cambridge, and published numerous books and essays, including *The Rise, Progress and Present State of Medicine* (1792), *A Prospect of Exterminating Smallpox* (Part I, 1800; Part II, 1802), and *The Botanist* (1811).

Although Waterhouse was not the first person to perform vaccination in North America, he was the first vaccinator to capture the attention of the public and the medical profession. Indeed, William H. Welch (1850–1934), a prominent pathologist and one of the founders of the Johns Hopkins School of Medicine, called Waterhouse the "American Jenner." Early in 1799, Waterhouse received a copy of Jenner's *Inquiry* from a friend. Under the heading "Something Curious in the Medical Line," Waterhouse published a brief note on vaccination in Boston's *Columbian Centinel* and appealed to local dairy farmers for information about the existence of "kine-pox" in their herds. After several frustrating attempts to obtain active vaccine, Waterhouse secured a sample in July 1800 and began experimenting on his own children and servants. Although he was later criticized for trying to establish a monopoly on vaccination in America, Waterhouse sent some of his vaccine to Thomas Jefferson, who vaccinated his entire household. In a letter sent to Jenner in 1806, Jefferson predicted: "Future generations will know by history only that the loathsome smallpox existed and by you has been extirpated." Although his prediction would not come true until the 1970s, Jefferson helped set the process in motion through his example and support.

Debates about the safety and efficacy of preventive vaccines have raged ever since the first experiments on smallpox inoculation and vaccination, long before the establishment of the sciences of microbiology and immunology. Many arguments about vaccination were more emotional than scientific: any interference with nature or the will of God is immoral; deliberately introducing disease matter into a healthy person is obscene; inoculations may appear to be beneficial, but the risks must ultimately outweigh the benefits. Other critics objected to the enactment of mandatory vaccination laws as an infringement on personal liberty. For example, the British philosopher Herbert Spencer (1820–1903) wrote: "Compulsory vaccination I detest, and voluntary vaccination I disapprove." On the other hand, Johann Peter Frank had no doubt that vaccination was "the greatest and most important discovery ever made for Medical Police." Frank predicted that if all states adopted compulsory vaccination, smallpox would soon disappear.

Early attempts to measure the impact of preventive immunizations lacked the rigorous controls that modern scientists demand. Indeed, results assembled from early clinical trials performed in hospitals, orphanages, and poorhouses were often little better than purely anecdotal evidence. When a disease is widespread, it is difficult to compare experimental and control groups because some people in both groups may have had the disease or, in the case of smallpox, may have contracted the disease just before the beginning of the experiment. Despite uncertainty and protests, during the 1850s, variolation was declared illegal and vaccination was made compulsory in the United Kingdom. The death rate from smallpox fell from the eighteenth century level of 3,000 to 4,000 per million to 90 per million after 1872, when enforcement of the vaccination laws became more common. Nevertheless, Alfred Russel Wallace (1823–1913), English naturalist and co-discover of evolution by natural selection, denounced vaccination as one of the major failures of the nineteenth century. According to Wallace, the public health authorities were not only guilty of incompetence and dishonesty in their use of statistics, but had conspired with the medical establishment to cover up numerous deaths caused by vaccination. Reflecting the views of many Englishmen, Wallace asserted that those who promulgated and enforced the vaccination statutes were guilty of a crime against liberty, health, and humanity.

Many Americans must have agreed with Wallace, because in the 1910s epidemiologists were still complaining that the United States was the least vaccinated industrialized nation in the world. Individual states were almost as likely to pass laws prohibiting compulsory vaccination as laws mandating vaccination. Surveys conducted between 1928 and 1931 found that more than 40 percent of U.S. residents had never been vaccinated. Enforcement of vaccination laws improved dramatically after World War II, and the risk of contracting smallpox within the United States eventually became so small that in 1971 the Public Health Service recommended ending routine vaccination. At that point, although the United States had been smallpox-free for over 20 years, six to eight children died each year from vaccination-related complications. Hostility to compulsory vaccination never entirely disappeared. Indeed, in the 1980s, opponents of immunization claimed that the global campaign for the eradication of smallpox was responsible for the AIDS epidemic.

Vaccinia virus made the eradication of smallpox possible, but the origin of vaccinia remains as great a puzzle as the nature of the relationships among smallpox, cowpox, and vaccinia viruses. As demonstrated in the 1930s, vaccinia is different from cowpox. Some virologists have defined vaccinia as a species of laboratory virus that has no natural reservoir. Smallpox, cowpox, and vaccinia viruses are all members of the genus

*Orthopoxvirus*, but they are distinct species and cannot be transformed into each other. Horsepox was extinct by the time immunological identification of particular strains was possible. Because cowpox and horsepox were rare and sporadic, virologists think that wild rodents were the natural reservoir of the ancestral poxvirus.

Since the 1960s, vaccines have been produced from three vaccinia strains maintained in England, America, and Russia. But the early trials of vaccination apparently involved an uncontrollable hodgepodge of viruses, with natural smallpox ever present. Inoculators took their material indiscriminately from cows and people, from primary pustules and secondary pustules of uncertain origin. The strength and duration of protection conferred by vaccination and inoculation were uncertain. Despite Jenner's optimistic declaration that vaccination, if properly done, produced life-long immunity, later research proved that immunity from vaccination, inoculation, and natural smallpox falls off with time and is variable in any population. Thus, it is not surprising that different patterns of morbidity and mortality have been found among different populations.

After World War II, smallpox was no longer considered endemic in Britain or the United States. Nevertheless, imported cases continued to touch off minor epidemics and major panics. Because the disease was so rarely seen in England, Europe, and the United States, smallpox patients often infected relatives, hospital personnel, and visitors before the proper diagnosis was made. Once a smallpox outbreak was identified, some cities launched heroic vaccination campaigns. During smallpox panics in the 1940s, newspaper and radio messages exhorted young and old: "Be Sure, Be Safe, Get Vaccinated!" In New York City, William D. O'Dwyer (1890–1964), who served as Mayor from 1945 to 1950, set a good example by having himself vaccinated in the presence of reporters and photographers five times during his years in office. Although vaccination was supposedly required before admission to the city school system, public health officials estimated that at the outset of the 1947 outbreak only about two million of New York's nearly eight million residents had any immunity to smallpox. Under the threat of an epidemic, five million New Yorkers were vaccinated within two weeks. This world record was achieved with the help of some 400 volunteers out of the city's 13,000 private physicians.

## THE GLOBAL ERADICATION OF SMALLPOX

Although smallpox killed more than 15 million people a year during the 1950s, by the 1960s, for most residents of the wealthy industrialized nations, the odds of suffering ill effects from vaccination became greater than the chance of encountering smallpox. However, given the extensive and rapid movement of people in the Jet Age, as long as smallpox existed anywhere in the world, the danger of outbreaks triggered by imported smallpox could not be ignored. For the United States, Great Britain, and the Soviet Union, the worldwide eradication of smallpox offered a humane and economical solution to the vaccination dilemma.

The World Health Organization adopted the Smallpox Eradication Program in 1958, but the intensive campaign for global eradication was not launched until 1967, when smallpox was endemic in 33 countries and another 11 reported only imported cases. Despite the availability of large stocks of donated vaccine, few public health specialists were optimistic about the possibility of eradicating smallpox from the world's least developed nations, with their negligible medical resources and overwhelming burden of poverty and disease. Surprisingly, within four years, eradication programs in West and Central Africa were successful. During this phase of the global campaign, public health workers learned to modify their strategy in ways appropriate to special challenges.

Originally, the smallpox eradication strategy called for mass vaccination using jet immunization guns that could deliver hundreds of doses per hour. In order to eradicate smallpox in any given nation, epidemiologists considered it necessary to vaccinate 80 to 100 percent of the population. Public health workers soon encountered virtually insurmountable difficulties in maintaining stocks of vaccine and injector guns under primitive conditions in hot, humid climates. Simpler equipment, like the bifurcated needle (two-pronged), proved to be more reliable and efficient. As a result of shortages of personnel and equipment in eastern Nigeria, public health workers discovered, almost by accident, that a strategy called "surveillance-containment" effectively broke the chain of transmission. By concentrating limited resources on the most infected areas, the new strategy was successful even when only 50 percent of the population had been vaccinated. In October 1977, Ali Maow Maalin of Somalia became the last person to contract smallpox outside a laboratory setting. The case might have spelled disaster for the containment program. Maalin worked as a cook in a busy city hospital and his disease was first misdiagnosed as malaria and later as chicken pox. During the most contagious stage of the disease, Maalin had more than 160 contacts, but no other cases of smallpox occurred.

Although humanitarian motives were not absent from the decision to declare a global war against smallpox, there is no doubt that economic factors loomed large in the choice of this target. Global eradication of smallpox cost billions of dollars, but, by eliminating the disease, sponsors of the campaign against smallpox were liberated from the threat of imported cases, without imposing the dangers of vaccination on their own people. For developing nations, malaria and other so-called tropical diseases caused more serious problems than smallpox. Most victims of smallpox die or recover within a matter of weeks, and in areas where the disease was endemic it was usually just one of many childhood illnesses. In contrast, malaria is a debilitating recurrent illness that reduces resistance to other infections, productivity, and the live birth rate.

The December 1979 Final Report of the Global Commission for the Certification of Smallpox Eradication solemnly declared that: "The world and all its peoples have won freedom from smallpox." At the end of the eradication program, WHO and a number of countries independently stored enough smallpox vaccine for 60 million people and a supply of the vaccinia virus that could be used to make vaccine. During the 1980s the practice of vaccination was essentially abandoned throughout the world, except for a few special cases, such as scientists conducting research on vaccinia or various poxviruses. In the United States, routine smallpox vaccinations for children ended in 1972; the military continued to recommend vaccinations until the late 1980s. In describing the successful completion of the Smallpox Eradication Program, Donald A. Henderson, director of the Eradication Program from 1966 to 1977, proposed the next logical step: what had been learned in the smallpox campaign should form the basis of global immunization programs for controlling diphtheria, whooping cough, tetanus, measles, poliomyelitis, and tuberculosis. Such global campaigns could transform the mission of health services "from curative medicine for the rich to preventive medicine for all."

After the terrorist attacks of September 11, 2001, Henderson became the director of the United States Office of Public Health Emergency Preparedness and Response. Finding the world in danger of "regressing" in the battle against a disease that was presumably eradicated in the 1970s, Henderson expressed the frustration and sorrow of those who had once envisioned an era of global disease control programs. In addition to a distinguished career in the Departments of Epidemiology and International Health in the School of Public Health at Johns Hopkins, Henderson became founding director of the Johns Hopkins Center for Civilian Biodefense Studies. His federal appointments include Associate Director of the Office of Science and Technology Policy, Executive Office of the President, Deputy Assistant Secretary and Senior Science Advisor to the Department of Health and Human Services on civilian biodefense issues, and Chairman of the National Advisory Council on Public Health Preparedness. His many awards and honors include the National Medal of Science, the Presidential Medal of Freedom, and the Royal Society of Medicine's Edward Jenner Medal.

At the time that global eradication of smallpox had been achieved, the only known reservoirs of smallpox virus were samples held, deliberately or inadvertently, by an unknown number of research laboratories. The danger of maintaining such laboratory stocks was exposed in 1978 when

Janet Parker, a 40-year-old medical photographer who worked in the Birmingham University Medical School, contracted smallpox. The virus apparently entered rooms on the floor above a virus research laboratory through air ducts. Parker was hospitalized and diagnosed 13 days after becoming ill; she died two weeks later. About three hundred people who had come in contact with her were quarantined. Her father died of a heart attack after visiting her. Parker's mother contracted smallpox, but she recovered. The accident also led to the death of Henry Bedson, the 49-year-old director of the virus research laboratory. After confirming the source of the virus that had killed Parker, Bedson wrote a note admitting that he had ignored safety precautions while conducting research. Overwhelmed by guilt, Bedson committed suicide. His laboratory was due to close at the end of the year, because inspectors considered it too old and unsafe to be used for smallpox research. Virologists have noted that, in addition to illicit laboratory stocks, potentially viable smallpox virus might still persist in ancient crypts and coffins, or in cadavers in the permafrost of the Siberian tundra.

With the threat of naturally occurring smallpox eliminated, fears have grown that the virus could be used as an agent of bioterrorism or germ warfare. Nations that were smallpox-free when the global campaign began generally abandoned their own vaccination programs in the 1970s, leaving new generations to confront the possibility that terrorists or rogue nations might obtain stocks of smallpox virus. Smallpox has been called the ideal agent for germ warfare because the virus is stable, easy to grow, easily disseminated, and, above all, causes a terrifying, highly contagious, and often fatal disease. Terrorists might utilize "human missiles" or "smallpox martyrs"—people infected and sent out to spread virus by coughing and sneezing in populous areas during the most infectious phase of the disease. Progress in molecular biology has added the possibility that terrorists might develop novel or genetically modified pathogens, including vaccine-resistant smallpox strains.

Revelations about the germ warfare programs carried out in the former USSR emphasized the potential dangers of weaponized pathogens. Information about the Soviet germ warfare program, including the development of weaponized smallpox, was provided by Kanatjan Kalibekov (also known as Ken Alibek), a scientist who defected to the United States in 1992. Alibek also warned that unemployed scientists might have sold stocks of the virus during the collapse of the Soviet Union. Later, Alibek attempted to reach a wider audience with his book *Biohazard* (1999), a landmark in the modern literature on biological weapons. A report released in 2002 suggested that a Soviet field test of weaponized smallpox might have caused an outbreak in Aralsk, a port city in Kazakhstan, in 1971. Ten people contracted smallpox and three unvaccinated people died of the hemorrhagic form of the disease. The seven survivors had previously received routine vaccinations.

Emergency teams quarantined hundreds of people and administered almost 50,000 vaccinations in less than two weeks.

In addition to worrying about the threat that bioterrorists might use smallpox as a weapon, virologists worry about the possible emergence of new or previously rare viral diseases, such as monkeypox, which was first discovered in the 1950s in monkeys from Zaire. The monkeypox virus is actually more commonly found in squirrels, mice, and other small rodents in western and central Africa. Although monkeypox virus is not readily transmitted to or among people, hundreds of sporadic human cases have been recorded; the fatality rate among reported cases is about 10 percent. Vaccination seems effective against monkeypox, but in areas of Africa where the virus occurs, AIDS is widespread today, which means many people could not be vaccinated. Until 2003, monkeypox had been reported only in Africa, but more than 70 suspected cases occurred in the United States in 2003. The virus reached the United States in Gambian giant pouched rats, which were shipped from Ghana to American pet stores. The demand for exotic pets has allowed the exchange of pathogens between different species and the subsequent infection of human beings. Since September 11 and the anthrax attacks, people tend to think that the sudden appearance of any exotic disease might be the result of bioterrorism, but the trade in exotic pets and live-animal-food markets must also be considered.

All stocks of the smallpox virus were supposedly destroyed by 1984, except for virus kept at two official depositories: the Atlanta headquarters of the Centers for Disease Control and Prevention and at a Russian government laboratory in Novosibirsk, Siberia. Since the eradication of smallpox, the WHO has debated the fate of the last official smallpox virus stocks. In the 1990s, the World Federation of Public Health Associations and the World Health Assembly called for the destruction of all remaining smallpox virus. The WHO planned to destroy the last official stocks of the virus in 2002, but the scheduled execution was delayed. Some scientists opposed destroying the last viral stocks because of the possibility that research might lead to new drugs and vaccines. Scientists thought that the smallpox virus could attack only humans, but in 2001 researchers were able to infect monkeys with a particularly virulent strain of the virus. With an animal model, scientists could conduct previously impossible studies of antiviral drugs, vaccines, biosensing systems, virulence factors, host specificity, and so forth.

Many experts on biological weapons believe that Iraq, Iran, North Korea, and perhaps other nations or terrorist groups might already have clandestine stocks of the virus. In response to the growing concern for bioterrorism since September 11, 2001, and the anthrax attacks in 2001, public health experts began to reconsider the need for vaccination, especially for potential "first responders" to terrorist attacks. Few public health experts favor a return to mass vaccinations, given the presumably small risk of uncontrollable outbreaks and the known risks of severe, even lethal, reactions to the vaccine. Perhaps one or two out of every million people vaccinated might die and a few hundred out of every million could have severe reactions. A vaccinated person could infect others, causing severe infections. Vaccination would not be recommended for people with AIDS and other conditions that damage the immune system, and people with skin disorders like eczema, atopic dermatitis, and acne. Scientists also fear that existing vaccines might not be effective against a new bioengineered strain of smallpox virus.

If terrorists wanted a weapon that rapidly killed large numbers of people, smallpox would be a poor weapon. But the fact that significant parts of the U.S. government and the post office were all but paralyzed in 2001 by a few envelopes containing anthrax spores, suggests that the *threat* of smallpox, even more than the reality of the disease, would make it an ideal tool for terrorists whose major objective is to frighten and demoralize people.

## SUGGESTED READINGS

Alibek, K., and Handelman, S. (1999). *Biohazard.* New York: Random House.

Altman, L. K. (1987). *Who Goes First? The Story of Self-Experimentation in Medicine.* New York: Random House.

Altschule, M. D. (1989). *Essays on the Rise and Decline of Bedside Medicine.* Philadelphia, PA: Lea & Fibiger.

Baxby, D. (2001). *Smallpox Vaccine, Ahead of Its Time: How the Late Development of Laboratory Methods and Other Vaccines Affected the Acceptance of Smallpox Vaccine.* Berkeley, England: Jenner Museum.

Bazin, H. (2000). *The Eradication of Smallpox: Edward Jenner and the First and Only Eradication of a Human Infectious Disease.* San Diego, CA: Academic Press.

Carpenter, K. J. (1986). *The History of Scurvy and Vitamin C.* New York: Cambridge University Press.

Carpenter, K. J. (2000). *Beriberi, White Rice and Vitamin B: A Disease, a Cause, and a Cure.* Berkeley, CA: University of California Press.

Copeman, W. S. C. (1964). *A Short History of the Gout and the Rheumatic Diseases.* Berkeley, CA: University California Press.

Dewhurst, K., ed. (1966). *Dr. Thomas Sydenham (1624–1689): His Life and Original Writings.* Berkeley, CA: University of California Press.

Fenner, F., Henderson, D. A., Arita, I., Jezek, Z., and Ladnyi, I. D. (1988). *Smallpox and its Eradication.* Geneva: WHO. (Out of print but available at http://www.who.int/emc/diseases/smallpox/Smallpoxeradication.htm.)

Frank, J. P. (1976). *A System of Complete Medical Police.* Selections from Johann Peter Frank. Edited with an Introduction by E. Lesky, Baltimore, MD: Johns Hopkins University Press.

Headrick, D. R. (1981). *The Tools of Empire: Technology and European Imperialism in the Nineteenth Century.* New York: Oxford University Press.

Honigsbaum, M. (2002). *The Fever Trail: In Search of the Cure for Malaria.* New York: Farrar, Straus & Giroux.

Hopkins, D. R. (2002). *The Greatest Killer: Smallpox in History.* Chicago, IL: University of Chicago Press.

Humphreys, M. (2001). *Malaria: Poverty, Race and Public Health in the United States.* Baltimore, MD: Johns Hopkins University Press.

Jarcho, S. (1993). *Quinine's Predecessor. Francesco Torti and the Early History of Cinchona.* Baltimore, MD: The Johns Hopkins University Press.

Kamminga, H. (2002). *Science, Food and Politics: The Making of Vitamins.* Burlington, VT: Ashgate.

Kiple, K. F., Ornelas, K. C., eds. (2000). *The Cambridge World History of Food.* New York: Cambridge University Press.

Koplow, D. (2003). *Smallpox: The Fight to Eradicate a Global Scourge.* Berkeley, CA: University of California Press.

Kors, A. C., ed. (2003). *Encyclopedia of the Enlightenment,* 4 vols. Oxford: Oxford University Press.

Lind, J. (1953). *Treatise on Scurvy. A Bicentenary Volume Containing a Reprint of the First Edition of "A Treatise of the Scurvy" by James Lind with Additional Notes.* Edited by C. P. Stewart and D. Guthrie. Edinburgh: University of Edinburgh Press.

Lloyd, C., ed. (1965). *The Health of Seamen: Selections from the Works of Dr. James Lind, Sir Gilbert Blane and Dr. Thomas Trotter.* London: Navy Records Society.

MacLeod, R., and Lewis, M., eds. (1988). *Disease, Medicine, and Empire: Perspectives on Western Medicine and the Experience of European Expansion.* London: Routledge.

Mather, C. (1972). *The Angel of Bethesda. An Essay on the Common Maladies of Mankind.* Reproduction of the 1724 manuscript. Edited by G. W. Jones. Barre, MA: American Antiquarian Society.

McKeown, T. (1976). *The Modern Rise of Population.* New York: Academic Press.

Morgani, G. B. (1980) *The Seats and Causes of Diseases.* 3 vols. (English trans. by B. Alexander). London, 1769. Facsimile reprint, Mount Kisco, NY: Futura.

Moss, R. W. (1987). *Free Radical. Albert Szent-Gyorgyi and the Battle Over Vitamin C.* New York: Paragon House Publishers.

Nestle, M. (2002). *Food Politics: How the Food Industry Influences Nutrition and Health.* Berkeley, CA: University of California Press.

Porter, R., and Rousseau, G. S. (1998). *Gout: The Patrician Malady.* New Haven, CT: Yale University Press.

Poser, C. M., and Bruyn, G. W. (2000). *An Illustrated History of Malaria.* Boca Raton, FL: CRC Press.

Preston, R. (2002). *The Demon in the Freezer: A True Story.* New York: Random House.

Rocco, F. (2003). *The Miraculous Fever-Tree. Malaria and the Quest for a Cure That Changed the World.* New York: HarperCollins Publishers.

Spielman, A., and D'Antonio, M. (2001). *Mosquito: A Natural History of Our Most Persistent and Deadly Foe.* New York: Hyperion.

Waterhouse, B. (1980). *The Life and Scientific and Medical Career of Benjamin Waterhouse: With Some Account of the Introduction of Vaccination in America*, 2 vols. Edited by I. Bernard Cohen. New York: Arno Press. Reprint.

World Health Organization (1980). *The Global Eradication of Smallpox. Final Report of the Global Commission for the Certification of Smallpox Eradication, Geneva, December, 1979.* Geneva: WHO.

# 10

# The Medical Counterculture: Unorthodox and Alternative Medicine

The nineteenth century was a period of transition in American medicine, a period especially marked by the proliferation of medical schools, medical societies, medical journals, controversial attempts to secure medical licensing laws, and the emergence of new medical sciences, such as bacteriology, immunology, and physiology. These developments helped create a consensus among physicians as to how medicine should be practiced, and by whom, but many patients rebelled against orthodox therapy and continued to demand freedom of choice in the medical marketplace.

## THE MEDICAL MARKETPLACE

Orthodox doctors constituted the majority of nineteenth-century medical practitioners, but popular health reformers and members of competing sects, generally known as irregular practitioners, did manage some effective challenges to their authority. Orthodox practitioners generally shared one view of alternative practitioners; they saw them as quacks, frauds, and deviants, even if such practitioners began their career as physicians. Quacks who really believe in their unconventional methods might be considered foolish, misguided, or deranged, while those who engaged in deliberate deceptions, were called charlatans. Orthodox doctors insisted that all quacks were harmful and that strict medical licensing laws were needed to remove them from the medical marketplace.

Despite being split into many groups that had different ideas about the nature of disease and therapy, irregular practitioners collectively agreed that regular medicine was both ineffective and dangerous. Of course, not all critics of orthodox medicine were healers with competing medical theories. For example, Thomas Jefferson (1743–1826) respected his good friend Benjamin Rush (1745–1813), but was quite sure that his enthusiasm for bleeding and purging had been very harmful. Followers of the approach epitomized by Rush were all too eager to treat victims of epidemic cholera (a disease that may cause death by dehydration) with ipecac, vomits of salt and water, frequent doses of calomel, castor oil, and enemas of spirits of turpentine. Although Rush never lost faith in his therapeutic system, many Americans were attracted to healers who offered remedies and regimens that were allegedly safe, natural, and effective.

Some irregulars were empirics or specialists—such as, herbalists, midwives, dentists, and oculists—who offered a limited range of services, without pretensions to learned medical theories. Other healers were members of medical sects or religious sects, such as Seventh Day Adventists and Christian Scientists. Some leaders of popular health crusades offered guides to dietetic regimens that would allegedly obviate the need for all drugs and doctors. Unorthodox healers might also be charismatic individuals, with or without medical training, who claimed to have discovered marvelous devices or drugs that were being suppressed by the dominant medical profession. Whatever their theories of health, disease, and therapy, unorthodox healers emphasized the dangers and expense of orthodox medicine. Many novel medical sects arose in the nineteenth century, but Thomsonianism, eclecticism, naturopathy, hydropathy, and homeopathy were the best known and most coherent. By the end of the century, many of the early medical sects had essentially disappeared, and homeopathic and eclectic practitioners faced growing competition from osteopaths and chiropractors, as well as the increasingly unified and powerful regular physicians.

In the 1830s and 1840s, the age of Jacksonian democracy, popular opinion favored egalitarianism, democratic ideals, and laissez-faire economics. The followers of Andrew Jackson (1767–1845), seventh president of the United States, denounced the creation of monopolies, restrictions on commerce, and all claims of expertise, professional privilege, and authority. In this context, Americans called into question the professional authority and legal monopoly demanded by regular physicians. As Mark Twain (1835–1910) explained, Americans believed that every man should be "free to choose his own executioner."

## HEALTH REFORM MOVEMENTS

Nineteenth-century physicians had little interest in disease prevention. Indeed, except for smallpox inoculation or vaccination, which involved a specific and somewhat dangerous operation, they had little to offer. But the prevention of disease was a major concern of the public and the promise of wellness through various hygienic regimens was irresistibly attractive. Health reformers and wellness advocates were a versatile and energetic group—juggling many good causes and dispensing avalanches of advice about health, exercise, diet, air, water, light, dress reform, sexual hygiene, family, community, temperance, tobacco, and drugs, in an endless recital of themes and variations. Disturbed by evidence of poor health and hygiene, and stimulated by new physiological knowledge, social reformers launched a moral crusade preaching the virtues of healthful living.

Converts to the health reform movement attended lectures, subscribed to health journals, adopted special diets, engaged in novel exercises, indulged in therapeutic baths, or sought out health resorts and spas. The popularity and influence of health reformers and newly emerging medical sects empowered health seekers to free themselves from medically approved purging, puking, and bleeding. Health reformers shared the belief that prevention is better than cure and they urged their followers to follow the path to optimum wellness. But the roads to wellness were many and diverse, even bizarre, although most emphasized control of the usual suspects—diet, exercise, sexual activities, personal hygiene, and so forth. Many of the most colorful and charismatic health reformers appealed to the latest findings of scientific research in support of their vision of a true physiological lifestyle, but they also assured their followers that their system of right living was mandated by God's laws of hygienic living. Cynics like H. L. Mencken (1880–1956), American editor and social critic, were annoyed by the evangelical enthusiasms of the health reformers. Mencken called hygiene "the corruption of medicine by morality" because it was "impossible to find a hygienist who does not debase his theory of the healthful with a theory of the virtuous."

Leaders of health crusades largely abandoned the old Hippocratic call for "moderation in all things" and substituted the concept of absolute prohibition, although different reformers adopted different prohibitions. Foods and behaviors were divided into moral categories of good things permitted, in moderation, and bad things—such as meat, alcohol, and other stimulants—that must be avoided altogether. Although vegetarianism is an ancient concept, the forms it has taken and the reasons for its adoption have varied considerably. Buddhists, Hindus, and Pythagoreans objected to the slaughter of animals for moral and religious reasons, but health reformers advocated vegetarianism as an absolute prerequisite for a healthy, harmonious life. The most influential leaders of the early nineteenth-century American health reform movement, William Andrus Alcott (1798–1859) and Sylvester Graham (1794–1851), claimed that their health advice, while in accord with Christian theology, was based on contemporary scientific knowledge about physiology and the nature of human beings. In addition to meat and other flesh foods, Alcott and Graham condemned alcohol, coffee, tea, tobacco, and spices because of their tendency to over stimulate the body's animal appetites and passions.

Presumably because of the eponymous graham cracker, Sylvester Graham is better known than William Alcott, his more prolific contemporary. Graham was an ordained Presbyterian minister, a temperance advocate, and a lecturer whose area of expertise was nothing less than "The Science of Human Life." Graham warned his followers of the destructive effects of intemperance, gluttony, sexual indulgence, flesh foods, mustard, pepper, and white bread made from "unnatural refined flour." In *Lectures on the Science of Life* and the *Graham Journal of Health and Longevity*, Graham offered advice about every aspect of hygienic living, from the need for fresh air, sunlight, loose clothing, and frequent bathing, to the preparation and proper consumption of bread. Graham bread was made from coarsely ground whole-wheat flour and eaten when slightly stale. Perhaps to compensate for the rather tough, lumpy quality of such bread, Graham conscientiously explained how it should be chewed slowly and thoroughly.

Many health reformers warned against excessive sexual activity, especially the "secret vice," but Graham believed that, except for absolutely necessary procreation within marriage, all sexual activity was unphysiological and unhealthy. The popularity of Graham's message led to the establishment of Grahamite health food stores, restaurants, health retreats, and boarding houses. Legions of critics, however, pointed out that the inventor of Grahamism was a sickly semi-invalid for much of his rather brief life. Meat eaters ridiculed the vegetarian banquets of Grahamites, which featured such unappetizing selections as "Graham bread, stewed squashes, wheaten grits, and pure cold water."

William Alcott earned a very respectable M.D. at Yale, but he became disillusioned with medicine and decided to rely on the healing power of nature rather than conventional therapeutics. After discovering that drugs could not cure him of tuberculosis, Alcott reformed his diet, abstained from alcohol, and acknowledged nature as the only true physician. Alcott devoted the rest of his life to developing and preaching his gospel of Physical Education and Christian Physiology. A prolific author, Alcott disseminated his message through books, journal articles, and self-help guides, such as *Lectures on Life and Health, The Laws of Health, The Physiology of Marriage*, and *Annals of Education*, but he was best known as the author of *The Vegetable Diet As Sanctioned by Medical Men and By Experience in All Ages*. Alcott warned that meat and other flesh foods caused nervous excitement, which led to self-abuse, and an unnatural desire for further stimulation. According to Alcott, a vegetarian diet was fundamental to all other reforms, "Civil, Social, Moral, or Religious."

In 1850, at a convention that established the American Vegetarian Society, William Alcott was elected President. When Alcott died,

William Metcalfe, founder of the Bible Christian Church, took his place. Metcalfe argued that the Bible, properly interpreted, demanded abstention from flesh foods. Graham and Alcott, in contrast, based their dietary regime on contemporary science, primarily the physiological studies of François J. V. Broussais (1772–1832) and the anatomical researches of Xavier Bichat (1771–1802). In the simplified form adopted by Alcott and Graham, Broussais's theory of pathology generally ascribed all disease to excessive stimulation of the digestive tract, which caused dyspepsia and generalized inflammation throughout the body.

Vegetarianism was promoted as a healthful, hygienic, and natural way of life, but health seekers also needed to find natural, hygienic relief from acute and chronic ailments. A healing system known as hydropathy, or the water-cure system, was virtually inseparable from the health reform doctrines taught by Alcott and Graham. When the water-cure system was popularized in America in the 1840s, it incorporated many elements of Grahamite physiology, with its emphasis on fresh air, sunlight, exercise, dietary regimen, and dress reform. Hydropaths established formal treatment centers and educational institutions to train practitioners, who created a new group of professional healers who competed with orthodox practitioners and other sectarian practitioners.

Hydropathy also represented a rejection of the long-held belief that excessive bathing or immersion in cold water was as dangerous as night air. For example, Benjamin Franklin (1706–1790) told fellow Americans that cold baths were very much in vogue in London as a tonic, but he thought the shock of cold water was too violent. As evidence of the dangers of cold baths, Franklin described the case of four young men who decided to cool themselves by plunging into cold spring water after working on a hot day. Two died immediately, the third was dead the next day, and the fourth barely recovered. To avoid the dangers of immersion in cold water, Franklin preferred air baths, which involved sitting in his room without any clothes for 30 minutes or so each morning. On the other hand, Franklin believed that swimming was "one of the most healthy and agreeable" forms of exercise in the world. Towards the end of his life, suffering from several illnesses, Franklin sought relief in warm baths in a special bathing vessel made of copper and shaped like a slipper.

Vincent Priessnitz (1799–1851), a Silesian farmer, is generally credited with the discovery of the fundamental water-cure methods. After an accident that left him with broken ribs and other injuries, Priessnitz claimed to have effected a miraculous recovery by drinking large quantities of cold water and wrapping himself in wet towels. The ingenious peasant then proved that the same methods also cured farm animals (which would tend to take the cure out of the realm of "mere suggestion"). Dr. Joel Shew (1816–1855), one of the early promoters of the American water-cure movement, insisted that exercise and a

388 A History of Medicine

strict vegetarian diet were essential adjuncts to hydropathic healing. Shew was soon overshadowed by Russell Trall (1812–1877), who was active in the temperance movement before discovering the remarkable health benefits of Hygienic Hygieo Therapy. In 1849, Shew, Trall, and others founded the American Hydropathic Society, which was renamed the American Hygienic and Hydropathic Society one year later. Trall was also an active participant in the American Anti-Tobacco Society and the American Vegetarian Society. Energetic and articulate, Trall enjoyed lecturing, debating, and challenging orthodox practitioners. In 1853, Trall founded the New York College of Hygieo-Therapy to instruct others in the use of water-cures, diet, and exercise regimens. Hydropaths generally rejected the use of drugs and claimed that the water-cure was a natural therapeutic system, effective in the treatment of acute and chronic ailments. Trall's *Hydropathic Encyclopedia* included advice about water-cure, exercise, diet, and sexual hygiene. He also published a hydropathic cookbook. When the *American Vegetarian and Health Journal* ceased publication in 1854, Trall agreed to reserve space in the *Water-Cure Journal* for articles written by members of the Vegetarian Society.

Vegetarians did not have to worry about finding suitable foods when seeking a cure at a hydropathic spa, because water-cure establishments typically prepared and sold "pure and proper" health foods, including grits, hominy, farina, oatmeal, Graham flour, and Graham crackers. Testimony from satisfied patients recalled how hydropathic treatments had cured them of complicated ailments such as "the horrors of dyspepsia, the depressions of nervous debility, the terrors of congestion of the brain." Some orthodox physicians, such as Simon Baruch Ward (1840–1921), believed that hydropathy had positive physiological effects and that it was useful in the treatment of typhoid and other febrile diseases. Ward taught hydrotherapy at Columbia College of Physicians and Surgeons from 1907 to 1913. Hydropathic spas were usually retreats for those with time and money, but Ward was particularly concerned with cleanliness and the need for public baths for the urban poor.

Many water-cure physicians and patients were women who were active in various reform movements who adopted the uplifting ideology of hydropathic living. Mary Gove Nichols (1810–1884), for example, was well known as a social reformer, pioneering feminist, utopian thinker, and an alternative medical practitioner. She lectured and wrote about women's health, anatomy, physiology, and sexuality, as well as equality in marriage, free love, the importance of happiness, and the benefits of the water-cure. Her second husband, Thomas Low Nichols (1815–1901) was a doctor, journalist, and social reformer. Mary and Thomas Nichols published several books, including *Lectures to Ladies on Anatomy and Physiology; With an Appendix on Water Cure, Nichols' Medical Miscellanies: A Familiar Guide to the Preservation of Health, and the Hydropathic Home Treatment of the Most Formidable Diseases,* and *Marriage: Its History, Character, and Results.*

Long after water-cure establishments ceased to exist as serious therapeutic institutions in the United States and Great Britain, water therapy spas continued to flourish in other parts of the world. German and Italian health seekers could enjoy therapeutic spas, knowing that at least half of the cost would be paid by their national health insurance system. In France, water-cure spas attained a prominent place within the medical establishment, and the treatment known as thermalism was included in the national health insurance system. In nineteenth-century France, the Academy of Medicine was involved in administrative supervision and scientific studies of mineral water spas. Elite and influential physicians promoted the development of the water-cure industry and hydrology became part of the curriculum of French medical schools. Patients sent to French spas typically remained under medical supervision for about 20 days. By the 1950s, however, the French government was struggling to reduce funding for thermal spas and medical school courses in hydrology. Most spas visitors hoped for relief from arthritic conditions, but others believed that thermalism cures a varity of digestive, respiratory, dermatological, circulatory, and nervous ailments. Critics of thermalism denounced it as a form of paid vacation, if not outright quackery.

One of the largest and most famous American water-cure sanitariums was the institution known as "Our Home on the Hillside," founded by Dr. Harriet Austin and James Caleb Jackson (1814–1895) in Dansville, New York. Jackson published many books and pamphlets with the usual advice about diet, alcohol, tobacco, hygiene, hydropathy, exercise, recreation, education, and sex, including *The Sexual Organism and Its Healthy Management.* In addition to selling Grahamite health foods, Jackson attempted to create a form of Graham bread with a longer shelf-life. His cold, ready-to-eat breakfast cereal, which he called Granula, did not receive much attention until it was discovered and adopted by Ellen G. White (1827–1915), the spiritual leader and prophetess of the Seventh Day Adventist Church, who visited "Our Home" when her husband was stricken with paralysis. Although White had great faith in the water-cure, James did not recover his health. Ellen White attributed this failure to the lack of an appropriate religious environment at Jackson's spa. In a divine vision that came to her on Christmas day in 1865, White learned that Seventh Day Adventists needed to create a health retreat and hospital in Battle Creek, Michigan.

The staggering burden of the Civil War eclipsed many aspects of the health reform movement, diverted attention and resources, and contributed to the disappearance of many hygienic institutions, spas, schools, and sanitariums. But as the story of Ellen White and Dr. John Harvey Kellogg (1852–1943) shows, new leaders and institutions sustained and reinterpreted fundamental ideals of the early health crusades—wellness, prevention, and right living.

While Graham and Alcott emphasized physiological science in support of their theories of healthful living, Ellen White, the Adventist prophetess of health, told her followers that she had received her messages from the Creator of the laws of hygiene. Initially, White's visions dealt with theological issues, but after 1848 many were about food, drink, clothing, and other remarkably practical aspects of healthful living. In 1863, White had a vision of the relation between physical health and spirituality, the importance of a vegetarian diet, and the benefits of nature's remedies—fresh air, sunshine, exercise, and pure water. In keeping with White's vision, Adventists launched a health education program with the publication of six pamphlets entitled *Health, or How to Live*. The fundamental principle that hygienic living was a religious duty was incorporated into Seventh Day Adventist doctrine. Critics of Ellen White, however, found her revelations less than wholly original and insinuated that a head injury sustained when she was young caused hallucinations, not divine visions.

In response to the vision that occurred after her visit to Jackson's hydropathic resort, White created a health spa and hospital where Adventists could benefit from natural therapies in an appropriate religious environment. The Adventist's Western Health Reform Institute of Battle Creek, Michigan opened in 1866 and offered natural methods of health and healing, through a vegetarian diet, hydrotherapy, exercise, light, fresh air, and instruction on the "right mode of living." Recognizing the need for serious medical leadership at the Institute, in 1876 White appointed her protégé John Harvey Kellogg to the position of Physician-in-Chief. It was Kellogg who transformed the struggling Institute into the highly successful Battle Creek Sanitarium.

In 1905, Ellen White published *The Ministry of Healing*, a book that summarized and clarified her teachings about the healing of body, mind, and soul. According to White, human beings became ill because they transgressed the laws established by God to govern health and life; they ignored the fact that improper eating, drinking, and licentiousness are sins that cause disease. Although White cited the Bible for directives about health and healing, she also provided remarkably detailed instructions that echo the advice of Alcott, Graham, and other health reformers. Modern "artificial civilization" was condemned as the source of customs, fashions, intemperance, crimes, and indulgences that contributed to an alarming and widespread decline in physical vigor and endurance. Artificial civilization, caused by rapid industrialization and urbanization, was condemned as the source of pollution, filth, overcrowding, corruption, vice, debility, and disease.

Health could, however, be restored by natural remedies, such as pure air, sunlight, rest, exercise, proper diet, pure water, and trust in divine power. Because regaining health through natural methods required time and patience, many people resorted to powerful drugs and patent medicines, without realizing that such preparations contained poisons and addictive intoxicants. Moreover, even though drugs seemed to provide temporary relief, they did not cure disease. Patent medicines, medicines legally sold without a physician's prescription, were very popular and widely used during the nineteenth century. Manufacturers and retailers advertised heavily and claimed that their products would cure virtually every disorder known to man and woman, from impotence, baldness, and female complaints to cancer, catarrh, tuberculosis, and arthritis. Patent medicines were fairly inexpensive compared to prescription drugs, but they were not necessarily innocuous. For the most part, their contents were secret and government regulation of such products was virtually nil, but popular pills and potions might contain cocaine, morphine, alcohol, or other addictive drugs. Until the Pure Food and Drug Act of 1906, there was little that could be done to regulate the marketing of patent medicines. Indeed most medical journals, including the *Journal of the American Medical Association*, relied on ads for such nostrums and many physicians prescribed them.

Like previous health reformers, White insisted that it was better to prevent disease than to treat the sick. Therefore, everyone should learn and obey the laws of life, study human anatomy and physiology, and understand the "influence of the mind upon the body, and of the body upon the mind, and the laws by which they are governed." Serious brain work, for example, was physically debilitating and called for balancing rest and exercise in order to build mental and physical endurance. Diseases caused by mental depression, anxiety, guilt, and other emotions that "break down the life forces," could be healed by contact with nature, White said, because the Creator had placed Adam and Eve in a garden, a place best adapted for human health and happiness.

Campaigns for dress reform, physical education for women, and frequent bathing, were often ridiculed and trivialized, but White incorporated these causes into her health message. Exercise promoted health and healing because it improved the circulation of the blood and brought pure, fresh air into the lungs. Dress reform was essential to health because tightly laced garments hindered the circulation of the blood and the movement of the lungs, while the weight of long skirts compressed the abdominal organs and the lungs. Scrupulous cleanliness of home, body, clothing, and frequent bathing were essential to both physical and mental health. Uncleanliness allowed the growth of germs, poisoned the air, and led to death and disease. Fashionable long skirts that swept the ground were, therefore, unclean, uncomfortable, inconvenient, and unhealthful, as well as extravagant.

While White agreed that food and drink were largely to blame for disease and suffering, she based her dietary advice on the Bible, rather than physiological science. Because God originally told Adam that he had been given the herbs and fruits of the Garden of Eden as his food, it followed that human beings should choose a diet of grains, fruits, nuts, and vegetables. After the Flood, when every green thing on the earth had been destroyed, human beings received permission to eat flesh, but this was, presumably, a short-term, emergency measure. Nuts and nut foods were meant to take the place of meat.

Biblical wisdom, White noted, was in harmony with scientific research that proved that the tissues of domesticated animals were swarming with parasites, including the germs that caused tuberculosis, cancer, and other fatal diseases. Like Graham, White rejected the use of refined white flour, but she also called for baking whole wheat bread very thoroughly in order to kill the yeast germs. She insisted that milk should be thoroughly sterilized to avoid contracting disease, but she considered cheese "wholly unfit for food." Members of the Church of Jesus Christ of Latter-day Saints also followed teachings on the preservation of health that were said to be divinely inspired. Many of the same kinds of dietary prohibitions were incorporated into Mormon traditions. Allegiance to the "words of wisdom" decreed in the 1832 Mormon health code has been credited for lower cancer and cardiovascular mortality among Mormons.

Like Ellen White, Mary Baker Eddy (1821–1910) became a health seeker after struggling with pain and illness in her youth. But the health message that Eddy imparted as the founder and leader of the Church of Christ, Scientist, commonly referred to as Christian Science, was very different from White's eminently practical advice. Eddy had experimented with many cures, from Grahamism to homeopathy, but found no lasting, meaningful relief until 1866 when she discovered the religious doctrine that she believed would totally reform and revolutionize medicine. She first published an account of the "healing Truth" of her Metaphysical Science in a pamphlet entitled, *The Science of Man, By Which the Sick are Healed* (1870). Five years later she published the first edition of *Science and Health with Key to the Scriptures*. By 1900, the Christian Science movement had spread throughout the United States and about five hundred congregations had been established.

The key to Eddy's Moral or Metaphysical Science was the fundamental concept that "all is mind and there is no matter." According to Eddy's teachings the remedy for disease is accepting the great "Truth ... that disease is *unreal*." Because matter "is a false mode of consciousness," sickness, evil, and death are only mistaken interpretations of reality created by our fallible mortal minds. When human beings fail to transcend the tendency to believe in matter, they mistakenly believe they are vulnerable to sickness, evil, and death. By steeping their daily thoughts in the principles of Christian Science, believers would elevate their minds above such errors.

Health seekers might not subscribe wholeheartedly to her metaphysics, but many became devoted followers after finding physical and spiritual relief though Christian Science healings. Eddy established the Massachusetts Metaphysical College in Boston in 1881 and many graduates found a profitable vocation as full-time Christian Science healers. Although Christian Scientists have demanded payments from insurance companies for their practitioners, they have lobbied intensively to exempt members of the church from medical legislation, such as compulsory vaccination for school children. Some members of the church have been charged with involuntary manslaughter or child endangerment for refusing to obtain conventional medical treatment for sick children.

Christian Science can be viewed as a particularly striking example of the putative relationship between religious doctrines and human health. Followers of Christian Science argue, however, that their practice is quite different from "faith healing" in Protestant and Catholic traditions. Christian Science healings exclude appeals to saints and symbolic acts just as strictly as they forbid the use of drugs and surgery. Nevertheless, the success of Christian Science stimulated other churches to establish ministries featuring religious therapeutics. The success of the health messages transmitted by Ellen White and Mary Baker Eddy might be seen as a resurrection of the healing role assumed by clergymen in Colonial America. Christian Science and Seventh Day Adventism offered views of health and healing that resonated with the search for spiritual and physical health.

John Harvey Kellogg grew up in a devout Seventh Day Adventist family that accepted the "healthy living" tenants advocated by the church. Kellogg had been a sickly child, but at age 14, he read the work of Graham and became a devout vegetarian. Under Ellen White's sponsorship, Kellogg studied at Russell Trall's Hygeio-Therapeutic College before earning a medical degree at New York's Bellevue Medical College. Unlike many vegetarian health crusaders, Kellogg had good credentials in regular medicine and surgery. Despite his enthusiasm for natural healing and his condemnation of conventional drugs, Kellogg was a skillful and innovative surgeon, with a special interest in abdominal surgery, and a member of the American College of Surgeons and the American Medical Association (AMA). During his long career, he performed more than 20,000 operations and published close to 50 books, including *Man the Masterpiece, The Home Hand-book of Domestic Hygiene and Rational Medicine*, which mainly dealt with his theories of "biological living" and the "Battle Creek Idea"—that good health and fitness were the result of good diet, exercise, correct posture, fresh air, and proper rest. Although he died of pneumonia a bit short of his 100-year goal, contemporaries said that at 91 he was still an excellent demonstration of the rewards of simple eating and healthy living.

Kellogg saw the Battle Creek Sanitarium, familiarly known as the "San," as a "University of Health," as well as a hospital and retreat for the rich and famous. John D. Rockefeller, Jr., Henry Ford, J. C. Penny, Montgomery Ward, S. S. Kresge, Richard Byrd, Thomas Edison, Harvey Firestone, Sarah Bernhardt, Amelia Earhart, and President William Howard Taft were among some three hundred thousand patients who came to the San in search of wellness. Kellogg used the San to train doctors, nurses, physical therapists, dietitians, and medical missionaries. A new fireproof San built after a fire destroyed the old building in 1902 accommodated several thousand guests a year. The stock market crash in 1929 had a disastrous impact on the San and Kellogg eventually sold the main building. In the 1940s, the former Sanitarium building was converted into the Percy Jones General and Convalescent Hospital, which served as an orthopedic hospital during World War II and the Korean conflict.

Although best known as a health reformer and proponent of vegetarianism, Kellogg also campaigned throughout his life for sexual temperance. Indeed, some of his critics said that Kellogg was opposed to all forms of sex; some even implied that he found his daily enemas more satisfying than conventional sexual activities. In his essays on the treatment of "self-abuse," Kellogg suggested extreme methods of punishment, such as circumcising boys (without the use of anesthetics). The pain caused by the operation, Kellogg explained, would "have a salutary effect upon the mind." For females who might be experiencing "abnormal excitement," Kellogg recommended applying pure carbolic acid (phenol) to the clitoris. (In a dilute form, carbolic acid is used as a disinfectant and antiseptic. Pure phenol is very caustic.)

A champion of vegetarianism, Kellogg would challenge his audiences: "How can you eat anything that looks out of eyes?" In addition to all the old arguments for vegetarianism, Kellogg shocked visitors to the San with a horror show of the microscopic germs and filth that could be found in meats coming from the slaughter house and warnings about the dire consequences of intestinal autointoxication. This theory was rather like Élie Metchnikoff's (1845–1916) concept of *orthobiosis*, which linked health and longevity to the organs of digestion. According to Metchnikoff, microbial mischief in the large intestine produced harmful fermentations and putrefaction. Intrigued by the possibility that it might be possible to reverse the aging process, Metchnikoff suggested disinfecting the large intestine with a hygienic diet to neutralize the deleterious effect of bacteria harbored by this perfidious and useless organ. Frustrated by evidence that traditional purges and enemas did more damage to the intestines than to the noxious intestinal flora, Metchnikoff recommended the consumption of large quantities of fresh yogurt as a means of introducing beneficial ferments into the digestive system.

Both Kellogg and Metchnikoff were obsessed by the threat of autointoxication, but Kellogg believed that the status of the colon was central to good health. To combat the menace of slow digestion, intestinal parasites, lack of bulk in the diet, intestinal kinks, constipation, and autointoxication, Kellogg advised a diet rich in roughage, bran at each meal, paraffin oil as an intestinal lubricant, and daily enemas. In pursuit of inner hygiene, patients were stuffed with bran cereals and dosed with laxatives, herbal cleansing kits, enemas, and high colonic irrigations. Fear of internal filth and decay, in both the real and the symbolic sense, can be traced back to the time of the Egyptian pharaohs, but Kellogg and other health crusaders embraced the old doctrine with unprecedented enthusiasm. Concern with inner hygiene coincided with growing concerns about urban filth, pollution, and dirt as the cause of epidemic disease. Many health reformers and social critics agreed that constipation was caused by the unnatural pressures associated with modern life in crowded, industrialized cites. In search of solutions to bowel problems, people turned to patent medicines, laxatives, mineral waters, bran cereals, yogurt, electrotherapy, calisthenics, abdominal exercises, enemas, intestinal irrigation, rectal dilation devices, or even surgery to remove intestinal kinks.

To make it possible for his followers to give up meat, Kellogg developed new foods made from grains and nuts. Kellogg held more than 30 patents for food products and processes, primarily health foods and coffee and tea substitutes, as well as exercise, diagnostic and therapeutic machines. He is credited with developing such diverse products as peanut butter, a menthol nasal inhaler, a mechanical horse, and the electric blanket. His ideas about health foods led to the establishment of more than 40 cereal companies that competed with the one established by Kellogg and his younger brother, William Keith Kellogg (1860–1951). In contrast to Dr. Kellogg, W. K. Kellogg lacked any formal education beyond the sixth grade when he was hired to work at the San as clerk, bookkeeper, manager, and assistant in the search for health foods. One of his most profitable discoveries was a process for making cereal flakes as opposed to the usual health food granules.

Entrepreneurs quickly copied the Kellogg process and over 40 rival food companies were soon selling their own ready-to-eat cereals. One of the most successful was established by Charles William Post (1855–1914) in 1895. Suffering from ulcers and other problems, Post came to the San because he was attracted to vegetarianism and the Adventist prohibitions on stimulants like coffee. Hoping to find a new highway to health after Kellogg's methods failed to cure him, Post turned to Christian Science. Convinced that coffee was a dangerous stimulant, Post developed and successfully marketed a replacement made of wheat, molasses, and bran that he called Postum. He also developed Grape Nuts and Post Toasties. Unfortunately, although Post made a fortune from health foods, neither vegetarianism nor Christian Science could cure his physical and spiritual ills, as indicated by his unsuccessful battle with depression and his suicide at the age of 59.

Dietary reformers advocated bizarre diets or fasts of every possible type, but it was Horace Fletcher (1849–1919), the "Great Masticator" and author of *Menticulture, or the A-B-C of True Living*, *The New Glutton or Epicure*, *The A.B.-Z. of Our Own Nutrition*, and *Optimism*, who tried to teach all of them how to actually eat their food. At age 40, the formerly robust and athletic Fletcher found himself suffering from dyspepsia, fatigue, obesity, and frequent bouts of influenza. Determined to regain his health, Fletcher turned to the study of hygiene and launched a new career as a health reformer. Through self-experimentation, he discovered that thorough chewing of each bite of food led to complete digestion, weight loss, strength, endurance, and perfect health. Of course, Fletcher was not the first to call attention to the American habit of eating too rapidly. In *Lectures on Life and Health*, William Alcott had ridiculed this vile habit and Sylvester Graham, Ellen White, and other health reformers had urged slower eating. In addition to promoting Fletcherism, or the "chew-chew" cult, Fletcher wrote and lectured on the importance of Menticulture, a system of positive thinking that would create Physiologic Optimism, fitness, and freedom from nervous exhaustion and neurasthenia.

By the end of the nineteenth century, the idealism of the health reform movement was increasingly subsumed by the entrepreneurial spirit of men like Bernarr Macfadden (1868–1955), self-proclaimed Professor of Kinesitherapy and Father of Physical Culture. According to Macfadden, Physical Culture would produce better as well as stronger people. Indeed, his magazine *Physical Culture* carried the motto "Weakness Is a Crime." In contrast to the sexual repression taught by Alcott, Graham, and Kellogg, Macfadden's writings, including his five-volume *Encyclopedia of Physical Culture*, glorified virility and healthy sexuality. His health advice appeared in *Building of Vital Power; Deep Breathing and a Complete System for Strengthening the Heart, Lungs, Stomach and All the Great Vital Organs*, *Constipation, Its Cause, Effect and Treatment*, *Fasting for Health*, *Home Health Manual*, and *The Virile Powers of Superb Manhood*.

The indefatigable Macfadden also published movie, romance, and detective magazines, including *True Story, True Confessions, True Detective*, and newspapers, and sponsored contests to select the World's most perfectly developed man. Charles Atlas (Angelo Siciliano, 1892–1972), former 97-pound weakling, who won the contest in 1922, claimed that he had transformed himself with "dynamic tension" exercises he invented after watching a lion at the zoo. By 1927 Charles Atlas, Ltd. was a very profitable enterprise—selling mail-order physical culture courses.

## DOMESTIC MEDICINE

Most families in Colonial America relied on their own resources or local healers and herbalists rather than professional physicians. Domestic medicine was preferred to imported drugs, which were either unavailable or expensive. Those who wanted to avoid doctors, or had no access to healers, depended on traditional remedies, popular herbals, and self-help books for information on how to maintain health and deal with illness and injuries. For example, *Every Man His Own Doctor: or, the Poor Planter's Physician* (1734) was written anonymously by John Tennent (ca. 1700–1760), a Virginia physician, who denounced other doctors for their exorbitant fees and for prescribing remedies that were as bad as the disease. Despite the attacks of fellow physicians, he offered advice, not for those who could afford "learned Advice," but for the poor, who needed to find the "cheapest and easiest ways of getting well again." The marshes and swamps of Virginia, he warned, generated many fevers, coughs, quinsies, pleurisies, consumptions, and other plagues. In addition to descriptions of the symptoms of each disease, Tennent provided advice on diet, prevention, and medicines. Some of his suggestions for preventing sore throat and similar disorders were as simple as washing the neck and behind the ears in cold water every morning, but other conditions required bleeding, blistering, poultices, syrup of peach blossoms, or even pills made of turpentine and "Deers Dung." Because the book was written for those who could not afford to "dye by the Hand of a Doctor," Tennent deliberately avoided references to mercury, opium, and Peruvian bark.

Many books offered advice to mothers about the health of their family and the physical and mental development of their children. Catharine Beecher (1800–1878), founder of the Hartford Female Seminary, advocated exercise and dress reform based on the science of physiology. The curriculum at Hartford Female Seminary included calisthenics and physical education. In *Suggestions Respecting Improvements in Education* (1829), Beecher insisted that the health and well being of children depended on teaching women about anatomy and physiology so that they would understand how diet, air, exercise, and modes of dress affect the body and promote good health. "The *restoration* of health is the physician's profession," Beecher explained, but preserving the health of children was primarily the responsibility of women.

By the end of the twentieth century, prestigious healthcare institutions and professional organizations were meeting the growing demand for domestic medical guides. Such texts include *The American Medical Association Family Medical Guide, Mayo Clinic Family Health Book, Johns Hopkins Family Health Book, Harvard Medical School Family Health Guide, American College of Physicians Complete Home*

*Medical Guide*, and *The Merck Manual of Medical Information: Home Edition*. In contrast to Tennent's 70-page pamphlet, modern guides to domestic medicine may approach 2,000 pages of advice on acute and chronic diseases, drugs, alternative medicine, medicinal herbs and nutraceuticals, diseases of unknown origin, death and dying, nutrition, and popular weight-loss diets.

Eighteenth-century Americans were actively involved in all aspects of medical practice, prevention, diagnosis, and treatment. By the onset of the Civil War, the influence of medical experts, whether orthodox or sectarian, on the management of disease was increasing. That is, practitioners were claiming professional privilege and expertise in the treatment of disease and warning potential patients and caregivers to defer to professionals. Many orthodox physicians believed that the widespread dissemination of information about diagnosing and treating disease increased the production and influence of competitors, such as Thomsonians, health reformers, homeopaths, and hydropaths. When writing health texts for laymen, regular physicians provided general guidance, but insisted that the management of disease required a well-qualified physician. The role of the patient was reduced to calling for a doctor and carefully following his advice. As sectarian practice became more organized and professional, they too advised patients to call for the expert.

## MEDICAL SECTS

The first wave of medical sectarianism in nineteenth-century America included Hydropaths, Thomsonians, Eclectics, Physio-Medicalists, Eclectics, and Homeopaths. Despite differences in their medical theories and therapeutic systems, members of these sects agreed that the allopaths, or so-called regular doctors, were the most dangerous quacks of all. Unorthodox practitioners saw themselves as reformers, healers, revolutionaries, professionals, and members of new philosophical schools, not as members of cults or sects. The true test of any medical system, they argued, should be patient satisfaction, especially in the case of chronic illnesses where allopaths had already failed. Critics of orthodox medicine argued that medical licensing laws infringed the rights of Americans to make their own decisions about health and healing.

Samuel Thomson (1769–1843), a New Hampshire farmer, created a system of medicine based on herbal remedies as substitutes for the harsh drugs prescribed by orthodox doctors, especially those that contained mercury, arsenic, antimony, and other toxic chemicals. Rejecting the therapeutics and the authority of regular physicians, Thomson became one of the most influential healers in America during the 1820s to the 1830s. Adopting what he called a wholly empirical approach,

Thomson advertised his system as the product of the "study of patients, not books—experience, not reading."

According to Thomson, he became an authority on herbal remedies by studying the methods of an old woman who practiced herbal medicine in rural New Hampshire, free of competition by any so-called real doctors. After losing loved ones to a combination of disease and the damage done by orthodox physicians, Thomson decided to abandon farming and became an itinerant botanical doctor. In his autobiography, Thomson noted that orthodox doctors called him a quack, but he asked: "which is the greatest quack, the one who relieves them from their sickness by the most simple and safe means... or the one who, instead of curing the disease, increases it by poisonous medicines which only tend to prolong the distresses of the patient, till ... death relieves him?" Unlike regular doctors who insisted on bleeding and purging with calomel and other dangerous drugs, Thomson offered a system that was cheap, safe, and easy to use. Following his system helped in avoiding the expense of consulting a doctor and the embarrassment of having male physicians examine female patients. While Thomson's remedies were not revolutionary, his marketing strategy was innovative and quite lucrative. By the early 1830s, millions of rural Americans were using his system and reading his books.

Basically, Thomson prescribed botanical substances and steam baths. Despite his empirical orientation, Thomson did express a simple theory of healing, which involved increasing internal and external bodily heat in order to eliminate disease. His botanical remedies included lobelia, a botanical emetic that cleansed the stomach and induced perspiration; cayenne pepper and steam baths to restore bodily heat; teas made from various roots, barks, and berries to improve the digestion; and botanical tonics made with wine or brandy to strengthen the patient. Followers of Thomsonism were taught to use a kit containing six numbered remedies that were given in a predetermined sequence. Thomson also gave practical advice about healthy living, and the harm caused by tainted meats and excessive alcohol consumption.

The first of many editions of Thomson's *New Guide to Health; or, Botanic Family Physician, Containing a Complete System of Practice, including A Narrative of the Life and Medical Discoveries of Samuel Thomson* was published in 1822. Some editions included the phrase *Learned Quackery Exposed* in the title. Before buying the book, subscribers had to purchase the "right" to a copy of the book and membership in a local Friendly Botanic Society. Members of Friendly Botanic Societies pledged to use the Thomsonian system and help other members "in times of need." Calling attention to the clear, simple language used in his book, Thomson warned readers against the deadly poisons prescribed in a dead language by regular doctors who deliberately used obscure Latin terminology in an attempt to confuse and intimidate simple people.

In many states, Thomsonism competed very successfully with regular medicine, but success led to the proliferation of agents marketing the authentic system, as well as the appearance of imitators and competitors. Some regular physicians surreptitiously adopted the Thomsonian system and unauthorized agents marketed drugs that were not approved by Thomson. Thomson fought to retain his vision of lay practice as a self-help movement, but the original system was subverted by "expert" practitioners who established their own drug regimens, established private clinics, trained students and apprentices, and warned patients against treating disease on their own. Thomsonism split into warring factions and no national conventions were held after 1838. By the 1840s, the Thomsonian movement had been fragmented and overshadowed by vigorous new competitors.

New sects known as physio-medicalists and eclectics adopted Thomson's botanic medicines and his condemnation of orthodox drugs, but in contrast to Samuel Thomson, members of these sects considered themselves professional physicians by virtue of their doctrines, education, schools, and professional journals. Alva Curtis (1797–1881), founder of physio-medicalism, was a botanical practitioner who attempted to compete with both Thomsonians and regular doctors by establishing a new professional identity. The first physio-medical school was founded in Columbus, Ohio, in 1836. Additional physio-medical colleges were established in Alabama, Georgia, Massachusetts, New York, Tennessee, and Virginia, but all of these schools disappeared by 1911.

The fundamental philosophy that united this otherwise contentious sect was the ancient belief in the body's inherent "vital force" or "internal physician." Physio-medicalists claimed that their botanical remedies enhanced the body's own healing force. Allopathic mineral drugs, those used by regular physicians, were condemned as dangerous and unnatural poisons. These fundamental principles were adopted by the Reformed Medical Association of the United States and the American Association of Physio-Medical Physicians and Surgeons. In addition to his lectures on medical science and botanical drugs, Curtis explained the advantages of physio-medicalism over other systems in his book *A Fair Examination and Criticism of All the Medical Systems in Vogue.* He also published responses to "provocation" from regular practitioners. Although the physio-medicalists constituted only a small fraction of American medical practitioners, and their medical schools were academically inferior, physio-medicalists demanded the right to compete for positions with the army and navy, as well as representation on state licensing and regulatory boards.

Wooster Beach (1794–1868), the founder of eclectic medicine, had no direct ties to Thomsonism, but he had studied with a botanical healer and published a book on domestic medicine. Beach considered himself a professional botanical physician, because he attended a medical school in New York and held a license issued by the county medical society. In *The American Practice of Medicine* (1833), Beach contended that the practice of orthodox medicine was "pernicious and dangerous to the extreme." The whole *materia medica* of orthodox medicine consisted of a few poisonous minerals that did more damage to the human body than the diseases for which they were prescribed. Eclectism, in contrast, was a philosophical school of thought that called for the reform of medicine. The new botanical medicine, according to Beach, was based on "immutable and eternal principles of truth." The principles of eclectic medicine had been proved by experiments, observation, and facts deduced from clinical practice. Texts published by eclectics included pathology, symptomatology, diagnosis, prognosis, and comparisons of the remedies used by allopathists, homoeopathists, hydropathists, and eclectics.

In 1830, Beach and several colleagues organized a medical college in Worthington, Ohio, that claimed to be the first chartered, degree-granting botanical medical school in the United States. Although Beach believed that the new school would establish a scientific foundation for botanical medicine, he called his therapeutic system "eclectic," because it lacked a unique medical philosophy. By the time the school closed in 1839, because of a dissection riot, it had graduated almost 100 eclectic physicians. The Eclectic Medical Institute in Cincinnati, Ohio, which was chartered in 1845, was the most important and successful eclectic school. By 1892 there were 10 eclectic medical schools. The curriculum of the eclectic schools was basically the same as that of orthodox medical schools. Courses included anatomy, pathology, materia medica, surgery, and obstetrics. Despite some resistance, eclectic schools were more willing to admit female students than regular medical schools.

As suggested by their name, eclectics adopted a flexible approach to therapeutics, although they emphasized remedies derived from native plants and new forms of so-called concentrated medicines, and categorically rejected bloodletting. Eclectics were fairly successful in competition with physio-medicalists and Thomsonians, but the sect remained small compared to regular medicine and homeopathy. Nevertheless, at the beginning of the twentieth century, the National Eclectic Medical Association had chapters in 32 states. John M. Scudder (1829–1894), a professor at the Eclectic Medical Institute, John Uri Lloyd (1849–1936), and others, attempted to elevate the status of Eclecticism by publishing textbooks and professional journals, developing new remedies, and improving the standardization of eclectic drugs. Their efforts failed and the Eclectic Medical Institute, the last eclectic school, closed in 1939. The Lloyd Library founded by John Uri Lloyd and his brothers, however, retains a valuable collection of books in phytopharmacy and its history. Despite the demise of eclecticism, Lloyd became a very successful pharmacologist and manufacturer of pharmaceuticals. Lloyd served as president of the American Pharmaceutical Association and was credited with helping to secure passage of the National Pure Food and Drug Act of 1906. A prolific author of works of fiction and nonfiction, Lloyd's books included *A Systematic Treatise on Materia Medica and Therapeutics, Dynamical Therapeutics*, and a study of the herb *Echinacea angustifolia* (which still is popular for colds and flu).

Homeopathy, one of the most successful of the nineteenth-century medical sects, was founded by the German physician Christian Friedrich Samuel Hahnemann (1755–1843). Although Hahnemann was a respected doctor and chemist, he withdrew from medical practice because of his conviction that conventional therapies were dangerous and ineffective. It was only in 1796 when he discovered his new system of healing, based on the principle *similia similibus curantur*—"like cures like"—that he felt capable of resuming his vocation. In 1810, Hahnemann published the first edition of his *Organon of Medicine*, which described the fundamental principles of homeopathy. In response to attacks on his system, Hahnemann published a *Defense of the Organon of Rational Medicine*.

"The physician's high and *only* mission," Hahnemann said in the *Organon*, "is to restore the sick to health." A true science of medicine must be built upon experience and advanced by "due attention to nature by means of our senses, by careful honest observations and by experiments." It was through his own experiments, using drugs of the highest degree of purity possible, that he discovered the principles of homeopathy. According to Hahnemann, when drugs are given to healthy people in large doses, they produce certain effects that are like the symptoms of disease in sick people. Hahnemann called his experimental program of testing drugs and determining what symptoms or effects they caused in healthy subjects "proving" the drug. The symptoms exhibited by patients were carefully noted, so that they could be given small doses of drugs known to produce the same symptoms.

In essence, Hahnemann's system of medical treatment was based upon the assumption that disease is not wrong but right action, that nature was doing its best, and that medicine should be given to help the body by increasing the existing symptoms instead of changing them. Hahnemann also believed that the less he helped or interfered with nature the better. Therefore, as soon as medicine had increased the existing symptoms, he stopped giving medicine. Hahnemann argued that members of the old school were simply members of a dangerous sect that practiced *allopathic medicine*, that is, treatment by opposites. In other words, allopaths belonged to a sect that believed in treating diseases with remedies that produce effects different from those caused by the disease itself. If true quacks existed, Hahnemann argued, they were practitioners who championed allopathic medical theories and methods.

In a scathing attack on the "old school," Hahnemann denounced allopathic medicine as "a pure nullity, a pitiable self-deception, eminently fitted to imperil human life by its methods of treatment." Allopathic doctors attacked the body with large and frequent doses of powerful medicines given as complex mixtures, including dangerous emetics, purgatives, sialagogues, diuretics, caustics, and then compounded the damages by massive bloodlettings that further weakened their unfortunate patients. As a result, in addition to the original disease, the body developed "new and often ineradicable medicinal diseases."

Allopaths had constructed "so-called systems" out of empty speculations about the unknowable nature of vital processes and the origin of diseases within the living organism. But, Hahnemann insisted that the physician could not expect to see the vital force or spiritual being that produced disease. For the homeopathic physician, the signs and symptoms presented to the senses constituted the "true and only conceivable portrait of the disease." By removing all the symptoms, the homeopath destroyed the internal, hidden cause of the disease. Ignoring the symptoms, allopaths engaged in a futile search for the hidden primary cause of disease. The goal of homeopathy, in contrast, was the complete annihilation of the disease by means of a cure that was rapid, gentle, reliable, and harmless. In order to determine the proper drugs and dosage, the homeopathic physician had to carefully assess the "physical constitution of the patient, his moral and intellectual character, his occupation, mode of living and habits, his social and domestic relations, his age, sexual function," and so forth.

The first law of homeopathy was the law of similars. The second fundamental principle was the law of infinitesimals. Because the sick were extremely sensitive to drugs, the homeopathic physician never used crude, undiluted drugs. To eliminate the possibility that even a small dose of the drug would aggravate the patient's symptoms, Hahnemann carried out a series of dilutions. In order to maintain the potency of the drug after dilutions that ordinary chemists thought would eliminate any trace of the original substance, Hahnemann diluted his preparations by a series of steps that he claimed reduced toxicity and increased the healing properties of his "high potency" dilutions. Each time he diluted his preparation he submitted it to a powerful series of shakes or succussions. According to Hahnemann, this process liberated the "essence" or "idea" of the drug from its inert material base or "substance." Drugs were diluted or attenuated by mixture with water, alcohol, or milk sugar, which according to painstaking provings were neutral substances.

Advocates of Natural Hygiene, naturopathy, and other drugless sects, preferred homeopathy to allopathy, but said that Hahnemann's theoretical basis was flawed because he assumed that medicines could help nature and cure disease. Naturopathy is the treatment of illness by "properly arranging the intake of foods," in order to eliminate toxins from the body and "build normal cells, blood, tissues, and secretions." Naturopaths do not use drugs for either healing or preventing disease. They attempt to establish a "health environment" through diet and proper mental attitude. In practice, homeopaths used such infinitesimal doses of drugs that they were unlikely to pose any danger to the patient. Allopaths and chemists ridiculed the claims made for the efficacy of extreme dilutions. Cynics proposed a homeopathic chicken soup recipe for particularly sensitive invalids, which was made by allowing the shadow of a chicken to fall into a pot of water.

Exploiting dissatisfaction with the harsh remedies of regular doctors, homeopaths enjoyed a tremendous wave of popularity in the United States. Epidemic diseases provided numerous opportunities for homeopaths to emphasize the safety and efficacy of their therapeutic system and the dangers of allopathic methods. According to homeopathic physicians Dr. William Holcombe and Dr. F. A. W. Davis, during a yellow fever epidemic in Natchez in 1835, only 33 of their patients died, while 430 died under the care of orthodox doctors. When homeopaths were put in charge of the Mississippi State Hospital in Natchez in 1854, they increased survival among their patients by forbidding the use of bloodletting, purgatives, calomel, blisters, and other allopathic methods.

Constantine Hering (1800–1880), one of the first homeopaths in America, established a successful practice and converted some allopaths to the new therapeutic system. Hering introduced an American edition of *Samuel Hahnemann's Organon of Homoeopathic Medicine*, which was issued under the auspices of the North American Academy of the Homoeopathic Healing Art, Allentown, PA. He also published *A Concise View of the Rise and Progress of Homoeopathic Medicine, Condensed Materia Medica*, and other works on the materia medica of homeopathic medicine.

When the Homeopathic Medical College of Pennsylvania was founded in 1848 most of the faculty members were graduates of regular medical schools who had adopted homeopathy. Disagreements within the faculty led to the creation of the rival Hahnemann Medical College, but the two schools merged in 1869. At the beginning of the twentieth century, there were about 40 homeopathic medical colleges in America, as well as homeopathic hospitals, dispensaries, medical societies, medical journals, and physicians, including many female practitioners. By the 1920s, however, only two homeopathic medical schools were still in existence. The successful development of bacteriology, pathology, physiology, and pharmacology tended to erode support for homeopathic theory. Hahnemann Medical College survived by modernizing its curriculum, abandoning the teaching of homeopathy, and eventually merging with the Medical College of Pennsylvania; the new entity was renamed the Allegheny University of the Health Sciences.

Women—as patients, advocates, and practitioners—played an important role in the growth and dissemination of homeopathic medicine among middle and upper class families. Popular female writers, such as Elizabeth Stuart Phelps (1844–1911), incorporated homeopathy into their work. Phelps, who said her personal causes were "Heaven, homeopathy, and women's rights," explored the affinity between women and homeopathy in her novel *Doctor Zay*. The protagonist of the novel was a female homeopathic doctor, Dr. Zaidee Atalanta Lloyd, a Vassar graduate with three years of medical school and one year of study abroad. Clearly, Dr. Lloyd was more highly educated and more sensitive to her patients than her allopathic rivals and detractors. Nevertheless, homeopathy did not always welcome female practitioners. In 1867, the American Institute of Homeopathy (AIH) rejected a woman's application for membership, but two years later the AIH voted to accept all candidates, male or female, who wanted to learn and practice homeopathy. Members of the AMA, which did not admit women until 1915, argued that the strong bonds between women and sectarian medicine provided further proof that women were unsuited to become physicians.

Some physicians were unsure where quackery pure and simple ended and eccentricity and innovation began, but Oliver Wendell Holmes (1809–1894) was sure he could tell the difference between true medicine and the "delusions" of homeopathy and other deadly errors that appealed to the fatal credulity of the public. While insisting on the superiority of orthodox medicine, Holmes admitted that probably 90 percent of the patients a physician might see would recover, sooner or later, if nature were not thwarted in effecting a cure. Therefore, he concluded, nature healed and the doctor claimed the credit and the fee. Holmes also famously declared that if all medicines, with a few important exceptions, were thrown into the sea, it would be better for humankind and worse for the fishes. Although William Alcott, John Harvey Kellogg, Wooster Beach, Andrew Taylor Still, and Samuel Hahnemann had credible medical credentials, despite their "delusions," Holmes charged the leaders of competing medical sects with misrepresenting themselves and their systems, claiming inventions and ideas that others had made, lying about their education and training, and other high crimes and misdemeanors.

Despite the disappearance of homeopathic medical schools, homeopathy remained popular in some populations and interest surged by the end of the twentieth century with the rising popularity of holistic and alternative medicine. Some states passed laws that gave certain alternative practitioners—homeopaths, acupuncturists, chiropractors, naturopaths, and so forth—equal status with traditional medicine for purposes of insurance reimbursement. A new homeopathy emerged

which emphasized spiritual and holistic doctrines rather than Hahnemann's principles of similars and infinitesimals.

Hahnemann's doctrine that the innermost workings of the body can
never be known and his rejection of the so-called reductionist doctrine
of specific diseases resonated with the belief that holistic homeopaths
treat the whole patient, while reductionists treat diseases. Purists object
to the use of homeopathy as a slogan applied to various preparations
sold in drug stores and health food stores. Nevertheless, like their
nineteenth-century predecessors, advocates of homeopathy and holistic
medicine seem to be calling for the breakdown of boundaries between
regular, reductionist medicine, and alternative practices.


## OSTEOPATHS AND CHIROPRACTORS

Andrew Taylor Still (1828–1917), the founder of osteopathy, was born
in Virginia, but his father, a Methodist minister, was assigned to frontier
communities in the Midwest. Like the early colonial preachers, Abram
Still attended to both the physical and spiritual needs of his people.
Although Andrew Still later claimed that he had attended medical
school in Kansas City and served as a surgeon during the Civil War,
he apparently became a doctor by assisting his father and reading textbooks. Following the example of Vesalius, Still furthered his knowledge
of anatomy by dissecting various animals and stealing bodies from
burial grounds. After three of his children died of spinal meningitis, Still
became profoundly dissatisfied with orthodox medicine. Religion, experience, and sectarian practitioners contributed to his belief that conventional drugs were dangerous and addictive. But he did not find the
rationale for contemporary alternatives to orthodox medicine entirely
convincing until he began to envision a connection between magnetic
healing and his studies of human mechanics. The body, he concluded,
was a machine through which invisible magnetic fluid flowed. Disease
was the result of disturbances or obstructions that interfered with the
normal healthy movement of this essential fluid. It should, therefore,
be possible to cure disease by restoring the harmonious flow of magnetic
fluid within the human machine.

In search of a new approach to medicine, Still came to the
conclusion that a just and loving God would have created the necessary
remedies for human sickness and suffering. In order to be sure that remedies were available when needed, God would have put all the remedies
that human beings would ever need within the body. What Still then discovered, at least to his own satisfaction, was osteopathy—an infallible
method of adjusting the mechanism of the body so that the pre-existing
remedies became available. By adjusting the bones, Still could cure disease without drugs. He experimented with various names for his new

approach to healing before discarding Magnetic Healer, Human Engineer, and Lightning Bone Setter. He finally decided to call his new science of natural healing *osteopathy*. Some critics, however, considered his manipulations a form of faith healing or the "laying on of hands."

Of course, Still did not invent the idea that the human body works like a machine, but he was ingenious in linking osteopathy to the popular concept of the "human motor." According to Still, osteopathy was a system for "engineering the whole machinery of life." The mechanical principle of leverage—manipulating bones as levers to relieve pressure on nerves and blood vessels—was the basis of osteopathic practice. Still compared the interdependence of all bodily organs to a great labor union. The body's parts "belong to the brotherhood of labor" and, when the body was healthy, they worked together perfectly and harmoniously, but if one member of the union was mistreated, the body as a whole was affected. At that point, osteopathy was needed to relieve pain and restore health by adjustments and manipulations that led to the proper integration of the body's structural components. Allopaths often described the female body as inherently weak and prone to sickness, in addition to pathological states, such as menstruation, pregnancy, labor, birth, and menopause. In contrast, osteopaths argued that the basic cause of disease was the same for men and women: mechanical displacements and the maladjustment of body parts.

In 1892, Still opened the American School of Osteopathy in Kirksville, Missouri, the first school to offer courses in osteopathic manipulative techniques, in addition to traditional classes in anatomy, diagnostics, chemistry, and so forth. Of the original class of 21 students, 5 were female. According to the Osteopathic Women's National Association, female students were welcome at osteopathic schools and female graduates practiced successfully in many states. As osteopaths incorporated bacteriology, pharmacology, and other aspects of regular medicine, divisions developed between practitioners who remained close to Andrew Still's views and those who adopted new theories, methods, and remedies. Nevertheless, osteopaths retained a general allegiance to the founder's doctrines and manipulative methods. Despite opposition from orthodox practitioners, osteopaths retained their independence and by the end of the 1970s had become legally eligible for unlimited practice licenses—as D.O.s—in every state. No longer in danger of being labeled quacks and cultists, osteopaths were transformed into members of a "parallel profession" struggling to avoid losing its unique identity.

By the end of the nineteenth century, as osteopaths gained a measure of professional recognition, they found themselves battling both medical doctors and "osteopathic imitators." Just as regular doctors tried to prosecute osteopaths for practicing medicine without a license, osteopaths charged their competitors with practicing unlicensed osteopathy. The most numerous and successful competitors, who called themselves chiropractors, argued that they were not practicing medicine or osteopathy. Chiropractic was founded by Daniel David Palmer (1845–1913). Canadian-born Palmer had been an itinerant tradesman and teacher before he settled down in Davenport, Iowa. An obsessive interest in human health and disease led him to experiment with spiritualism, phrenology, and osteopathy before he began to practice magnetic healing, which skeptics considered a crude form of hypnotism. Palmer became convinced that there must be one specific cause of disease and, therefore, one true method of healing.

In 1895, Palmer was sure that he had discovered the key to health and healing. According to Palmer's account of this landmark event, when he examined Harvey Lillard, who had been deaf for 17 years, he discovered a subluxated (misaligned) vertebra. By applying pressure to Lillard's spine and adjusting the vertebral column, Palmer reduced the subluxation and restored Lillard's hearing almost instantly. Examining a patient with heart trouble, Palmer found another subluxation and successfully cured this patient by adjusting the spine. Just as displaced bones caused painful bunions and corns, Palmer reasoned, luxated bones in the spine must press against nerves, increasing vibration, creating tension and heat, altering tissue, modifying nerve impulses and causing abnormal functions in the affected tissues and organs. Palmer then constructed his own anatomical charts of the relationship between spinal nerves and the organs and tissues they affected and began treating a variety of problems, including heart disease, asthma, kidney problems, and cancer.

One of Palmer's satisfied patients suggested the name *chiropractic*, from the Greek *cheiro* and *praktikos*, for "done by hand" to designate Palmer's new system of treatment. Chiropractic theory ascribed disease to a deficiency of nerve function caused by spinal misalignment or subluxation. The line of reasoning developed by Palmer was remarkably similar to that recounted by Andrew Taylor Still, the founder of osteopathy. Palmer reasoned that the body had its own supply of natural healing power and that this power was transmitted throughout the body by the nervous system. If a specific organ did not receive its proper nerve supply, it would become sick. Like osteopathy, chiropractic was a way of providing relief and healing through physical manipulation of the spinal column and other body structures.

Palmer provided very specific details about his theory of disease and the effects of chiropractic manipulation, but many modern practitioners prefer to avoid scientific arguments and simply say that there is empirical evidence that chiropractic works, although understanding the physiological effects of spinal manipulation requires more research. One all-purpose explanation that is used to explain a myriad of therapies, conventional and unconventional, is that treatment may affect the release of chemicals that influence pain and pleasure sensations, such as substance P and endorphins.

In 1906, Palmer and several colleagues were jailed and fined for practicing medicine without a license. A year later, one of Palmer's former students was arrested in Wisconsin for practicing medicine, surgery, and osteopathy without a license, but the judge and jury agreed that he was not practicing medicine, surgery, and osteopathy—he was practicing chiropractic. Chiropractors fought hard, state by state, to secure limited medical practice licensing. Although practitioners with such licenses are called "doctor," the scope of their practice does not include the whole range of functions and activities granted to medical doctors. Podiatrists, for example, have limited practice licensing by virtue of their scope of practice, not their fundamental philosophy. A license that prohibits prescribing drugs or performing surgery is not a troublesome restriction for chiropractors, because these activities are not part of chiropractic. In 1913, Kansas became the first state to license chiropractors. Currently, all 50 states have statutes recognizing and regulating the practice of chiropractic.

In 1897, Daniel David Palmer offered the first classes in chiropractic medicine at the Palmer School and Cure, later known as the Palmer Infirmary and Chiropractic Institute. Palmer's son, Bartlett Joshua Palmer (1881–1961), was one of the school's first students and instructors. Many rival schools opened and closed, but none could compete with "the Fountainhead " established by the Palmers. Although Bartlett Joshua always claimed total confidence in the theory and efficacy of chiropractic, his critics noted that he went to medical doctors when he was sick and X-rays of his spine allegedly revealed "advanced degenerative arthritis with marked curvature."

In chiropractic tradition, D. D. Palmer is known as "The Discoverer," Bartlett Joshua as "The Developer," and David D. Palmer (1906–1978) as "The Educator." Bartlett Joshua was a successful businessman and the school, which he described as a business that "manufactured chiropractors," flourished under his administration. Bartlett Joshua's wife, Mabel Heath Palmer (1881–1949), another Palmer graduate, taught anatomy and served as the treasurer of the School. Bartlett Joshua was particularly interested in the mysterious X-rays that had been discovered in 1895, the year in which his father discovered chiropractic adjustment. Chiropractors were soon using X-ray machines to create pictures of the spine as part of the search for subluxations.

Since chiropractic became successful, there have been ideological divisions within the field. Chiropractors who objected to any methods other than spinal adjustments were called "straights." Those who employ additional methods—such as nutritional therapy, massage, colonic irrigation, and even drugs—were called "mixers." In reality, however, chiropractors have embraced a spectrum of beliefs rather than two separate and distinct schools of thought. Many chiropractors give advice on diet, nutrition, and exercise. Most visits to chiropractors are for musculoskeletal complaints, and almost half are for back pain. Diagnostic procedures such as X-ray, computed tomography, magnetic resonance imaging, and thermography may be used, followed by treatment with ice packs, heat packs, massage, guided movement, friction, traction, electrical current, ultrasound therapy, and Rolfing. Not all practitioners of Rolfing (also known as structural integration or somatic ontology), the technique developed by Ida P. Rolf (1896–1979), are chiropractors, but Rolfers also believe that health problems are caused by misalignments.

Rolf earned a Ph.D. in Biological Chemistry from Columbia University, New York, in 1920. After 12 years at the Rockefeller Institute, Rolf went to Europe where she studied homeopathic medicine. Disillusioned by orthodox medicine, Rolf experimented with osteopathy, chiropractic, yoga, and other healing techniques before developing her own approach, which she called structural integration. According to Rolf, stiffness and thickening of the tissues surrounding the muscles lead to musculoskeletal dysfunction and misalignment of the body. Rolfing involves deep tissue massage, which is supposed to relieve stress and improve mobility, posture, balance, muscle function and efficiency, energy, and overall well being.

According to chiropractors, since D. D. Palmer opened his first school, the AMA selected chiropractic as a prime target of ridicule and harassment. Despite attempts by the medical profession to portray chiropractic theory as "voodoo or witchcraft" or a "scientific fairy tale" and the profession as a form of "licensed medical superstition," chiropractors have enjoyed considerable success in the healthcare marketplace. Some chiropractors have attempted to provide scientific evidence that spinal adjustment is effective in the treatment of various conditions, but, for the most part, support for chiropractic has come from testimonials rather than controlled clinical trials or animal experiments. Chiropractors have reported treating migraine and tension headaches, low back pain, herniated lumbar disks, neck pain, asthma, carpal tunnel syndrome, ulcers, fibromyalgia, colic, jet lag, bed-wetting, AIDS-HIV, whiplash, and so forth, but the results of clinical studies have been ambiguous. Outside the chiropractic community, the safety, as well as the effectiveness of spinal manipulative therapy remains controversial. Critics warn of increased risk of stroke, bleeding, and blood clots in the spine, fractures, nerve damage, muscle strains, sprains, spasms, and the risks of postponing conventional treatment for life-threatening diseases. Skeptics note that chiropractors are unlikely to win support from scientists and physicians when they insist that even cancer is caused by nerve blockage, or that manipulation affects "bio-energetic synchronization" or the flow of the "life forces" that heal the body, and that germ theory is wrong or irrelevant.

When Congress passed the Medicare Act in 1967, it asked the Secretary of the Department of Health Education and Welfare (HEW) to study the question of whether certain types of practitioners who were not medical doctors should be included in the program. HEW's report, entitled "Independent Practitioners Under Medicare," recommended against the inclusion of chiropractors and naturopaths. In 1971, the Director of the AMA Department of Investigation and the Secretary of its Committee on Quackery (COQ), submitted a memo to the AMA Board of Trustees stating that the Committee's prime mission was to contain the cult of chiropractic and, ultimately, to eliminate it. The AMA fought coverage of chiropractic under Medicare law, and the recognition of any chiropractic accrediting agency by the U.S. Office of Education. The Council on Chiropractic Education (CCE) adopted national standards in 1974, which are now recognized by the U.S. Department of Education. Since 1975, the CCE has accredited all U.S. chiropractic colleges and Medicare has reimbursed for chiropractic since 1972.

After chiropractors filed and won a series of antitrust lawsuits against the AMA from the 1970s to the 1980s, the AMA has generally censored its references to chiropractic, at least in public. A lawsuit initiated in 1976 against the AMA, the American College of Radiology, the American College of Surgeons, and other critics, charged the defendants with conspiring to destroy chiropractic and illegally depriving chiropractors of access to laboratory, X-ray, and hospital facilities. In 1987, a federal court judge ruled that the AMA had engaged in an illegal boycott.

Chiropractors claimed that the decision was a triumph for chiropractic therapy, but the trial was decided primarily in response to evidence that the AMA had attempted to eliminate chiropractic as a competitor in the health care system. The AMA was, therefore, guilty of engaging both "overtly and covertly" in a conspiracy "to contain and eliminate the chiropractic profession," in violation of the Sherman Antitrust Act. The judge ordered a permanent injunction against the AMA to prevent such behavior in the future. In addition, the AMA was forced to publish the judge's decision in the *Journal of the American Medical Association*. During the 1990s, several attempts by the AMA to overturn the injunction were unsuccessful. Continuing the litigious approach into the twenty-first century, chiropractic associations filed lawsuits against Blue Cross and Blue Shield for discriminating against chiropractors by limiting reimbursements for chiropractic procedures. In filing lawsuits against medical insurance companies, chiropractors demanded a "level playing field" with medical doctors and osteopaths.

## ALTERNATIVE, COMPLEMENTARY, AND
## INTEGRATIVE MEDICINE

The challenges represented by popular health reform movements and medical sects were among the factors that eventually forced regular practitioners to explore the therapeutic systems of their competitors. Even though late nineteenth-century science led to improved means of diagnosing and explaining the mechanism of disease through germ theory, cellular pathology, and physiology, the scope of therapeutic medicine remained limited. Physicians gradually abandoned calomel, bleeding, and purging, and turned to laboratory research, controlled clinical trials, and more rigorous medical education to validate the superiority of orthodox medicine. As the medical profession improved its image and power, as well as the efficacy of its therapeutics and the safety of surgical operations, physicians were confident that the challenge of unorthodox practitioners and their systems would disappear.

Until the last decades of the twentieth century, historians and social scientists of medicine, as well as medical policy analysts, generally assumed that medical sectarianism, unorthodox healers, and traditional or folk practices were disappearing as modern, scientific medicine became increasingly effective and powerful. Unorthodox practitioners, whether advocates of antiquated medical theories or leaders of novel cults, seemed to have little relevance to the medical marketplace, except as sources of colorful anecdotes. It came as a surprise to the medical community when surveys conducted during the 1990s revealed that more than 30 percent of all Americans had utilized some form of alternative medicine, creating a multibillion dollar market. Further studies demonstrated that public interest in and usage of alternative medicine was increasing rather than decreasing.

A major survey conducted in the early twenty-first century indicated that over 40 percent of Americans had used or were using some form of alternative medicine; about 75 percent believed in the healing power of prayer and 85 percent believed that certain foods could cure disease or enhance health. The survey included questions on 27 types of alternative or unconventional therapies. Unconventional healing approaches included acupuncture, aromatherapy, Ayurvedic medicine, herbs, botanical products, enzymes, deep breathing exercises, meditation, energy healing, yoga, homeopathy, medical magnets, chiropractic, massage, reflexology, naturopathy, special diets, megavitamin therapy, prayer, and even the ancient practice of dowsing. Moreover, polls indicate that educated people in search of optimum health are the most likely to seek out holistic or alternative medicine. Seventy percent of Canadians have used alternative medicine and one-third of the population uses it on a regular basis. In France, where homeopathic medicine is popular, 75 percent say they have tried alternative medicines. In China, 95 percent of hospitals have folk medicine wards.

Popular demand for choices in approaches to wellness, healing, and medical care, transformed the relationship between orthodox medicine and forms of healing once denounced as sectarianism, superstition, and quackery. As physicians attempted to incorporate rather than eradicate competing healing approaches, unorthodox medicine was subsumed into complementary, alternative, or integrative medicine. From the perspective of mainstream medicine, alternative medicine included osteopaths and chiropractors, as well as folk and religious healers, naturopaths, homeopaths, acupuncturists, diet and fitness programs, reflexology, therapeutic massage, magnetic devices, self-help systems promising natural healing, and herbalism.

Proponents of complementary or integrative medicine tend to be interested in herbal remedies, vitamins, and other so-called dietary supplements. When Congress passed the Dietary Supplement and Health Education Act of 1994, it allowed significant differences between the marketing of prescription medicines and dietary supplements. Prescription drugs must provide proof of safety and efficacy to secure Food and Drug Administration (FDA) approval, but the agency cannot recall products sold as dietary supplements from the market unless the FDA can prove that they are harmful. Supplement manufacturers are permitted to use advertisements and testimonials claiming that their products are "all natural" and "completely safe." Stores specializing in dietary supplements, herbs, and vitamins sell products that purportedly boost metabolism, improve cardiovascular health, prevent heart attacks, and so forth. Food and beverage companies have experimented with "functional" or "nutraceutical products" containing ingredients more commonly associated with dietary supplements and traditional herbal medicines. Skeptics have noted that such supplements are present in such low doses that they probably pose no risk at all, but it might be appropriate to market them as homeopathic rather than functional foods. Some of the most popular herbal remedies include ephedra for energy and weight loss, echinacea for colds, black cohosh for hot flashes, kava for nerves, saw palmetto for benign prostate enlargement, St. John's wort for depression, and ginkgo biloba for memory loss. Pharmacologists, however, emphasize the potentially toxic effect of various herbs, such as ephedra, comfrey, germander, Indian snakeroot, lobelia, pennyroyal, wormwood, yohimbe, and even chamomile. Even though these herbs have been used for many centuries, a low incidence of adverse reactions, or toxic effects on the liver or fetus, may go unnoticed among the small numbers of patients seen by a traditional healer.

Critics of attempts to integrate alternative medicine and mainstream medicine warn that this amalgamation would undermine the foundations of modern medicine and obstruct the progress of biomedical science. Defenders of integrative medicine argue that throughout the world patients are turning to alternative healers because of dissatisfaction with conventional medicine. Patients are particularly interested in nutritional influences on health and skeptical about the excessive use of drugs and surgery. Critics of conventional medicine note that prescription drugs and medical errors directly cause many thousands of deaths in hospitals. Moreover, many practices and beliefs associated with conventional medicine are not necessarily based on randomized clinical trials.

In 1998, under pressure from Congress, the National Institutes of Health upgraded the Office of Alternative Medicine, which had been funded by Congress in 1991, and established the National Center for Complementary and Alternative Medicine (NCCAM). The new institute was charged with evaluating alternative medicine, supporting clinical trials, and providing information and advice to the public. In 2002, the White House Commission on Complementary and Alternative Medicine Policy released a report on alternative therapies calling for increased research spending, more coverage by insurance companies and more Medicare coverage of such treatments. In response to popular and government attention to alternative therapies, medical schools and prestigious university hospitals developed programs for research on alternative therapies and programs in integrative medicine. Even the American Veterinary Medical Association has accommodated forms of alternative medicine. Members of the American Holistic Veterinary Medical Association recommend herbal remedies, acupuncture, acutherapy, homeopathy, and chiropractic treatments for animals.

Attempts to subject traditional and alternative remedies to rigorous testing have often produced ambiguous results that fail to satisfy critics or proponents. In 1996, for example, Emily Rosa designed an experimental test of a widely used alternative technique known as "therapeutic touch." Her fourth grade Science Fair project was published in the *Journal of the American Medical Association* in 1998. Proponents of therapeutic touch claim that by passing their hands over a patient's body, without actual physical contact, healers can relieve the symptoms of disease by manipulating and rebalancing defective energy fields. However, when separated from the investigator by a screen, the 21 practitioners who participated in Rosa's study were unable to identify the investigator's energy field any better than by chance. Practitioners objected to the conclusion and pointed out that the study's authors included skeptics from the National Therapeutic Touch Study Group and Quackwatch.

Leaders of Quackwatch warn that the growing acceptance of integrative medicine epitomized by the establishment of NCCAM might not co-opt alternative medicine as the mainstream hopes. Perhaps, skeptics warn, accommodation might encourage the resurgence of unregulated, uncontrolled medical diversity, and quackery. Nevertheless, hospitals, academic medical centers, and medical schools are attempting to attract new patients and consumers by offering programs for wellness, stress reduction, yoga, meditation, massage, biofeedback, Shirodhara (warm herbalized sesame oil dripped onto the forehead), acupressure, aromatherapy, and so forth. The American Hospital Association found that more than 15 percent of all hospitals were offering alternative therapies, including walk-in complementary medicine centers.

In response to a rapid increase in the use of alternative medicine, in 2002 the World Health Organization (WHO) created the first global strategy to analyze traditional and alternative therapies and help integrate them into healthcare services. It was also noted by WHO that it was important to ensure that traditional remedies would not be appropriated and patented by pharmaceutical companies and that medicinal plants would not be eradicated by overharvesting. In many parts of the world, the vast majority of people depend on traditional therapies. In Mozambique, for example, there was 1 medical doctor for every 50,000 people as compared to 1 traditional healer for every 200. Officials of WHO plan to advise nations on how to ensure the quality of traditional remedies and practices through the regulation of drugs and the training and licensing of healers. Unless traditional healers practice nontraditional antiseptic techniques, they can spread diseases by using dirty syringes, knives, razor blades, glass shards, or porcupine quills.

Skeptics warn that the growing interest in alternative medicine encouraged by WHO might allow insidious and dangerous forms of quackery to emerge and flourish within a more welcoming, less skeptical environment that awards "equal time" to any and all ideas. When diseases are serious, chronic, and incurable, people are very vulnerable to quackery. Those who have waged war against cancer quackery and AIDS quackery warn against social and legislative changes that make unconventional medicine more acceptable and may make it possible for a global "army of quacks" to thrive and prosper.

## SUGGESTED READINGS

Baer, H. A. (1991). *Biomedicine and Alternative Healing Systems in America: Issues of Class, Race, Ethnicity, and Gender.* Madison, WI: University of Wisconsin Press.

Bauer, H. H. (2001). *Science or Pseudoscience: Magnetic Healing, Psychic Phenomena, and Other Heterodoxies.* Urbana, IL: University of Illinois Press.

Berman, A., and Flannery, M. A. (2001). *America's Botanico-Medical Movements: Vox Populi.* Binghamton, NY: Pharmaceutical Products Press.

Brenneman, R. J. (1990). *Deadly Blessings: Faith Healing on Trial.* Buffalo, NY: Prometheus Books.

Cayleff, S. E. (1987). *Wash and Be Healed: The Water-Cure Movement and Women's Health.* Philadelphia, PA: Temple University Press.

Coulter, H. L. (1994). *Divided Legacy: A History of the Schism in Medical Thought.* Washington, DC: Center for Empirical Medicine.

Crellin, J. K., and Philpott, J. (1997). *A Reference Guide to Medicinal Plants: Herbal Medicine Past and Present.* Durham, NC: Duke University Press.

Dinges, M., ed. (2002). *Patients in the History of Homoeopathy.* Sheffield, U.K.: EAHMH Publications.

Donegan, J. B. (1986). *Hydropathic Highway to Health: Women and Water Cure in Antebellum America.* Westport, CT: Greenwood Press.

Engs, R. C. (2000). *Clean Living Movements: American Cycles of Health Reform.* Westport, CT: Praeger Publishers.

Ernst, R. (1991). *Weakness is a Crime: The Life of Bernarr Macfadden.* Syracuse, NY: Syracuse University Press.

Flannery, M. A. (1998). *John Uri Lloyd: The Great American Eclectic.* Carbondale, IL: Southern Illinois University Press.

Frohock, F. M. (1992). *Healing Powers: Alternative Medicine, Spiritual Communities, and the State.* Chicago, IL: University of Chicago Press.

Fuller, R. C. (1989). *Alternative Medicine and American Religious Life.* New York: Oxford University Press.

Gardner, M. (1993). *The Healing Revelations of Mary Baker Eddy: The Rise and Fall of Christian Science.* Buffalo, NY: Prometheus Books.

Gevitz, N., ed. (1988). *Other Healers. Unorthodox Medicine in America.* Baltimore, MD: The Johns Hopkins University Press.

Gevitz, N. (1991). *The D.O.'s. Osteopathic Medicine in America.* Baltimore, MD: The Johns Hopkins University Press.

Gijswijt-Hofstra, M., Marland, H., and de Waardt, H., eds. (1997). *Illness and Healing Alternatives in Western Europe.* New York: Routledge.

Goldstein, M. S. (1999). *Alternative Health Care: Medicine, Miracle, or Mirage?* Philadelphia, PA: University Press.

Hafner, A.W., Carson, J. G., and Zwicky, J. F., eds. (1992). *Guide to the American Medical Association Historical Health Fraud and Alternative Medicine Collection.* Chicago, IL: American Medical Association Division of Library and Information Management.

Haller, J. S., Jr. (1994). *Medical Protestants: The Eclectics in American Medicine, 1825–1939.* Carbondale, IL: Southern Illinois University Press.

Haller, J. S., Jr. (1997). *Kindly Medicine. Physio-Medicalism in America, 1836–1911.* Kent, OH: Kent State University Press.

Haller, J. S., Jr. (2000). *The People's Doctors: Samuel Thomson and the American Botanical Movement, 1790–1860.* Carbondale, IL: Southern Illinois University Press.

Helfand, W. H. (2002). *Quack, Quack, Quack: The Sellers of Nostrums in Prints, Posters, Ephemera, and Books.* Chicago, IL: University of Chicago Press.

Jütte, R., Eklof, M., and Nelson, M. C., eds. (2002). *Historical Aspects of Unconventional Medicine: Approaches, Concepts, Case Studies.* Sheffield, U.K.: EAHMH Publications.

Jütte, R., Risse, G. B., and Woodward, J., eds. (1998). *Culture, Knowledge, and Healing: Historical Perspectives of Homeopathic Medicine in Europe and North America.* Sheffield, England: EAHMH Publications.

Kaufman, M. (1971). *Homeopathy in America: The Rise and Fall of a Medical Heresy.* Baltimore, MD: The Johns Hopkins University Press.

Moore, J. S. (1993). *Chiropractic in America. The History of a Medical Alternative.* Baltimore, MD: The Johns Hopkins University Press.

Murphy, L. R. (1991). *Enter the Physician. The Transformation of Domestic Medicine, 1760–1860.* Tuscaloosa, AL: University of Alabama Press.

Nicholls, P. A. (1988). *Homeopathy and the Medical Profession.* London: Croom Helm.

Nissenbaum, S. (1988). *Sex, Diet, and Debility in Jacksonian America: Sylvester Graham and Health Reform.* Chicago, IL: University of Chicago Press.

Numbers, R. (1992). *Prophetess of Health: A Study of Ellen G. White and the Origins of Seventh-Day Adventist Health Reform.* Knoxville, TN: University of Tennessee Press.

Numbers, R. L., and Amundsen, D. W. (1998). *Caring and Curing: Health and Medicine in the Western Religious Tradition.* Baltimore, MD: Johns Hopkins University Press.

O'Connor, B. B. (1995). *Healing Traditions: Alternative Medicine and the Health Professions.* Philadelphia, PA: University of Pennsylvania Press.

Peel, R. (1989). *Health and Medicine in the Christian Science Tradition: Principle, Practice, and Challenge.* New York: Crossroad Publishing.

Randi, J. (1987). *The Faith Healers.* New York: Prometheus Books.

Risse, G. B., Numbers, R. L., and Leavitt, J. W., eds. (1977). *Medicine without Doctors: Home Health Care in American History.* New York: Science History Publications.

Rogers, N. (1998). *An Alternative Path: The Making and Remaking of Hahnemann Medical College and Hospital.* New Brunswick, NJ: Rutgers University Press.

Rosenberg, C. E., ed. (2003). *Right Living: An Anglo-American Tradition of Self-Help Medicine and Hygiene.* Baltimore, MD: Johns Hopkins University Press.

Rothstein, W. G. (1992). *American Physicians in the Nineteenth Century. From Sects to Science.* Baltimore, MD: The Johns Hopkins University Press.

Salmon, J. W., ed. (1985). *Alternative Medicine. Popular and Policy Perspectives.* New York: Tavistock.

Sampson, W., and Vaughn, L., eds. (2000). *Science Meets Alternative Medicine: What the Evidence Says About Unconventional Treatments.* Amherst, NY: Prometheus Books.

Schnucker Robert, V., ed. (1991). *Early Osteopathy in the Words of A.T. Still.* Kirksville, MO: Thomas Jefferson University Press at Northeast Missouri State University.

Schoepflin, R. B. (2002). *Christian Science on Trial: Religious Healing in America.* Baltimore, MD: Johns Hopkins University Press.

Silver-Isenstadt, J. L. (2002). *Shameless: The Visionary Life of Mary Gove Nichols.* Baltimore, MD: Johns Hopkins University Press.

Smith, R. (1984). *At Your Own Risk: The Case Against Chiropractors.* New York: Simon and Schuster.

Smith-Cunnien, S. L. (1998). *A Profession of One's Own: Organized Medicine's Opposition to Chiropractic.* Lanham, MD: University Press of America.

Trowbridge, C. (1991). *Andrew Taylor Still, 1828–1917.* Kirksville, MO: Thomas Jefferson University Press.

Walter, G. W. (1994). *Women and Osteopathic Medicine: Historical Perspectives.* Kirksville, MO: Kirksville College of Osteopathic Medicine.

Ward, P. S. (1994). *Simon Baruch: Rebel in the Ranks of Medicine, 1840–1921.* Tuscaloosa, AL: University of Alabama Press.

Wharton, J. C. (1982). *Crusaders for Fitness. The History of American Health Reformers.* Princeton, NJ: Princeton University Press.

Whorton, J. C. (2002). *Nature Cures: The History of Alternative Medicine in America.* New York: Oxford University Press.

Whorton James, C. (2000). *Inner Hygiene: Constipation and the Pursuit of Health in Modern Society.* New York: Oxford University Press.

Young, J. H. (1992). *American Health Quackery: Collected Essays.* Princeton, NJ: Princeton University Press.

# 11

# Women and Medicine

## PUERPERAL OR CHILDBED FEVER

During the second half of the eighteenth century, the population of Europe began a steep increase, unprecedented in extent, duration, and permanence. The eighteenth century, a period of particular interest to philosophers, political scientists, demographers, and historians of medicine, has been called the age of enlightenment and revolution. Within this context of social and intellectual change, medical men first made significant inroads into the traditionally female domain of childbirth. Epidemics of the previously rare and sporadic disease known as puerperal or childbed fever apparently became more common during this period, especially in the lying-in hospitals that accommodated poor women in cities and towns throughout Europe. The death of new mothers was of special interest to social reformers and physicians like Johann Peter Frank (1745–1821), who believed that the greatest wealth of the state should be measured in terms of the number, health, and productivity of its subjects. The state could not afford to lose its peasants, workers, sailors, and soldiers to disease. It could not, therefore, afford to lose fertile women through diseases associated with childbirth. In an ideal state, the health of mothers would be properly valued so that they could continue to produce healthy new workers. Frank believed that each nation should establish a Supreme Medical Board to collect and analyze lists of births and deaths from each village, town, district, and province in order to discover the local causes of excessive mortality, especially the factors responsible for the deaths of pregnant women, women in childbirth, postpartum women, infants, and children.

It has been a tenet of historical demography and of many feminist scholars that there must have been a causal relationship between the apparent rise of epidemic puerperal fever and the development of a new medically oriented obstetrics, characterized by the "man midwife" and the lying-in ward of the urban hospital. Puerperal fever, or childbed fever, is generally and nonspecifically defined as a severe, generalized

infection that occurs within 11 days of childbirth. In addition to the
raging fever and pus emanating from the birth canal, victims often
developed painful abscesses in the abdominal cavity and chest, and fatal
septicemia. The reason for the vulnerability of puerperal women to life-
threatening infections had been recognized by the great seventeenth-
century physician and physiologist William Harvey (1578–1657): after
childbirth the site of placental detachment constituted a large internal
wound. Except for burns, which often become infected, wounds are
rarely very large. Although the term puerperal fever implies a causal
link to childbirth, the definition provides no specific information about
the etiology of the disease. Not all postpartum fevers and infections
should be called puerperal fever, a condition now typically attributed
to Group A hemolytic streptococcus. Streptococcal disease can also
appear as scarlet fever, septic sore throat, erysipelas, and rheumatic fever.
This makes the task of tracing the history of childbed fever and its possible causal connection to changes in patterns of fertility, use of lying-in
hospitals, and the evolution of gynecology and obstetrics very difficult.

In addition to its place within the larger history of women and
medicine and the professionalization of the healing arts, the battle
against puerperal fever can be seen as part of the story of the development of antiseptic surgery, because puerperal fever is essentially equivalent to wound infection. Unfortunately, although an understanding
of the etiology, contagiousness, and prevention of puerperal fever preceded the development of antiseptic surgery, acceptance of the principles
of asepsis and antisepsis in the nineteenth century did not lead to the universal adoption of practices that could have prevented most cases of puerperal fever. Even in the 1930s, before the introduction of sulfanilamide,
puerperal fever remained the most important illness threatening parturient women. In the maternity wards of even the best American teaching
hospitals, it was not unusual for at least 20 percent of the women to
develop fevers after giving birth and for patients to die of puerperal
infections. Once puerperal fever set in, there was little that medical intervention could accomplish, although doctors confidently administered
mercurochrome via vaginal instillation during labor and intravenously in
infected patients, along with other useless and dangerous treatments,
such as intramuscular injections of cow's milk, intravenous injections
of alcohol, blood transfusions, and hysterectomy.

Case histories in the Hippocratic texts indicate that puerperal
infection was rare, but not unknown in ancient Greece. The transformation of a rare, private tragedy into a well known, frequent, and much
feared epidemic disease of lying-in hospitals apparently took place in
the eighteenth century. Epidemics occurred at the Hôtel Dieu in Paris
and the newly established lying-in hospitals of Great Britain. Several
doctors suggested that puerperal fever might be contagious, but Alexander
Gordon (1752–1799) of Aberdeen and Charles White (1728–1813) of

Manchester were probably the first to realize that doctors could carry the fever from patient to patient. White boasted that he had never lost a patient to puerperal fever, while colleagues who performed autopsies often lost several patients in succession.

It was the relationship between autopsies and childbed fever that led the American poet and physician Oliver Wendell Holmes and the Hungarian obstetrician Ignaz Philipp Semmelweis to their understanding of the contagiousness of the disease. Not all historians award major honors to Oliver Wendell Holmes for his essays on puerperal fever. Physician and educator Sir William Osler (1849–1919), for example, praised Holmes for his logical and convincing arguments, but did not believe that Holmes had actually discovered the cause and prevention of puerperal fever. Osler agreed with British clergyman and satirist Sydney Smith (1771–1845) that credit for a discovery did not belong to the first man to say something, but to the one who says it "so long, so loudly, and so clearly that he compels men to hear him."

## OLIVER WENDELL HOLMES

In 1843, Oliver Wendell Holmes (1809–1894) read a paper to the Boston Society for Medical Improvement entitled "The Contagiousness of Puerperal Fever." The audience response ranged from indifference to hostility, although the paper is now generally regarded as a clear, convincing, and logical argument concerning the transmission and prevention of puerperal fever. Holmes, the father of U.S. Supreme Court justice Oliver Wendell Holmes Jr. (1841–1935), spent several years "yawning over law books" before taking up the study of medicine. After completing his medical studies in Europe, Holmes combined private practice with various academic positions, including professorships at Dartmouth and Harvard. He first gained national attention with the publication of "Old Ironsides," the poem that gave him a taste of the "intoxicating pleasure of authorship."

A report on a fatal case of childbed fever presented at a meeting of the Boston Society for Medical Improvement piqued Holmes's curiosity about the disease. The physician who conducted the autopsy died of "pathologist's pyemia" (septicemia) within a week. Before his own demise, the doctor attended several women in labor; all of these patients were stricken with puerperal fever. Such a pattern suggested to Holmes that puerperal fever was a form of contagion that could be transmitted from one patient to another by the attending physician. To confirm this hypothesis, Holmes needed the kind of data that doctors were understandably reluctant to share—a record of patients who had died under their care, perhaps *because* of their care. Ultimately, Holmes gathered evidence that should have been more than sufficient to convince a

"Committee of Husbands" to demand that a practitioner should be banished from obstetrics "after five or six funerals had marked the path of his daily visits." Even a superficial acquaintance with statistics and the laws of probability would suggest that Holmes had good circumstantial evidence when he asserted: "It is not chance that accounts for a single practitioner having 16 fatal cases in a single month."

Nevertheless, Holmes was distressed to find that America's foremost authorities on obstetrics consistently rejected the doctrine of the contagiousness of puerperal fever. Holmes's critics defended the "value and dignity" of the medical profession and denied the possibility that a physician could become a "minister of evil" carrying disease to his patients. Rather than acknowledge a personal role in the transmission of puerperal fever, doctors attributed the disease to chance or to God. But, because the disease followed particular physicians and spared women attended by other practitioners, Holmes argued that childbed fever must be transmitted by contagion rather than miasma. Physicians used the term *contagion* to denote an agent that transmitted infectious disease through touch or direct contact. The term *miasma* referred to poisonous vapors that were thought to infect the air and cause disease. In other words, Holmes contended, puerperal fever was transmitted by a particular *person*, who obviously had a vested interest in "denying and disbelieving the facts." Eventually, enraged by the intransigence of his colleagues, Holmes denounced them as self-righteous, ignorant men guilty of "professional homicide" and thundered a warning that for their voluntary blindness, interested oversight, and culpable negligence each of these pestilence carriers of the lying-in chamber "must look to God for pardon, for man will never forgive him."

For many and complex theoretical reasons, given the longstanding debate about the nature of the transmission of disease, physicians generally rejected the possibility that puerperal fever could be transmitted by contagion. Still, it is difficult to ignore Holmes's charge that at least in part the learned debates about contagion could be reduced to a self-serving refusal to believe that a gentleman with apparently clean hands could be the agent of death. Steeped in prevailing miasmatic doctrine, doctors were a source of grave danger to their patients. This point is well illustrated by Holmes's account of how Dr. Warrington performed five deliveries shortly after conducting an autopsy on a victim of puerperal fever in which he had scooped out the contents of the abdominal cavity with his bare hands. All five women were stricken with puerperal fever. Another example cited by Holmes involved an ardent opponent of the doctrine of contagion who participated in the autopsy of a victim of puerperal fever. For the edification of his students, Dr. Campbell "carried the pelvic viscera in his pocket to the class-room." That evening, without changing his clothes, he attended a woman in labor. That patient died. The next day he delivered another patient with the obstetrical forceps.

That patient also died, as did many others during the next few weeks. A few months later, after participating in another autopsy, Dr. Campbell attended two patients before he found time to wash his hands or change his clothes. Both of these patients died of puerperal fever.

Having presented his case for the contagiousness of puerperal fever, Holmes outlined methods of prevention. He thought it best that obstetricians avoid active participation in all postmortems. If a physician had been an observer at an autopsy, he should wash thoroughly, change every item of clothing, and allow 24 hours to pass before attending women in labor. A physician who had two cases of puerperal fever among his patients should give up obstetrics for at least one month and try to rid himself of the contagion. Finally, when a "private pestilence" appeared in the practice of one physician, it should be seen as a crime rather than a misfortune. Professional interests, Holmes insisted, must then give way to the physician's duty to society.

Even admirers of Holmes's ability to present a logical case in luminous prose have been dubious of his claim to the discovery of the cause and prevention of puerperal fever. His observations were not wholly original and his logic failed to compel the medical community to accept his doctrine. Critics dismissed him as merely a poet-physician who had restated observations already made by Gordon and White without coming any closer to an understanding the specific etiology of puerperal fever. Holmes fought the battle against puerperal fever with no weapons other than logic and his eloquent pen, but no one ever accused his Hungarian counterpart, Ignaz Philipp Semmelweis, of excessive eloquence. In contrast to Holmes, Semmelweis, a man apparently lacking even a rudimentary sense of tact and diplomacy, fought childbed fever with the blunt club of statistical and empirical evidence.

## IGNAZ PHILIPP SEMMELWEIS

The life of Ignaz Philipp Semmelweis (1818–1865) encompasses elements of heroism and tragedy more appropriate to treatment by a novelist than a historian. But some historians have argued that Semmelweis's contributions to medical history have been grossly exaggerated because mortality from childbed fever actually increased after his work was published. Moreover, Semmelweis was all but forgotten by the time the doctrine of antisepsis was accepted. It is true that both Semmelweis and Holmes had little or no impact on obstetrical practice among their contemporaries, but this unfortunate reality has generally been considered part of the tragedy of puerperal fever.

A native of Budapest, Hungary, Semmelweis was sent to Vienna in 1837 to study law, but he soon transferred to the school of medicine. At

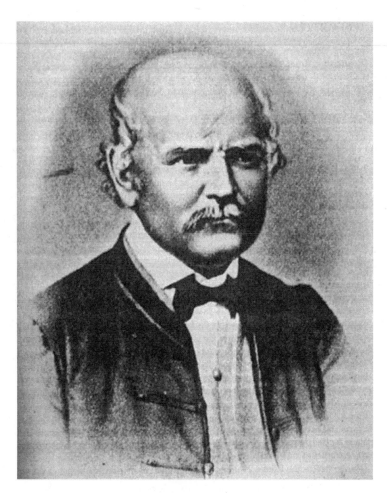

**Ignaz Philipp Semmelweis.**

the time, the University of Vienna, especially the medical school, was aptly described as a hotbed of revolutionary activity, where senior, well-entrenched professors with close ties to the conservative government were being confronted by younger faculty members with opposing views of politics, society, and scientific research. Indeed, it was often said that the great physician-scientists of Vienna were more interested in scientific research than surgery and patient care. Semmelweis came under the influence of three of the leaders of the new approach to pathological and clinical investigation: Karl von Rokitansky (1804–1878), Josef Skoda (1805–1881), and Ferdinand von Hebra (1816–1880). While serving as professor of pathological anatomy, Rokitansky had personally conducted some 30,000 autopsies. Rudolf Virchow (1821–1902), the founder of cellular pathology, called Rokitansky the "Linnaeus of pathological anatomy."

After earning his medical degree, Semmelweis remained in Vienna for further training in midwifery and surgery. He also studied diagnostic and statistical methods with Skoda. In 1846, Semmelweis became titular house officer of the First Obstetrical Clinic at the Vienna General Hospital, under the direction of Professor Johann Klein (1788–1856). The Vienna General Hospital had been quite large even in the eighteenth century when Johann Peter Frank described it as having many advantages over other hospitals in terms of space and suitable divisions for the isolation of contagious diseases. Although the Vienna Hospital did not have all the special departments that Frank recommended, it did have a lunatic tower, wards for contagious diseases, small rooms for paying customers and pregnant women, and large sickrooms, with 20 or more beds. The purposes of the ideal hospital, according to Frank, were: curing poor, sick people, perfecting medical science, and educating good practitioners. Eighteenth- and nineteenth-century hospitals were generally far from ideal. Contagious diseases became a major threat to patients and staff in a general hospital because of overcrowding and the lack of resources, which made it impossible to keep the wards clean and well ventilated. Such conditions were especially dangerous to women during labor and the postpartum period.

To protect new mothers from acquiring contagious diseases, Frank stipulated that the lying-in ward should be quite separate from the general hospital. Ideally, the lying-in ward should have three departments: one where pregnant women could rest and prepare for the ordeal of childbirth; the second should be dedicated to women giving birth; and the third should have small rooms with only two or three beds reserved for postpartum women. Women who needed surgical intervention during childbirth should not be kept in the common labor room, Frank warned, because the sights and sounds of such "artificial births" would have a bad effect on women in labor. The lying-in ward did not need rooms for the sick, because postpartum women who became ill should be transferred to the general hospital. Hospital managers and physicians, however, considered such elaborate precautions unnecessary, irrational, and, most of all, too costly for a largely charitable enterprise.

In the 1840s, the Vienna Hospital provided medical researchers and teachers with a plethora of "clinical material"—patients forced by poverty, if not expectation of a cure, to use the hospital. Doctors and students could anticipate thousands of childbirth cases and hundreds of autopsies annually. Vienna was, therefore, a magnet for foreign medical students. The founder of the Vienna Obstetrical Department, Lucas Boër (1788–1822), established the enviable record of a 1.25 percent maternal mortality rate among some 70,000 patients. Boër restricted medical students to practicing their skills on the "phantom" (a mannequin with a uterus and birth canal), but his successor, Johann Klein, let students take an active role in examinations and deliveries. In support of the doctrine that even dead patients could serve educational purposes, Klein allowed the bodies of women and infants who died in the hospital to be used for demonstrations of the birth process. Klein's methods gave medical students better clinical experience, but maternal mortality soared to about 10 percent and above.

During a period of expansion and reorganization, Klein divided the obstetrical service into two separate divisions: one was supervised by midwives training midwifery students. In the other division, medical students practiced under the supervision of physicians. Women in the First Clinic, the teaching division for medical students, were sometimes examined by five or more different students, who moved freely between the wards and the adjoining dissection room. From 1841 to 1846, the maternal mortality rate was about 10 to 13 percent; but during particularly virulent epidemics, 20 to 50 percent of the maternity patients died of the fever. In contrast, the mortality rate in the Second Obstetrical Clinic, the section dedicated to the instruction of midwives, was usually about two to three percent. Some studies of maternal mortality suggest that, in contrast to hospital childbirths, about five women per thousand died in deliveries that took place at home.

Unable to explain the high death rate of his patients, Semmelweis became obsessed by the problem of childbed fever. Each day he examined every patient in his ward, demonstrated the proper methods for examining patients in labor, and performed operations. Before beginning work in the wards, Semmelweis conscientiously dissected the bodies of puerperal fever victims. During the first few months of his assistantship, the mortality from puerperal fever actually increased to about 18 percent.

Ironically, it was not the systematic study of mortality rates, observations of patients, or diligent work in the dissection room that gave Semmelweis his flash of insight into the cause of puerperal fever; it was the death of his friend Jakob Kolletschka (1804–1847), professor of forensic medicine at Vienna. While Semmelweis was away on vacation Kolletschka died of pathologist's pyemia from a minor wound incurred during a postmortem examination. Pyemia (blood poisoning) was a well-known risk to anatomists. A small injury on the hands incurred during dissection might go unnoticed until redness, throbbing pain, and red streaks up along the arm announced the presence of a potentially fatal infection. When Semmelweis studied the results of the autopsy conducted on Kolletschka's body, he realized that the findings were nearly identical to those characteristic of death from puerperal fever.

Obviously, Kolletschka's massive infection had been triggered by the introduction of "cadaveric matter" into a small wound caused by a dissection knife. Therefore, Semmelweis concluded, *cadaveric matter must also be the cause of puerperal fever*. Few maternity patients underwent any surgical interventions, but after childbirth, women were especially vulnerable to infection because, in addition to the trauma of the passage of the infant through the birth canal, a large internal wound was created by the detachment of the placenta from the wall of the uterus. Just as the dissecting knife introduced cadaveric matter into the anatomist's blood stream, the contaminated hand of the examining physician carried cadaveric matter from the autopsy room to the laboring woman. As demonstrated by the persistence of cadaveric odor on the hands of the anatomist, ordinary washing with soap and water did not entirely remove the contamination carried from the autopsy room.

The insight gained from Kolletschka's tragic death was the foundation on which Semmelweis constructed what he called his doctrine: puerperal fever was identical to pathologist's pyemia and was caused by the introduction of cadaveric matter or morbid poison into the body. In opposition to almost all medical authorities, Semmelweis asserted that only his doctrine was consistent with the statistics and facts observed at the Vienna Lying-In Hospital. His major argument was that none of the prevailing theories could explain away the threefold difference in mortality rates between the First Division, staffed by medical students, and the Second Division, staffed by midwives. Actually, the difference was greater than threefold, because, whenever possible, women with puerperal fever were transferred to wards in the General Hospital and their deaths were not included in the reports of the First Division. Very few patients in the Second Division were transferred to other wards unless they had a contagious disease like smallpox.

According to prevailing medical dogma, childbed fever was caused by "atmospheric-cosmic-tellurgic influences" or an "epidemic constitution" that peculiarly affected puerperal women because of internal predisposing conditions, such as milk fever, or a peculiarity of the blood associated with childbirth and lactation. Many complicating factors were suggested to explain away the differences between Division I and Division II. Some physicians blamed overcrowding, but Division II was actually more crowded. Semmelweis drew attention to another interesting difference between the two sections: in the midwives' ward long labors were not more life-threatening than short labors, but in Division I, women with long labors were especially prone to puerperal fever. Moreover, women brought into the hospital after so-called street births seemed to be immune to the fever. This anomaly could be explained by remembering that hospital charity was formally extended to women and their infants in return for their use as "teaching material." Generally, the hospital accepted women after childbirth only if the patient could convince the authorities that she had intended to be delivered in the hospital but the birth occurred before she could get there. To avoid being used for "public instruction," some women

employed a midwife and then appeared at the hospital claiming to be
victims of street births.

Hospital administrators blamed high mortality rates on the
miserable condition of the poor, desperate, unmarried women who
needed the services of the maternity ward. While such a theory might
explain the difference between charity patients in hospitals and private
patients giving birth at home, it could not explain the difference between
Divisions I and II. Another explanation attributed differential mortality
to the shame women experienced when attended by male physicians and
students. Ironically, delicate upper-class ladies were able to employ physicians, rather than midwives, without dying of shame. The fear inspired
by the bad reputation of Division I was also cited as a possible factor in
the genesis of disease. Semmelweis proved that statistical differences in
mortality rates between the two divisions preceded the recognition that
such differences existed. He also dismissed the idea that fear could produce the anatomical findings characteristic of both puerperal fever and
pathologist's pyemia as patently absurd.

Foreign medical students had been singled out for being particularly rough and coarse in their treatment of patients and, therefore,
responsible for a high incidence of injuries during physical examinations. Semmelweis protested that compared to the birth of a baby, manual examination, even by the most uncouth medical student, hardly
constituted a major trauma. Nevertheless, reducing the number of
foreign medical students in the ward and the number of manual
examinations per patient did produce a temporary decline in maternal
mortality rates. Here again, Semmelweis explained, his doctrine
was consistent with the observations. The attempt to improve medical
education by giving students clinical experience and anatomical instruction had produced ideal conditions for the transmission of
puerperal fever. The foreign medical students, who had come to Vienna
at great trouble and expense, were especially eager to take advantage of
access to the cadavers and the "clinical material" available only in the
great teaching hospitals of European cities.

To eliminate the transmission of cadaveric particles, Semmelweis
insisted that all medical students and hospital staff wash their hands
with a solution of chlorinated lime each time they left the autopsy room
to examine patients. Within a month the mortality from puerperal fever
decreased from about thirteen to three percent. Contrary to popular
belief, hand washing was not an unknown custom among nineteenth-
century doctors. However, the soap and water wash that might bring
hands to a state of socially acceptable cleanliness did not remove all
the dangerous cadaveric matter. In 1848, the first full year of rigorous
hand washing, the mortality rate in Division I fell below two percent.
Transient increases in puerperal fever cases were traced to patients
with other forms of infections, which indicated that the autopsy room

was not the only source of the deadly contamination. Gradually, Semmelweis realized that disinfection procedures should be extended to include all the instruments that came in contact with patients in labor. Although the decrease in mortality in Division I was undeniably dramatic, the disinfection procedures that Semmelweis demanded were not thought appropriate for a charity hospital. Even in the absence of rigorous hand washing, fluctuations in the rate of puerperal fever were not uncommon and, skeptics argued, it is a very old adage in clinical medicine that correlation need not indicate causation. Professor Klein, who remained a bitter enemy of Semmelweis and his doctrine, accused his assistant of insubordination and other crimes.

For Semmelweis, the discovery of the cause and prevention of puerperal fever was complete by the autumn of 1847. All further observations, including some experiments on laboratory animals, simply confirmed and extended the doctrine. Ironically, the discovery of the cause and prevention of puerperal fever brought him a terrible burden of guilt. Driven by concern for his patients and the desire to understand the disease, Semmelweis had pursued pathological studies more diligently than any of his colleagues. Therefore, every day when he entered the clinic after his work in the autopsy room, he had carried with him the deadly cadaveric particles that caused the fever.

Unfortunately, Semmelweis was unwilling to assume the burden of bringing his doctrine to the attention of the medical community, either through lectures or publications. His friend and mentor, Ferdinand von Hebra, published two articles about the etiology of puerperal fever and the use of chlorinated lime, but his accounts failed to generate significant attention. Skoda, who was impressed by Semmelweis's statistical data, presented a lecture on puerperal fever to the Royal Academy of Sciences and urged the creation of a commission to investigate Semmelweis's results. Although Hebra, Skoda, and Rokitansky supported Semmelweis, they did not fully understand his procedures and their presentations were not totally accurate. Primarily, Semmelweis's doctrine was a victim of the defeat of the liberal movement of 1848 and his own failure to present a compelling case to the medical community. Because of his political activities in support of the liberal movement and Klein's resentment of a doctrine that was fundamentally an indictment of his management of the clinic, Semmelweis found himself unemployed.

Although Semmelweis had provided a practical system of antisepsis that could have mitigated the burden of postsurgical infection as well as puerperal fever, his discovery had little or no immediate impact on medical practice. Just as the term "classic" is generally applied to a book that nobody reads, the term "landmark" is often applied to an insight that was generally ignored. To say that Semmelweis's discovery was a "breakthrough" would imply that after it was made, maternity wards were significantly safer places for women. In reality, Semmelweis lost his sanity and his life in the battle against puerperal fever and prevailing medical opinion. Unwilling to compromise with those he saw as corrupt and ignorant, and lacking any talent for diplomacy, public speaking, or literary exposition, Semmelweis ruined his own career and made few converts to his doctrine. He also displayed a perverse sense of timing by establishing his doctrine in 1848 as a wave of liberal revolutions swept through Europe. The time was quite appropriate for making a revolutionary discovery, but not a convenient time for a foreigner in Vienna to achieve the official recognition that might win the support of the medical establishment.

When Semmelweis finally received an appointment as a Privatdozent in midwifery, the official decree stipulated that he could only teach obstetrics using a mannequin. Angry, discouraged, and without hope of professional advancement in Vienna, Semmelweis abruptly left the city and returned to Hungary. Not surprisingly, misfortune followed him—poverty, professional rejection, and two broken limbs within a year. The only ray of hope to fall into Semmelweis's life was his marriage to Marie Weidenhofer, a woman 20 years his junior. Their first child died within 48 hours of hydrocephalus; the second died when 4 months old of peritonitis, but two daughters and a son survived. Fortunately, Semmelweis obtained an appointment as chair of theoretical and practical midwifery at the University of Pest and an honorary position at Pest's St.-Rochus Hospital. Despite initial resistance by the hospital staff, Semmelweis enforced his system of disinfection and eventually reduced the mortality rate in the maternity ward to less than one percent. A textbook on childbirth and gynecology published by Johann Baptist Chiari (1817–1854), Ritter von Fernwald Braun (1822–1891), and Joseph Späth (1823–1896) in 1855, was the first to include information about Semmelweis's doctrine of rigorous hand washing as a means of preventing puerperal fever. Chiari, who had worked at the first obstetrical clinic in Vienna under Professor Klein from 1842 to 1848, died of cholera before the text was published.

Even among his friends, Semmelweis's doctrine was generally misunderstood as a simplistic attempt to link childbed fever to cadaveric matter. Thus, some rather half-hearted attempts to test the Semmelweis doctrine were failures because of the lack of attention to related factors, such as the disinfection of instruments, linens, dressings, and the isolation of patients with purulent infections. Indeed, after Semmelweis had explained the doctrine to a visiting obstetrician, his skeptical colleague replied that this was certainly not new. All English doctors washed their hands when they left the hospital.

The resistance and apathy that greeted Semmelweis's doctrine were due in part to medicine's conservative traditions, but his reluctance to publish his observations also played a role. Declaring himself pathologically averse to writing, Semmelweis left the task of publicizing the doctrine to colleagues who overemphasized the problem of cadaveric matter. Since some hospitals were plagued by high maternal mortality rates despite the absence of routine autopsies, the doctrine appeared to be irrelevant to their problem. Moreover, hand washing seemed too simple an answer to epidemics supposedly spawned by the ineluctable cosmic forces that ostensibly absolved the doctor of responsibility for the fate of his patients.

In 1861 Semmelweis finally overcame his aversion to writing, and published *The Etiology, Concept, and Prophylaxis of Childbed Fever*. Semmelweis explained that he had developed his doctrine and written the book "in order to banish the terror from lying-in hospitals, to preserve the wife to the husband, and the mother to the child." Unfortunately, by the 1860s, many physicians who knew of the doctrine from vague, secondhand accounts assumed that it had been discredited since the 1840s. Critics dismissed the book as the obsolete ravings of the "Pester Narr" (the fool from Budapest). Having finally accepted the burden of authorship, Semmelweis launched a flood of vitriolic pamphlets and open letters accusing his critics of having massacred mothers and infants. Citing the names of his enemies, he denounced them "before God and the world" as medical Neros, guilty of willful homicides. His depression deepened as he brooded upon the deaths that could have been prevented had his doctrine been accepted in 1848. His condition continued to deteriorate until his wife agreed to send him to a mental asylum where he died two weeks later. His death was originally attributed to septicemia caused by an infected dissection wound, but there is some evidence that suggests the unfortunate Semmelweis was suffering from dementia, syphilitic psychosis, or Alzheimer's disease when he was beaten to death by keepers at the asylum.

Despite demonstrations of the value of the doctrine in the hospitals of Vienna and Budapest, few physicians were aware of or interested in the work of Semmelweis. Rudolf Virchow, the German "Pope of Pathology," initially rejected the doctrine in favor of the theory that pregnant women were predisposed to inflammations. Not until 1864 did Virchow accept the concept of the contagiousness of puerperal fever. Shortly after Semmelweis died, Joseph Lister (1827–1912) began to publish a series of papers describing his antiseptic system. By 1880, as part of the Listerian antiseptic system, rather than the work of Semmelweis, the doctrine was more or less incorporated into obstetrical practice throughout Europe. Although Lister later graciously acknowledged Semmelweis as his "clinical precursor," Lister's immediate inspiration was the work of the great French chemist Louis Pasteur (1822–1895) on the diseases of wine and beer. Nevertheless, the concept of a special epidemic constitution of parturient women was still blamed for puerperal fever when Pasteur announced his discovery of the probable causative agent of puerperal fever at a meeting of the Paris Academy of Medicine in 1879.

Actually, the role of germ theory in the transformation of obstetrics and surgical practice is problematic. Oliver Wendell Holmes, for example, did not think that the germ theory of disease was prerequisite to the acceptance of his theory of the contagiousness of puerperal fever. Indeed, in the 1880s, he reminded his colleagues that he had given his warning and advice long before the advocates of germ theory had marshaled their "little army of microbes" in support of the doctrine he shared with Semmelweis. Moreover, despite the general adoption of antisepsis and asepsis in surgery, the mortality rate from puerperal fever remained quite high until the introduction of sulfonamide and penicillin. Maternal mortality rates remained higher in the United States and Great Britain than in continental Europe.

## MIDWIVES AND MEDICAL MEN

Of course, puerperal fever was not always an epidemic disease and childbirth did not always fall within the province of medical men. While women were almost universally excluded from the medical profession, the province of midwifery was once exclusively theirs. Until very recent times, childbirth was considered a natural, rather than a medical event. When labor began, a woman remained at home and sent for her female friends, relatives, and a midwife. This "social childbirth" provided a support system in which women comforted the laboring woman, shared experience and advice, provided witnesses against accusations of infanticide, and helped the new mother through the lying-in period.

Throughout much of European history, religious authorities exerted considerable influence over the selection of midwives; character and piety were essential criteria for obtaining approval. Midwives were forbidden to perform abortions or conceal a birth. They were expected to make the mothers of illegitimate infants reveal the name of the father. If an infant seemed likely to die before proper baptism, a qualified midwife could perform an emergency baptism. Should the mother die in labor, the midwife might attempt baptism in utero or cesarean section. According to the Dominican inquisitors Heinrich Krämer and Jakob Sprenger, the authors of the infamous *Malleus Maleficarum* (*The Hammer of Witches*, 1486), midwives were among the most pernicious of all witches. Midwives were accused of inducing miscarriages and offering newborn infants to Satan. The products of miscarriages and abortions, stillborn infants, the umbilical cord, and the afterbirth (placenta) played a notorious role in the pharmacology of witchcraft. Given the midwife's low status and wretched fees, the temptation to engage in magic, sell forbidden materials, or accept bribes for family planning through abortion

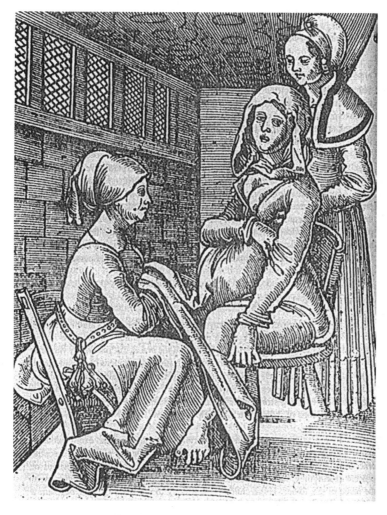

**Midwives Attending a Delivery.**

or infanticide, must have been overwhelming. While there were few prosecutions for the crime of witchcraft in England after 1680, the witchcraft statutes were not repealed until 1736 and there is evidence that the belief in witches persisted into the late eighteenth century. Because of the biblical curse on Eve, midwives were forbidden to use drugs or magical practices to ease the pain of childbirth. Nevertheless, midwives trafficked in charms, amulets, and drugs said to relieve pain and facilitate labor. When discovered, the patient and the midwife might face heavy penalties.

As women became increasingly disadvantaged in terms of legal opportunities to study and practice medicine, those women who had served as healers were extirpated from historical memory. One example of this process is the treatment of Trotula of Salerno in histories of medieval medicine. There has been considerable disagreement as to whether Trotula was a professor at the University of Salerno during the twelfth century and the author of major treatises on obstetrics and gynecology, or a mythical, and somewhat ludicrous figure sometimes referred to as Dame Trots. Simplified translations of gynecological texts attributed to Trotula were treasured by generations of women. The *English Trotula*, for example, contains complex and bizarre remedies, advice about conception, pregnancy, childbirth, "wind in the uterus" and other female problems. For readers who were skeptical about certain prescriptions, the author helpfully suggested testing them on chickens or roosters.

By the middle of the fifteenth century, secular authorities were beginning to displace the church in regulating the practice of midwifery. When labor did not proceed normally, the midwife, who was prohibited by law from using surgical instruments, was required to send for a doctor. Although the penalty for disobedience might be death, midwives apparently adapted common tools to suit their needs, as indicated by accusations that midwives used hooks, needles, spoons, and knives in difficult deliveries. Many midwives were probably illiterate or too poor to buy books, but medical men objected to the publication of midwifery texts in the vernacular. The earliest printed textbook for midwives, Eucharius Rösslin's (d. 1526) *Garden of Roses for Pregnant Women and Midwives* (1513), was still in use in the 1730s. The German text, which was mainly a compilation of Greek and Latin works, included 20 illustrations. An English translation published in 1540 was entitled *The Byrth of Mankynde*.

A few women were able to emerge from the largely anonymous ranks of female practitioners and issue strong calls for improvements in the training and status of midwives. In France, Louise Bourgeois (1563–1636) gained fame as midwife to the French court. In writings addressed to her daughter, Bourgeois described the difficulties of a career as a midwife. Patients took the midwife for granted when childbirth was normal, but blamed her for complications and stillbirths. Elizabeth Cellier, a seventeenth-century London midwife, was known to contemporaries as an "ingenious, and energetic woman," but nineteenth-century male obstetricians called her efforts to raise the status of midwives "unscrupulous." In a petition submitted to King James II in 1687, Cellier argued that unskilled birth attendants were responsible for the deaths of many infants and mothers. To reduce infant and maternal mortality and improve the status of midwives, Cellier proposed the establishment of a College of Midwives and a royal hospital. Cellier hoped the king would support and fund her proposal, but the College of Physicians easily suppressed this scheme. Despite the notoriety associated with Cellier's trials for high treason and libel, little is known about her life. After she was acquitted of involvement in the

"Meal-Tub Plot" of 1680, she published an account of the affair, under the title *Malice Defeated; or a brief relation of the Accusation and Deliverance of Elizabeth Cellier*, which led to a trial for libel. Found guilty of libel, Cellier was ordered to pay a fine and stand in the pillory. Cellier's willingness to petition the king and her ability to write and debate her critics demonstrate that some seventeenth-century midwives were literate and active in public life. Indeed, studies of the hundreds of women who practiced midwifery at the time indicate that many were well trained, successful, and respected.

Despite evidence that eighteenth-century doctors were displacing female midwives as birth attendants, at least for wealthy women, Marguerite Le Boursier du Coudray (1715–1794), the "king's midwife," enjoyed a long and successful career. In 1740, du Coudray was certified to practice midwifery in Paris after passing an examination administered by a panel of royal surgeons and experienced midwives. Her successful practice and political skills resulted in her appointment as the king's midwife. In this capacity, she traveled throughout France to teach midwives and surgeons about the latest methods of delivery. The ingenious du Coudray designed an elaborate "teaching machine" that consisted of a life-sized model of the female pelvis with a fetus, placenta, and umbilical cord and published an illustrated textbook on the art of midwifery. A survey conducted in 1786 suggests that du Coudray or her assistants trained at least half of the midwives, surgeons, and doctors who were delivering babies at the time.

Soranus of Ephesus (98–138) was considered an authority on obstetrics and gynecology, but the birth attendant he described in the *Gynecology* was a midwife—literate, familiar with medical theory, free from superstition, strong, sober, respectable, dexterous, and female. Although physicians from Hippocrates to William Harvey were interested in obstetrics and gynecology, they took it for granted that the practice of midwifery belonged to women. Even in the seventeenth century, the man-midwife was a controversial, menacing, yet somewhat ridiculous figure. Doctors or surgeons were only called for in cases of difficult or obstructed labor. When the man-midwife appeared, the death of the mother or the infant was the most likely outcome. As doctors became more successful at managing difficult births, women were more willing to call on them before complications occurred. By the eighteenth century, wealthy women were increasingly likely to choose male attendants, hoping for a safer delivery. Doctors who used obstetrical instruments began to replace the surgeons who had extracted dead fetuses and the midwives who were not allowed to use surgical instruments.

Ancient misconceptions about the female reproductive system were closely linked to medical theories about conception, gestation, sex determination, and childbirth. Of special significance in the management of birth was the idea that the fetus, rather than the mother, was the active participant in the process. Since the laboring woman was regarded as the obstacle, the doctor's task was to employ whatever tools were necessary to assist the poor little prisoner in its struggle to escape from the womb. Nevertheless, as medical men challenged midwives for control of childbirth, their claims were heavily based on their alleged possession of superior knowledge of female reproductive anatomy and physiology. Renaissance anatomists had certainly rejected many myths about the human reproductive system, such as the ancient Greek description of the uterus as a mobile, restless, two-chambered organ with an innate hunger for childbearing. Still, even in the early twentieth century, there was considerable controversy over the morphology of the uterus, the function of the cervix, and the mechanism of labor.

A good example of the way in which writers create rather than recreate the past can be found in two books written by James Hobson Aveling (1828–1892), Physician to the Chelsea Hospital for Women and Examiner of Midwives for the Obstetrical Society of London. Aveling's hagiography, *The Chamberlens and the Midwifery Forceps* (1882), was written to demonstrate the great contributions of medical men to midwifery. In contrast, the stated purpose of Aveling's *English Midwives: Their History and Prospects* (1872) was to call attention to female midwives and show the misery and damage that had resulted from their ignorance. Aveling used a picture of Elizabeth Cellier at the pillory as the frontispiece of his history of midwives, as if her crime had been medical malpractice rather than libel of a political nature. Trying to explain just how low the midwife's status was, Aveling noted that a midwife might even be called to attend cows that were experiencing a difficult delivery. In impoverished rural households, however, where a cow might be considered more valuable than a wife, such a request was probably not taken as an insult.

Aveling claimed that William Harvey had rescued English midwifery from its place as the most despised part of the medical profession. But it would be more accurate to say that it was a monopoly on the obstetrical forceps and other surgical implements, as well as large claims of specialized professional knowledge, that was responsible for male domination of the field rather than Harvey's remarkable studies of embryology. The origins of the obstetrical forceps are obscure, although the instrument seems simple enough in form and function. All that is known with certainty is that the "hands of iron" evolved from instruments of death. Before surgeons adopted the obstetrical forceps, they could do little more than kill and extract an impacted fetus with knives, hooks, perforators, and lithotomy forceps, or attempt cesarean section on a moribund woman. By the early eighteenth century, medical men had several versions of the obstetrical forceps, with which they could deliver a live, if somewhat squashed baby. The original version of the instrument, however, had been invented at least one hundred years before by a member of the Chamberlen family. Between 1600 and 1728, while famously boasting that their skills in managing difficult labors far exceeded those of any member of the Royal College of Physicians, four generations of Chamberlens enjoyed a lucrative midwifery practice.

Just which of the Chamberlens invented the obstetrical forceps is uncertain because of the family's obsessive secrecy and strange penchant for naming almost all sons Peter or Hugh. In 1598, Peter Chamberlen the Elder (1560–1631) was inducted into the guild of barber-surgeons. Peter the Elder was probably the inventor of the first practical obstetrical forceps. Using his secret instrument, Peter the Elder was able to deliver babies who would otherwise die. Although he was only a barber-surgeon, Peter the Elder had royal patrons, including Queen Anne, wife of King James I. The Chamberlens claimed that it was Peter's remark-able skill in midwifery that led to a series of prosecutions by the Royal College of Physicians. In addition to fines and censures, Peter the Elder was sent to Newgate Prison for the crime of practicing medicine without a license.

Like his older brother Peter the Elder, Peter Chamberlen the Younger (1572–1626) was a barber-surgeon who specialized in mid-wifery and feuded with the Royal College of Physicians. Hoping to ter-minate a long series of prosecutions by elite London physicians, Peter the Younger attempted to join the College. He presented himself for examination in 1610, but apparently failed to satisfy the examiners that he was sufficiently learned in medicine. Members of the College, includ-ing the eminent Robert Fludd (1574–1637), had previously accused Peter the Younger of insulting the College. Dissatisfied patients had also complained that Peter had taken large fees, promised complete cures, and then gave them medicines that made them worse. In 1616, Peter the Younger became involved in efforts to organize an official corpor-ation for the midwives of London. The College of Physicians rejected the petition. In 1634, Chamberlen's eldest son, Peter Chamberlen Jr. (1601–1683) revived the proposal, but it was again rejected.

Peter Chamberlen Jr., studied medicine at several prestigious Italian medical schools and became the first member of the family to obtain a bona fide medical degree. In 1628, Doctor Peter Chamberlen became a member of the Royal College of Physicians, the prestigious organization that had persecuted and harassed his father and uncle. Doctor Peter was physician-in-ordinary to three Kings and Queens of England and several foreign princes. Like the previous Peters, the first Doctor Chamberlen boasted of his success as an obstetrician and quarreled with the College of Physicians.

Three of Doctor Peter Chamberlen's sons—Hugh Senior, Paul, and John—became obstetricians and continued to profit handsomely from the family monopoly. Doctor Hugh Chamberlen (1630–1720) served as midwife to Catherine, wife of Charles II. In the preface to his translation of a French treatise on midwifery, Hugh acknowledged that women were invariably afraid of seeing a doctor enter the lying-in room, because they were sure that when "the man" came, mother or child would die. But, he revealed, this need not be the case. The Chamberlens had, "by God's Blessing" and their own genius and industry, discovered a way of safely delivering the infants of women in difficult cases where any other practitioner "must endanger, if not destroy one or both with Hooks." Apologizing for not sharing the secret of his success, Hugh explained that he could not do so without financial injury to his family. Eventually, however, he betrayed the family secret by offering to sell the instrument.

In 1818, a collection of obstetrical instruments was discovered in a hidden compartment in a house once owned by the Chamberlens. The original obstetrical forceps had separable, curved, and fenestrated blades. After the blades had been inserted into the birth canal, one at a time, they were positioned around the head of the infant. The crossed branches were then joined and fastened with a rivet or thong, so that the doctor could grasp the instrument and exert traction. The instrument looked somewhat like salad tongs grasping a head of lettuce. In his hagiography of the Chamberlens, Aveling made the startling claim that among the forceps discovered in Dr. Peter's house was "doubtless the first midwifery forceps constructed by the Chamberlens, and from which sprung all the various forms now in use." How these instruments could have *sprung* from such a well-kept secret is something of a mystery. In any case, by the mid-eighteenth century, several versions of the obstetrical forceps had been independently invented. Over the years, many variations on the basic instrument were introduced—some trivial, some futile, and some dangerous. Perforators and hooks on the handles of the instrument were employed when a forceps delivery was unsuccessful. Not all doctors were convinced that the instrument was invariably a blessing to women in labor. The great English surgeon, obstetrician, and anatomist William Hunter (1718–1783), for example, cautioned practitioners that "Where they save one, they murder twenty."

An early warning of the threat medical men would pose to midwives and their patients was issued by the English midwife, Jane Sharp, author of *The Midwife's Book; or, The Whole Art of Midwifery Discovered* (1671). Sharp's text, the first midwifery manual written by a British woman, was an accessible, practical guide for midwives, based on her experience and available medical information about the female body and its reproductive functions. The text included descriptions of the female and male "generative parts," discussions of conception, sterility, labor, miscarriage, illnesses and diseases related to pregnancy, postpartum care, wet nurses, the newborn infant, and common childhood diseases. Sharp argued that female midwives were sanctioned by the Bible, whereas male midwives were not, and that women should place greater

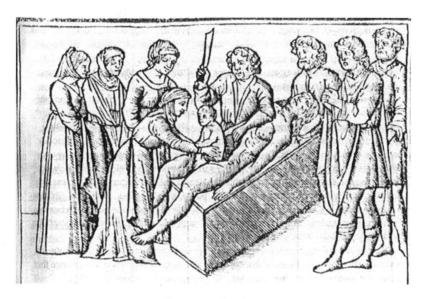

**Cesarean Section.**

reliance on God than the College of Physicians. Although Sharp acknowledged that infant and maternal mortality rates were distressingly high, she refused to let midwives bear all the blame. Emphasizing the poverty and misery endured by the majority of women, she insisted that poor women needed meat more than they needed the services of physicians and surgeons.

Poorly trained midwives and surgeons contributed to infant and maternal mortality, but malnutrition, crowded and unsanitary housing, contaminated food and water, bad air, and occupational hazards deserved equal honors, as demonstrated by the work of the leaders of the nineteenth-century sanitary reform movement. Although infant mortality averaged about 150 per 1,000 live births for England as a whole, in working class areas the rate was much higher. Where mothers were employed and drugs were used as "babysitters," infant mortality rates soared to 200–260 per 1,000 live births. Apothecaries sold hundreds of pounds of opium per year in the form of pills, elixirs, and soothing cordials. While mothers worked in fields or factories, their tranquilized babies were left at home to die of drugs, dysentery, and malnutrition.

Eighteenth-century moralists and journalists found the man-midwife controversy a wonderful source of salacious and titillating stories. Social critics warned that French dances, French novels, and male midwifery would lead to the complete corruption of female virtue, social chaos, and the end of civilization. The man-midwife was also the object of scorn within the medical profession, where all forms of specialization were regarded with suspicion. The College of Physicians was reluctant to allow obstetricians the rights and privileges of membership, because midwifery was a manual operation, foreign to the ways of learned gentlemen who should not stoop to participating in the "humiliating events of parturition." But to keep the spoils within the family, leaders of the College of Surgeons suggested that midwifery should be conducted by the wives, widows, and daughters of surgeons and apothecaries.

Critics charged the man-midwife with deliberately exaggerating the dangers of childbirth in order to turn a natural event into a surgical process for self-serving motives. Doctors were also accused of misusing instruments to save time and justify large fees. According to one English midwife, the man-midwife hid his mistakes in a cloud of scientific jargon so that confused patients thanked the man who had killed the infant and maimed the mother. Obstetricians cynically shared tricks for impressing the patient and avoiding blame. For example, if the doctor left during the early stages of labor, he should poke the patient intravaginally and tell her he was doing something to help the progress of labor. Thus, even if he was not present when the child was born, he could claim the credit if all went well, and blame the nurse for any problems.

Some doctors admitted that factors other than the sex of the birth attendant might determine the outcome of labor. Dr. Charles White (1728–1813) of Manchester, for example, noted that sick, half-starved, impoverished, rural women, served only by the worst sort of midwives might actually have a lower maternal mortality rate than city women delivered in lying-in hospitals, or wealthy women attended by male doctors. Critics of female midwives argued that women were totally unable to master scientific knowledge or use medical instruments. Since problems could develop suddenly, even in apparently normal labors, all cases should be attended by male practitioners.

Many doctors were willing to accept a class of midwives who would relieve them of unprofitable cases, but they would not tolerate women who might offer real competition. Members of the Obstetrical Society saw a clear division between the role of the midwife and that of the obstetrician. Midwives were suitable for poor women, because they were less delicate than rich women and, therefore, less in need of sophisticated medical assistance at childbirth. Midwives should be restricted to "the hard, tedious, ill-paid work appropriate for women" while medical men maintained a "manly and dignified position" in service to wealthy clients. Midwives were supposed to call for a doctor when confronted by abnormal labor, but doctors might refuse to see a patient who had chosen to use a midwife. Even in notorious cases where women died because obstetricians would not respond to a midwife's appeal for assistance, many doctors argued that such fatalities would teach the improvident to mend their ways, save their money, and call a doctor first. When potential patients realized that doctors would not "cover" for midwives, these archaic female competitors would disappear.

The outcome of the rivalry between midwives and medical men was already obvious by the end of the nineteenth century. The promise of total victory was apparent in Aveling's claim that the sordid history of the ignorant and incompetent midwife was drawing to a close. Nevertheless, the triumph of the medical man in the nineteenth century is an enigma. Certainly, science had not yet entered the lying-in chamber. The transition from midwifery to obstetrics occurred at a time when intervention was often performed by rough, inexperienced, surgically-oriented practitioners, still concerned with strength and speed, uninhibited by considerations of asepsis. Moreover, the transition occurred in a period obsessed with female modesty. The proper Victorian lady was expected to prefer death to a discussion of "female complaints" with a male physician. Women entering the medical profession in the late nineteenth century also tended to disapprove of traditional midwives. Struggling for a place in the medical community, they generally accepted Victorian conventions of female modesty and argued that female doctors were a better choice for childbirth than midwives or male doctors.

Paradoxically, the most prudish societies of all were those that most completely accepted the new male-dominated obstetrics. It has been argued that the medicalization of birth reflected a deeper concern for the welfare of women. Alternatively, the paradox can be explained as a reflection of hostility towards women which generated a desire to punish them for their sexuality by the ultimate degradation: taking away their female support system and substituting the control of the male doctor who would transform the dangerous, unpredictable process of childbirth into a routine surgical process. Certainly, the argument that birth was a pathological process, and that perhaps nature deliberately intended for women to be "used up in the process of reproduction, in a manner analogous to that of salmon," suggests a deep-seated contempt for women, or at least a lack of sympathy.

As the role of the hospital expanded in the eighteenth and nineteenth centuries, physicians in the major cities were able to gain the clinical experience that made it possible for the "hands of iron" to emerge as the "imperishable symbol and weapon" with which the battles between traditional female-centered births and the medicalization of birth would be fought. With the introduction of obstetrical anesthesia in the 1850s, the physician could add the promise of pain-free labor to his monopoly on obstetrical instruments. Forceps and anesthesia could make childbirth more rapid and less painful, but the resultant burden of injury and infection was a heavy price for women to pay. Critics warned that when the mother was under anesthesia, the forceps could be used brusquely and unnecessarily, causing profound damage to mother and infant. Often the damage was done simply because the doctor had not troubled himself to be sure that maternal tissues were not trapped within the locking mechanism of the forceps. On the other hand, doctors who took the precaution of passing a finger around the locking mechanism—a finger ungloved and perhaps unwashed—also endangered the patient.

Although the poor and desperate women who served as clinical material in the hospitals of the nineteenth century had little choice in birth attendants, wealthy women increasingly chose physician-attended home delivery in hopes of safer and less painful deliveries. During the mid-twentieth century, childbirth moved out of the sphere of women's domestic culture and into the hospital. To improve the status of obstetrics as an area of specialization, Joseph B. DeLee (1869–1942) and other leading obstetricians considered it essential to eliminate competition from general practitioners as well as midwives. According to DeLee, childbirth was a surgical procedure that should be managed by an obstetrician in a hospital operating room where forceps deliveries and episiotomies were routine. The Chicago Maternity Center, founded by DeLee, provided "clinical material" for an intensive course in obstetrics where students from Wisconsin, Marquette, and Northwestern University were taught DeLee's principles of scientific obstetrics.

The trend towards hospital delivery had been accelerating since the 1920s. Before 1938, in the United States, half of all babies were still born at home; by 1955, about 95 percent of all births took place in hospitals where the laboring woman found herself "alone among strangers." This transition has been called the most significant change in the history of childbirth, but it occurred *before* the medicalized hospital birth had actually become statistically safer than home births. Nevertheless, women chose hospital delivery with the expectation that the hospital offered expertise, new technology, freedom from pain, and increased safety for both mother and infant.

Ever since medical men gained a monopoly over the "hands of iron" and the "potions of oblivion," the midwife has been an endangered species. Unlike chiropractors, optometrists, podiatrists, and dentists, the midwife never had a chance at the title "doctor." In the 1960s and 1970s, interest in natural approaches to health care and the Woman's Rights Movement led to calls for a return to "woman-centered childbirth," but the trend towards medicalization of birth had become so powerful that in the 1980s more than 25 percent of all babies born in some American hospitals were brought into the world by cesarean section. In this context, the history of puerperal fever and midwifery are clearly only part of a complex transformation that encompassed changes in medical institutions, professional roles, social expectations, and beliefs about the nature of woman. The man-midwife entered the female-dominated world of social childbirth as a lowly surgeon, transformed childbirth into a surgical event in the physician-dominated world of the hospital, and created highly valued professional roles for obstetricians and gynecologists.

The increased use of anesthesia—ether and chloroform in the second half of the nineteenth century and "Twilight Sleep," a combination of morphine and scopolamine, in the early decades of the twentieth century—also increased the status of the obstetrician. Women learned that the benefits of painless childbirth were only available in a hospital setting with a trained obstetrician. Twilight Sleep was often combined with the "prophylactic forceps operation," episiotomy, and other routine surgical interventions. Episiotomy was promoted as part of obstetric practice in the 1920s, supposedly as a means of preventing serious lacerations of the perineum during childbirth, but probably its main effect was to make it easier to insert forceps and expedite delivery. By the 1980s, however, researchers began to realize that the risks associated with episiotomy were significantly greater than the alleged benefits. Other forms of surgery on the female reproductive organs were also quite common in the late nineteenth and early twentieth centuries. Such surgery included what was called "normal ovariotomy" because it was carried out on normal healthy ovaries. Gynecologists argued that this operation could correct the behavior of women exhibiting signs of insanity, neurosis, mental instability, menstrual irregularities, and so forth. Clitoridectomy was done for similar reasons.

Critics of the "over medicalization of modern life" warn about the dangers of treating normal female functions, including pregnancy and menopause, as pathological states. For example, since the 1960s, some gynecologists have argued that menopause is an estrogen-deficiency disease and that estrogen replacement therapy is needed to prevent defeminization, hypertension, high cholesterol, osteoporosis, arthritis, and serious emotional disturbances. Despite claims that hormone replacement therapy (HRT) was completely safe, by 1975 researchers had evidence of a relationship between postmenopausal estrogen therapy and endometrial cancer. Other reports of damage caused by medical devices and prescription drugs furthered feminist criticism about medical interventions in women. The abuse of diethylstilbestrol (DES), a synthetic estrogen first produced in 1938, demonstrated that the medicalization of pregnancy and childbirth could also be dangerous to the next generation. Diethylstilbestrol was prescribed for menopause, diabetes, amenorrhea, dysmenorrhea, genital underdevelopment, infertility, morning sickness, toxemia, suppression of lactation, and to prevent spontaneous abortion. Many obstetricians considered DES part of the routine management of pregnancy. In some clinics that were engaged in tests of DES, pregnant women were not told that the "vitamin pills" they were given contained an experimental drug.

In 1970, when a rare form of malignant vaginal cancer (clear cell adenocarcinoma) in young women was linked to intrauterine exposure to DES, the FDA ruled that DES was "contraindicated for use in the prevention of miscarriages." The question of whether DES actually prevented miscarriage remains controversial, but researchers found significant evidence that the synthetic hormone is embryopathic, teratogenic, and carcinogenic. Neonatologists noted that DES was only one of many ineffectual and dangerous treatments that were supposed to improve pregnancies or help newborns. For example, thalidomide, the most notorious teratogenic agent of the twentieth century, was prescribed as a remedy for morning sickness during pregnancy and as a sleeping aid.

In many parts of the world, midwives continued to have a major role in caring for pregnant women and delivering babies, but efforts to improve the status of midwifery in the United States were generally unsuccessful. In the interests of public health, some American reformers attempted to replace traditional direct-entry midwives with registered nurses who had taken advanced training in midwifery. The Frontier Nursing Service (FNS), initiated by Mary Breckinridge (1881–1965) in 1925, provided a demonstration of the value of nurse-midwifery, as well as the ability of the American medical community to suppress such programs. Breckinridge became interested in midwifery training programs while serving as a volunteer nurse in Europe. As part of her plan to bring nurse-midwifery to impoverished areas in the South, she studied public health nursing at Columbia Teachers' College and midwifery at hospitals in England and Scotland. Women in the Kentucky mountain region selected for the demonstration program were usually attended by midwives who learned the art from other midwives. Doctors, if available, charged at least ten times as much as "granny" midwives and expected cash rather than payment in-kind.

Frontier Nursing Service nurse-midwives provided prenatal care, administered inoculations for typhoid, diphtheria, and smallpox, and treatments for parasitic infections. Although most of their patients lived in poverty-stricken homes, accessible only by horseback, the FNS achieved mortality rates well below those of the general population of Kentucky and the United States as a whole. Although the FNS was largely successful in fulfilling its goals, it did not establish an autonomous professional role for nurse-midwifery in the United States. Neither did the any of the other midwifery training programs in rural or urban America.

Nevertheless, nurse-midwifery did not entirely disappear. The American College of Nurse-Midwives was founded in 1955 to represent certified nurse-midwives, that is, birth-attendants educated in both nursing and midwifery. Even though certified nurse-midwives are trained to care for healthy women and newborns, they can only practice legally if they are affiliated with a physician. The American College of Obstetricians and Gynecologists adopted the policy that cooperation between doctors, nurse-midwives, and other health personnel was possible, if all concerned acted within "medically directed teams." Although statistical studies repeatedly demonstrated that when nurse-midwives care for pregnant women, there are fewer premature and underweight babies, the medical community remained indifferent or hostile to nurse-midwives. The American Nurses' Association and the National League for Nursing were also ambiguous about nurse-midwifery. The Midwives' Alliance of North America, which was founded in 1982, took the position that nursing was not a necessary prerequisite for midwifery.

Interest in midwifery began to grow again in the 1970s among women who wanted to avoid aggressive medical techniques like induced labor, epidural blocks, episiotomies, and cesarean sections. Women who were troubled by the impersonality and medicalization that typified hospital births began to see midwife-attended home births as a possible alternative. By 2000, every state allowed certified nurse-midwives to practice, however, state laws concerning lay-midwives and home births vary considerably. According to the National Center for Health Statistics, in 1976, certified nurse-midwives attended just one percent of births in America. In 2002, certified nurse-midwives attended almost eight percent of births, but midwifery was in decline by 2004. In New York City, certified nurse-midwives attended about 12 percent of births in 1997, but by 2002, that had fallen to 9.7 percent, according to the City's Department of Health and Mental Hygiene. Midwives, doctors, hospital executives, and patients generally attribute the declining use of midwives to insurance issues and the threat of lawsuits. Malpractice insurance premiums increased more steeply for midwives than for obstetricians. Only two of the four freestanding birthing centers run by midwives in New York City in 2002 were still in business the next year. Hospitals that had established birthing centers staffed by midwives to attract patients limited the work of midwives by classifying more patients as "high risk."

Even in the twenty-first century, where women's access to medical care and education is restricted, maternal and infant mortality may approach premodern levels. Studies of Afghanistan revealed remarkably high rates of both infant and maternal mortality. Millions of women across rural Afghanistan live in a constant cycle of pregnancy and birth through most of their adult lives with little or no medical care. A study conducted in 2001 by the World Health Organization estimated that there were more than two thousand maternal deaths per one hundred thousand live births. Babies whose mothers die in childbirth have only a one in four chance of surviving to their first birthday. Almost half of the deaths of Afghan women of childbearing age are caused by complications during pregnancy, or by childbirth itself. Researchers suggested that almost 90 percent of the maternal deaths could have been prevented with better medical care.

## THE EVOLUTION OF THE NURSE

It was often said that every woman is a nurse. After nursing adopted the Nightingale model, it could be said that "every nurse is a woman." (A man who performed similar hospital work was typically called an orderly.) Nursing, whether in the sickroom or in the hospital ward, was considered part of woman's natural role. While accepting many aspects of the traditional division between male and female roles, Florence Nightingale (1820–1910) and other nursing reformers attempted to transform nursing from another form of unskilled drudgery into a profession suitable for educated, middle-class women. Before Nightingale was called to nursing, religious women—nursing sisters—were involved in the development of nursing and the establishment of hospitals. Nevertheless, by the nineteenth century, hospitals were generally infamous for their miserable conditions and the incompetence of their nursing staff. Thus, although Nightingale did not invent nursing, she was certainly a key figure in reforming the image and training of the modern nurse.

Without excessive exaggeration, Nightingale often said that the benefits of medicine were uncertain, but the value of good nursing care was beyond dispute. Well-trained Nightingale nurses emphasized obsessive cleanliness in hospitals wards, even before surgeons adopted antisepsis and asepsis. Although the work carried out by nurses has changed in many ways since the Nightingale era, studies conducted in the 1990s confirmed Nightingale's dictum. Patients treated at hospitals with a higher proportion of registered nurses suffered lower rates of complications and were released sooner than patients in hospitals with relatively low numbers of registered nurses. Longer hospital stays were associated with higher rates of complications like urinary infections, pneumonia, gastrointestinal bleeding, shock, cardiac arrest, and deaths that might have been prevented by rapid intervention. The American Nurses Association has long insisted that maintaining appropriate levels of registered nurses is critical to insuring good patient care.

In 1921, when American hospital administrators celebrated the first National Hospital Day, they acknowledged the coevolution of the modern hospital and the trained nurse by selecting May 12, Florence Nightingale's birthday, for the festivities. In the United States, efforts to establish nursing schools were inspired by Nightingale and the experiences of the Civil War. Long before hospitals assumed a significant role in the education of doctors, hospital administrators found it rewarding to establish schools for the training of nurses. The number of nurse training schools in the United States grew rapidly after the first such schools were founded in the 1870s. By 1930, over two thousand hospitals were staffing their wards and selling the services of their own student nurses. As the number of nursing schools expanded, competition for the limited number of hospital positions and private duty assignments diminished the professional expectations of all trained nurses. Following the Nightingale model, early nursing reformers hoped to recruit from a select pool of "lady pupils" who would see nursing as a special calling. As the number of hospital nursing schools expanded, however, selectivity declined and nurses were seen as merely useful, reliable workers, who were expected to remain subordinate and deferential to doctors. While attempting to create a standardized curriculum for nursing schools, nursing leaders also struggled to establish a professional identity for trained nurses. Well aware of the fact that the term "nurse" was used indiscriminately, nursing associations worked for licensing laws that would differentiate between trained and untrained nurses. By World War II, nursing practice had essentially established its modern form as graduate nurses replaced student nurses in hospital wards.

Mary Adelaide Nutting (1858–1948) and Lavinia Lloyd Dock (1858–1956), nursing reformers and educators, insisted that the primary obligation of the nurse was the patient, not the doctor and urged nurses to control their own profession. As advocates of the Progressive worldview, Dock and Nutting saw their work as part of women's mission to achieve social reform and progress. In addition to teaching and writing, Dock expressed her commitment to social reforms and public health concerns through her work in the settlement house movement. Dock worked as a public health nurse with her colleague Lillian Wald (1867–1940), the founder of the Henry Street Settlement, in New York City. Convinced that books and journals written by and for nurses were essential elements in the battle for professional autonomy, Dock and Nutting spent many years gathering material for their four-volume *History of Nursing* (1907–1912). Recent studies indicate that nurses are still working towards Dock's goal of the control of nursing by nurses.

Following the model of Nightingale's district nursing experiments, during the 1880s charitable organizations throughout the United States sponsored visiting nursing organizations. Nurses cared for the sick poor, providing help in bathing, dressing, feeding, and cleaning the home, as well as giving medicines, taking vital signs, teaching family members how to care for the patient and avoid contagion. Nurses in major cities also attempted to Americanize the immigrant families they visited. Some nurses and social reformers believed their work would also help reform the social conditions that led to illness, filth, and poverty. During the early twentieth century, the expanding public health movement offered trained nurses a field with the promise of more professional autonomy than routine hospital work or private duty nursing. Public health nurses were involved in visiting nurse services, settlement houses, school nursing, child welfare, anti-venereal disease campaigns, factory dispensaries, first aid stations, preventive medicine, and health education. By having an approved protocol and standing orders from a doctor, the nurse avoided legal problems and enjoyed considerable autonomy. The National Organization for Public Health Nursing was founded in 1912, but most local governments did not respond to the idea that nursing services were essential aspects of public health work. Visiting nurse associations were, however, profoundly impacted by changes in the medical system as the role of hospitals expanded. After World War II, the organization of health services underwent changes that once again thwarted the professional aspirations of the nurse. Eventually, hospitals, official government agencies, and physicians found ways to take over work previously done by voluntary social service agencies and public health nurses.

### "WOMAN'S NATURE" AND WOMEN DOCTORS

The "Woman Question" was the theme of endless books by nineteenth-century physicians, scientists, and philosophers. Using so-called scientific arguments to rationalize and legitimate traditional social and economic patterns, doctors portrayed themselves as scientists with special knowledge of female physiology. American physicians argued that women were condemned to weakness and sickness, because female physiology, including the menstrual cycle, was inherently pathological. In the 1870s, doctors increasingly focused on the threat that education posed to the health of girls and women. Woman's whole being, especially her central nervous system, was said to be controlled by her uterus and ovaries. Brainwork during puberty, especially in a coeducational setting, therefore, would interfere with the development of the female reproductive system. The best-known proponent of this rationale was Edward H. Clarke (1820–1877), author of an influential book entitled *Sex in Education: or, a Fair Chance for the Girl*s (1874).

In addition to his large private practice in Boston, Clarke was a Harvard professor and a leader in the battle to prevent the admission of female students to Harvard. Clarke subscribed to the prevailing idea that the human body was a closed system with a limited "energy bank." In other words, the body was a battlefield where all organs fought for a share of limited energy resources. The struggle between the brain and the female reproductive system was particularly dangerous. "Nature has reserved the catamenial week for the process of ovulation," Clarke insisted (quite incorrectly), "and for the development and perfection of the reproductive system." Total mental and physical rest during the menstrual period was essential for the proper development of the female reproductive system.

According to Clarke, women who graduated from college, if they survived the ordeal at all, were doomed to become sterile, sickly invalids, subject to amenorrhea, dysmenorrhea, leucorrhoea, chronic and acute ovaritis, prolapsus uteri, anemia, constipation, headaches, hysteria, neuralgia, and other horrors. The "intellectual force" expended by girls studying Latin or mathematics destroyed significant numbers of brain cells in addition to decreasing fertility. Educated women who escaped sterility would face dangerous pregnancies and deliveries because they had smaller pelvises and their babies had bigger brains. They would be unable to nurse their own babies, because they had "neither the organs nor nourishment requisite." As evidence, Clarke presented the sad case of the flat-chested Miss D., who entered Vassar at 14. By the time she graduated, she was the victim of dysmenorrhea, hysteria, nervousness, headaches, chronic invalidism, and constipation. Another unfortunate student died soon after graduation; the postmortem revealed a worn-out brain. Even Martha Carey Thomas (1857–1935), founder and president of Bryn Mawr College, remembered being terrified when she read such warnings as a girl.

Tests of the Clarke hypothesis demonstrated that college women were as healthy as other women and studies of motor and mental skills found no special effects associated with the menstrual cycle. Critics of the Clarke hypothesis argued that doctors who shared his beliefs were simply prejudiced and influenced by the fact that the women they saw as patients were indeed sickly. Female doctors argued that girls were often sickly because of bad diet, lack of fresh air, tight corsets, restrictive clothing, and the lack of education and exercise. Some skeptics argued that, because of the great oversupply of doctors, practitioners were eager to find chronic, but nonfatal "female complaints" among delicate upper-class women. Servants, factory workers, and other poor women did not seem to need a week of rest during their menses.

Mary Putnam Jacobi (1842–1906), an eminent physician and medical writer, explicitly asserted that women were diagnosed as perpetual invalids because doctors saw them as lucrative patients. Her book *The Question of Rest for Women During Menstruation*, which was written to answer the question "Do women require mental and bodily rest during menstruation, and to what extent?," won the Boylston Prize from Harvard University in 1876. Jacobi's work demonstrated that education and professional work did not damage women's health. Indeed, educated women were healthier than any other group of women. Certainly, many women were not as healthy as they could be, but the true remedy for them was more education, not less. Sickly women were most likely the victims of alcoholic fathers, husbands with venereal diseases, and "bad social arrangements," but hysteria and other debilitating "nervous diseases" supported doctors like Clarke quite well, because they were "never fatal, impossible to cure, but always in need of medical attention." Jacobi, one of the founders of the Women's Medical Association of New York City, was an active crusader for women's access to medical education. Jacobi graduated from the Female Medical College of

Pennsylvania in 1864. She spent a year as an intern in the New England Hospital. To improve her medical training she went to Paris and was the first woman admitted to the Paris School of Medicine. She graduated in 1871 with high honors.

Representatives of many colleges studied Clarke's claims and argued that their women students were very healthy. The Resident Physician at Vassar College insisted that no one who knew how wrong Clarke was about Vassar could trust the rest of his book. No evidence of Clarke's unfortunate "Miss D." could be found at Vassar, an outstanding school that did not accept 14-year-old girls. Julia Ward Howe (1819–1910), American feminist and author of the "Battle Hymn of the Republic" (1862), published a collection of critical responses entitled *A Reply to Dr. E. H. Clarke's "Sex in Education."* After carefully reviewing *Sex in Education*, Howe concluded that it was not a work of science, literature, philosophy, or a treatise on health, but simply a polemic against education for women. Contrary to Clarke's ominous predictions, women were not becoming sick and sterile just because some wished to enter Harvard College. Clarke's warnings about the dangers of education during female development had no more validity than ancient "old wives' tales" that attributed female complaints to wet feet, silk stockings, horseback riding, dancing, or winter parties. The true remedy for female disabilities was more education, not less, especially education about physiology. While Clarke generalized from his own observations of sick women, he failed to note that women did not become sick until after graduation when they stopped studying and succumbed to intellectual starvation.

Clarke was not alone in his campaign against female education. Horatio Storer (1869–1872), a Boston gynecologist and publisher of the *Journal of the Gynaecological Society of Boston*, also used the "menstrual difficulties" argument. Another American gynecologist advised girls to "spend the year before and two years after puberty at rest." Each menstrual period, he added, should be endured in "the recumbent position." American neurologist S. Weir Mitchell (1829–1914) asserted that excessive brainwork before a girl was fully mature would damage her "future womanly usefulness" and turn her into an invalid. The well-known American psychologist G. Stanley Hall (1844–1924) agreed that excessive mental stimulation was a danger to girls and women. Girls should, therefore, attend special schools that accommodated the female cycle of disability.

When the American Medical Association (AMA) debated admitting female physicians, the arguments offered in the 1870s included the assertion that women could never become physicians because they lacked rational judgment, that physiological evidence proved that the brain size of females was insufficient for medical education, and that their judgment varied daily "according to the time of the month." In the great debate about the "woman question" in Great Britain, editorials in the *Lancet* proclaimed that women were too encumbered by "physical disqualifications" to become physicians, although they could serve as nurses and midwives for the poor. Many doctors agreed with the doctrines proposed by Edward H. Clarke in *Sex and Education*, but a few argued in favor of accepting women as professional colleagues. One doctor complained that if the AMA would not recognize female physicians, he would be unable to consult with the "most highly educated" women physicians, even though he was free to consult "with the most ignorant masculine ass in the medical profession."

Women did not necessarily turn to medical men like Dr. Clarke for their special "female complaints." Indeed, most people relied on domestic medicine, folk remedies, and patent medicines rather than physicians. Nursing the sick was part of "woman's natural sphere." However, some women were able to turn female modesty and the womanly art of healing into flourishing businesses. The most famous example was Lydia E. Pinkham (1819–1883) and her Vegetable Compound, an herbal remedy supposedly effective for dozens of female complaints related to the reproductive organs and functions, but not excluding headache and fatigue. The success of the Vegetable Compound reflected widespread dissatisfaction with orthodox medicine, especially among women, and the genius for marketing and advertising displayed by the Pinkham family. Pinkham's "female weakness cure" was a forty proof herbal tonic containing life root, unicorn root, black cohosh, pleurisy root, and fenugreek seeds. Thousand of letters from satisfied customers supported her belief that the Vegetable Compound was more effective and certainly less dangerous than the medicines prescribed by doctors. Pinkham's Compound was still popular in the 1940s when modern "miracle drugs" displaced Lydia Pinkham's herbal elixir.

During the nineteenth century, many medical practitioners had earned the title "doctor" by apprenticeships or a few months of dreary lectures at a medical school—orthodox or sectarian—with dubious credentials. In this context, it is important to remember that although Elizabeth Blackwell is often called the first woman doctor, this is not strictly true. Other women had practiced medicine before Blackwell, but she was a pioneer in opening the orthodox medical profession to women. Throughout history, female practitioners were typically described as midwives and herbalists even if their training and their work was essentially the same as that of male practitioners. Harriot Hunt (1805–1875), for example, practiced medicine in Boston for about 40 years, after completing a medical apprenticeship. At the time, only a minority of medical practitioners had graduated from a medical college. Nevertheless, in her autobiography, Hunt described being shunned by the male medical establishment as if she had some terrible disease.

In her autobiography Elizabeth Blackwell (1821–1910) said that she decided to become a doctor because of a friend who died of a painful disease of a "delicate nature"—probably uterine cancer. Confiding that her "worst sufferings" were caused by having to be treated by a male physician, this woman suggested that Blackwell become a doctor. Overcoming her initial disgust at the thought of studying anatomy, physiology, and all the afflictions of the human body, Blackwell decided that becoming a doctor was a necessary moral crusade. In 1847, when Blackwell began to apply to medical schools, none of the regular schools admitted women. Eventually, she was accepted by Geneva Medical College, New York, a mediocre, but orthodox medical school. In January of 1849, Blackwell was awarded her diploma and the title Doctor of Medicine.

To gain clinical experience in surgery and obstetrics, Blackwell went to Europe. An eye infection, contracted while caring for a patient at La Maternité in Paris, almost destroyed her career. Treatment of the infection included cauterization of the eyelids, application of leeches to the temples, cold compresses, ointment of belladonna, footbaths, mustard plasters, and a diet limited to broth. With the sight in one eye permanently destroyed, Blackwell gave up the idea of specializing in surgery. While in England, Blackwell met Florence Nightingale and became aware of the importance of sanitation and proper hospital administration. In 1859, Elizabeth Blackwell became the first woman listed in the Medical Register of the United Kingdom. Blackwell gave several lectures on medical education for women and helped establish the London School of Medicine for Women, the first medical school for women in Great Britain.

Hopeful that opportunities for medical women were improving, Blackwell returned to America. Her sister Emily Blackwell (1826–1910), who had graduated from Cleveland Medical College in 1854, studied obstetrics with James Young Simpson (1811–1879), Professor of Midwifery at Edinburgh and one of Scotland's leading surgeons and obstetricians. In 1857, the Blackwells and Marie Zakrzewska (1829–1902) established a dispensary and a hospital to serve the poor. The Woman's Medical College of the New York Infirmary for Women and Children provided instruction and clinical experience for female students until 1899. Zakrzewska, originally a professor of midwifery at the Berlin School for Midwives, immigrated to America and earned a medical degree from the Cleveland Medical College. After working with the Blackwells, she moved to Boston and established the New England Hospital for Women and Children.

When Elizabeth Blackwell assessed the progress of women in medicine in 1869, she was entirely optimistic about the future. Blackwell asserted that, at least in the northern states, "the free and equal entrance of women into the profession of medicine" had been achieved. Twentieth-century women, who venerated Blackwell as a role model, had to admit that she was obviously better at being a pioneer than a prophet. Similarly, although Blackwell served as an inspiration to generations of American girls, her life was often presented as the inevitable long, lonely struggle that a woman would have to wage if she chose a professional life instead of marriage and family. A closer study of the pioneering generation of female physicians reveals a broad range of personal and professional relationships. Many little known nineteenth-century women physicians married, raised children, and practiced medicine. Excluded from full participation in the medical community, other female physicians found their niche in public health, the settlement house movement, well-baby clinics, industrial hygiene, and laboratory medicine.

In 1859, while visiting her sister in London, Elizabeth Garrett (1836–1917) met Elizabeth Blackwell at one of her lectures on "Medicine as a Profession for Ladies." Blackwell's example stimulated Garrett's determination to become a physician. When one doctor asked Garrett why she wanted to be a doctor instead of a nurse, she retorted: "Because I prefer to earn a thousand rather than twenty pounds a year!" The logic of her answer won the complete and total support of her father, Newson Garrett, a prosperous businessman.

No British medical schools were open to women and the Medical Register had been closed to women with foreign degrees after Blackwell secured a place on the list. Friends suggested that Garret work as a nurse at Middlesex Hospital for six months to test her endurance and dedication before attempting to study medicine. After a three-month probationary period, Garrett abandoned the pretense of being a nurse and simply assumed the role of a medical student, making rounds in the wards, working in the dispensary, helping with emergency patients, attending lectures, and taking examinations. Although Garrett received a Certificate of Honor in each of the subjects covered by her lecture courses, she was not allowed to become an official student. Her applications were rejected by Oxford, Cambridge, and the University of London, which according to its charter provided education for "all classes and denominations without distinction whatsoever." She was told that women were neither a class nor a denomination.

Determined to secure a qualifying diploma in order to have her name on the Medical Register, Garret decided to obtain the degree of Licentiate of the Society of Apothecaries (L.S.A.). The L.S.A. was not as prestigious as the M.D., but holders of the license granted by the Apothecaries' Hall could become accredited physicians. To qualify, an applicant had to serve a five-year apprenticeship under a qualified doctor, take lecture courses with recognized university tutors, and pass the qualifying examination. The Hall of Apothecaries was certainly not an advocate of equal opportunity for women, but its charter stated that it would examine "all persons" who had satisfied the regulations. According to legal opinions obtained by Mr. Garrett, "persons" included women. In 1865, Garrett finally forced the Society of Apothecaries to accept her credentials and administer the qualifying examination. One year later, Garrett's name was enrolled in the Medical Register. The Society of Apothecaries immediately changed its charter to require graduation from an accredited medical school as a prerequisite for the L.S.A. degree. Of course, all such schools excluded women. For another 12 years, no women's names were added to the Medical Register.

In 1866, Garrett opened the St. Mary's Dispensary for Women in London. Six years later, the dispensary became the New Hospital for Women and Children. (When Elizabeth Garrett Anderson died, the hospital was renamed the Elizabeth Garrett Anderson Hospital.) In 1869, Garret met her future husband, James George Skelton Anderson, who was serving as a member of the board of directors of the Shadwell Hospital for Children. Despite marriage and the birth of three children, Garrett Anderson continued to practice medicine. Moreover, she earned the degree of M.D. from the University of Paris, successfully passing examinations and defending a thesis on "Migraine." Garrett Anderson and other women doctors established the London Medical College for Women. As dean and professor, Anderson opposed the idea that women planning work as missionaries should come to the school and acquire a little medical knowledge. Medicine, she believed was a profession and not a charity. Moreover, she thought that the willingness of women to sacrifice themselves was too easily exploited. During World War I, Garrett Anderson's daughter Dr. Louisa Garrett Anderson (1873–1943) served as organizer of the women's hospital corps and chief surgeon of the military hospital at Endell Street.

Some women doctors carved out unique careers by entering fields closely allied with social reform movements that were of little interest to established male practitioners. Alice Hamilton (1869–1970), American pioneer of industrial hygiene, decided to study medicine because she considered it the only profession open to women that would allow her to support herself while doing useful and independent work. When she received her M.D. in 1893 from the medical department of the University of Michigan, she was one of 13 women in a class of 47. Hamilton interned at the Northwestern Hospital for Women and Children in Minneapolis and the New England Hospital for Women and Children in Boston. More interested in research than private practice, Hamilton studied bacteriology and pathology at the Universities of Leipzig and Munich, the Pasteur Institute in Paris, and the Johns Hopkins School of Medicine.

While teaching pathology at the Woman's Medical School of Northwestern University, Hamilton became a resident of Hull House, the settlement house founded by American social reformer Jane Addams (1860–1935). When the Woman's Medical School closed in 1902, Hamilton joined the new Memorial Institute for Infectious Diseases. Hamilton's studies of typhoid fever in Chicago called attention to the role of the fly in transmitting germs, the relationship between disease and sanitation, and the need for public health reforms. Through her experiences at Hull House, Hamilton realized that many workers became incurable invalids because of exposure to poisonous substances in factories, foundries, and steel mills. Although industrial medicine was already an established discipline in Europe, in the United States occupational diseases were essentially ignored. Medical men, she discovered, seemed to consider the study of occupational disease somewhat "tainted with Socialism or with female sentimentality for the poor."

As managing director of the Illinois Commission on Occupational Diseases, Hamilton combined field studies of industrial poisons, such as lead, with laboratory research. As a result of her survey, Illinois passed a workmen's compensation law requiring safety measures in factories and medical examinations of workers. In 1911, Hamilton became an unpaid special investigator for the United States Bureau of Labor. When Hamilton began her studies of industrial diseases, doctors and employers argued that industrial poisoning could be prevented by having workers keep their hands clean. Hamilton tried to convince them that "a lead worker eats only three times and day and even then he does not wash his hands in his soup or coffee, but he breathes sixteen times a minute and when there is lead in the air, he will get it no matter how often he scrubs his nails." Having established the dangers of lead dust, Hamilton went on to investigate the hazards of arsenic, mercury, organic solvents, radium, and many other toxic materials, especially in the rubber industry and munitions plants. Hamilton wrote that she was often successful in negotiating with factory owners, because she was pragmatic, persistent, and "fair but not too fair."

After World War I, interest in industrial hygiene increased, but because the field was new and still somewhat suspect, it was of limited interest to medical men. Hamilton readily admitted that she became assistant professor of industrial medicine at the Harvard Medical School, because she was the only candidate available. Harvard attached three stipulations to her appointment as the university's first female professor. She was not to enter the Harvard Faculty Club, march in the commencement procession, or claim her quota of football tickets. In 1935, Hamilton retired from Harvard with the title of Assistant Professor Emeritus of Industrial Medicine. Throughout her life, Hamilton was an advocate of protective legislation, child labor laws, pacifism, birth control, and other social reforms. She was 101 when she died of a stroke at her home.

In the United States, 19 female medical schools were established between 1850 and 1895. The schools that survived until the end of the century were the Boston Female Medical College (New England Female Medical College), Woman's Medical College (Kansas City, Missouri),

Woman's Medical College of the New York Infirmary for Women and Children, Women's Hospital Medical College of Chicago, the New York Free Medical College for Women, Woman's Medical College of Baltimore, the Woman's Medical College of Pennsylvania, and the New York Woman's Medical College and Hospital for Women. Only the last three schools were still open in 1909. The others closed or merged with coeducational schools. The Woman's Medical College of Pennsylvania was initially staffed by male physicians who supported medical education for women. By the 1890s, the Woman's Medical College was staffed by both women and men. Generally, the professors of obstetrics and of gynecology and the dean of the school were women. After first admitting male students in 1969, the school became the Medical College of Pennsylvania.

In 1899, when Cornell University admitted women as medical students, the Blackwells closed the Woman's Medical College of the New York Infirmary. Many leaders of the campaign for opening the medical profession to women saw coeducational schools as proof that separate women's schools were no longer needed. After the struggle to gain admission to American medical schools, the 1890s seemed to represent a "golden age" for women physicians. The Blackwells believed that the doors to all medical schools were opening to women. Unfortunately, it did not take long for the doors to slam shut once again. During the first half of the twentieth century, the number of "places" allotted to female medical students was so small that it was difficult for girls to believe that women had ever constituted a significant fraction of medical students.

Some nineteenth-century sectarian schools were more accessible to women than orthodox medical schools, but most of those schools disappeared by the turn of the century. A few survived by abandoning the philosophy of their founders or merging with orthodox institutions. The College of Medical Evangelists, for example, was founded by Ellen G. White to promote the Adventist health message and protect the modesty of female patients by including female teachers and students. Four of the first 10 students were female. The Adventist College of Medical Evangelists in Loma Linda, California, began as a hydropathic school, although White expected the college to attain full accreditation. As White's influence diminished, the college's leaders were able to change the balance between religious doctrine and the medical sciences. White's goal of training women to serve women patients was quickly abandoned, along with the "modesty doctrine" that had rationalized the role of women as students and teachers. By the 1920s, the Adventist school had transformed itself into an orthodox medical school and abandoned its commitment to the education of women physicians.

A century after Blackwell optimistically declared that the battle for women's access to medical education was all but won, Congressional hearings provided ample evidence of what women had long known: American medical schools discriminated against women. Some school administrators, however, argued that a five percent quota of "women's places" was actually more than sufficient. In 1970, the Women's Equity Action League (WEAL) filed a class action complaint against all medical schools in the United States, alleging abuses in admission and challenging the quota system. From 1905 to 1955, about four to five percent of medical students were female. In 1969, women made up nine percent of medical students. In 1971, in response to the lawsuit filed by the WEAL, the U.S. Public Health Service announced that medical schools accepting federal funds could not discriminate against women in admissions or salaries. By 1975, the number of female medical students had tripled.

## SUGGESTED READINGS

Apple, R. D., ed. (1992). *Women, Health, and Medicine in America. A Historical Handbook*. New Brunswick, NJ: Rutgers University Press.

Ashley, J. A. (1976). *Hospitals, Paternalism, and the Role of the Nurse*. New York: Teachers College Press.

Aveling, J. H. (1967). *English Midwives: Their History and Prospects*. London: Elliott. (Reprint of the 1872 edition.)

Aveling, J. H. (1977). *The Chamberlens and the Midwifery Forceps, Memorials of the Family, and an Essay on the Invention of the Instrument*. New York: AMS Press. (Reprint of the 1882 edition.)

Barker-Benfield, G. J. (1976). *The Horrors of the Half-Known Life: Male Attitudes Toward Women and Sexuality in Nineteenth-Century America*. New York: Harper & Row.

Blackwell, E. (1977). *Pioneer Work in Opening the Medical Profession to Women: Autobiographical Sketches by Dr. Elizabeth Blackwell. Introduction by Dr. Mary Roth Walsh*. New York: Schocken. (Reprint of the 1914 edition.)

Blustein, B. E. (1976). *Educating for Health and Prevention: A History of the Department of Community and Preventive Medicine of the (Woman's) Medical College of Pennsylvania*. Canton, MA: Science History Publications.

Bonner, T. N. (1992). *To the Ends of the Earth. Women's Search for Education in Medicine*. Cambridge, MA: Harvard University Press.

Borst, C. G. (1995). *Catching Babies. The Professionalization of Childbirth, 1870–1920*. Cambridge, MA: Harvard University Press.

Breckinridge, M. (1981). *Wide Neighborhoods: A Story of the Frontier Nursing Service*. Lexington, KY: University Press of Kentucky.

Buhler-Wilkerson, K. (2001). *No Place Like Home: A History of Nursing and Home Care in the United States*. Johns Baltimore, MD: Johns Hopkins University Press.

Bullough, B., Bullough, V. L., and Stanton, M., eds. (1990). *Nightingale and Her Era*. New York: Garland.

Bullough, V. L., Church, O. M., and Stein, A. P., eds. (1988). *American Nursing: A Biographical Dictionary*. New York: Garland Publishing.

Caton, D. (1999). *What a Blessing She Had Chloroform: The Medical and Social Response to the Pain of Childbirth from 1800 to the Present*. New Haven, CT: Yale University Press.

Clarke, E. H. (1972). *Sex in Education; or, A fair Chance for the Girls*. New York: Arno Press. (Reprint of the 1873 edition.)

DeVries, R. G. (1985). *Regulating Birth: Midwives, Medicine and the Law*. Philadelphia, PA: Temple University Press.

Djerassi, C. (2001). *This Man's Pill: Reflections on the 50th Birthday of the Pill*. New York: Oxford University Press.

Donegan, J. B. (1978). *Women and Men Midwives: Medicine, Morality, and Misogyny in Early America*. Westport, CT: Greenwood Press.

Doyal, L. (1995). *What Makes Women Sick. Gender and the Political Economy of Health*. New Brunswick, NJ: Rutgers University Press.

Drachman, V. G. (1984). *Hospital with a Heart: Women Doctors and the Paradox of Separatism at the New England Hospital, 1862–1969*. Ithaca, NY: Cornell University Press.

Evenden, D. (2000). *The Midwives of Seventeenth-Century London*. Cambridge: Cambridge University Press.

Fee, E., and Krieger, N., eds. (1994). *Women's Health, Politics, and Power: Essays on Sex/Gender, Medicine, and Public Health*. Amityville, NY: Baywood Publishing.

Fraser, G. J. (1998). *African American Midwifery in the South. Dialogues of Birth, Race, and Memory*. Cambridge, MA: Harvard University Press.

Furst, L. R., ed. (1997). *Women Healers and Physicians: Climbing a Long Hill*. Lexington, KY: University Press of Kentucky.

Gelbart, N. R. (1998). *The King's Midwife: A History and Mystery of Madame du Coudray*. Berkeley, CA: University of California Press.

Hamilton, A. (1985). *Exploring the Dangerous Trades: The Autobiography of Alice Hamilton, M.D. Foreword by Barbara Sicherman*. Boston, MA: Northeastern University Press. (Reprint of the 1943 edition.)

Hibbard, B. (2000). *The Obstetrician's Armamentarium: Historical Obstetric Instruments and their Inventors*. San Anselmo, CA: Norman Publishing.

Howe, J. W. (1972). *Sex and Education; A Reply to Dr. E. H. Clarke's "Sex in Education"*. New York: Arno Press. (Reprint of the 1874 edition.)

Kaufman, M., Hawkins, J. W., Higgins, L.P., and Friedman, A.H., eds. (1988). *Dictionary of American Nursing Biography*. Westport, CT: Greenwood Press.

Koblinsky, M., Timyan, J., and Gay, J., eds. (1993). *The Health of Women: A Global Perspective*. Westview Press.

Leavitt, J. W., ed. (1999). *Women and Health in America: Historical Readings.* Madison, WI: University of Wisconsin Press.

Leighow, S. R. (1996). *Nurses' Questions/Women's Questions: The Impact of the Demographic Revolution and Feminism on the United States Working Women, 1946–1986.* New York: Peter Lang.

Loudon, I. (2000). *The Tragedy of Childbed Fever.* New York: Oxford University Press.

Magner, L. N., ed. (1997). *Doctors, Nurses, and Medical Practitioners: A Bio-Bibliographical Sourcebook.* Westport, CT: Greenwood Press.

Marland, H., and Rafferty, A.M., eds. (1997). *Midwives, Society and Childbirth. Debates and Controversies in the Modern Period.* New York: Routledge.

McGregor, D. K. (1998). *From Midwives to Medicine. The Birth of American Gynecology.* New Brunswick, NJ: Rutgers University Press.

Melosh, B. (1982). *"The Physician's Hand": Work Culture and Conflict in American Nursing.* Philadelphia, PA: Temple University Press.

More, E. S. (1999). *Restoring the Balance: Women Physicians and the Profession of Medicine, 1850–1995.* Cambridge, MA: Harvard University Press.

More, E. S., and Milligan, M. A., eds. (1995). *The Empathic Practitioner: Empathy, Gender, and Medicine.* New Brunswick, NJ: Rutgers University Press.

Nuland, S. B. (2003). *The Doctors' Plague: Germs, Childbed Fever and the Strange Story of Ignác Semmelweis.* Norton/Atlas Books.

Nutting, M. A., and Dock, L. L. (2000). *A History of Nursing.* (With a new introduction by L. Williamson.), 4 volumes. Bristol, UK: Thoemmes Press.

O'Dowd, M. J. (2001). *The History of Obstetrics and Gynaecology.* Boca Raton, FL: CRC Press.

Oakley, A. (1984). *The Captured Womb: A History of the Medical Care of Pregnant Women.* Oxford: Basil Blackwell.

Peitzman, S. J. (2000). *A New and Untried Course: Woman's Medical College and Medical College of Pennsylvania, 1850–1998.* New Brunswick, NJ: Rutgers University Press.

Reverby, S. M. (1987). *Ordered to Care: The Dilemma of American Nursing, 1850–1954.* New York: Cambridge University Press.

Rooks, J. P. (1997). *Midwifery and Childbirth in America.* Philadelphia, PA: Temple University Press.

Rosser, S. V. (1994). *Women's Health—Missing from U.S. Medicine.* Bloomington, IN: Indiana University Press.

Sandelowski, M. (2000). *Devices and Desires: Gender, Technology, and American Nursing.* Chapel Hill, NC: University of North Carolina Press.

Semmelweis, I. (1983). *The Etiology, Concept, and Prophylaxis of Childbed Fever.* (Trans., ed., Introductory Essay by K. Codell Carter.) Madison, WI: University of Wisconsin Press.

Sharp, J. (1999). *The Midwife's Book; or, The Whole Art of Midwifery Discovered*. Edited by E. Hobby. Oxford: Oxford University Press.

Sicherman, B., ed. (1984). *Alice Hamilton: A Life in Letters*. Cambridge, MA: Harvard University Press.

Stage, S. (1979). *Female Complaints. Lydia Pinkham and the Business of Women's Medicine*. New York: Norton.

Thompson, L. (1999). *The Wandering Womb: A Cultural History of Outrageous Beliefs About Women*. Amherst, NY: Prometheus Books.

Ulrich, L. T. (1990). *A Midwife's Tale: The Life of Martha Ballard, Based on Her Diary, 1785–1812*. New York: Knopf.

Walsh, M. R. (1977). *"Doctors Wanted: No Women Need Apply": Sexual Barriers in the Medical Profession, 1835–1975*. New Haven, CT: Yale University Press.

Williamson, L., ed. (1999). *Florence Nightingale and the Birth of Professional Nursing*, 6 Vols. Bristol, UK: Thoemmes Press.

Wilson, A. (1995). *The Making of Man-Midwifery: Childbirth in England, 1660–1770*. Cambridge, MA: Harvard University Press.

# 12

# The Art and Science of Surgery

Modern surgery has evolved from one of the most despised branches of medicine into one of the most respected, powerful, and best compensated areas of medical specialization. The transformation seems to have occurred with remarkable speed once surgeons were given the tools to overcome pain and infection, two of the greatest obstacles to major operative procedures. General anesthesia was introduced in the 1840s and antisepsis in the 1870s.

A closer examination of the evolution of surgery, however, suggests a more complex explanation for the remarkable changes that occurred in the nineteenth century. First of all, surgeons could point to a long history of successes, if not in major operative procedures, then at least in the treatment of wounds, ulcers, skin diseases, fractures, dislocations, and so forth. In comparison to the treatment of internal diseases by physicians, the surgeons who treated traumatic injuries, urinary disorders, and broken bones had good reason to boast of the efficacy of their methods. Indeed, it could be argued that, as surgeons used their claims of expertise and knowledge to close the gap between medicine and surgery, they established the basis for the professionalization and modernization of a powerful, unified, and inclusive medical profession.

Taking a broader view of surgery, the developments that took place from the time of Ambroise Paré (1510–1590) to the early nineteenth century can be largely attributed to the work of inventive surgeons, better education and practical training, and anatomical and physiological researches. Even when allegiance to humoral pathology was all pervasive, the surgical point of view had to focus more narrowly and pragmatically on localized lesions. As the study of correlations between the course of disease in the living and pathological lesions in the dead gained support, physicians increasingly accepted the validity of a localized pathology. Surgery not only gained much from the researches of physicians, but also contributed an empirical, anatomically based point of view that was to have important ramifications for medicine as a whole.

461

## ANESTHESIA

During the eighteenth century, progress in anatomical investigation, and the acceptance of a localized, lesion-based, or solidistic approach to pathology, provided an intellectual framework for surgical innovations. From the patient's point of view, however, pain was a powerful reason for avoiding even the most desperately needed operation. Physiologists define pain as an "unpleasant sensory and emotional experience associated with actual or potential tissue damage," which, nevertheless, is important to the maintenance and preservation of life. Pain provides an essential warning about trauma and injury, but it can also have strong negative effects on health. Usually, pain motivates behaviors that help prevent further injuries, but fear of pain kept patients from accepting the advice of surgeons and dentists.

Despite the fact that narcotics have been used for rituals and recreation for thousands of years, Oliver Wendell Holmes (1809–1894) reflected conventional medical wisdom when he said that nature offered only three natural anesthetics: sleep, fainting, and death. Experimentation with mind- and mood-altering substances is older than agriculture, but the potions prepared for ceremonial, religious, or social purposes were rarely used for the relief of surgical pain. Perhaps the powerful religious associations of intoxicants militated against their use as secular anesthetics. On the other hand, the magical agents used in ceremonies culminating in ecstasy and self-mutilation might have worked primarily through the power of suggestion. If the potion did not work, the person using the drugs was to blame for lack of faith. If someone died as a result of an overdose, it was the will of the gods.

Thus, it is unreasonable to assume that the preparations used to induce ceremonial intoxication would satisfy the essential criteria for surgical anesthetics: relief of pain must be *inevitable, complete*, and *safe*. Drugs that are appropriate for ceremonial purposes might cause unpredictable and dangerous effects in a person undergoing surgery. As statistics for deaths due to drug overdoses indicate, people are willing to take risks with recreational drugs that they would not find acceptable in medical procedures. In the religious context, death was in the hands of the gods; in the operating room, the responsibility belonged to the surgeon.

If anesthetics are "tamed inebriants," then alcohol should have been the drug of choice for surgery. Alcoholic preparations have been used as the "potion of the condemned" and in preparation for ceremonial tribal rites, such as circumcision and scarification. Unfortunately, the large doses of alcohol needed to induce stupefaction are likely to cause nausea, vomiting, and death instead of sleep. Healers could also try to induce what might be called a state of psychological anesthesia by means of mesmerism, hypnotism, shamanistic rituals,

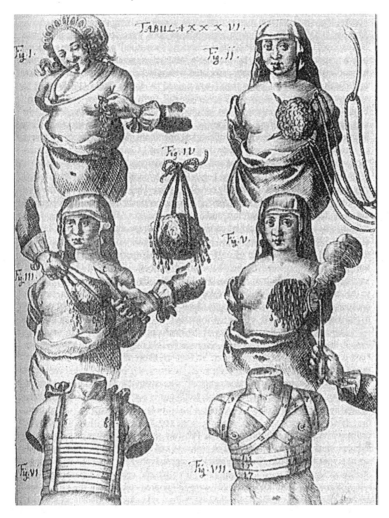

**Mastectomy procedures depicted in a 1666 text by Johann Schultes (1595–1645).**

prayers, and the symbolic transference of pain to an animal or inanimate item. Such methods might not be inevitable and complete, but a mixture of hope and faith is likely to be safer than complex, impure mixtures of drugs and alcohol.

Various forms of self-hypnosis were used in India, but these practices require high levels of training, concentration, and self-discipline. The best known European version of psychological anesthesia was developed by the Austrian physician Friedrich Anton Mesmer (1734–1815). Although Mesmer's methods were criticized by physicians and exposed as fraudulent by skeptical scientists, including American scientist and statesman Benjamin Franklin (1706–1790) and French chemist Antoine Laurent Lavoisier (1743–1794), sensitive patients were easily put into a somnambulistic state by Mesmer's "animal magnetism." Not surprisingly, physicians and scientists were generally suspicious of mesmerism, because of its close association with quackery. James Braid (1795–1860) coined the term *hypnotism* to separate the scientific study of mesmerism or "nervous sleep" from spiritualism and quackery. According to Braid, hypnosis was a subjective condition that depended on the suggestibility of the patient. Nevertheless, in sensitive subjects, the hypnotist could induce a state of somnambulism deep enough to overcome the pain of surgical operations. To demonstrate the power of this technique, a notorious French "midwifery-mesmerist" mesmerized women in a lying-in hospital and a lion at the zoo.

By the time European physicians began to take hypnotism seriously, the triumph of inhalation anesthesia was virtually complete. Somewhat out of phase with the tides of history, John Elliotson (1791–1868), lecturer on medicine at the University of London, founded a hospital for studies of mesmerism. He reported that even amputations at the thigh could be carried out under hypnotism. James Esdaile (1808–1859), who became interested in mesmerism while working in India, claimed that the mortality rate for more than two hundred operations he had performed using mesmerism as an anesthetic was less than six percent. Unfortunately, when he returned to Scotland in 1851, he found that mesmerism did not work as well there as it had in India. Eventually, hypnotism proved to be more significant in the development of psychoanalysis than in surgical anesthesia. The Parisian neurologist Jean Martin Charcot (1825–1893) used hypnotism in his clinical studies of hysteria, but considered the hypnotic state pathological in itself. Recent studies of the neuroendocrinology of pain may help explain the mechanism of hypnotism. Surprisingly, although hypnotism has generally been denigrated as "mere suggestion," it is more likely to ameliorate "real" pain than "imaginary" pain.

Surgeons experimented with many methods of distracting the patient from the pain of an imminent operation. A direct, but crude way of inducing a state of insensitivity was to knock the patient unconscious with a blow to the jaw. This technique is not very specific or complete, but the surgeon might be able to extract a bullet before his patient recovered from the shock. Distraction could also be achieved by rubbing the patient with counterirritants such as stinging nettles. Pressure applied to nerves or arteries could induce insensitivity to pain, but it could also result in asphyxia and death. Even phlebotomy could act as a painkiller when it was carried out aggressively enough to induce fainting. Such bleedings were used in preparation for childbirth, reducing dislocations, and setting fractures. Such methods were too unpredictable to fit the criteria for surgical anesthesia.

Mythology and folklore are rich in allusions to wondrous potions such as the potion used by Helen of Troy to quench pain and strife. Unfortunately, the ingredients in the perfect painkillers of mythology were secret and mysterious. More accessible recipes for sleep potions typically contained so many dangerous ingredients that it was safer to inhale them than to ingest them. With inhalation, the amount of the active ingredients need not be calculated too precisely, because the inhalant could be withdrawn as soon as the patient was sufficiently affected. In contrast, an overdose of drugs swallowed or injected could not be recalled.

The medieval prototype of the "sleep apple" that appears in the story of Snow White usually contained opium, mandrake, henbane, hemlock, wine, and musk. Usually, the user was expected to inhale the fumes of the apple rather than eating it. The "soporific sponges" recommended by medieval surgeons contained similar mixtures. By the sixteenth century, surgeons were describing old favorites like mandrake as poisonous drugs that lulled the senses and made men cowards. In Shakespeare's *Antony and Cleopatra*, Cleopatra safely used mandrake to sleep away the hours before Antony's return. Shakespeare alludes to various soporific agents, such as poppy, mandragora, and "drowsy syrups," but these agents were unreliable at best. In the real world, surgeons found that drugged patients who slept like the dead during surgery often failed to awaken afterwards. Opium retained its favored status long after mandrake was discarded. Eminent physicians like Thomas Sydenham (1624–1689) and John Hunter (1728–1793) saw opium as a powerful drug and proof of God's mercy. As Hunter told a colleague seeking advice about treating a patient with a painful malignant cancer, the only choice was "Opium, Opium, Opium!" In large doses, opium generally causes drowsiness and depression, but excitation, vomiting, headaches, and constipation are not uncommon side-effects. Opium and other opiates do not prevent breathing, but they do reduce the sensitivity of the respiratory center to carbon dioxide. Because the automatic drive to breathe is reduced, a person who falls asleep after taking such drugs may die. Opiates may also cause constipation, severe sedation, nausea and vomiting, repression of the cough reflex, or bronchospasm. Despite such problems, opium was used in cough medicines, sleeping potions, and soothing elixirs for crying babies. Some critics recognized the dangers of drug dependence, but opium remained widely available into the twentieth century. Soporifics and narcotics were also prepared from marijuana, hellebore, belladonna, henbane, jimsonweed, and enough miscellaneous greens to make a very exotic salad. Henbane, which was known as the poor man's opium, was recommended for insomnia, toothache, and pain.

Poisonous substances are present throughout the tissues of the ubiquitous jimsonweed, but the powerful alkaloids atropine and scopolamine are concentrated in the seeds. Reports of atropine-like poisoning in people who have eaten the seeds and washed them down with alcohol are not uncommon. Long used as a hypnotic and sedative, scopolamine became popular with twentieth-century obstetricians, who claimed that the so-called twilight sleep induced by a combination of scopolamine and morphine allowed scientific management of painless childbirth. Critics argued that twilight sleep was more effective as an amnesiac than an anesthetic. When this method was used, women experienced labor pains, but later forgot them and thought that the birth had been painless. Even though she knew that women had to be restrained when given scopolamine–morphine anesthesia, Dr. Bertha Van Hoosen (1863–1952) praised twilight sleep as "the greatest boon the Twentieth Century could give to women." Van Hoosen devised a special crib to confine women undergoing this allegedly painless form of childbirth in order to prevent injury as they thrashed about and screamed. In 1915, Van Hoosen founded and became first president of the American Medical Women's Association. By the 1920s, skepticism about twilight sleep and the availability of other drugs ended the era of scopolamine–morphine anesthesia. Scopolamine has even been marketed for relief of seasickness, despite the fact that it can produce dangerous hallucinations.

Hemlock was the active ingredient in the infamous death potion given to the Greek philosopher Socrates (470–399 B.C.E.), who was condemned for corrupting the minds of the youth of Athens. Although clearly a dangerous drug, hemlock was sometimes used in anesthetic concoctions. The drug depresses the motor centers before the sensory centers are affected; this may be good for the surgeon, but bad for the patient. Surgeons were eager to find drugs that would produce muscle relaxation as well as analgesia. Curare, an arrow poison used by South American Indians, was brought to the attention of European scientists by naturalist and explorer Alexander von Humboldt (1769–1859), who came close to killing himself in the course of this research. Curare does not relieve pain, but it is useful in surgery because it prevents movement and provides profound muscle relaxation. Since the state of paralysis induced by curare can be fatal without artificial respiration, it would not have been useful in nineteenth century surgery. Many decades later, surgeons would redefine the "classical triad" of anesthesia as: unconsciousness (or amnesia), analgesia, and muscle relaxation (where appropriate).

## LAUGHING GAS, ETHER, AND SURGICAL ANESTHESIA

Despite the wealth of soporific agents available in nature's medical garden, the remarkable products of the eighteenth-century chemical revolution eventually eclipsed the ancient anodynes. Joseph Priestly (1733–1804), British theologian, educator, writer, and political theorist, is best known as the discoverer of oxygen, but as Sir Humphry Davy (1778–1829) said of this indefatigable chemist, "no single person ever discovered so many new and curious substances." Most curious of all was the gas known as nitrous oxide, or laughing gas. As he was in the habit of testing the effect of new gases on himself, Priestley might have discovered the anesthetic properties of laughing gas if his research had not been interrupted by the political and religious conflicts that forced him to emigrate to America in 1794.

The ingenious discoveries of the first pneumatic chemists provided new opportunities for quacks and charlatans. Conscientious experimentalists could not compete with charlatans promising miraculous cures for asthma, catarrh, consumption, and cancer through the inhalation of oxygen, hydrogen, and other "factitious airs." Some physicians, however, attempted to find legitimate medical uses for the new gases. Fascinated by pneumatic chemistry, Thomas Beddoes (1760–1808) persuaded his friends Thomas Wedgwood (1771–1805) and James Watt (1736–1819) to help him establish the Pneumatic Institute, a hospital in which the inhalation of factitious airs was used in the treatment of lung disease. Many scientists, including Humphry Davy, were intrigued by his work. While suffering from toothache in 1795, Davy began inhaling nitrous oxide. In addition to feeling giddy, relaxed, and cheerful, Davy noted that the pain caused by his wisdom teeth had almost disappeared. Soon after the exhilaration wore off, the pain returned, worse than ever. Nevertheless, Davy suggested that nitrous oxide might be useful during surgical operations. Davy's associate, Michael Faraday (1791–1867), discovered the soporific effect of ether vapor during experiments on various gases. In comparing the effects of ether and nitrous oxide, Faraday found that both chemicals produced similar responses. Most subjects found inhalation of ether or nitrous oxide very pleasant, but, occasionally, people who inhaled ether or nitrous oxide experienced frightening and bizarre effects, such as loss of sensations, prolonged lethargy, hallucinations, and fainting. Other eighteenth-century chemists recommended ether for fits, headaches, gout, rheumatism, asthma, deafness, whooping cough, and other disorders.

Even the valiant attempts of Henry Hill Hickman (1801–1830) to validate the safety and efficacy of inhalation anesthesia failed to arouse the interest of the medical profession. Unlike many pioneers of anesthesia, Hickman did not simply sniff at various chemicals. Dogs and mice placed in a sealed glass vessel were subjected to various test gases until they were in a state of "suspended animation." In this state, animals were insensitive to pain, but were at risk of circulatory collapse during surgery. Unsuccessful in his attempts to call attention to surgical anesthesia, Hickman apparently succumbed to an overwhelming sense of failure and committed suicide.

The story of the development of surgical anesthesia in the 1840s involves a most unlikely cast of characters more suited to farce than historical drama. Moreover, the major events took place not in the prestigious medical colleges and hospitals of Europe, but at the periphery of the medical and scientific world. The chief characters were peripatetic professors, show-business chemists, and dentists, who at the time were regarded as closer to quacks than to doctors. Bitter priority disputes consumed and even destroyed the lives of several of the participants in the discovery of surgical anesthesia. The cast of characters includes Horace Wells (1815–1848) and William Thomas Green Morton (1819–1868), dentists who had shared a successful partnership before Wells recognized the anesthetic properties of nitrous oxide and Morton demonstrated the value of ether. Charles Thomas Jackson (1805–1880), chemist and physician, later claimed that he rather than Morton discovered ether anesthesia. While the priority battle between Morton and Jackson raged in New England, Georgia physician Crawford Williamson Long (1815–1878) announced that he had discovered ether anesthesia before Morton.

During the nineteenth century, medicine shows and philosophical lectures by self-appointed professors brought edification and entertainment to the citizens of cities and towns throughout America. "Professors of chemistry" enlivened lectures on the amazing properties of newly discovered gases by breathing fire with hydrogen and encouraging volunteers to make fools of themselves after inhaling nitrous oxide. Students of dentistry, medicine, and chemistry did not have to wait for the itinerant professors; they could enjoy "laughing gas parties" and "ether frolics" whenever they wished. Indeed, the "champagne effect" of these substances was so well known that when Jackson attempted to claim priority, Morton's defenders noted that one could hardly find a school or community in America where the boys and girls had not inhaled these drugs.

Dentists were probably more highly motivated than any other practitioners to discover novel and powerful anesthetics. Until the excruciating pain of a rotting tooth exceeded the anticipated agony of extraction, the victim of toothache was unlikely to submit to the services of a dentist. Throughout history, dentists claimed to possess potions that would remove bad teeth and eliminate pain. Ancient tooth-dressings included everything from honey and opium to sour apples, powdered beetles, and even rattlesnake venom in vinegar. Kissing a donkey, biting off the head of a mouse, inserting a live louse in the bad tooth, and applications of powdered crow dung were among the most peculiar treatments for toothache.

In France, dentistry evolved as an area of specialization in surgery. Textbooks written by and for surgeons typically included descriptions of the teeth, diseases of the teeth and gums, tooth extraction, the construction of artificial teeth, materials for filling teeth, and other methods of treating disorders of the teeth and gums. Although the status of those who only pulled teeth was lower than that of barber-surgeons, even master surgeons performed dental procedures. Texts devoted to dentistry had been published in the sixteenth century, but *Le chirurgien dentiste* (1728), a comprehensive, two-volume treatise by surgeon-dentist Pierre Fauchard (1678–1761), is considered a landmark in the history of dentistry. Surgeons who treated the dental problems of eighteenth century French aristocrats enjoyed considerable prestige.

Chapin Aaron Harris (1806–1860), a founder of American dentistry, began the study of medicine, surgery, and dentistry as apprentice to his brother. In 1833, Harris passed an examination administered by the Maryland State Medical Board and was awarded the M.D. Although Harris began his career as a doctor, he decided to specialize in dentistry and spent many years as an itinerant practitioner before he received a license to practice dentistry from the Medical and Chirurgical Faculty of Maryland and settled in Baltimore. Harris published many articles and books about dentistry, including *The Dental Art: A Practical Treatise on Dental Surgery, Principles and Practice of Dental Surgery*, and *Dictionary of Dental Science: Bibliography, Biography and Medical Terminology*. Harris was a cofounder of the first dental school in the world, the Baltimore College of Dental Surgery (1840), and established the first national dental society, the American Society of Dental Surgeons.

As nineteenth-century American dentists introduced improved dental appliances and instruments, their professional and economic advancement was limited by the fears of prospective patients and the disdain of the medical profession. These obstacles were especially galling to men like Horace Wells and his business partner William Morton. Wells and Morton had developed improved sets of false teeth and dental solder, but potential customers were reluctant to accept their "money-back-if-not-satisfied" deal because it required extraction of all remaining teeth and roots. Thus, Wells and Morton were keenly interested in any agent that could reliably achieve painless dentistry.

On December 10, 1844, Wells attended a lecture by Dr. Gardner Quincy Colton, during which the remarkable properties of nitrous oxide were demonstrated. Wells was struck by the fact that, while under the influence of laughing gas, a volunteer remained in a state of euphoria even though he fell off the stage and injured his leg. Wells asked Colton to bring laughing gas to his office for an experiment. The next morning, Colton administered the gas to Wells and John M. Riggs, a dental student, extracted a tooth. When Wells regained consciousness, he was elated to realize that he had not experienced any pain during the operation. Within a month, Wells had used nitrous oxide on over a dozen patients. At Morton's request, Dr. John Collins Warren (1778–1856), Professor

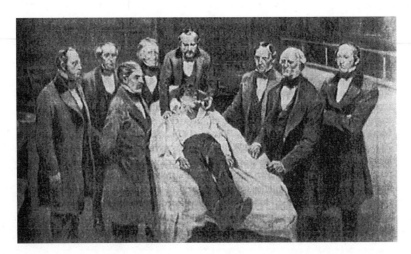

**Surgical anesthesia at Massachusetts General Hospital, 1846.**

of Anatomy at Harvard Medical School, allowed Wells to address a class in surgery. However, Warren's skeptical attitude toward painless dentistry was evident in his introductory remarks. "There's a gentleman here," Warren warned his students, "who pretends he has something which will destroy pain in surgical operations." When the medical student who "volunteered" to have a tooth extracted groaned during the operation, Wells and Morton were ridiculed and humiliated by the hostile audience. Ironically, the patient later admitted that he had felt no pain.

In 1848, when he evaluated the anesthesia controversy, Henry J. Bigelow (1818–1890) argued that Wells had not satisfied the criteria for surgical anesthesia. Surgeons needed an anesthetic agent that was inevitable, complete, and safe. Behaviors elicited by nitrous oxide inhalation were unpredictable and suggestion played an important role in determining the effect of the gas. Those who inhaled for amusement almost always became exhilarated; those well prepared for surgery became drowsy and lost consciousness. During the priority battle that followed the acceptance of inhalation anesthesia, Morton complained that he was the only person involved in the discovery who had suffered a "pecuniary loss." His colleague Horace Wells, however, paid a higher price for his part in the controversy; he lost his sanity and his life. Failing to find professional recognition, Wells resorted to sniffing ether and chloroform to cope with depression. Less than four years after his humiliating experience at Massachusetts General Hospital, Wells was arrested for allegedly accosting a young woman and throwing something, which might have been acid, ether, or chloroform, at her. Two days later, Wells was found dead in his cell, with an empty vial of chloroform, a penknife, a razor, and a suicide note. Thus, Wells would never know that nitrous oxide, mixed with oxygen, would become an important anesthetic agent in dentistry.

Only a short time after Wells's dismal performance reassured the Boston Brahmins that a mere dentist could not teach them the secret of painless surgery, Morton convinced the same elite physicians that inhalation anesthesia was "no humbug." Like nitrous oxide, ether had been used for recreational purposes. Moreover, during its long history as a chemical oddity, several investigators came tantalizingly close to discovering its anesthetic properties. The honor of being first to synthesize ether has been attributed to several Renaissance alchemists, but the nature of these alchemical preparations is obscure. The starting materials (sulfuric acid and alcohol) would have been widely available, but careful temperature regulation is needed to enhance the production of ethyl ether as opposed to other possible reaction products. Certainly, early preparations of ether would have been impure, and, as Morton discovered, purity was critical when ether was used as an anesthetic agent. Even though ether had been used as a sedative in the treatment of tuberculosis, asthma, and whooping cough, its anesthetic potential was rarely exploited. Extrapolating from the pleasant experience of an ether frolic to dental and surgical operations was not a simple, self-evident step before practitioners deliberately set forth on a quest for inhalation anesthetics.

According to family tradition, Morton graduated from the Baltimore College of Dental Surgery in 1842. There is, however, no proof that Morton ever matriculated at any dental school. Although dentistry was hardly recognized as a profession at that time, practitioners were working to improve the training and status of dentists by establishing journals, professional societies, and schools, such as the Baltimore College of Dental Surgery (later the School of Dentistry, University of Maryland). Whatever their education and training may have been, both Wells and Morton were apparently skillful and inventive dentists who specialized in "mechanical dentistry," or "plate work." Because of the suffering of his patients, and their tendency to prefer death to dentistry, Morton was obsessed with finding a way to mitigate the pain of dental operations. Like surgeons, dentists could offer their patients only unreliable soporifics. Moreover, the nausea caused by alcohol and laudanum was especially dangerous during dental procedures because vomiting could lead to suffocation and death.

Despite the financial success of the Wells–Morton partnership, Morton became one of Jackson's private pupils in order to make the transition from dentistry to medicine. In a discussion of toothache, Jackson recommended using ether as "toothache drops." Jackson later claimed that he had known about ether anesthesia since the early 1840s, but when Morton performed tooth extractions on Jackson's wife and aunt, Jackson merely encouraged the ladies to be brave. Therefore, during the priority battle over the discovery of anesthesia, Morton argued that his former mentor had never thought of going beyond the application of liquid ether *"in the same manner that laudanum and other narcotics have always been applied to sensitive teeth."* Always on the alert for pain-relieving agents, Morton consulted the medical literature and found that ether had been used as an antispasmodic, anodyne, and narcotic. Noting that when ether was applied to a rotten tooth, the gums became numb, Morton wondered whether ether could numb the whole body. Taking elaborate precautions to ensure secrecy, Morton tested the effects of ether inhalation on various animals. Disconcerted by the variability of his results, Morton sought Jackson's advice and learned that the ether sold by pharmacists was rarely pure enough for special uses.

On September 30, 1846, Morton saturated a handkerchief with ether, looked at his watch, and inhaled deeply. He regained consciousness about 8 minutes later with no ill effects other than mild exhilaration, followed by headache. That evening Morton tested the effect of ether while extracting a patient's firmly rooted bicuspid. After the painless operation, the patient gave Morton a written testimonial. Convinced of the validity of his discovery, Morton again approached Dr. Warren to ask for an opportunity to demonstrate his method of producing insensibility to pain. Thinking that inhaling ether through some special apparatus might produce more reliable results than the "rag-and-gag" method previously employed, Morton sought the assistance of a well-known scientific instrument-maker.

By October 16, 1846, the day of the hospital demonstration, Morton was in a state of terrible anxiety and his inhalation apparatus was still unfinished. The patient was already strapped to the table in preparation for his ordeal when Morton rushed in with his new inhaler and administered his secret "Letheon gas." Amazed by the patient's complete quiet and tranquility during the extirpation of a large tumor from his mouth and tongue, Warren graciously announced: "Gentlemen, this is no humbug." Witnesses later recalled this demonstration as "the most sublime scene ever witnessed in the operating-room." The operation performed by Warren at Massachusetts General Hospital under ether anesthesia was seen as the beginning of a new age for the ancient art of surgery. It also marked the beginning of a vicious priority battle that found its way into petitions, patent applications, pamphlets, testimonials, and learned articles in professional journals and encyclopedias.

According to Morton, the first intimation of the trouble to come was a visit from Jackson on October 23, 1846. Jackson had heard that Morton intended to take out a patent for surgical anesthesia and expected to make a good deal of money. Dentists routinely patented their inventions, but physicians supposedly answered to a higher code of ethics. However, Jackson demanded fees for professional advice, his name on the patent, and 10 percent of the net profits. Shortly after presenting his demands to Morton, Jackson sent a sealed report to the Academy of Sciences of France in which he claimed that he had discovered ether anesthesia and had instructed a certain dentist to use ether when extracting teeth. Jackson's sealed report was his insurance policy; if ether proved to be dangerous, his report could be destroyed, but if it was successful, he intended to use it to claim priority. As soon as the success of ether anesthesia seemed assured, Jackson presented himself as its sole discoverer and denounced Morton as a "stooge" acting under his direction. When Jackson spoke to the Massachusetts Medical Society, most of his audience accepted the claims of the eminent physician, chemist, and geologist against his rival, the "quack dentist." Not everyone was convinced that Jackson deserved credit for the discovery. Indeed, Jackson was asked whether he would have accepted the blame if Morton's patient had died. Jackson's critics saw this as an example of the old adage: success has many fathers, failure is a bastard.

On the grounds that the Massachusetts Medical Society's ethics code did not allow doctors to use secret remedies, when Morton offered his services for another operation, hospital surgeons refused to employ him until he revealed the identity of Letheon. They also assured him that the patient would die if her leg was not amputated, and would probably die of shock if the operation was conducted without anesthesia. It was not easy for Morton to envision the greater good of humanity while his dreams of fame and fortune evaporated even more quickly than ether itself. Opportunities to profit from his discovery continually eluded him. In 1868, shortly after consulting his lawyer about issues related to his 20-year conflict with Jackson, Morton died of a cerebral hemorrhage. An inscription on Morton's tomb, composed by Dr. Jacob Bigelow, honors him as the inventor of inhalation anesthesia. Jackson survived Morton by 12 years, but he did not enjoy a peaceful old age. According to a story probably too good to be true, after considerable drinking, Jackson wandered into the Mount Auburn Cemetery and was overcome by a frenzy while reading the inscription on Morton's tomb. Declared hopelessly insane, Jackson was confined to a mental asylum for the rest of his miserable life.

While Wells, Morton, and Jackson were disputing the discovery of inhalation anesthesia, Crawford Long emerged from his obscure existence in rural Georgia with testimonials documenting his own priority claim. Like Wells, Long came to an appreciation of the medical potential of a drug from casual observations of its recreational uses. When a traveling chemist sparked local interest in laughing gas, Long had suggested that ether would be just as exhilarating. According to Long, sniffing ether became a popular form of entertainment at local social events. After these ether frolics, participants sometimes discovered bruises and

other injuries acquired while "under the influence." Long concluded
that ether might be used to induce insensitivity to pain during surgery,
but he apparently had more opportunities to stage ether frolics than surgical operations. In March of 1842, Long persuaded James M. Venable
to have a tumor on his neck surgically removed. Knowing that Venable
was afraid of the knife but fond of ether, Long suggested that he sniff
ether prior to the operation. It was not until 1849 that Long published
an account of his discovery in the *Southern Medical and Surgical Journal.* Technically, Long established his priority, but as Sir William Osier
said: "In science the credit goes to the man who convinces the world,
not to the man to whom the idea first occurs."

Despite warnings from the Philadelphia *Medical Examiner* that the
physicians of Boston would soon constitute one fraternity with the
quacks, ether anesthesia quickly spread from Massachusetts to Paris
and London. Although anesthesia was certainly an important factor
in the surgical revolution, more subtle and complex factors were also
involved. Indeed, given the increased use of the knife that accompanied
the decline of humoralism and the rise of morbid anatomy during the
period from about 1700 to the 1830s, the rapid acceptance of anesthesia might have been the result of the increasing role of surgery rather
than the reverse. Potentially useful anesthetic agents had obviously been
available before the 1840s. In any case, with the rapid dissemination
of surgical anesthesia, advances in the art were inevitable; so too were
iatrogenic accidents and deaths. Anesthesia so transformed the art
of surgery that Henry J. Bigelow urged reform of the curriculum at
Harvard Medical School to inculcate humanity and sensitivity back into
medical students. Within two years of Morton's first public demonstration of inhalation anesthesia, ether, nitrous oxide, chloroform,
and other anesthetic agents were widely used in dentistry, obstetrics,
and surgery. Physicians also prescribed these powerful anesthetic agents
for convulsions, asthma, whooping cough, menstrual cramps, vaginis-
mus, neuralgia, insomnia, and insanity.

Inspired by his successful use of ether, James Young Simpson
(1811–1879), Professor of Midwifery at Edinburgh and one of Scotland's leading surgeons and obstetricians, initiated a search for an anesthetic without ether's disadvantages. Using himself and his friends as
guinea pigs, Simpson began a systematic but dangerous search for a
volatile anesthetic agent with a better aroma and more rapid action than
ether. Having asked for advice from chemists and sniffed his way
through samples of acetone, benzene, benzoin, and a variety of organic
solvents, Simpson tested chloroform. This dense, colorless liquid produced a sense of euphoria as well as loss of consciousness. Within a
week, Simpson's patients were enjoying the benefits of chloroform analgesia. Chloroform was easier to administer than ether, but it also seemed
to be more dangerous. Indeed, it was fortunate that the principle of

surgical anesthesia had been established with ether, because the relatively high mortality rate with chloroform might have inhibited development of this branch of the healing art. Emphasizing the more unpleasant aspects of using ether, Simpson noted that it irritates the respiratory tract and is highly inflammable, which would be very dangerous to anyone operating by candlelight. In 1868, chemists found that chloral hydrate, which was used in the synthesis of chloroform, also acted as a soporific agent. Instead of releasing chloroform, however, chloral hydrate formed trichloroethanol in the liver. Chemists synthesized more useful analogues of chloral hydrate in the 1870s and 1880s.

The safety of anesthesia was not the only point of contention, as demonstrated by the ferocity of the attack on the use of anesthetics in obstetrics. Clergymen, doctors, and assorted amateur moralists argued that pain had a God-given, and therefore holy role to play in the lives of men, and especially in the lives of women. Midwives had been put to death for the blasphemous, sinful, unnatural crime of attempting to alleviate the pains of childbirth. Clergymen denounced Simpson and commanded women to endure the pains of childbirth with patience and fortitude. Did the Bible not say that Eve was condemned to bring forth children in sorrow? Obstetricians warned women that labor contractions were identical to labor pains. Therefore, without pain there would be no contractions and normal delivery could not occur. Suffering was inherent in female physiology and labor pains enhanced woman's capacity for tenderness, femininity, and maternal feelings.

Saddened by the controversy, Simpson met his critics on theological as well as scientific grounds. Using the Bible to substantiate his work, Simpson asserted that the curse in Genesis had been revoked by a passage in Deuteronomy that promised: "The Lord will bless the fruit of the womb and the land." Moreover, the word translated as "sorrow" in the case of Eve's punishment was really the word for "labor," which referred to both farming and childbirth. Furthermore, God established the principle of anesthesia when he caused a deep sleep to fall upon Adam before operating on his rib. When John Snow (1813–1858) administered chloroform to Queen Victoria in 1853 during the birth of her eighth child, the issue of whether a proper lady would accept anesthesia was settled. When one of her daughters gave birth, Queen Victoria said: "What a blessing she had chloroform." Unlike his American counterparts, Simpson died rich in honors and respect. He was knighted, appointed Physician in Scotland to the Queen, awarded an honorary doctorate by Oxford University, received the Freedom of the City of Edinburgh, and, after his untimely death at age 59, academic and commercial activities in Scotland were suspended to accommodate one of the largest funerals ever to honor a Scottish doctor.

The priority battle in America became part of a broader contro-versy about which agent, ether or chloroform, was better, as well as arguments about the relative value of Simpson's work and that of the Americans who had discovered inhalation anesthesia. When the *Edinburgh Daily Review* called the introduction of chloroform for anes-thesia "the greatest of all discoveries in modern times," Bigelow complained that Simpson was ignoring his American predecessors and claiming too much credit for surgical anesthesia. In response, Simpson informed Bigelow that he saw the use of chloroform and ether as anesthetic agents not as great discoveries in themselves, but as steps in a long history that included Sir Humphry Davy, as well as the Greek, Roman, and medieval surgeons who had used various soporific vapors. For Simpson and his British colleagues, the discovery of chloroform was the climax of a sweeping historical narrative. Infuriated, Bigelow insisted that it was wrong to call chloroform the "greatest discovery" in any account of surgical anesthesia. Ether had been used successfully and safely for many years before chloroform anesthesia caused "hundreds of cases of disaster and death." According to Bigelow, Simpson's self-aggrandizing historical account was nothing but "antiquarian dust" that was used "to obscure the truth." Bigelow wanted the world, especially the British, to acknowledge the difference between "the mod-ern discovery of anesthesia and the less important use of chloroform." Even after Simpson and Bigelow were dead, the controversy continued. Jacob Bigelow's son, Dr. Henry J. Bigelow, wanted to make it perfectly clear that Americans had discovered the first surgical anesthetic agent that was *"inevitable, complete, and safe."* That agent was ether, not chloroform.

The changing nature of surgical practice must have been rather painful to those who had established their reputation through speed and strength and now saw surgeons developing a deliberate and subtle touch. Practitioners who had struggled to attain the professional detach-ment (or callousness) needed to operate in the pre-anesthetic era had taken great pride in their achievements. Like the librarian who objects to people taking books from neatly ordered shelves, the master surgeon might resent the trick that obviated the need for his painstakingly acquired skills. Some doctors believed that inhalation of anesthetic agents would poison the blood, promote hemorrhages, cause convul-sions, nausea, intoxication, prolonged stupor, cerebral excitement, asphyxia, bronchitis, pneumonia, inflammation of the brain, paralysis, insanity, depression, local or systemic infection, miscarriage, or damage to the fetus. Anesthetics might damage nerves and muscles or interfere with wound healing. Many sectarians, such as hydropaths, homeopaths, and naturopaths, opposed the use of all powerful, chemical agents, including anesthetics. Some temperance advocates denounced Demon Anesthesia as well as Demon Rum.

While some practitioners denounced anesthesia as a dangerous and blasphemous novelty and others adopted it without reservations, most doctors cautiously accepted it as a mixed blessing that had to be used selectively. The risks and benefits of anesthesia had to be evaluated by a new "utilitarian calculus" that took into consideration a host of variables, such as age, sex, race, ethnicity, the seriousness of the operation, and so forth. The rapid spread of anesthetic techniques was unprecedented in medical history, but not all patients received the blessings of painless surgery, even for major limb amputations. Some surgeons justified anesthesia by arguing that pain itself was dangerous, because it caused shock, depleted precious stores of vital energy, and damaged the body. Moreover, anesthesia encouraged patients to accept operations and allowed surgeons to refine their skills. Advocates of universal anesthetization accused doctors who insisted on the selective use of anesthetics of exaggerating potential risks in order to maintain exclusive control over anesthesia. The American Medical Association's Committee on Medical Science warned that chloroform and ether should only be used by physicians; with respect to anesthesia, even dentists should defer to physicians. To put this concern in context, note that doctors also warned patients that bathing could prove fatal unless prescribed by a physician instead of a hydropath.

Many nineteenth century critics of anesthesia sincerely believed that pain was God's punishment for human failures and wickedness. William Henry Atkinson, M.D., the first president of the American Dental Association, contended that anesthesia was a Satanic plot to deprive men of the capacity to reason and endure the pain that God intended them to experience. Certainly doctors were influenced by religious dogma, but professional norms also conditioned them to be suspicious of an innovation that challenged centuries of medical experience in which insensitivity to pain (as in coma, shock, or brain damage) was a harbinger of death. Pain, life, and healing had always been inextricably linked.

Opponents of the new surgery pounced upon reports of deaths after anesthesia, ignoring the fact that it was not uncommon for patients to die after operations performed without anesthesia. Some critics feared that anesthetics gave doctors excessive power over patients. Anesthetic agents could be used to subdue and tranquilize uncooperative patients into unnecessary, experimental operations. It was even possible that the relief of pain was an illusion; the patient might actually suffer pain but be rendered incapable of expressing or recalling the experience. Although many of these fears were obviously exaggerated, further experience proved that anesthetics, like any potent drug, could cause serious side effects: fatal cardiac arrhythmias, circulatory failures during surgery, postsurgical pneumonia, vomiting that could cause suffocation or tissue damage, and more subtle effects on the liver, brain, fetus, or newborn infants. As a modern medical specialty, anesthesiology includes the administration of surgical anesthesia, acute and chronic pain relief, postoperative care, the management of intensive care, respiratory intensive care, chronic pain management, resuscitation, and emergency medicine. Some departments of anesthesia have become departments of anesthesia and perioperative medicine. Nevertheless, even under optimum, fully modern conditions, the dangers of anesthesia should never be underestimated. In many cases, general anesthesia may be the most dangerous part of an operation.

With proper management, inhalation anesthesia was generally safe, complete, and inevitable. Complete insensibility, however, is not suitable for all operations. Although some of the drugs and instruments involved in the development of local, regional, and spinal anesthesia predate Morton's demonstration, the development of special techniques for their use began in earnest after the acceptance of inhalation anesthesia. In 1803, Friedrich Wilhelm Sertürner (1783–1841) isolated crystals of a powerful analgesic agent from crude opium. Sertürner named this chemical *morphine*, for Morpheus, the Greek god of dreams. Morphine paste could be introduced locally with the point of a lancet, or a solution of morphine could be instilled into a wound. In the 1850s, Charles Gabriel Pravaz (1791–1853) and Alexander Wood (1817–1884) independently invented the modern type of hollow metal needle. (The device known as a hypodermic syringe in the United States and England is called a Pravaz syringe on the Continent.) Injections of morphine were generally used for the relief of localized pain, but some surgeons administered morphine in preparation for surgery under general anesthesia in the belief that it prevented shock, delirium, nausea, and lessened the amount of inhalant needed. Heroin, a derivative of morphine first synthesized in 1874, was widely marketed in the 1890s as a pain reliever that was allegedly safer than morphine. After the chemical structure of morphine was elucidated in 1923, many other derivatives of morphine were tested, but very few had any particular advantages.

The ancient Incas had successfully exploited the anesthetic qualities of the coca leaf as well as its mood-altering properties, and their Peruvian descendants continued to use coca leaves to drive away pain, hunger, nausea, fatigue, and sorrow. While Europeans quickly took up the native American custom of smoking tobacco, they ignored coca leaves until nineteenth-century chemists isolated interesting alkaloids, including cocaine. After reading a report on the physiological effects of cocaine, Sigmund Freud (1856–1939) decided that the drug might serve as a tonic in the treatment of mental and physical diseases. Using himself as guinea pig, Freud discovered that cocaine banished his depression and increased his energy. Freud urged Carl Koller (1857–1944), a physician who specialized in eye disorders, to try cocaine for the relief of eye diseases such as trachoma and iritis. When a solution of cocaine was instilled into the eye of a frog, Koller could touch the cornea without eliciting any reaction. Following successful tests on rabbits and humans, Koller announced his discovery at the 1884 Ophthalmologic Congress in Heidelberg. Freud credited his colleague Carl Koller with discovering the local anesthetic properties of cocaine, but some scholars think that Freud should be considered one of the founders of psychopharmacology for his own studies of cocaine. By the end of the nineteenth century, many popular ointments, snuffs, suppositories, cigarettes, cigars, patent medicines, and beverages contained cocaine. The best known is Coca-Cola, a patent medicine introduced in 1886 as a therapeutic agent and general tonic. In addition to coca leaf extract, Coca-Cola contained an extract of the kola nut, which is high in caffeine. By 1906 when the Pure Food and Drug Law was passed in the United States, the makers of Coca-Cola were using decocainized coca leaves, but the caffeine remained.

William S. Halsted (1852–1922), one of New York's leading surgeons, realized that Koller had barely begun to exploit the possible range of cocaine anesthesia. Impressed with the drug's effects, Halsted performed a series of tests on himself, his medical students, and experimental animals. Because cocaine constricts blood vessels, it seemed to be the ideal local anesthetic for surgery in highly vascularized areas. Halsted developed a technique that he called conduction anesthesia or nerve block anesthesia—a means of specifically anesthetizing various parts of the body by injecting cocaine solutions into the appropriate nerves.

When using cocaine, Halsted enjoyed feelings of increased energy and creativity, as well as freedom from pain and fatigue, but when he stopped taking cocaine he experienced vertigo, cramps, anxiety, insomnia, and hallucinations. When his addiction to cocaine interfered with his ability to operate, Halsted was sent to an asylum for the mentally ill. He was quite a different person when he emerged a year later, cured of the cocaine habit, but addicted to morphine. Encouraged and supported by his colleagues William Osler (1849–1919) and William Henry Welch (1850–1934), Halsted continued his distinguished career as the first professor of surgery at Johns Hopkins. A century later, descriptions of the symptoms of cocaine abuse included intense anxiety, depression, acute psychosis, paranoid delusions, auditory or visual hallucinations, and seizures followed by respiratory or cardiac arrest.

The history of anesthesia is closely related to studies of the meaning and mechanism of pain. While scientific understanding of the mechanism of pain is far from complete, the problem can now be reformulated in terms of neuroendocrinology and the discovery of the opiate receptors and the endorphins, the body's own endogenous morphine-like substances, in the 1970s. Given the fact that opium and morphine are not natural constituents of the nervous system, scientists reasoned that there must be opiate receptors that play a role in the control of pain via some endogenous narcotic. Avram Goldstein (1919–), one of the pioneers of this field, said that when thinking about the effects of morphine he asked himself "why would God have made opiate receptors unless he had also made an endogenous morphine-like substance?" Just as enzymes and substrates fit together like locks and keys, so too might natural opiates interact with the receptors on nerve cells that apparently interacted with morphine and morphine-like drugs. In 1973, Solomon Snyder (1938–) and Candace Pert (1946–) identified the opiate receptors in the brain. Within the year, scientists at several other laboratories confirmed their discovery. By 1975, scientists had discovered the endogenous opiates, neurotransmitter peptides called endorphins or enkephalins that mimic the action of morphine. Several families of endorphins were found in the brain, pituitary gland, and other tissues. Through studies of the endorphin system, neurobiologists and pharmacologists expect to find ways to control the production of endorphins, develop safe endorphin-like drugs, and modulate acute and chronic pain.

Although patients and lay people tend to believe that the relief of suffering is one of the primary goals of medicine, pain and suffering have received relatively little attention in medical education and training. Subjective pain, and the cultural contexts in which patients experience pain are not necessarily considered aspects of the "functional impairments" and disabilities that fall into the domain of medicine. Pain was traditionally regarded as a symptom, rather than a diagnosis, and thus, of little interest in and of itself. Control of surgical pain presumably raised expectations that all forms of pain could be controlled by appropriate analgesics. However, success in the development of surgical anesthesia was not readily extended to the broader problem of acute and chronic pain. Since the 1960s, patients and patient advocates have become increasingly vocal about the problem of pain, particularly chronic pain, which was not a major concern of surgeons. Chronic pain, in particular, has been called one of the most intractable of modern epidemics. In response, many hospitals and medical centers have established multidisciplinary pain clinics.

## POSTSURGICAL INFECTIONS

The impact of anesthesia on the frequency of operations has been a matter of debate, but careful analyses of patterns of surgery in nineteenth century hospitals indicate a positive correlation between the development of anesthesia and the number and range of surgical operations. In part, the rise in surgical cases was an outgrowth of urbanization and industrialization, but the increase in gynecological surgery, especially ovariotomy was dramatic; many of these operations were done to treat nonspecific "female complaints" and emotional problems. Those who harbored suspicions that surgeons were driven by a "savage desire for cutting" were convinced that surgeons operated on moribund accident victims not because they expected to save them, but because doctors saw them as "teaching material" or experimental specimens. Sir John Bell (1774–1842), eminent surgeon, physiologist, and neurologist, said that the ideal surgeon had the "brain of an Apollo, the heart of a lion, the eye of an eagle, and the hand of a woman," but his contemporaries were more likely to see the surgeon as an "armed savage."

A striking upsurge in novel operations occurred in the post-anesthetic, pre-antiseptic period, but there is some evidence that the notoriously high rates of post-surgical infections associated with this era had more to do with changing patterns of urbanization, industrialization, poverty, and malnutrition than anesthesia. The deplorable conditions of hospitals, the misery of the typical hospital patient, and the growing evils of poverty and industrialization provide an explanatory framework for the prevalence of hospital infections in the nineteenth century.

Ideally, surgery should be judged in terms of the survival and rehabilitation of the patient, but the drama of the operation tends to overwhelm the mundane details of post-surgical management. In the pre-anesthetic era, the dazzling speed, strength, and daring of the master surgeon were displayed to good advantage in a limited range of operations. The legendary surgeon who amputated a leg at the thigh, along with two fingers of his assistant, and both testes of an observer, represented the epitome of this genre of surgery. Better authenticated heroes of this era were men like William Cheselden (1688–1752) who could perform an operation for bladder stones in less than one minute, and James Syme (1799–1870), who amputated at the hip joint in little more than 60 seconds. Surgeons were as obsessed with setting speed records as modern athletes, but their goal was the reduction of the stress, pain, and shock endured by the patient. In this context, surgical anesthesia might be seen as a prerequisite for the standardized antiseptic ritual, because it would have been virtually impossible for the lightening-quick surgeon to carry out such procedures while coping with a screaming, struggling, conscious patient.

When the art of anesthesia had been mastered, the surgeon was no longer damned as the "armed savage," but, in the crowded, filthy wards of the typical nineteenth-century hospital, wound infection was transformed from a sporadic event into an array of epidemic conditions generically referred to as *hospitalism*. Although surgeons might admit that the patient on the operating table in a hospital was more likely to die than a soldier on the battlefield, the poor prognosis did not inhibit rising interest in surgical intervention. The cause of wound infection was not clearly understood until the elaboration of germ theory, but "uncleanliness" had been a prime suspect since the time of Hippocrates. Hippocratic physicians knew that it was preferable for a wound to heal by first intention, that is, without suppuration (pus formation). Surgeons could only hope that if a wound was washed with wine, vinegar, freshly-voided urine, or boiled water, cleansed of foreign objects, and covered with a simple dressing, healing would proceed without complications. Wound infection was, however, such a common occurrence that by the medieval period, surgeons had developed elaborate methods to provoke suppuration. The theoretical rationalization for these procedures is known as the doctrine of "laudable pus." According to this offshoot of humoral pathology, recovery from disease or injury required casting off putrid humors from the interior of the body. The appearance of nice creamy white pus in a wound was, therefore, a natural and necessary phase of healing.

Assessing the relationship between changing surgical practice and post-surgical mortality rates in the nineteenth century is complicated by the simultaneous shift to hospital-based medical practice. Crude statistics, such as the 74 percent mortality rate among Parisian hospital patients who had undergone amputation at the thigh in the 1870s, however, seems to speak for itself. Knowing how often successful operations were followed by fatal infections, doctors were famously among those who refused to submit to the knife. For example, when the great French surgeon, diagnostician, and anatomist Guillaume Dupuytren (1777–1835) faced death, he rejected the possibility of an operation, saying he would rather die by God's hand than by that of the surgeon. The motto so popular with anatomists, medical examiners, and pathologists, "*Hic locus est ubi mors gaudet succurrere vitae*" (This is the place where death delights to help the living), would certainly not be comforting to a surgeon who found himself in the role of the patient. Respect for the sick was, however, reflected in another Latin maxim often found in hospitals: "*Praesent aegroto taceant colloquia, effugiat risus, namque omnia dominatur morbus.*" (In the presence of the sick, all conversation should cease, laughter should disappear, because disease reigns over all.)

Despite the reputation of hospitals as places where people went to die, perhaps comforted by an atmosphere imbued with compassion and piety, the annual reports of some hospitals suggest a respectable success rate. For example, the 1856 annual report of Philadelphia's Children's Hospital claimed that of 67 children admitted that first year, 41 were discharged as cured, and none had died. In contrast, in 1870, when Dr. Abraham Jacobi (1842–1906) publicly revealed the appalling mortality rate at a children's hospital in New York, he was forced to resign. Hospital administrators had refused to institute reforms suggested by Jacobi, one of the founders of American pediatrics. The philanthropists who controlled many hospitals often considered moral guidance more important to the mission of the institution than medical science.

Physicians and surgeons knew all too well that even a pinprick opened a doorway to death. The doctor was no more immune to the danger than his patient; minor wounds incurred during dissections or operations could lead to death from a massive systemic infection known as pathologist's pyemia. With but slight exaggeration, doctors warned that it was safer to submit to surgery in a stable, where veterinary surgery was routinely and successfully performed, than in a hospital. When miasmata generated by ineluctable cosmic influences permeated the hospital, patients in the wards inevitably succumbed to hospital gangrene, erysipelas, puerperal fever, pyemia, and septicemia. Physicians endlessly discussed the nature of these disease entities, but all of these hospital fevers can be subsumed by the term *hospitalism*. When epidemic fevers were particularly virulent, the only way to prevent the spread of infection was to burn down the hospital.

Ironically, the evolution of the hospital into a center for medical education and research may have been a major factor in the appalling mortality rates of the large teaching hospitals. Changes in the hospital's social role may also have contributed to the pandemic of hospitalism. By the nineteenth century, the reputation of many urban hospitals was so low that no horror story seemed too implausible. Impoverished slum dwellers were convinced that hospital patients were doomed to death and dissection to satisfy the morbid curiosity of doctors. Hospital managers in France were confronted by terrifying rumors of secret dissection rooms where human fat was collected to light the lamps of the Faculty of Medicine.

Descriptions of major hospitals invariably refer to the overcrowding, stench, and filth of the wards. Surgeons complained that nurses were rarely sober enough to work; patients complained that they were being starved to death. Blood, pus, expectorations, excrement, and urine covered hospital floors. Operations were often performed in the center of the ward when a separate operating room was unavailable. The same washbasin, water, and sponge were used to treat a whole row of patients, and the pus-saturated dressings were collected in the common "pus-bucket." On a more positive note, pus-saturated surgical bandages provided the cells that Johann Friedrich Miescher (1844–1895), physician and chemist, used in the research that led to the discovery of nucleic acid. Moreover, the great quantity and diversity of patients provided invaluable clinical experience for young surgeons, physicians, and pathologists. Hospitals began as places of refuge and charity that cared for the sick and comforted the dying. Changing medical theory, training, practice, and intense interest in pathological anatomy, as well as socioeconomic factors, created new roles for this institution. But the hospital remained embedded in a matrix of poverty and charity in which the virtues of economy and efficiency were more important than cleanliness. Philanthropists, administrators, and physicians, as members of the "better classes," expected their "lower class" patients to be conditioned to crowding, discomfort, and filth; excessive cleanliness might even shock and distress such people.

Surgeons began operations without any special preparation, although a brief hand wash was considered appropriate when leaving the dissecting room. During operations, surgeons protected their clothes with an apron or towel, or wore an old coat already covered with blood and pus. Patients were "worked up" for surgery by the removal of their outer clothing and a swish of a well-used sponge. Observers were often invited to probe and examine interesting wounds. After the introduction of anesthesia, the pace of surgery became less frantic, but certainly not leisurely. Habits acquired in the pre-anesthetic era were not easily broken. A surgeon took pride in his ingenious methods for saving time, such as holding a knife in his mouth while operating. Using the same coat for all operations was convenient, because needles, sutures, and instruments could be kept handy in the lapel, buttonhole, and pockets.

It would be wrong to extrapolate from the epidemics of infection that swept through nineteenth-century hospitals to the problem of surgical infection in other ages. Indeed, it has been suggested that fluctuations in hospital mortality rates reflected the level of distress in the community. Famine, scurvy, and disease would certainly affect resistance to infection. This hypothesis is consistent with the observation that veterinary surgery was relatively free of the problem of wound infection, although it was carried out under rather primitive conditions with little concern for asepsis. Hospitalism might, therefore, have been a unique nineteenth-century plague, perhaps caused by the effects of the Industrial Revolution, rather than a reflection of surgical practice from Hippocrates to Lister.

## JOSEPH LISTER AND THE ANTISEPTIC SYSTEM

Nineteenth-century surgery is so inextricably associated with epidemic hospitalism that modern surgery seems to be a direct product of the introduction of Joseph Lister's (1827–1912) antiseptic system. The factors involved in the evolution of modern surgery were certainly more complex, but the importance of Lister's obsession with preventing infection by attention to both the surgical operation and the quality of post-surgical care should not be underestimated.

Lister's father, Joseph Jackson Lister (1786–1869), was a wine merchant whose scientific interests included the development of the achromatic microscope. Joseph Lister attended Quaker schools in London and University College before going to Edinburgh to study surgery. As a protégé of the great Scottish surgeon James Syme (1799–1870), Lister learned to love the most "bloody and butcherly department of the healing art." Happily married to his mentor's daughter, Lister established his reputation as a surgeon, scientist, and teacher. In keeping with his father's interests, Lister supplemented his clinical work with microscopic studies of inflammation, infection, and blood clotting. His success as a teacher and assistant surgeon at the Royal Infirmary in Edinburgh led to an appointment in 1860 as Regius Professor of Surgery in Glasgow where Lister developed his antiseptic techniques. Lister's ideas and methods continued to develop, especially when he returned to Edinburgh in 1869 to replace Syme as professor of clinical surgery. Lister returned to London in 1877 as professor of surgery at King's College Hospital.

Unlike Ignaz Philipp Semmelweis (1818–1865), Lister was an experimental scientist who shared Louis Pasteur's (1822–1895) insights into the relationship between theory and practice. Like most of his contemporaries, Lister initially believed that infection might be caused by the entry of noxious air into a wound. When his attention was drawn to Pasteur's research on the diseases of wine and beer, however, Lister reached an understanding of the applicability of germ theory to surgical infection. Although few physicians were willing to believe that what occurred in the chemist's laboratory was relevant to medicine, Lister began a study of inflammation in which he used various animal models. Insights gained through these experiments and in hospital wards provided the basis for the development of the antiseptic system.

In attacking the problem of hospital infections, Lister deliberately chose compound fractures for his critical tests, because "disastrous consequences" were frequent with open or compound fracture (a fracture in which the broken ends of the bone protrude through the skin), in contrast to the uncomplicated healing characteristic of simple fracture (a fracture in which the skin remains unbroken), although the trauma involved and the possibility of deformity were similar. Infection often claimed more than 60 percent of patients with compound fractures. Surgeons traditionally probed and enlarged the opening of the wound, but the prognosis was so poor that immediate amputation was considered a reasonable course of treatment. Nevertheless, as Ambroise Paré (1510–1590) demonstrated when he managed his own broken leg, amputation and/or death were not inevitable consequences of compound fracture. According to experienced surgeons, any blockhead could perform an amputation, but great skill was needed to heal a compound fracture without primary amputation.

The search for antiseptics and disinfectants has been part of folk medicine and surgery throughout history. As Florence Nightingale (1820–1910), pioneer of modern nursing and sanitary reform, often said, most of these agents were useless, except when they overwhelmed the nose and forced people to open the windows. Carbolic acid (a solution of phenol) was one of many chemicals used in the nineteenth century as

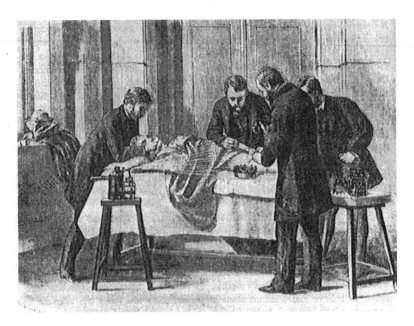

**Antiseptic surgery in 1882.**

a general disinfectant for cesspools, outhouses, stables, and drains. After reading about the beneficial effects the town of Carlisle enjoyed after adding carbolic acid to its sewage works, Lister tested it in animal and human experiments. Several cases ended in failure, but suggested ways in which Lister could improve his techniques. In 1865, an 11-year-old boy with a compound fracture of the leg was admitted to the Glasgow Royal Infirmary. The limb was splinted and the wound was washed and dressed with carbolic acid. Within six weeks, the bones were well united and the wound had healed without suppuration. Between August 1865 and April 1867, Lister treated 11 patients with compound fractures using the antiseptic technique; nine survived. Further refinements of the antiseptic system led to successful treatments for a variety of life-threatening conditions. Moreover, when the antiseptic system was fully incorporated into the hospital routine, the overall rate of hospitalism declined dramatically. Although Lister published an account of the antiseptic system in *The Lancet* in 1867, English surgeons generally ignored his work. In order to convert English surgeons to the antiseptic system, in 1877, Lister accepted the chair of clinical surgery at King's College, London. His surgical demonstrations at King's College Hospital eventually won over many skeptical surgeons, despite continuing resistance to germ theory in the English medical community.

Surgeons who worked with Lister brought his ideas and methods back to their own medical communities where they were able to expand their repertoire and range of operations. Rather than confining themselves to interventions deemed absolutely necessary to preserve life, they could perform operations previously considered unsafe or even impossible. By the time Lister retired in 1892, his methods were finally winning due recognition and many honors. Lister was the first medical man elevated to the British peerage (he became Baron Lister of Lyme Regis in 1897). He was an ardent supporter of medical research at a time when antivivisectionists were very active. Theoretical reasons for resistance to the germ theory were emphasized in professional debates, but, as in the battle against puerperal fever, much of the opposition came from hospital managers who were reluctant to assume the costs of improving operating rooms and hospital wards.

Lister attributed his success to his appreciation of Pasteur's argument that the "septic property of the atmosphere" was due to germs suspended in the air and deposited on surfaces. To attack the germs in the air directly, Lister experimented with devices that sprayed carbolic acid into the air of the operating room. His favorite pump—known as the mule—dispensed a fine mist that his patients and assistants found extremely irritating. Eventually, Lister acknowledged that he had overemphasized the problem of airborne germs. Focusing his attention on improvements in the disinfection of hands, instruments, and wound dressings, he reluctantly abandoned the spray. Unfortunately, surgeons who thought that the "antiseptic system" was simply a matter of sloshing carbolic acid on wounds assumed that the system had failed if wounds became infected.

Although few Americans today are familiar with the work of Joseph Lister, some vague memory of "Lister the germ killer" survived in advertisements for Listerine. The name of this product added the suggestive value of Lister's name to the ancient tradition of strong-smelling wound disinfectants. Since the 1870s, when Listerine the "germ fighter" was sold to doctors and dentists as a general antiseptic and mouthwash, the secret formula has retained its strong flavor and odor. Since the 1920s, Listerine has been advertized to the public as a "germ killer" for the prevention of colds, sore throats, and bad breath.

## ANTISEPSIS AND ASEPSIS

By the end of the nineteenth century, many surgeons had joined microbiologists in using improved methods of sterilization and were full participants in the debates concerning the relative merits of heat versus chemical sterilization, and antiseptic versus aseptic methods. The goal of *antisepsis* is to kill the germs in and around a wound by means of germicidal agents. The goal of *asepsis* is to prevent the introduction of germs into the surgical site. Because almost all wounds contain some microbial contaminants, the concept of aseptic wounds is essentially an oxymoronic microbiological myth. On the other hand, antiseptics alone cannot guarantee uncomplicated healing; the immunological status of the patient and the pathogenic burden are important factors. Lister generally preferred his own antiseptic methods and, despite his admiration for Louis Pasteur, insisted on keeping his instruments in carbolic acid, even after Pasteur and his colleague Charles Chamberland (1851–1908) demonstrated that heat sterilization was superior to chemical disinfection of surgical instruments. Chamberland's autoclave, a device for sterilization by moist heat under pressure, was in general use in bacteriology laboratories in the 1880s.

The relationship between Listerian antisepsis and the acceptance of asepsis by nineteenth-century surgeons involves a complex web of motives, prejudices, loyalties, and theories. What has been called the "full aseptic ritual" never became part of Lister's routine. Lister himself had little enthusiasm for some of the later additions to the surgical ritual, such as white gowns, masks, and gloves. After adopting the aseptic ritual, some of Lister's disciples recalled that Lister, operating in his old coat under a cloud of carbolic acid spray, had had just as much success with much less fuss. As surgeons adopted asepsis and antisepsis with increasing rigor, operations that had once been the miraculous achievements of truly gifted or unusually lucky performers became a matter of routine. The conversion of surgeons to the gospel of antisepsis and asepsis was, however, not rapid or universal, nor were all hospitals capable of providing a supportive staff and environment. Even at the turn of the century, indifference toward antiseptic procedures was not uncommon. Advocates of asepsis adopted the habit of answering the question "What is new in surgery?" with the declaration: "Today we wash our hands *before* operations!"

Surprisingly, the last of the critical factors considered in the battle against infection was the surgeon's hand. William Stewart Halsted (1852–1922), a pioneer of local anesthesia, was also a leader in the battle for aseptic surgery. The great French chemist Louis Pasteur said that if he had been a surgeon, he would not only use perfectly clean instruments and heat-sterilized water and bandages, he would willingly submit his hands to a rapid flaming after washing them with the greatest care. It is difficult to imagine surgeons agreeing to a routine "flaming" of their hands, but the antiseptic solutions used for scrubbing were almost as unpleasant. When Halsted came to terms with the fact that the human hand could not be sterilized, he decided that it should be covered by flexible gloves, resistant to harsh disinfectants. Initially, Halsted asked the Goodyear Rubber Company to make rubber gloves for Miss Caroline Hampton, head nurse in the surgical division, because she was very sensitive to disinfectants. The experiment was successful, except for the fact that Johns Hopkins lost an efficient nurse when

Miss Hampton married Halsted. In the 1890s, the use of rubber gloves was added to the surgical ritual at Johns Hopkins. Doctors had previously used gloves to protect themselves from patients, especially those who might be syphilitic, but surgical rubber gloves were an innovation designed to protect the patient from the surgeon.

Halsted attempted to instill in his associates an understanding of antiseptic and aseptic principles and an operating style that minimized injury and insult to the tissues. In treating patient with breast cancer, however, Halsted insisted that his radical mastectomy was needed to save lives and cure the disease. Halsted paid little attention to the patient's future "quality of life" and the disfiguring and crippling effect of radical surgery since he thought that was not very important in such cases. A famous portrait of the surgeon D. Hayes Agnew, painted by Thomas Eakins (1844–1916), depicts the conditions under which mastectomy was conducted in 1889. Like Leonardo da Vinci, Eakins was intensely interested in science and medicine. He often attended medical lectures and surgical demonstrations and taught anatomy at the Pennsylvania Academy of the Fine Arts. Nineteenth-century audiences were shocked by his highly realistic portraits of surgeons at work, but today "The Gross Clinic" (1876) and "The Agnew Clinic" (1889) are regarded as masterpieces. "The Gross Clinic" shows Dr. Samuel Gross in a blood-stained frock coat operating on a patient's leg. The portrait of Agnew depicts surgeons in clean, white gowns conducting a mastectomy on an anesthetized woman. The mortality rate for this operation was very high and surgeons acknowledged that few patients actually benefited from the procedure. Surgery did not cure the disease and, in many cases, it probably shortened the patient's life.

Recalling the surgical technique taught at Johns Hopkins in the 1890s, Halsted's students described it as "rigorous and even painful to the staff if not to the patient." For the sake of asepsis, some surgeons even trimmed their magnificent beards and mustaches and refrained from talking to observers and yelling at their assistants during operations. Eventually, the full aseptic ritual included special surgical gowns, caps, masks, and the banishment of spectators from the operating room. Some hospitals installed special mirrors or glass domes so that observers could watch without contaminating the operating room. When properly applied, antisepsis, asepsis, and anesthesia transformed the operating room from the doorway to death into an arena of quiet routine.

To explore the achievements of the many famous surgeons of the post-Listerian period would be an impossible task, and rather like compiling a catalog of all the parts of the body. It is more important to recognize the fact that the surgical revolution involved much more than the obvious technical triumphs of anesthesia and antisepsis. More subtle, but fundamental factors involved changes in the status and training of the surgeon, which made it possible for practitioners of a once lowly craft to integrate advances in pathological anatomy, medical instrumentation, and the life sciences into the science and art of surgery.

Since the late nineteenth century, progress in controlling the three major obstacles to successful surgery—pain, infection, and bleeding—has been remarkable. Understanding of the immunological basis of blood-group substances and practical methods for the storage and transfusion of blood and blood products have made it possible for the patient to survive even when accidents or surgical errors cause catastrophic blood loss. Knowledge of the most hidden parts of the body has grown via the classical pathway of anatomical study and through the introduction of new instruments and techniques for visualizing, exploring, and sampling body parts and products. The surgeon is no longer engaged in single-handed combat, but is part of a team of specialists in anesthesia, pathology, radiology, bacteriology, immunology, and so forth. Surgical triumphs had become so routine by the 1960s that gaining an international reputation, or at least a cover story in *Time* magazine, required nothing less than a return to the stuff of myth: the transplantation of human hearts.

Not all of the factors that determine the success of surgery are, strictly speaking, a part of medical science. Some of the major postoperative threats to the patient are so humble that it would have been an insult to the dignity of the medical profession to take notice of them. For example, hospital bandages were generally made of rags that had gone through a laundry process that scarcely inconvenienced their microbial passengers. Rags were a major item of international trade and a good vehicle for the exchange of disease. No matter how skillful the surgeon, no matter how clean the operating room might be, if the patient was later bandaged with contaminated dressings, and put into soiled bedding, infection and death could claim another victim.

## FROM HOSPITALISM TO NOSOCOMIAL INFECTIONS

Surgeons no longer fear the old hospital fevers, but few patients realize that *nosocomial infections* are still a very significant threat. Probably few patients know that nosocomial infection simply means hospital-acquired infection. Although it is difficult to assess the morbidity and mortality directly due to nosocomial infections, according to the National Nosocomial Infections Surveillance System, the overall infection rate is highest in large teaching hospitals and lowest in non-teaching hospitals. Based on a representative sample of American hospitals, investigators calculated that five to six percent of hospitalized patients developed nosocomial infections, which cause or contribute to many thousands of deaths each year. The true incidence of nosocomial infections was presumably much higher, because many cases were not properly reported. In response to calls for cost-containment, hospital infection-control departments are often neglected, because they use resources, but do not generate revenue. In all hospitals, the incidence of nosocomial infections was highest in the surgery department, followed by the medicine and gynecology wards. Semmelweis and Lister would be dismayed to find that the most common and most preventable cause of nosocomial infections is a general neglect of hand washing, the most fundamental aspect of infection control, by many doctors and healthcare professionals. Many healthcare practitioners think that hand washing is a nineteenth century technique that has been superseded by modern methods, such as the use of disposable gloves, despite the fact that bacteria can contaminate gloves as well as hands. A 1999 report by the Institute of Medicine found that medical mistakes in hospitals killed an estimated 44,000 to 98,000 patients a year. Theoretically, operating teams keep track of everything used during surgery and make sure that anything that went into the patient was taken out before the conclusion of the operation. Surgeons acknowledge that leaving objects inside a patient occurs occasionally and that it is a dangerous error that can lead to severe infections, organ damage, and even death. Researchers estimate that sponges or instruments are left behind at least 1,500 times a year in the United States; the total number of operations exceeds 28 million. Objects left behind after surgery include sponges and various instruments, like clamps, retractors, or electrodes. These mistakes have caused deaths, sepsis, further surgeries, and prolonged hospital stays.

Although there is no doubt that nosocomial infections significantly add to morbidity and mortality rates and increase the costs of hospital care, it is difficult to determine the actual risk assumed when a patient enters a hospital. The proportion of extremely sick and vulnerable patients found in today's hospitals—transplant patients, premature infants, elderly patients with multiple disorders, cancer patients, burn victims, AIDS patients—has dramatically increased. Such patients would not have lived long enough to contract hospital infections in the not so distant past.

## SUGGESTED READINGS

Baszanger, I. (1997). *Inventing Pain Medicine: From the Laboratory to the Clinic.* New Brunswick, NJ: Rutgers University Press.

Bending, L. (2000). *The Representation of Bodily Pain in Late Nineteenth-Century English Culture.* New York: Oxford University Press.

Cassell, J. (1991). *Expected Miracles: Surgeons at Work.* Philadelphia, PA: Temple University Press.

Caton, D. (1999). *What a Blessing She Had Chloroform: The Medical and Social Response to the Pain of Childbirth from 1800 to the Present.* New Haven, CT: Yale University Press.

Cole, F. (1965). *Milestones in Anesthesia: Readings in the Development of Surgical Anesthesia, 1665–1940.* Lincoln, NE: University Nebraska Press.

Ellis, H. (2001). *A History of Surgery.* San Francisco, CA: Greenwich Medical Media.

Eaulconer, A., and Keys, T.E., eds. (1965). *Foundations of Anesthesiology.* 2 Volumes. Springfield, IL: C.C. Thomas.

Fenster, J. M. (2001). *Ether Day: The Strange Tale of America's Greatest Medical Discovery and the Haunted Men Who Made It.* New York: HarperCollins.

Fisher, R. B. (1977). *Joseph Lister, 1827–1912.* London: Macdonald and Jane's.

Gaw, J. L. (1999). *"A Time to Heal": The Diffusion of Listerism in Victorian Britain.* Philadelphia, PA: American Philosophical Society.

Gootenberg, P., ed. (1999). *Cocaine: Global Histories.* London: Routledge.

Keys, T. E. (1963). *The History of Surgical Anesthesia.* New York: Dover.

Lawrence, C., and Lawrence, G. (1987). *No Laughing Matter: Historical Aspects of Anaesthesia.* London: Wellcome Institute for the History of Medicine.

Livingston, W. K. (1998). *Pain and Suffering.* Seattle, WA: IASP Press.

Ludovici, L. J. (1961). *The Discovery of Anaesthesia.* New York: Thomas Y. Crowell.

Mann, R. D., ed. (1988). *The History of the Management of Pain: From Early Principles to Present Practice.* Park Ridge, NJ: Parthenon Publishing.

Meldrum, M., ed. (2003). *Opioids and Pain Relief: A Historical Perspective.* Seattle, WA: IASP Press.

Organ, C. H., and Kosiba, M. M. eds. (1987). *A Century of Black Surgenos: The U.S.A. Experience*, 2 Volumes. Norman, OK: Transcript Press.

Pernick, M. S. (1985). *A Calculus of Suffering: Pain, Professionalism, and Anesthesia in Nineteenth-century America.* New York: Columbia University Press.

Pert, C. B. (1997). *Molecules of Emotion: Why You Feel the Way You Feel.* New York: Scribner.

Ravitch, M. M. (1982). *A Century of Surgery. 1880–1980.* 2 Volumes. Philadelphia, PA: J.B. Lippincott Co.

Rey, R. (1995). *The History of Pain.* Cambridge, MA: Harvard University Press.

Rosai, J., ed. (1997). *Guiding the Surgeon's Hand: The History of American Surgical Pathology.* Washington, DC: Armed Forces Institute of Pathology.

Rutkow, I. M. (1992). *The History of Surgery in the United States, 1775–1900.* Vol. 1, *Textbooks, Monographs, and Treatises.* Vol. 2, *Periodicals and Pamphlets.* San Francisco: Norman Publishing.

Rutkow, I. M. (1998). *American Surgery: An Illustrated History.* Philadelphia, PA: Lippincott-Raven.

Snyder, S. H. (1989). *Brainstorming: The Science and Politics of Opiate Research.* Cambridge, MA: Harvard University Press.

Spillane, J. F. (2000). *Cocaine: From Medical Marvel to Modern Menace in the United States, 1884–1920.* Baltimore, MD: Johns Hopkins University Press.

Sykes, W. S. (1982). *Essays on the First Hundred Years of Anaesthesia.* 3 Volumes. Chicago, IL: American Society of Anesthesiologists.

Thomas, V. T. (1985). *Pioneering Research in Surgical Shock and Cardiovascular Surgery. Vivien Thomas and His Work with Alfred Blalock.* Philadelphia, PA: University Pennsylvania Press.

Volpitto, P. P., and Vandam, L. D., eds. (1982). *The Genesis of Contemporary American Anesthesiology.* Springfield, IL: Charles C. Thomas.

Wall, P. (2000). *Pain: The Science of Suffering.* New York: Columbia University Press.

Wangensteen, O. H., and Wangensteen, S. D. (1978). *The Rise of Surgery. From Empiric Craft to Scientific Discipline.* Minneapolis, MN: University Minnesota Press.

Wolfe, R. J. (2001). *Tarnished Idol: William Thomas Green Morton and the Introduction of Surgical Anesthesia: A Chronicle of the Ether Controversy.* San Anselmo, CA: Norman Publishing.

Worboys, M. (2000). *Spreading Germs: Disease Theories and Medical Practice in Britain, 1860–1900.* New York: Cambridge University Press.

Younger, S. J., Fox, R. C., and O'Connell, L. J., eds. (1996). *Organ Transplantation: Meanings and Realities.* Madison, WI: University of Wisconsin Press.

# 13

# Medical Microbiology and Public Health

Despite the antiquity of concepts that seem to be associated with the germ theory of disease, microbiology was not established as a scientific discipline until the end of the nineteenth century. In the process, scientists and medical reformers often cast their arguments in terms of an opposition between *contagion theory* and *miasma theory*. Although the miasma theory of disease was the primary stimulus to the public health campaigns of the nineteenth century, closer inspection of the evolution and usage of these terms in earlier periods suggests that they were not necessarily seen as mutually exclusive. Sharp distinctions between contagion and miasma models might be considered rather misleading and anachronistic when applied to the period between Girolamo Fracastoro's *On Contagion* (1546) and triumph of microbiology at the end of the nineteenth century. That is, Renaissance authors and those who followed them often switched back and forth between the two terms. When contagion was defined loosely enough to include harmful material that was indirectly, as well as directly transmitted, it was not incompatible with equally vague definitions of miasma as disease-inducing noxious, contaminated air. Thus, when nineteenth-century bacteriologists expressed their interest in Fracastoro as the precursor of germ theory, they were probably interpreting his views in a manner very different from the way in which Fracastoro and other Renaissance physicians saw them.

During the seventeenth century, microscopists established the existence of tiny "animalcules," infusoria, the capillary network, and certain kinds of cells. Antoni van Leeuwenhoek (1632–1723), one of the most ingenious microscopists of that period, described molds, protozoa, bacteria, sperm cells, and other "little animals." Nevertheless, most physicians and natural philosophers regarded the notion of "disease-causing animalcules" as little better than ancient superstitions about elf-shot, worms, and flying venom. Moreover, there was little evidence available to decide between the hypothesis that the minute entities

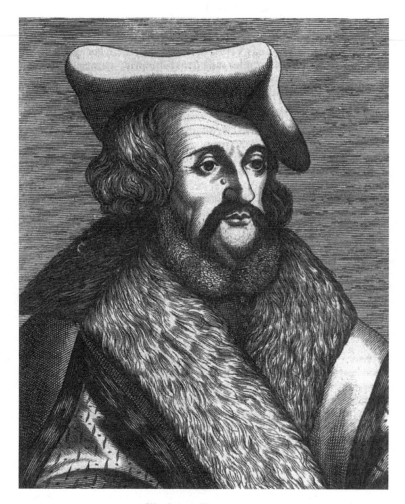

**Girolamo Fracastoro.**

observed by microscopists were the *product* of disease, putrefaction, and fermentation and the alternative hypothesis that they were the *cause* of these phenomena.

The idea that disease, impurity, or corruption can be transmitted by contact is an ancient folk belief. *On Contagion* (1546) by Girolamo Fracastoro is generally regarded as the earliest exposition of germ theory, but it was Giovanni Cosimo Bonomo (1663–1696) who provided the first convincing demonstration that a contagious human disease was caused by a minute parasite close to the threshold of invisibility. Bonomo proved that scabies, commonly known as "the itch," was caused by a tortoise-like mite (now known as *Sarcoptes scabiei* var. *hominis*) just barely visible to the naked eye. When the female mite burrows into the skin and lays her eggs, the unfortunate host develops a rash and intense itching. The mites can be transferred directly from person to person or by means of bedding or clothing used by "itchy" persons. *Sarcoptes scabiei* can also affect cats, dogs, horses, cattle, pigs, and wild animals, but the condition is generally referred to as mange. The itch mite, however, was regarded as an interesting curiosity rather than an example that might apply to other diseases.

Further evidence for contagion theory appeared in studies of silkworm diseases. Agostino Bassi (1773–1857) found that he could transfer the disease called muscardine to healthy silkworms by inoculating them with material taken from worms that had died of the disease. According to Bassi, muscardine was caused by a minute living plant or parasitic fungus. Bassi suggested that other contagious diseases might be caused by similar parasites. The fungus that causes muscardine was later named *Botrytis bassiana* in honor of Bassi. Johann Lucas Schönlein's (1793–1864) search for the cause of ringworm was influenced by Bassi's work on muscardine. In 1839, Schönlein, a professor of medicine at Zurich, reported finding a fungus in the pustules of ringworm. Unlike the prolix Bassi, Schönlein set forth his case for a causal relationship between parasite and disease in barely two hundred words.

When Jacob Henle (1809–1895), Professor of Anatomy at Zurich, published *On Miasmata and Contagia* in 1840, several examples of microparasites as putative agents of disease had been added to scabies and muscardine. Critically evaluating the experimental evidence, Henle discussed the nature of the proofs that would be required to establish a causal relationship between microbes and disease. Although it is possible to link Fracastoro's account of contagion and miasma to Henle's hypothesis, the context in which they worked and the centuries that separated them infused very different meanings into their use of the terms miasma and contagion.

Henle argued that physicians blamed disease on miasma, which they defined as something that mixed with and poisoned the air, but no one had ever demonstrated the existence of miasma with scientific instruments. Miasma was only presumed to exist, by exclusion, because no other cause could be demonstrated.

According to Henle's hypothesis, *contagia animata* (living organisms) caused contagious diseases because whatever the morbid matter of disease might be, it obviously had the power to increase in the afflicted individual. Given the fact that a small inoculum of pus from smallpox pustules could be used to infect a multitude of people, the contagion must be an animate entity that multiplies within the human body. Chemicals, toxins, and venoms remain fixed in amount. By definition, only living things have the power of growing and multiplying.

One could most logically explain the natural history of epidemics by assuming that a living agent excreted by sick individuals was the cause. If this agent were excreted by the lungs, it might easily pass to others through the air. If excreted by the gastrointestinal system, it would enter sewers and wells. Acknowledging the lack of rigorous evidence for the germ theory of disease, Henle argued that science could not wait for unequivocal proofs, because scientists could only conduct research in "the light of a reasonable theory." Although Henle's theory was generally ignored by his contemporaries, after the establishment of microbiology, his essay on contagion was awarded the status of a landmark.

## LOUIS PASTEUR

Microbe hunting was not uncommon in the first-half of the nineteenth century, and Louis Pasteur (1822–1895) was not the first to argue that infectious diseases were caused by germs, but his work was of paramount importance in demonstrating the relevance of germ theory to infectious disease, surgery, hospital management, agriculture, and industry. Pasteur's work illuminated many areas of the nineteenth-century science, including stereochemistry, fermentation, biogenesis, the germ theory of disease, immunology, virology, disinfection, sterilization, and the preparation of protective vaccines. Generally, Pasteur and his associates were involved in several research problems simultaneously. The interaction between Pasteur's many interests makes it impossible to discuss his work as an orderly chronological progression, but this complexity reflects his belief that "the sciences gain by mutual support." His career can also serve as a case study for the interplay between researches devoted to practical problems and so-called pure or basic scientific knowledge.

As a youth, Pasteur was a diligent student and talented artist, but his high school work in chemistry was rated only mediocre. (Stories about such ludicrous errors in judgment by teachers of the gifted and talented seem to be a required part of the hagiography of great scientists, perhaps to give hope to underachieving students and to make teachers more humble.) Pasteur's first attempt at student life in Paris in 1838 led to homesickness so acute that he had to return to his family. Portrait painting during this period seemed to provide a form of therapy and the energy to return to his studies. Eventually, Pasteur decided to abandon art in order to devote all his energies to science. He went on to study chemistry and physics with distinction, but the most important lesson he learned from his studies at the prestigious École Normale Supérieure of Paris was a willingness to apply the experimental approaches he had learned in chemistry to a broad range of problems in biology and medicine, areas in which he had no specific training.

The research problems and methods that Pasteur assimilated as a doctoral student led to studies of many different problems. Nine specific

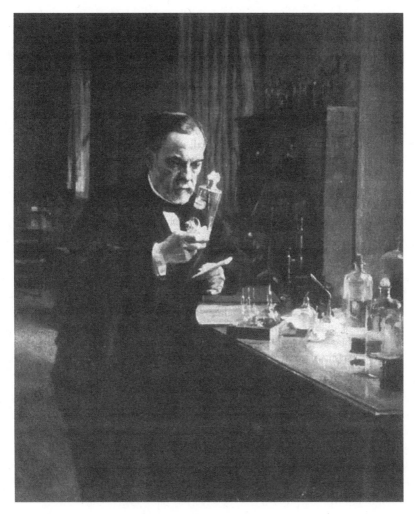

**Louis Pasteur studying rabies.**

aspects of his work were carved into the marble walls of the chapel at the Pasteur Institute in Paris where he was buried: molecular dissymmetry, fermentations, studies of so-called spontaneous generation, studies of wine, diseases of silkworms, studies of beer, contagious diseases, protective vaccines, and the prevention of rabies. Although Pasteur was actually more interested in broad philosophical questions and basic scientific issues than specific medical problems, in terms of the history of medicine, he is primarily remembered for the practical aspects of his work that are most directly related to understanding and preventing infectious diseases.

Studies of crystal structure, stereoisomerism, and molecular dissymmetry seem remote from medical microbiology, but this work provided the unifying thread that guided Pasteur through the labyrinth of research. Pasteur discovered that certain organic molecules could exist as mirror images, that is, as right-handed and left-handed versions, rather like gloves or mittens. As Pasteur pursued this remarkable trait from the behavior of crystals to that of microorganisms, he came to see molecular dissymmetry as a fundamental criterion that distinguished the chemical processes of vital phenomena from those of the inanimate world.

Among the aphorisms of Louis Pasteur, the most quoted have to do with the importance of theory and the role of chance in discovery. He insisted that the theoretical was as important as the practical, although he accepted the idea that, for the good of the state, scientific education should be made relevant to industrial and commercial needs. "Without theory," Pasteur argued, "practice is but routine born of habit." When asked the use of a purely scientific discovery, Pasteur liked to pose the question: "What is the use of a newborn child?" By chance, Pasteur discovered that mold growing in solutions of certain organic chemicals fermented the right-handed form but not the mirror image. In keeping with his conviction that "in the field of observation, chance favors only the mind that is prepared," Pasteur followed the implications of this observation on to fundamental studies of the role of microorganisms in fermentation.

When Pasteur was appointed Professor of Chemistry and Dean of Sciences at the University of Lille, he was urged to assist local industries. Applying the methodology he had used in his studies of crystals to fermenting vats of beet juice, Pasteur observed microorganisms and optically active products of fermentation. His stereochemical studies led him to the hypothesis that the fermentation process was dependent on living germs or ferments. Previous speculations about the role of yeasts in fermentation had been ridiculed by Justus von Liebig (1803–1873), Jöns Jacob Berzelius (1779–1848), and Friedrich Wöhler (1800–1882), the most illustrious organic chemists of the period, who argued that fermentation was a purely chemical process and that microorganisms were the *product* rather than the *cause* of fermentation. Although today Pasteur is universally known, Liebig has been called the greatest organic chemist of the nineteenth century. Like Pasteur, Liebig was known for his combative personality, quarrelsome nature, productivity, and his ability to pursue many projects simultaneously.

Further experiments on a variety of fermentations led Pasteur to the conclusion that all fermentations are caused by specific, organized ferments. Changes in environment, temperature, acidity, composition of the medium, and various poisons affected different ferments in particular ways. Moreover, Pasteur suggested that living ferments might be the cause of infectious diseases as well as fermentation. Although Joseph Lister's work on the antiseptic system of surgery owed a great deal to Pasteur's fermentation studies, most physicians rejected the idea that the diseases of wine and beer were related to human disease. Nevertheless, Pasteur's fermentation studies made it possible to improve the production of wine, beer, vinegar, and so forth. Establishing controlled conditions for fermentation, partial sterilization (pasteurization), and the preparation of pure inocula were developments that were immediately applicable to many industrial problems of substantial economic importance.

Studies of fermentation led Pasteur to a declaration of war on the ancient doctrine of spontaneous generation. Friends warned him against being drawn into a contest that could not be won, for one cannot prove a universal negative. That is, one cannot prove that spontaneous generation never occurred, never occurs, or never will occur. Certainly, Pasteur did not enter the battle with an open mind. Although his private notebooks reveal that he was fascinated by the doctrine, in public he was passionately dedicated to destroying advocates of the doctrine of spontaneous generation and their allies in the medical profession. Building on an experimental approach that can be traced back to Francesco Redi's (1626–1698) studies of the alleged spontaneous generation of flies in rotting meat, Pasteur set out to prove that microbes do not spontaneously arise in properly sterilized media and that all the so-called evidence in support of the contrary proposition was the result of careless technique and experimental artifacts.

Philosophical arguments about the origin of life, materialism and atheism, or religion and spiritualism were irrelevant to the daily concerns of wine-makers and surgeons. The practical point established in the context of the spontaneous generation controversy was that, under present conditions, fermentation, putrefaction, infection, and epidemic diseases were caused by specific microbes found in the air and on surfaces, including instruments, bandages, sponges, and the hands of the surgeon. The germ-carrying capacity of air could be measured by sucking air through cotton filters to trap the germ-laden dust particles. The numbers and kinds of germs in the air depended on many environmental factors; for example, the germ content of hospital air was quite high compared with that of mountain air.

One of Pasteur's simplest and most convincing experiments involved the use of specially constructed swan-neck flasks. When liquids were properly sterilized in flasks with long necks drawn out into an S-shaped curve under a flame, the medium remained sterile even though ordinary air could enter the flask. Critics could not argue that some mysterious life force had been tortured out of the medium, because if the flask was tipped so that sterile medium mixed with the germ-laden dust particles trapped in the bend of the swan neck, the medium was soon teeming with microbial life. Although almost all kinds of media could be sterilized by fairly simple means, certain apparent exceptions were eventually traced to the existence of heat-resistant spores that gave rise to microbes under appropriate conditions. Convinced that a revolution in medicine would only become possible when the defenders of spontaneous generation were totally defeated, Pasteur and his disciples created the sterile techniques that made modern microbiology and surgery possible. Despite the apparent futility of jousting with the advocates of spontaneous generation, Pasteur warned that the development of rational methods for the prevention and treatment of disease depended on annihilating the erroneous doctrine of spontaneous generation.

Well aware of the skepticism with which the conservative medical profession regarded his theories, Pasteur was apparently reluctant to begin a direct assault on the diseases of higher animals. However, in 1865, at the request of his friend Jean Baptiste Dumas (1800–1884) and the Minister of Agriculture, Pasteur became involved in studies of silkworm diseases. By 1870, Pasteur had demonstrated the existence of two microbial diseases in silkworms. The condition that was threatening the silkworm industry of France, however, was the result of complex interactions among environmental factors, nutritional deficiencies, and microbes. Research on silkworms provided a transition between Pasteur's studies of fermentation and his studies of the microbial agents that cause anthrax, chicken cholera, swine erysipelas, puerperal fever, cholera, and rabies. As Pasteur became more confident of the general applicability of the germ theory of disease, he acquired collaborators with the skills that made it possible to carry out experiments on higher animals and even human patients. Contrary to the Pasteur mythology, not all of these studies were successful. For example, his studies of a microbe found in victims of childbed fever led him to warn hospital personnel that they carried the microbe from infected women to healthy women, but, like Oliver Wendell Holmes and Ignaz Philipp Semmelweis, he failed to convince physicians of the need to change their approach to obstetrics and gynecology. Indeed, an outraged opponent challenged Pasteur to a duel for this assault on the honor of the medical profession. Such violent and personal animosity was not characteristic of the entire medical and public health community. Many of France's statistically based hygienists, for example, enthusiastically accepted Pasteur's work as an asset to their own public health reform campaigns. Although some French physicians resisted Pasteur's ideas because they anticipated a new form of preventive medicine that would threaten the profession and practice of medicine, by about 1895 this opposition was essentially disarmed by the prospects of powerful new therapeutic tools that strengthened the medical profession. Ultimately, of course, Pasteur and the research institute dedicated to him became icons of French science. According to Nobel Laureate Françoise Jacob (1920–), when a Cabinet minister suggested making some changes to the Collège de France, General de Gaulle (1890–1970) retorted: "There are three things in

France that are inviolable: the Collège de France, the Pasteur Institute, and the Eiffel Tower."

Rabies, a rare but fatal human disease, and its invisible microbe provided Pasteur's most famous triumph. In his development of a protective vaccine against rabies, Pasteur provided ample proof of his contention that microbiology was a demonstration of how the role of the "infinitely small in nature is infinitely great." The first step in all his previous studies of specific diseases had been to find the microbe, but all efforts to identify the causative agent for rabies proved futile. At a time when scientists were just beginning to formulate the technical and theoretical problems of immunization, Pasteur was able to make the intellectual leap of developing a vaccine against an invisible virus. During this period, the term *virus* was traditionally used in a nonspecific sense in referring to an unknown disease-causing agent or poison. In terms of modern virology, rabies is an acute fatal encephalitis caused by neurotropic viruses in the genus *Lyssavirus*, family Rhabdoviridae. The majority of rabies cases are caused by bites by rabid mammals. After an incubation period of several weeks to months, the virus makes its way to the central nervous system where it replicates. Rabies virus can then be disseminated to the salivary glands and other organs via the nerves. Modern medicine has provided an unanticipated mechanism for the transmission of rabies from person to person. Three people died of rabies in 2004 after receiving infected organs (lungs, kidneys, liver) from the same donor. The donor had shown no symptoms of rabies before his death from a brain hemorrhage. Previous reports indicate that at least eight people have contracted the rabies virus through cornea transplants.

Given the difficulties involved in pursuing this project, Pasteur's decision to study a disease as rare as rabies when there were so many common diseases that might have been easier to work with seems puzzling. Several answers have been offered. Perhaps it really was the haunting memory of the howls of the mad wolf that had invaded Arbois when Pasteur was a boy and the screams of its victims as their wounds were cauterized. Alternatively, the choice may have reflected Pasteur's ambition and his flair for the dramatic. However, Pasteur had done enough to achieve immortality before embarking on what was obviously a dangerous project, for research on rabies must begin with one of the most feared of all creatures, the mad dog.

Another factor influencing Pasteur's choice may have been the tension between his condemnation of experimentation on human beings and his desire to prevent human disease. Human experimentation, Pasteur believed, was not only immoral, but also criminal. Moreover, his entry into the study of human diseases was apparently inhibited by a deep antipathy for vivisection and his ambivalence towards physicians. To reconcile these conflicts, Pasteur needed a disease shared by humans and animals that was invariably fatal so that an experimental treatment could not make the outcome any worse. Whatever the motive might have been, Pasteur had chosen well; the success of his quest for a rabies vaccine was greeted throughout the world as the greatest achievement of microbiological science. (Those old enough to remember the fear aroused by polio might reflect upon the similar outbursts of joy, hope, and gratitude that greeted Jonas Salk (1914–1995) and the polio vaccine in the 1950s.) The real Pasteur, a great scientist who certainly had his faults and failures, all but disappeared under the weight of myth, romanticism, and adoration. Venerated by the public as genius, hero, and saint, Pasteur, or the mythic Pasteur, became the target of late twentieth-century historians of science.

The difficulty of predicting the outcome of the bite of a rabid animal is a complicating factor in assessing Pasteur's rabies vaccine. That is, rabies was invariably fatal if contracted, but not all encounters with mad dogs result in human rabies; and not all "mad dogs" are actually rabid. Moreover, the incubation period for rabies is so variable that in some cases the association between bite and disease was difficult to assess. The English surgeon John Hunter (1728–1793) noted a report of a dog that allegedly bit 21 people. None of these people received any medical attention, but only one became ill. If all of them had been treated, the attending doctors would have claimed 20 cures. Nevertheless, physicians were unlikely to forego treatment, even if their remedies did more harm than good. For example, the distinguished medieval physician Arnau de Villanova (c. 1235–1311) believed that wounds resulting from the bites of mad dogs should not be allowed to heal. Leeches, cupping vessels, and noxious dressings should be applied to the open wound for at least 40 days. The notion that like cures like was the basis for remedies containing either the worms found under a mad dog's tongue or the heart of a hound. According to Anglo-Saxon folklore, even mad dogs had medical virtues. Mixing a powder made from the head of a mad dog with wine was said to produce a cure for scrofula (a form of tuberculosis that affects the lymph nodes of the neck).

In order to isolate the rabies virus and prepare a vaccine, Pasteur needed a laboratory culture of the causative agent. Obviously, it was difficult to find rabid dogs on a routine basis and even harder to secure their cooperation. Not surprisingly, kennels for rabid dogs were as welcome in any neighborhood as an AIDS clinic in the 1980s or a toxic waste dump. A reliable and relatively safe system of transmitting rabies, which involved trephining experimental animals and inoculating infectious material through the dura mater, was used to study the disease in rabbits and other animals. Rabies was transmitted from rabbit to rabbit so that "fixed virus" with a reproducible degree of virulence and a shortened incubation period was always available. Finally, Pasteur and his colleagues discovered that when the isolated spinal cord of a rabid animal was subjected to increasing periods of air-drying, the rabies virus became progressively weaker. To test the use of the air-dried material as a preventive vaccine, dogs were inoculated daily with suspensions of increasingly virulent preparations of spinal cord. At the end of this procedure, dogs were resistant to rabies even if the most virulent preparations were inoculated directly into the brain. By 1885, Pasteur was satisfied that he could reliably induce immunity to rabies in dogs.

The question of the safety and effectiveness of this vaccine in human beings could not be avoided once the results on dogs became known. Protecting people by immunizing all the dogs in France was surely an impossible task; moreover, wild animals served as an infinite reservoir of disease. Obviously, rabies vaccine was not a candidate for mass immunizations because human rabies was too rare a condition to justify a dangerous series of painful injections. However, Pasteur's vaccine was the only hope against the pain, suffering, and death that were inevitable for those who contracted the disease. On July 6, 1885, nine-year-old Joseph Meister was brought to Pasteur's laboratory. He had sustained at least 14 wounds, some very deep, when attacked by a mad dog two days before. Physicians who examined the boy did not doubt that he would contract rabies and that death was inevitable. After consultation with colleagues at the Academy of Medicine, Pasteur initiated the immunization procedure. Despite the discomfort entailed by the long course of injections, Joseph made a complete recovery. The next well-known patient was a 15-year-old boy who had been savagely bitten by a rabid dog six days before treatment began. News of the apparently successful use of Pasteur's vaccine created both bitter criticism and excessive hope. Pasteur was attacked by physicians, veterinarians, antivivisectionists, and antivaccinators, while terrified victims of the bites of rabid (or presumably rabid) animals besieged his laboratory.

The uncertainties inherent in the course of human rabies and the crudeness of the vaccine led to tragic failures and successes. Successful immunization depends on how soon the inoculations are begun and the individual's reaction to the vaccine. A certain number of deaths due to reactions to the vaccine were inevitable. Critics could always charge that success measured only by the failure of patients to die of rabies was meaningless. When some patients developed paralysis, Pasteur's critics called him an assassin and charged him with infecting human beings with "laboratory rabies." However, when victims of dog bites compared the risks of the Pasteur treatment to rabies, thousands decided that the vaccine was a great victory in the battle between science and disease and chose the vaccine. Throughout the world, people echoed Joseph Lister's tribute to Louis Pasteur: "Truly there does not exist in the whole world a person to whom medical science owes more than to you." Perhaps Pasteur's German counterpart Robert Koch would have quarreled with that assessment. The hostility between Koch and Pasteur was due, at least in part, to nationalistic rivalries inflamed by the Franco-Prussian War, but there were also major differences in their goals, objectives, scientific style, and personalities.

Pasteur's account of Joseph Meister's treatment was presented to the Academy of Science of Paris, in October 1885. Newspapers and journals quickly disseminated news of the rabies vaccine and generated interest in the germ theory of disease and expectations of imminent cures for other deadly diseases. Victims of bites by rabid dogs and wolves were soon appealing to Pasteur for treatment. For example, when a rabid dog bit seven dogs and six children in Newark, New Jersey, the boys were sent to France, where they received the Pasteur vaccine. When the boys returned, they were widely exhibited, which created additional interest in Pasteur's work and his germ theory of disease. During the twentieth century, efforts to prevent rabies in the United States were largely directed at domestic animals, which represented most reported cases before 1960. Because of the success of such campaigns, by 2000, only 10 percent of rabies incidents were attributed to domestic animals. Rabies-related human deaths dropped from more than one hundred a year in the early 1900s to about two a year. However, about 40,000 people in the United States are treated for rabies exposure annually, primarily because of contact with rabid raccoons, coyotes, and bats. Federal and state officials have attempted to eradicate raccoon rabies by dropping bait containing oral rabies vaccine from aircraft. Switzerland and France used oral vaccine to become rabies-free. Statistically, however, rabid bats pose a greater danger than raccoons.

In public, Pasteur insisted on a rational scientific method, but in private he pursued a more empirical approach, often guided by theories that might be considered irrational. His colleague, the clinician Emile Roux, urged more caution and was critical of Pasteur's approach to human experimentation. Some historians of science have depicted Pasteur as "authoritarian, politically reactionary, self-deceiving, overly concerned with priority and credit, ungenerous to his assistants, ruthless with his adversaries, and recklessly overconfident in putting human patients at risk." However, other scholars and scientists argue that Pasteur took calculated risks that were appropriate to the information available to him and the dangers that his human subjects were already facing. Pasteur was a public figure and a scientist and he was very adept at attracting attention and converting people to his views. Pasteur apparently chose to conceal ambivalent or unfavorable aspects of his work on rabies and anthrax. At least two patients had been inoculated with rabies vaccine before Joseph Meister, but the results were considered inconclusive and they were not published. Not surprisingly, Pasteur's critics called his rabies vaccine dangerous and his defenders insisted on the relative safety of the vaccine in the face of a deadly disease. Pasteur's advocates emphasized the fact that there are unknown risks inherent in all medical therapies and known risks inherent in the diseases that scientists selected for their research. Historians of science have also subjected Pasteur's work on vaccines to scathing criticism, but, it should be noted, many of the difficulties and uncertainties that Pasteur and his contemporaries faced in attempting to develop safe and effective vaccines remain unresolved.

## ROBERT KOCH

In contrast to Louis Pasteur, whose road to microbiology began with chemistry, Robert Koch (1843–1920) came to bacteriology as a physician, and his research was primarily motivated by medical and methodological questions. Lacking Pasteur's flair for the dramatic, Koch's gift was for attention to detail and simple, but ingenious techniques that made modern microbiology possible. To his contemporaries, Koch was "a man of genius both as technician and as bacteriologist."

Robert Koch was the third of 13 children born to Mermann Koch, a mining administrator, and his wife Mathilde. When Koch began his medical studies at the University of Göttingen, the faculty included many eminent scientists, but in the 1860s not even Jacob Henle seemed to have any interest in the possible relationship between bacteria and disease. In 1866, Koch received his doctor's degree and passed the state medical examination. He spent several months in Berlin, observing medical care at the Charité hospital and attending a course of lectures by Germany's most famous physician, Rudolf Virchow (1821–1902), the founder of cellular pathology. Given to romantic dreams, despite his rather phlegmatic personality, Koch originally hoped for a career as a ship's doctor or military surgeon, but he abandoned this goal in order to become engaged to Emmy Fraatz. His first position as a medical assistant at the Hamburg General Hospital gave him some practical experience in working with cholera, a disease he would return to later. In 1867, after finding another position and establishing a modest private practice, he married Emmy and appeared to be doomed to spending his life in rural isolation as a general practitioner and district medical officer. A brief interruption occurred during the Franco-Prussian War of 1870 when Koch enlisted in the medical corps. Like many other doctors, Koch found that war was indeed the ultimate medical school. His experience with typhoid fever and battle wounds would later prove valuable in his research.

Despite his official duties and busy practice, Koch found time for hobbies such as natural history, archaeology, photography, and for research concerning hygiene, public health, and bacteriology. A trip taken in 1875 to attend medical meetings and visit various scientific

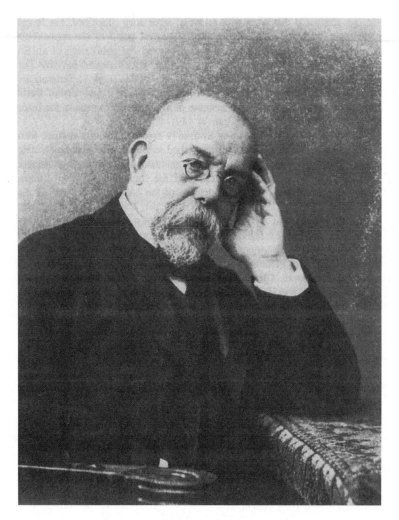

**Robert Koch.**

laboratories encouraged his commitment to scientific research. Thus, when anthrax appeared in his district, Koch began a serious study of the relationship between bacteria and disease. Anthrax is primarily a disease of sheep and cattle, but several forms of the disease can occur in human beings: severe, localized skin ulcers known as malignant pustules, a dangerous condition known as gastric anthrax, and a virulent pneumonia known as woolsorter's disease. Proponents of the germ theory were particularly interested in anthrax and the relatively large bacilli associated with it. Franz Pollender (1800–1879) had observed bacteria in the blood of anthrax victims as early as 1849, but he did not publish his findings until 1855. Pierre Rayer (1793–1867) claimed to have seen the bacillus in the blood of sheep he had inoculated with blood from animals that had died of anthrax. However, it was Casimir Joseph Davaine (1812–1882) who first presented good, albeit circumstantial evidence of a link between the bacillus and the disease. Davaine demonstrated that inoculations of blood from anthrax victims transmitted the disease to experimental animals. In 1863, Davaine published several papers on the infectivity of the "filiform bodies" that appeared in the blood of animals dying of anthrax. Identical bacilli could be found in the malignant pustules of human victims. These experiments were suggestive but not compelling; Davaine had not isolated and purified the anthrax bacillus nor had he satisfied the criteria of proof suggested by Jacob Henle.

By 1876, Koch had obtained cultures of *Bacillus anthracis* and had worked out the life cycle of the bacillus and the natural history of the disease. Like Davaine, Koch transferred anthrax from infected cattle to rabbits and mice. Going beyond his predecessors, Koch discovered that he could grow anthrax bacteria outside the body of living animals. Using the aqueous humor of rabbits or cattle as his growth medium, Koch was able to establish and purify bacterial cultures, which could then be injected into experimental animals. These laboratory cultures produced anthrax just as if a sample of blood from a naturally infected farm animal had been used. In order to have fresh anthrax material continuously available and determine whether the bacilli would change after a certain number of generations, Koch conducted a series of mouse-to-mouse inoculations. Even after the bacilli had been passed through a series of 20 mice, they remained true to form. These experiments ruled out the possibility that some poison or toxin from the original animal caused the disease in the experimental animals. Only an agent capable of multiplying within the bodies of infected animals could create such a long chain of transmission.

While observing anthrax bacilli on microscope slides, Koch saw thread-like chains of bacteria become bead-like spores. When fresh medium was added, the spores were transformed into active bacilli, which began to multiply again. The extreme hardiness of the spores explained many of the mysteries surrounding the persistence of anthrax in contaminated pastures. Because spores were resistant to harsh conditions, a carcass deposited in a shallow grave could furnish enough spores to infect other animals for many years. Thus, an understanding of the natural history of anthrax immediately suggested measures for controlling the disease through proper disposal of contaminated carcasses.

Convinced that he had solved the riddle of anthrax, Koch sent an account of his work to Ferdinand Cohn (1828–1898), the eminent botanist who was Germany's leading expert on bacteriology. Despite some initial skepticism, Cohn invited Koch to come to the University of Breslau to demonstrate his experiments. Certainly, Koch was not the first amateur to invade the academic community claiming to have found a solution to the problem of contagion. In this case, however, Cohn and his associates found the experimental results and demonstrations absolutely convincing. Under Cohn's sponsorship, Koch's paper "The Etiology of Anthrax, Based on the Life Cycle of *Bacillus anthracis*" was published in *Contributions to Plant Biology*.

On the basis of his work with anthrax, Koch confidently predicted that bacteriological science would lead to control over infectious diseases. To overcome the opposition of conservative physicians and scientists, Koch urged advocates of the germ theory of disease to learn to cultivate pure strains of microbes, abandon careless and speculative work, and demonstrate the value of microbiology in the prevention or treatment of disease. In the long run, Koch's predictions were richly validated, but it was Pasteur who produced an anthrax vaccine to prevent the disease in sheep and cattle. Moreover, Pasteur explained how earthworms participated in the natural chain of transmission by bringing anthrax spores to the surface of pastures where they were ingested by grazing animals. Although quantity is not necessarily a sign of quality, it is interesting to note that Pasteur published 31 papers on anthrax to Koch's total of 2. Such differences in approaching a problem, as well as achieving practical solutions, aggravated the conflict between Koch and Pasteur. Attacking Pasteur's work openly and directly, Koch called the results of his rival into question for his alleged failure to produce pure cultures and emphasized the obvious and well-known fact that Pasteur was not a physician. Responding to those who had praised Pasteur as a "second Jenner," Koch contemptuously noted that Edward Jenner's work had involved humans, not sheep.

Establishing a safe and effective vaccine for anthrax in humans remained a problem into the twenty-first century, although the possibility of the use of anthrax spores as a terrorist weapon gained plausibility. During the 1990s, anthrax vaccinations were blamed for Gulf War Syndrome among American soldiers who had been subjected to mandatory vaccinations. Although the effectiveness of the anthrax vaccine was already controversial, critics argued that modifications of the vaccine had been made without sufficient testing and insufficient safeguards were applied to production. The dangers of the large-scale production of weaponized anthrax spores were revealed by an anthrax epidemic that occurred in 1979 in Sverdlovsk, Russia, near a Soviet Biopreparat plant that was doing research on chemical and biological weapons. Initially, Soviet officials blamed the outbreak on contaminated meat. Problems with livestock and meat processing had been responsible for many cases of anthrax in Russian history. However, the 62 deaths that occurred during the 1979 outbreak were clearly due to inhalation anthrax, not gastric anthrax. Revelations about the nature and extent of the Biopreparat program appeared in the 1990s.

Having demonstrated the etiology of a specific disease, Koch turned to the general problem of wound infection, which the British surgeon Joseph Lister had begun to master through the antiseptic system. Many investigators had observed bacteria in traumatic infective diseases, but they could not determine whether bacteria were nonspecific entities, the cause of disease, or the product of some pathological processes. In part, Koch's work on wound infection was meant to support the concept that bacteria existed as distinct, fixed species. Karl von Nägeli (1817–1891), the eminent Swiss botanist, who holds a special place in the history of genetics for his failure to appreciate Gregor Mendel's (1822–1884) theory of inheritance, had attacked the concept of specific bacterial species. If bacteria did not exist as separate species, it made no sense to say that a specific microbe—such as *Bacillus anthracis*—caused a specific disease. Many critics of the doctrine of specific etiology claimed to have "seen" transformations between various types of bacteria. Convinced that such observations were invariably the result of sloppy laboratory techniques, Koch realized that scientists needed simple, reliable methods of establishing pure cultures and standardized means of preparing bacteria for microscopic examination.

Studies of experimentally induced traumatic infective diseases led Koch to believe that a different microorganism caused each septic condition. He also demonstrated that bacteria were not found in the blood or tissues of healthy animals. Unfortunately, the medical community misinterpreted Koch's general proof of the applicability of germ theory to wound infection as a series of laboratory curiosities involving gangrene and septicemia in mice. Although Koch excelled in the rigorousness of his techniques, he lacked Pasteur's flair for choosing and staging dramatic, attention-getting events. Koch's colleagues would have been more impressed if he had demonstrated the relationship between his work on sepsis in mice and human disease. In this case, the disadvantages of working in rural isolation, instead of an urban medical center with access to clinical material were critical. However, Joseph Lister understood the implications of Koch's work and was instrumental in having Koch's *Aetiology of Traumatic Infective Diseases* translated into English.

After years of struggling to pursue his research while maintaining a private practice, Koch finally obtained a position as head of a newly established laboratory for bacteriological research with the Imperial Health Office in Berlin. In 1885, he became Professor of Hygiene at the University of Berlin and Director of the University's Institute of Hygiene, a title he held until 1891 when the Institute for Infectious Diseases was created for him. Despite his professional success, Koch's private life was evidently quite unsatisfactory until he met 17-year-old Hedwig Freiberg and divorced his first wife. By this time, Koch's daughter Gertrude had married Koch's research associate Eduard

Pfuhl. The romance between the eminent scientist and the young artist's model raised a "moral storm" in the medical and scientific community. At the 1892 Congress of German Physicians there was more excitement about Koch's escapades than the scientific papers. Koch was almost 50 and Hedwig was 20 years old when they married in 1893.

Frustrated by the skepticism with which the medical community viewed germ theory, Koch became convinced that finding reliable methods of obtaining pure cultures was the key to progress. The animal body might well be the optimum apparatus for cultivating pathogenic bacteria, but bacteriologists had to cultivate pure strains outside the body in order to establish the role of bacteria in causing disease. Finding it impossible to construct a universal medium suitable for all bacteria, Koch sought a method that would convert the usual nutrient broths into a solid form on which bacterial colonies would stand out like islands, rather like the colonies of mold often found on old bread or

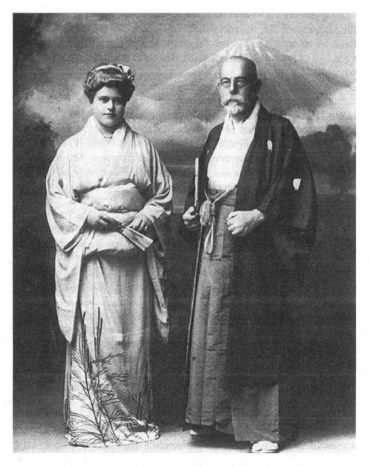

**Robert Koch and his second wife in Japanese costume (1903).**

potatoes. Ancient kitchen lore solved this problem when Koch substituted agar-agar, a polysaccharide derived from seaweed that is used in Asian cooking, for gelatin. (Gelatin liquefies at normal body temperature, 37°C, and is digested by many bacteria; gels made with agar are inert to bacterial digestion and remain solid up to 45°C.) Use of agar gels to isolate bacterial colonies was called "Koch's plate technique." Koch argued that the pure culture was the essential foundation for work on infectious diseases. A special plate for use with agar cultures was invented by Richard Julius Petri (1852–1921), who worked at Koch's Institute of Hygiene. Thanks to the universal adoption of the Petri dish, Petri's name is generally more familiar to biology students than that of Robert Koch. Another technical problem addressed by Koch and his associates at the Imperial Health Office was a re-examination of various public health measures, such as disinfection. Microbiology made it possible to understand the difference between disinfection (killing vegetative cells, but not necessarily all spores) and sterilization (completely killing both spores and vegetative cells). In testing the activity of reputed antiseptics, Koch discovered that many old favorites had virtually no disinfecting powers, whereas other supposedly antiseptic agents inhibited the growth of bacteria but did not kill them.

When Lister, Pasteur, and Koch met in London at the Seventh International Medical Congress in 1881, Koch enjoyed the opportunity to demonstrate his plate technique in Lister's laboratory. Shortly after returning from this triumphant visit, Koch began his work on tuberculosis. Committing all his energies to the task of identifying the causal agent of tuberculosis and finding a cure for this ubiquitous malady, Koch worked indefatigably in strict secrecy. In March 1882, at a meeting of the Berlin Physiological Society, Koch announced his discovery of the tubercle bacillus, *Mycobacterium tuberculosis*. News of Koch's discovery caused great excitement throughout the world. British physicist John Tyndall (1820–1893), one of Pasteur's most dedicated supporters, published an English summary of Koch's paper as a letter to the London *Times*. A few weeks later Tyndall's letter was published in the *New York Times*. News reports and editorials immediately took up the theme that Koch's discovery would soon lead to a cure for tuberculosis.

During the golden age of bacteriology, Koch reflected, the bacterial agents of many infectious diseases seemed to fall into the hands of microbiologists "like ripe apples from a tree," but the tubercle bacillus did not fall so easily. Of all the microbes studied by Koch, the tubercle bacillus was the most difficult to identify, isolate, and culture. On appropriate nutrient agar, most bacteria produce large colonies within two days; the tubercle bacillus took two weeks to form visible colonies. In these investigations, superb microbiological technique, special media and staining techniques, and appropriate experimental animals were indispensable. But so too were Koch's conviction that tuberculosis was a contagious bacterial disease, his strong faith that the causative agent could be isolated, and his almost infinite patience. The discovery of the tubercle bacillus and Koch's proof that it could be found in diseased tissue swept away the confusion that had so long thwarted efforts to understand tuberculosis in all its many forms. Because *M. tuberculosis* can attack virtually every part of the body, it produces a bewildering array of clinical patterns known as phthisis, consumption, scrofula, miliary tuberculosis, meningitis, and so forth. Identification of the tubercle bacillus proved that the various forms of tuberculosis were manifestations of the work of a specific pathogen.

To understand the profound effect of Koch's discovery requires an appreciation of the ways in which this disease permeated the fabric of life in the nineteenth century. Tuberculosis was, in terms of the number of victims claimed, more devastating than the most-dreaded epidemic diseases, including smallpox and cholera. Even in the seventeenth century, Richard Morton (1637–1698), author of *Phthisiologia: A Treatise of Consumptions* (1694), found it difficult to believe that anyone could reach adulthood without at least a touch of consumption. Well known as the "captain of the men of death," in the nineteenth century tuberculosis was the cause of about one in seven deaths. Its devastating impact on society was amplified by the fact that tuberculosis was particularly likely to claim victims in their most productive adult years. The tragic deaths of young artists, writers, composers, and musicians supported the myth that tuberculosis was related to artistic genius. Robust artists complained that it was fashionable for poets to suffer from consumption and die before reaching the age of 30 years. The brief life of John Keats (1795–1821) reflects the romantic view of tuberculosis and the medical mismanagement that often accelerated the inevitable. Although the poet's mother and brother had died of tuberculosis, his illness was misdiagnosed as "gastric fever" and Keats was subjected to a debilitating regimen of bleeding and starvations diets. A definitive diagnosis of pulmonary tuberculosis was finally made at autopsy; the lungs were almost totally destroyed.

Victims of most infectious diseases died or recovered too quickly to indulge in the deep, dark meditations of consumptive artists brooding on the slow, but inexorable, progress of their disease. To Austrian novelist Franz Kafka (1883–1924), tuberculosis was not an ordinary disease but the "germ of death itself." In Romantic imagery, consumptives were possessed by a nervous force that drove them to artistic accomplishments. However, with the disease running rampant in city slums and impoverished villages, the connection was obviously fortuitous, not causal. Perhaps the threat of early death, the chronic mild fever, and the opiates taken to control coughing intensified the creative drive of consumptives who were artists and enhanced the allure of tubercular women. Only an "angel of phthisis" fit the Romantic ideal of femininity: young, pale, thin, with eyes bright from fever, discreetly coughing up blood into her lace handkerchief before her inevitable, but redemptive death. As Keats lamented: "Youth grows pale, and specter thin, and dies."

After Koch's discovery of the tubercle bacillus, the perverted sentimentalism associated with the disease was gradually superseded by acceptance of the fact that it was more intimately linked to poverty and filth than to genius and art. Worse yet, as Koch noted in his early papers on tuberculosis, the tubercle bacillus was very similar in form, size, and staining properties to the microbe that caused leprosy. Medical thinking about the cause and management of tuberculosis reflected peculiar regional differences. Consumptives from northern climates, seeking a cure in the south, were shocked to find themselves quite unwelcome in sunny Spain and Italy, where people assumed that tuberculosis was contagious. Physicians in northern Europe generally believed in a noncontagious, hereditary "tubercular diathesis" (which essentially means that people who are susceptible to tuberculosis are susceptible to tuberculosis). It was common knowledge that the disease "ran in families," sometimes for several generations. Moreover, the fact that only certain individuals developed the disease, although almost everyone was exposed to it, was used to argue against contagion. This is rather like saying that bullets do not kill, because not every soldier on the battlefield was killed by a barrage of bullets.

Koch was not the first scientist to argue for the "unitary theory" of tubercular disease, nor even the first to demonstrate that consumption was contagious. William Budd (1811–1880), an English epidemiologist best known for his classic treatise on typhoid fever, argued that the epidemiology of tuberculosis among blacks in England and Africa indicated that it was a contagious disease. The distinguished French physician, Jean Antoine Villemin (1827–1892), attempted to demonstrate the contagiousness of tuberculosis by inoculating rabbits and guinea pigs with sputum and other materials from victims of tuberculosis. The transmission of human tuberculosis to rabbits allowed Villemin to demonstrate the infectiousness of sputum, blood, and bronchial secretions. He even argued that tuberculosis in humans was identical to that occurring in cattle. However, Villemin's work had little immediate impact and attempts by other physicians to repeat his experiments were inconclusive. Indeed, Rudolf Virchow argued that pulmonary tuberculosis and miliary tuberculosis were different diseases, although René Laënnec (1781–1826), the inventor of the stethoscope, had shown that tuberculosis caused morbid effects throughout the body. In some individuals, tuberculosis infection resulted in the acute miliary pattern, whereas others exhibited the symptoms of pulmonary tuberculosis. Despite the brilliance of Virchow's work in cellular pathology, his views on tuberculosis may have been distorted by nationalistic pride and prejudice. Just as Koch belittled French microbiology, Virchow denigrated the combination of clinical observation and autopsy studies that characterized the work of René Laënnec and French investigators of pathological anatomy. Of course, Virchow's resistance was not entirely a matter of nationalism. Even after inspecting Koch's demonstrations, Virchow continued to speak of the "so-called tubercle bacillus."

Having cultured a specific microbe apparently associated with tuberculosis in all its manifestations, Koch provided unequivocal evidence that *B. tuberculosis* was the specific cause of the disease. In doing so, Koch formalized the criteria now known as "Koch's Postulates," a series of steps that must be performed in order to prove that a particular microbial agent is the cause of a particular disease. In a general way, these criteria had been suggested previously by Jacob Henle and others, but Koch provided the most rigorous demonstrations of the germ theory of disease. To satisfy Koch's postulates, the investigator must prove that a specific microorganism is invariably associated with the disease. Combining such observations with evidence that the microbe was not found in healthy individuals or in those suffering from other diseases was suggestive, but not compelling. To establish unequivocal proof, the investigator had to isolate and culture the microbe in the laboratory in order to separate it from contaminating tissue and other organisms. After the putative pathogen had been transferred through a series of cultures, it should be inoculated into healthy animals. If pure laboratory cultures induced the disease in experimental animals, the investigator should isolate the microbe from those animals in order to prove that a causal relationship existed between microbe and disease. For many human diseases, such as cholera, typhoid, and leprosy, it was impossible to satisfy Koch's postulates, because scientists had not found any suitable experimental animal model. To provide unequivocal evidence in such cases would require unethical human experimentation. Koch's postulates were formulated for studies of infectious disease, but his general approach has been extended to guide studies of other disorders, such as the health hazards posed by asbestos and other chemicals.

Even though Koch's discovery of the tubercle bacillus was not immediately followed by a preventive vaccine or specific therapeutic agent, it stimulated hope that conscientious patients might recover their health through appropriate medical guidance. Nevertheless, Koch was under considerable pressure to match the achievements of his great French rival. In 1889, after devoting several years to his official duties and travels, Koch began to work in the laboratory again, with great intensity and complete secrecy as to the nature of the experiments that produced such large numbers of dead guinea pigs. One year later, at the

Tenth International Congress of Medicine in Berlin, Koch seemingly implied that he had discovered a cure for tuberculosis. A close examination of what Koch actually said should have prevented the excess of hope and the sense of betrayal that followed distorted newspaper accounts of his tentative assessment of the prospects for a cure. In his speech, Koch discussed a substance that arrested the growth of the tubercle bacillus in the test tube and in living bodies. The living bodies, however, were those of guinea pigs, not human beings. This was an important point, because guinea pigs do not acquire tuberculosis naturally, although they become infected when properly inoculated. Nevertheless, Koch incautiously referred to the agent he had discovered as a remedy. Press reports immediately labeled the mysterious agent "Koch's lymph," "Kochin," or "Koch's fluid." Koch called his preparation "tuberculin." Based on Koch's preliminary results in guinea pigs, large-scale human trials were obviously premature, but desperate consumptives were not willing to wait for controlled clinical tests to validate tuberculin's promise.

Despite the fact that Germany had a law prohibiting "secret medicines," Koch refused to reveal the nature of tuberculin. He did, however, provide the name and address of a doctor who was preparing tuberculin under the direction of Koch's son-in-law, Eduard Pfuhl. As reported by Sir Arthur Conan Doyle (1859–1930), who came to Berlin to learn about the alleged German remedy, hundreds of thousands of consumptives were begging for treatment. Even Joseph Lister, who brought his niece to Berlin for treatment, had to wait a week before Koch had time to see him. Impressed by the work on tuberculin, as well as the new therapeutic methods for diphtheria and tetanus developed by Emil von Behring (1854–1917) and Shibasaburo Kitasato (1852–1931), Lister complained that German science was far ahead of British science.

Within a year, thousands of people had received tuberculin treatment, but Koch's associates had little or no interest in rigorous clinical trials. Tuberculin seemed to help some patients in the early stages of tuberculosis of the skin, bone, or joints, but physicians and patients were often misled by subjective signs of improvement induced by hope rather than specific therapeutic interventions. Unfortunately, in patients with pulmonary tuberculosis, further experience indicated that tuberculin was useless, or even dangerous. For example, Dr. Edward L. Trudeau (1848–1915) who directed an important tuberculosis sanatorium at Saranac Lake, New York, discovered that tuberculin did not provide the miraculous cures that he and his patients had anticipated. Throughout the world, disappointed and disillusioned patients and physicians bitterly condemned Koch and his secret remedy. A study prepared for the German government found remarkably little evidence to justify the claims made for tuberculin. Nevertheless, anecdotal reports of cures and improvements led government officials to continue support for tuberculin, which was used in prisons and in the army.

When Koch finally described the nature and preparation of his remedy, scientists and physicians were surprised to learn that tuberculin was simply a glycerin extract of tubercle bacilli. Critics cynically noted that Koch had revealed the great secret after it had become obvious that tuberculin was worthless. In his own defense, Koch argued that preparing tuberculin was very difficult. Therefore, he had been afraid that doctors and quacks all around the world would attempt to prepare and inoculate harmful imitations, causing great damage to patients and to the reputation of German science. As condemnation mounted, Koch undertook a visit to Egypt, leaving his son-in-law in charge of tuberculin and the Institute for Infectious Diseases. After 1896, Koch essentially gave up research on tuberculosis and tuberculin. Turning to the study of tropical diseases, Koch finally realized his old dreams of traveling to exotic locations. Despite his pioneering role in the history of medical microbiology, it was not until 1905 that Koch was awarded a Nobel Prize for his work on tuberculosis and bacteriology.

Experience with a wide variety of diseases led Koch to the conclusion that it was probably impossible to achieve immunity to tuberculosis by the methods successfully used for other bacterial diseases. Nevertheless, Koch never completely gave up hope that an improved form of tuberculin would serve as an immunizing agent or cure. This dream was never realized, but at least the medical community could agree that tuberculin was a valuable diagnostic aid in the detection of early, asymptomatic tuberculosis. In the heroic tradition of the time, Koch had tested tuberculin on himself. His strong reaction indicated that, like most of his contemporaries, he had not escaped a "touch of tuberculosis." What Koch had actually stumbled upon was the complex immunological phenomenon later called delayed-type hypersensitivity. Where tuberculosis was considered a shameful disease, an obstacle to marriage, or a condition excluded from life insurance policies, many individuals and their families might not find an accurate diagnosis particularly desirable.

Tuberculin was not a cure, but the discovery of the tubercle bacillus and tuberculin provided the basic weaponry for a crusade against tuberculosis. The tuberculin test could detect asymptomatic cases of tuberculosis, and microbiology laboratories could help the physician monitor the patient's status by analyzing throat cultures or sputum samples. The need for caution and for critical clinical trials should have been a major part of the lessons taught by the tuberculin fiasco. Widespread support for abandoning the whole apparatus of double-blind clinical trials in the search for AIDS remedies one hundred years later suggests that such lessons are quickly forgotten. AIDS in the 1980s, like tuberculosis in the 1880s, was perceived as a mysterious, dreaded, shameful, and fatal illness. Withholding a drug that might cure, or at least slow, the progress of a fatal illness is, doubtless, a cruel and unethical act. The history of phantom remedies indicates that it is more difficult to come to grips with the pressures that lead to dispensing ineffectual drugs and unjustified optimism when treating a disease with as complex and uncertain a natural history as AIDS or tuberculosis.

Expressing the despair caused by tuberculosis, the British writer Charles Dickens (1812–1870) characterized consumption as the disease that medicine never cured and wealth never warded off. Nevertheless, tuberculosis morbidity and mortality rates declined significantly well before the advent of specific antibiotic therapy. Progress in controlling tuberculosis was gradually achieved, as physicians and public health workers assimilated the idea that it was a preventable disease and began to think in terms of a complex web of causation. Detecting early cases and accurately measuring the incidence of infection were made possible by the development of more sensitive tuberculin skin tests and X-ray examinations of the lungs. Even though the tubercle bacillus remained ubiquitous, the incidence of sickness declined with changes in living standards, as more people gained access to fresh air, sunlight, and improved nutrition. Scientists suggested that with biological wisdom directing social and individual behavior, the disease could be eradicated without vaccines. However, medical and public health authorities have rarely reached a workable consensus as to the nature of "biological wisdom."

According to surveys conducted during the 1920s and 1930s, tuberculin skin tests indicated that 50 to 60 percent of undergraduates in northeastern colleges and about 80 percent of students in the southwest were infected. Medical and nursing students had even higher rates of infection. Some schools reported that by graduation all the students were tuberculin positive. At the same time, tuberculosis was declining in the general population. Because tuberculosis was associated with poverty, these findings among the relatively privileged college population were disconcerting. Women's colleges, in particular, made the preservation of student health a top priority. This was essential to counteract the medical warnings about how detrimental education was to female health and development.

When marked variations in the virulence of different varieties of tubercle bacilli were discovered, scientists hoped that a particular strain could play the role cowpox served in preventing smallpox. However, evaluating tuberculosis vaccines is very difficult; in some areas, almost everyone has been exposed to the bacillus and many have long-standing, but dormant, infections. The tubercle bacillus can remain dormant in the human host for many years. It effectively evades immune attack and protects itself with a thick coat of complex lipids. The most widely used vaccine against tuberculosis is derived from the live, attenuated strain produced by Albert Léon Charles Calmette (1863–1933) and co-workers. Since the 1920s, Bacille Calmette-Guérin (BCG) has been used as a vaccine against childhood tuberculosis. Despite recurring questions about the safety and efficacy of BCG, preventive vaccination remains the basis of antituberculosis efforts in many developing nations.

Recognition of the danger posed by contaminated milk played an important part in efforts to control tuberculosis. Some scientists thought that tuberculosis originated in domesticated cattle and had been transmitted to humans through milk and meat, but the relationship between human and bovine tuberculosis became very controversial. In 1901, at the First British Congress of Tuberculosis in London, Koch announced that bovine and human tuberculosis were two distinct diseases. Counter to prevailing opinion at the time, Koch declared that humans could not be infected with the bovine tubercle bacillus. This announcement was stunning, not just because it was absolutely wrong, but because in his early work on tuberculosis Koch had said that bovine and human tuberculosis were caused by the same microbe. If true, Koch's new ideas about bovine tuberculosis had tremendous public health implications. Bacteriologists, therefore, rushed to confirm or disprove his proclamation. A British Commission reached the conclusion that bovine tuberculosis was a public health menace, but a German Commission agreed with Koch. Emil von Behring (1854–1917), however, argued that contaminated milk was the major source of infection for children. This view was confirmed by American bacteriologist Theobald Smith (1859–1934). Children between the ages of one and five years of age were particularly susceptible to infection from the "pale cultures of tuberculosis" sold as milk. Smith, therefore, campaigned for the destruction of tuberculous dairy cattle as a necessary public health measure.

Veterinarians and public health workers tended to emphasize the dangers of bovine tuberculosis to human health. Koch was criticized for his emphasis on pulmonary tuberculosis and his suggestion that bovine tuberculosis was an insignificant issue. American pediatrician Abraham Jacobi said: "The lives of the thousands of babies in the world are far more important than the reputation of one scientist." Although the vast majority of deaths from tuberculosis were the result of active pulmonary tuberculosis, about 10 percent of the deaths of infants and young children in urban America could be blamed on diseases transmitted by milk. Theobald Smith argued that "the whole machinery of public health" was at risk if the battle against contaminated milk and water was undermined by Koch and others.

While pursuing his early work under primitive and difficult conditions, Koch had been a patient and conscientious worker. After achieving his greatest victories, he seems to have become increasingly opinionated, arrogant, and dogmatic. Many critics pointed to the militaristic and authoritarian environment of German science as a factor. Perhaps even Koch fell victim to the Koch mythology and was swept away by official and public adulation and pressure. When a scientist of Koch's standing was wrong, his oracular pronouncements could endanger the public health.

In 1908, the major issue of contention at the International Tuberculosis Congress was the problem of bovine tuberculosis. To the delight of America's "anti-pasteurizers," Koch focused on pulmonary tuberculosis. According to Koch, the question of the intestinal infection of children was essentially irrelevant, because pulmonary tuberculosis accounted for 11 out of every 12 deaths from tuberculosis. Whatever the mortality and morbidity rates for the various forms of tuberculosis might have been, ignoring preventable infections caused by contaminated dairy products revealed a very strange approach to childhood illness. Critics contended that Koch had taken this position to shield the German government and the German meat industry. When Koch returned to Berlin after the bitter 1908 meeting, he tried to resume his research on tuberculosis, but his health deteriorated rapidly and he died of a heart attack in 1910. Two years later, the Institute for Infectious Diseases was renamed the Robert Koch Institute.

Since the time of Hippocrates, consumptives have been subjected to bizarre diets, noxious remedies, and a soothing elixir of "opium and lies." Probably, the most colorful cure was the ritual of the Royal Touch, performed by kings of England and France from the Middle Ages to the eighteenth century. Because the scrofulous wretches selected for the ceremony received a coin as a souvenir, records of the alms disbursed during such rituals provide estimates of the number of touches. Perhaps a few skeptics like Michael Servetus (1511–1553) could see that many were touched and few were cured, but because of the unpredictable nature of the disease, the Royal Touch might have worked as well as any other remedy.

Depending on the shifting tides of medical fashion, physicians have prescribed rest, exercise, starvation diets, rich foods, fresh air, sunshine, tonics, and tranquilizers for their consumptive patients. Many standard remedies were useless, and some, like gold salts, actually exacerbated the illness. Folk remedies for phthisis included wolf's liver boiled in wine, weasel blood, pigeon dung, and essence of skunk. Eating live snails was said to prevent the disease. Twentieth-century physicians prescribed creosote, digitalis, opium, cod-liver oil, heavy metals, gold salts, and Fowler's solution (a tonic rich in arsenic). Public and private agencies established tuberculosis dispensaries and sanatoriums. Some physicians prescribed mountain air, hiking, horseback riding, and carefully graduated work programs, whereas others warned that exercise placed too much stress on the lungs. Complete rest for the afflicted lung was produced by artificial pneumothorax or "collapse therapy." Collapsing the lung by injecting air into the pleural cavity was supposed to rest a tuberculous lung and allow it to heal. Artificial pneumothorax, which had been demonstrated in the 1890s, was widely practiced in the 1930s and 1940s. Injections were repeated at regular intervals until the lung healed or the patient died.

During the early decades of the twentieth century, tuberculosis remained the "captain of the men of death." The work of Koch and the scientific hygiene movement made it possible to believe that tuberculosis could be controlled, perhaps ultimately eradicated, by new medical techniques, institutions, administrative structures, and the authority of the state. However, twentieth-century campaigns against the disease emphasized individual responsibility while neglecting the deep-seated social and economic problems that forged close links between poverty and tuberculosis. Many physicians ignored the implications of Koch's work and minimized the role of the microbe and the contagiousness of the disease. Old ideas about the hereditary nature of the disease, or an innate predisposition, were not abandoned. The social and environmental factors responsible for the association between poverty and tuberculosis, such as malnutrition, crowding, lack of fresh air and sunlight, were neglected. Victims of the disease were isolated, shunned, and confined in sanatoriums in a manner reminiscent of the medieval leper.

The romantic notion of the tuberculosis sanatorium as a peaceful place on a "Magic Mountain" that offered rest, sunshine, nourishing food, and a healing atmosphere has been largely dispelled by further studies of the suffering endured by patients who experienced the isolation, rigidity, and degradation characteristic of many of these institutions. In the nineteenth and twentieth centuries, the sanatorium regimen evolved from a benign program of fresh air and rest to more rigid and medicalized programs involving strict prescriptions of graduated work, drug trials, and surgery. The criteria used to measure success were remarkably low, as indicated by claims of success for gold salts in which nine out of 42 patients died. Many patients were subjected to artificial pneumothorax, although, in some institutions, the mortality rate for this operation was about 50 percent. The analysis of such disappointing results convinced many investigators that it was impossible to find a specific chemotherapeutic agent for a disease as intractable and unpredictable as tuberculosis.

For complex reasons that are still the subject of heated debate, by the time effective antibiotics were available, tuberculosis, the "white plague," was already subsiding. All detailed studies of tuberculosis reveal that a significant decrease in tuberculosis mortality occurred before the introduction of specific antibiotic therapy in 1947. As in the case of leprosy, the history of tuberculosis, when considered in a broad social and global context, reminds us that the pattern of human suffering and death associated with a specific disease cannot be reduced to a description of its microbial agent. The tubercle bacillus did not, however, disappear.

Epidemiologists at the Fourth World Congress on tuberculosis (2002) warned that about two billion people were infected with tuberculosis and that the disease killed about two million people a year. About one thousand cases of tuberculosis were reported in New York City in 2002, but about 5 to 10 percent of New Yorkers tested positive for exposure to the disease. The machinery for dealing with tuberculosis had been essentially dismantled by the time tuberculosis became associated with AIDS and drug-resistant strains became common. Drug-resistant tuberculosis outbreaks were reported in the 1980s in New York City prisons and shelters. By 1991, 20 percent of those diagnosed with tuberculosis in New York City were resistant to the antibiotics commonly used to treat the disease (rifampin and isoniazid). Case fatality rates for drug-resistant tuberculosis were as high as 40 to 60 percent, which is essentially the same as that for untreated drug-susceptible tuberculosis. Epidemiologists estimated that, on a global basis, about three hundred thousand new cases of drug-resistant tuberculosis occurred each year, but reliable data were lacking for many poor countries with high rates of HIV/AIDS. Drug-resistant cases are more common in countries where patients have received inadequate treatment, a situation that favors the development of drug-resistant strains. In some countries, tuberculosis drugs are sold over the counter and often misused.

The successful introduction of penicillin during World War II led to hope that other antibiotic agents would be effective against tuberculosis. Unfortunately, drugs that were effective against experimental tuberculosis in laboratory animals were not necessarily useful in the treatment of the disease in humans. Reports that streptomycin, an antibiotic discovered by Selman A. Waksman (1888–1973) in 1943, was effective against tuberculosis in guinea pigs were soon followed by evidence of its efficacy in humans. The early, impure preparations of streptomycin, however, caused serious side effects, including deafness. In some trials, only 51 percent of the treated patients improved after six months of treatment. Eventually, *para*-aminosalicylic acid, isoniazid, rifampin, and other drugs were added to the antituberculosis arsenal. Alone and in various combinations, these chemotherapeutic agents transformed the management and treatment of tuberculosis patients and virtually emptied the sanatoriums. Efforts to evaluate the contribution antibiotics made to the decrease in the mortality rate for tuberculosis are complicated by the fact that BCG vaccine was widely adopted shortly before the introduction of streptomycin.

From the public health standpoint, even a partial course of treatment is useful in arresting an active tuberculosis infection and breaking the chain of transmission. A complete cure may, however, take many months. As in the case of leprosy, the long course of treatment is costly and creates ideal conditions for the proliferation of drug-resistant bacteria. Although tubercle bacilli grow slowly, they are remarkably persistent; bacilli have been cultured from surgical and autopsy specimens immersed in formalin solutions for many years. With proper treatment, however, the disease was entirely curable. By the 1960s, global eradication of tuberculosis was regarded as well within the technical possibilities of medical science. Nevertheless, for complex socioeconomic and political reasons, in the 1980s epidemiologists acknowledged that eradication was a very remote possibility. In the United States, for example, public health authorities detected localized increases in the incidence of tuberculosis in areas marked by poverty and HIV/AIDS. Drug-resistant tuberculosis, often associated with AIDS, highlights the vast chasm between what medical science and public health programs expected to achieve and the heavy toll taken by old and new epidemic diseases.

By the end of the nineteenth century, microbiology was a well-established discipline that had sprouted several specialized branches. Textbooks, journals, institutes, and courses in microbiology multiplied almost as rapidly as bacteria. In 1879, Pasteur's associate Émile Duclaux (1840–1904) established a course in microbiology at the Sorbonne. Koch introduced a course in medical microbiology at the University of Berlin in 1884. By the 1890s, even American medical schools and agricultural colleges were beginning to include bacteriology in their curricula. Medical microbiology was an important stimulus for the emerging acceptance of the laboratory-based curriculum that the 1910 Flexner Report on medical education in the United States and Canada presented as an absolute necessity.

While most physicians and surgeons learned to reconcile medical practice with the germ theory of disease, some continued to challenge germ theory well into the twentieth century. For example, Charles Creighton (1847–1927), British pathologist, epidemiologist, medical historian, and anti-Jennerian, argued that miasmata, climatological disturbances, and soil poisons were the most significant factors in the generation of epidemics. Although Creighton acknowledged the fact that bacteria were associated with some diseases, he did not accept them as causal agents. Many of those who rejected germ theory were actively involved in sanitary or hygienic reform movements, which had significant successes in improving the health of cities. In practice, an all-out attack on filth, contamination, and pollution may be even more effective in the long-range control of epidemic and endemic diseases than an attack on specific pathogens, because of the general improvements in hygienic conditions.

The indomitable Max von Pettenkofer (1818–1901), a man who had little sympathy for the germ theory of disease, established the first Institute of Hygiene. After seriously considering a career in acting,

Pettenkofer decided to study physiology, chemistry, and medicine. In 1843, he was awarded his medical degree at Munich. Four years later, he was appointed professor of medicinal chemistry, but in 1878, in honor of his pioneering work on hygiene and epidemiology he became Munich's first professor of hygiene. Pettenkofer believed that the science of hygiene would reveal the origin of infectious diseases and the most effective means of preventing them. His approach to medicine was sanitarian or what would now be called environmental medicine.

Rejecting the major conclusions drawn by Pasteur, Koch, and other germ hunters, Pettenkofer continued to argue that poisonous miasmata, soil conditions, and climatological disturbances were primarily responsible for the generation and dissemination of disease. For example, while minimizing the discovery of the microbe that causes cholera, Pettenkofer developed his own "ground-water theory" of the development of cholera-producing miasmata. On the basis of this theory, he led a very successful campaign for the improvement of Munich's sewage systems. As a consequence of these sanitary reforms, Munich enjoyed a significant reduction in the burden of intestinal diseases. Challenging Koch's claim that the causal agent of cholera was the so-called comma bacillus or cholera vibrio, in 1892, in the presence of unimpeachable witnesses, Pettenkofer swallowed a broth culture of cholera vibrios. Later, Pettenkofer confessed that he had experienced some intestinal discomfort, but he refused to diagnose this as cholera.

Improvements in water systems and sewers undertaken in response to cholera also diminished the threat of other water-borne diseases, such as typhoid fever. William Budd (1811–1880), author of the classic *Typhoid Fever; Its Nature, Mode of Spreading, and Prevention* (1873), demonstrated that water contaminated by the excrements of typhoid fever patients transmitted the disease from household to household. Victims of the disease may suffer from fever, rash, headaches, bloating, diarrhea, stupor, delirium, coma, or peritonitis and gastrointestinal hemorrhages. After *Salmonella typhi* was discovered in the 1880s, Robert Koch proposed practical means of preventing the spread of the disease. The isolation of "healthy carriers" became one of the most controversial aspects of the public health battle against enteric fevers.

Mary Mallon (1870?–1938), the woman who became known as "Typhoid Mary," has been called an icon of public health history. Mallon was an Irish immigrant who supported herself as a cook. Unfortunately, she was also an asymptomatic carrier of *S. typhi*. Her cooking led to the infection of 47 people and caused three deaths. Public health authorities were particularly concerned about the role of food-handlers in the transmission of disease. Some typhoid outbreaks were traced to carriers working at dairy farms, a discovery that added to demands for the pasteurization of milk. Mallon was identified as a carrier in 1907, after her employers became ill. New York City public health officials had her confined, but she was released in 1910 and warned against working as a cook. After a typhoid outbreak in 1915, officials discovered Mallon working as a cook at Sloane Maternity Hospital. She was confined again to North Brother Island where she died in 1938. Social historians have attributed Mallon's draconian treatment to gender, ethnicity, and class, rather than her bacteriological status.

Asiatic cholera was apparently unknown to Europeans until the nineteenth century when it escaped its ancestral home in India. European trade, commerce, travel, and military incursions presumably broke down regional barriers that had previously confined cholera to limited areas of India. The disease spread westward, becoming endemic in new areas, and generating major pandemics. Cholera was present in 75 countries and on all continents at the beginning of the twenty-first century.

Compared with pandemics of bubonic plague or influenza, cholera generally traveled slowly along major trade routes, until railroads and steamboats expedited the movements of goods, armies, and microbes. Although in terms of total mortality cholera was much less significant than tuberculosis and malaria, cholera became the most feared epidemic disease of the nineteenth century. The terror provoked by cholera played a major role in forcing many cities to deal with water purity and other fundamental public health projects.

The onset of symptoms was often sudden and violent, although some patients initially noticed intestinal discomfort, dizziness, and lassitude. Many cases began with severe vomiting and diarrhea, thirst, painful cramps, and so forth. The catastrophic loss of body fluids led to the characteristic "rice water stools" that reflected loss of bits of the intestinal lining. In a matter of hours, healthy adults could become as desiccated as ancient mummies. Debilitated survivors experienced muscle cramps, chills or fever, and profound weakness.

By the beginning of the twentieth century, Western Europe was essentially free of the disease, but cholera remained a serious public health problem in Russia, the Middle East, Africa, and Asia. Since World War I, cholera outbreaks in the most impoverished areas of the world have claimed the lives of 50 to 60 percent of its victims. Death occurs primarily from dehydration and its complications. Where intravenous infusion of liquids can be arranged, almost all patients recover, but treatment requires fairly sophisticated medical resources. Victims of severe dehydration cannot ordinarily be restored to normal by means of liquids taken by mouth, because water cannot be absorbed quickly enough to make up for such profound losses. However, where intravenous infusion is not available, oral administration of appropriate solutions of salts and glucose can reduce the mortality rate to about 5 percent. This simple and effective form of treatment provides a remarkable contrast to the methods advocated by many nineteenth-century physicians.

With estimates of mortality rates ranging from 30 percent to 80 percent, it is likely that many less serious diarrheal diseases were misdiagnosed as cholera and gave rise to miraculous "cures." Many doctors urged early and vigorous interventions at the first signs of intestinal disturbance. Treatments included bleeding, calomel, opium, laudanum, brandy, naphtha, valerian, phosphorous, and magnesium carbonate or castor oil as gentle laxatives. Warm baths, hot blankets, mustard and linseed poultices, bags of hot salt and bran, and friction and counter-irritants applied to the skin were thought to fight circulatory collapse and debility. Some doctors favored immersion in ice water, tobacco smoke enemas, and intravenous injections of salt water. Many patients rejected orthodox medicine and turned to Thomsonian herbal remedies, patent medicines, water cure doctors, and homeopaths. Hospital doctors who applied the "numerical method," that is, a statistical analysis of different treatments, began to realize the futility of their remedies. Faced with the threat of cholera outbreaks, public health officials warned that only common sense, fresh air, and personal and public cleanliness could ward off the disaster. In some cites, the threat of cholera provoked such unprecedented fits of cleanliness that residents discovered cobblestones emerging from traditionally filth-covered streets.

Physicians and public health officials engaged in endless debates about the nature and transmission of cholera. Florence Nightingale (1820–1910) argued that experience in India, where cholera was endemic, proved that the disease was not communicable from person to person. Doctors who examined the sick or performed autopsies rarely contracted the disease, because they washed their hands afterwards and did not eat in the sickroom. In impoverished households, all members of the family might have to eat in the sickroom and had little opportunity to wash.

The classic epidemiological study of cholera was conducted by the British physician John Snow (1813–1858). Snow argued that the cholera "poison" must be introduced into the alimentary canal via the mouth in food, water, and on contaminated fingers. Direct contact between the sick and new victims was not required, because the disease was transmitted by water contaminated with cholera "evacuations." Some aspects of the story of John Snow and the 1854 Broad Street cholera outbreak have assumed a mythic status in the history of public health, epidemiology, cartography, and medical geography. Snow published his theory that cholera was transmitted through contaminated drinking water in 1849 in a work entitled *On the Mode of Communication of Cholera*. A second edition of the book published in 1855 included new investigations and evidence.

The discovery of the cholera vibrio is generally associated with Robert Koch and his coworkers in the 1880s, although earlier studies had been carried out by the Italian histologist Filippo Pacini (1812–1883). Bacteriologists found the cholera vibrio in dirty linens and in water used for drinking, bathing, and washing clothes. After Koch isolated the cholera vibrio, Elie Mechnikoff confidently predicted that "the fight against cholera will soon result in relegating this disease to the archives of history." Unfortunately, Mechnikoff was too optimistic.

The sanitary reforms pioneered in Europe and America have essentially precluded the possibility of major, sustained epidemics of cholera in the wealthy, industrialized nations. Cholera has not disappeared; it is only kept in check by modern sanitary control of water and sewage. Sporadic cases have appeared along the Gulf Coast in Texas and Louisiana, but because Americans have become so unfamiliar with cholera, the disease may be mistakenly diagnosed as food poisoning. There are many different strains of cholera vibrios and confusion about the virulence of different strains. Cholera vibrios persist in oceans and brackish water, where they are widely associated with shellfish, crustaceans, and zooplankton. Cholera vibrios have been found in the raw sewage of various towns in Louisiana, and cases of cholera have been traced to the ingestion of raw oysters and steamed crabs. Global climate change might affect the distribution of the cholera vibrio. Changes in ocean temperature affect various blooms of plankton, and blooms precede cholera outbreaks.

Cholera remains a danger in many parts of the world. The true extent of the problem is probably unknown because governments prefer to list deaths from cholera as food poisoning, gastroenteritis, intestinal flu, or other euphemisms for "diarrheal diseases." In the 1990s, significant outbreaks occurred in South America, primarily in poor, rural areas in Peru. Some cases, however, were associated with foods served in airplanes, proving again that any disease anywhere is just a plane ride away from any other point on the globe.

Despite detailed scientific knowledge about the cholera vibrio, its genome, and its toxin, at the end of the twentieth century the disease remained a threat to hundreds of thousands of people in the developing world. As many as three hundred thousand people in developing countries contract cholera every year. In 2002, scientists discovered that cholera vibrios appear to become more infectious as they pass through the human intestinal tract, which complicates attempts to develop a vaccine based on laboratory cultures. Cholera bacteria isolated from the stool of patients in Bangladesh after an epidemic were 10 to 100 times more infectious than laboratory strains when injected into mice.

Despite chlorination, the water available in many of the world's overpopulated cities is probably worse than that studied by John Snow. Microbial contaminants found in water samples taken in Karachi, the capital of Pakistan, in 2004, for example, included campylobacter, *E. coli*, shigella, giardia, rotovirus, hepatitis A, and hepatitis E. In the 1950s, the population of Karachi was about 435,000; in 2002 there were about 14 million residents.

If Pettenkofer could have investigated the status of water-borne diseases in much of the world today, he would claim vindication of the sanitarian doctrine that contamination, poverty, and the lack of hygienic conditions were the most significant factors in generating and disseminating epidemic disease. Nevertheless, despite the ostensible conflict between Pettenkofer's miasmatic theory and Koch's germ theory, both physicians were dedicated to the idea that the scientific study of hygiene would have a great and beneficial impact on the battle against infectious diseases. However, it was the work of Pasteur, Koch, and their disciples, grounded in microbiology, or the "gospel of the germ" that generated interest in public and private hygiene and sanitary reform. Some historians have argued that germ theory and medical microbiology deflected attention from the real socioeconomic roots of disease and reinforced industrial capitalism, racism, and moralistic victim blaming. Certainly, poverty, overcrowding, poor sanitation, and lack of access to medical care are associated with the public and private burden of disease. Microbiologists and epidemiologists note, however, that specific microbes are still necessary factors in the development of specific diseases.

## INVISIBLE MICROBES AND VIROLOGY

Long before scientists could define the nature of specific viruses, viral diseases—smallpox and rabies—had provided the most significant and dramatic examples of the potential of preventive inoculations. Because the meaning of the Latin word *virus* has undergone many changes in two millennia of usage, the modern reader is likely to be confused upon finding the term in ancient texts. The first and most general meaning of virus was slime, presumably unpleasant, but not necessarily dangerous. However, Latin authors increasingly used the term with the implication of poison or venom, something menacing to health, or a mysterious, unknown infectious agent. Thus, both the Roman writer Celsus (ca. 14-37) and Louis Pasteur could speak of the virus of rabies.

Medieval scholars generally used virus as a synonym for poison. In medical treatises of the sixteenth and seventeenth centuries, translators usually replaced the Latin term virus with the English word venom. Seventeenth-century writers referred to a *virus pestiferum* or *virus pestilens* in discussing infectious diseases. Eighteenth-century medical writers applied the term virus to the contagion that transmitted an infectious disease, as in Edward Jenner's discussion of the "cow-pox virus" in the pustular lymph that transmitted the disease. For medical writers in the early nineteenth century, virus stood for the obscure causative principles of infectious diseases. The vagueness of the term made it particularly attractive.

After the establishment of germ theory in the late nineteenth century, virus was used in the general sense of "an agent with infectious properties." When submicroscopic filterable infectious agents were discovered in the 1890s, the term virus was applied to these mysterious entities. Even if the causative agent for an infectious disease had not been identified, Pasteur argued that "Every virus is a microbe." Speculating about the still unknown causes of various infectious diseases, Koch suggested that pathogenic organisms different from bacteria might be discovered. The exceptional agents that were known at the time were larger than bacteria, most notably the protozoan that causes malaria, but there was no theoretical reason to rule out the existence of smaller parasites. Among microbiologists, however, respect for Koch's postulates might have inhibited virology, as well as protozoology, because it was virtually impossible to culture such entities in artificial media. Koch himself did not let bacteriological dogma inhibit his work on tropical medicine even where the microbes could not be cultured in the laboratory.

By the end of the nineteenth century, the techniques of microbiology were sufficiently advanced for scientists to state, with a high degree of confidence that certain diseases were caused by specific bacteria or protozoa. However, the infectious agents of some diseases refused to be isolated by conventional techniques. Eventually, exotic, but visible, pathogens (rickettsias, chlamydias, mycoplasmas, and brucellas) joined the classical fungi, bacteria, and protozoa. Because some of the exotic pathogens had complicated life cycles and were difficult to culture in vitro, it seemed possible that members of these groups might be the undiscovered agents of various infectious diseases.

Therefore, in the early twentieth century, the term virus was generally restricted to the class of "filterable-invisible" microbes. Such microbes were defined operationally in terms of their ability to pass through filters that trapped bacteria and their ability to remain invisible to the light microscope. The criterion of filterability was the outcome of work conducted by Pasteur's associate Charles Chamberland (1851–1908), who discovered that a porous porcelain vase could be used to separate visible microorganisms from their culture medium. This technique could be used in the laboratory to prepare bacteria-free liquids and in the home to prepare pure drinking water. Chamberland was also instrumental in the development of the autoclave, a device for sterilizing materials by means of steam heat under pressure. However, technique-based criteria provided little insight into the genetic and biochemical nature of viruses. As scientists closed in on the invisible-filterable-viruses, they discovered that their operational criteria were not necessarily linked. The failure of infectious agents to grow in vitro was not a satisfactory criterion either, because scientists could not exclude the possibility that exotic microbes might need special media and growth conditions. A more radical explanation for the failure to identify the causative agents of some apparently infectious diseases was that some microbes might be obligate parasites of living organisms that could not be cultured in vitro on any cell-free culture medium.

Although for the sake of human health, it would have been better if viruses had totally destroyed all tobacco plants, progress in virology owes a great deal to this pernicious product of the New World, because it was the tobacco mosaic virus (TMV) that established Adolf Eduard Mayer, Martinus Beijerinck, and Dimitri Ivanovski as the founders of virology. The study of plant virology can be traced to 1886 when Adolf Eduard Mayer (1843–1942) discovered that tobacco mosaic disease (TMD) could be transmitted to healthy plants by inoculating them with extracts of sap from the leaves of diseased plants. Unable to culture a tobacco mosaic disease microbe on artificial media, Mayer filtered the sap and demonstrated that the filtrate was still infectious. Mayer was certain that his microbe must be a very unusual bacterium. In 1892, Dimitri Iosifovitch Ivanovski (1864–1920) demonstrated that the infectious agent for tobacco mosaic disease could pass through the finest filters available, but all attempts to isolate or culture the "tobacco microbe" were failures.

Apparently unaware of Ivanovski's work, Martinus Willem Beijerinck (1851–1931) also reported that a filterable agent caused TMD. Thinking about the way in which a small quantity of filtered plant sap transmitted the disease to a large series of plants, Beijerinck concluded that TMD must be caused by a *contagium vivum fluidum* that could pass through filters and reproduce within the living plant tissues. On the basis of reports in the botanical literature, Beijerinck thought soluble germs could cause many other plant diseases.

Similar observations were made by Friedrich Loeffler (1862–1915) and Paul Frosch (1860–1928) in their studies of foot-and-mouth disease (FMD), the first example of a filterable virus disease of animals. Attempts to culture bacteria from lesions in the mouths and udders of sick animals were unsuccessful. Even after passage through a Chamberland filter, however, the apparently bacteria-free fluid from FMD lesions could transmit the disease to cattle and pigs. Filtered fluids from these animals could transmit the disease to other experimental animals. Their experiments and calculations suggested that only a living agent, capable of reproducing itself could continue to cause the disease after passage through a series of animals. Loeffler and Frosch suggested that other infectious diseases, such as smallpox, cowpox, and cattle plague, might be caused by similar filterable microbes. Nevertheless, they continued to think of the infectious agent as a very small and unusual microbe rather than a fundamentally different entity.

Scientists later demonstrated that FMD is a highly infectious, airborne viral disease that attacks cloven-hoofed livestock animals like cows, sheep, goats, and pigs. The FMD virus is a member of the picornavirus family, which includes many important human pathogens, such as poliovirus, hepatitis A virus, and rhinovirus. Picornaviruses are characterized by a small RNA genome. FMD is generally not regarded as a threat to humans who consume meat or pasteurized milk from affected animals, but people in close contact with infected animals can acquire the disease. In the 1830s scientists apparently infected themselves with FMD by inoculation and by drinking milk from infected cows. Proven cases of FMD in humans have occurred in several countries in Europe, Africa, and South America. Nevertheless, human cases appear to be extremely rare, even when large numbers of farm animals are affected.

Foot-and-mouth disease was introduced into the Americas in 1870. The disease was soon reported in parts of the United States, Argentina, Chile, Uruguay, Brazil, Bolivia, Paraguay, and Peru. Known outbreaks of FMD occurred in the United States from the 1870s to the 1920s, from New England to California. In the 1950s, the disease was reported in Venezuela, Colombia, Ecuador, and Canada. A Pan-American Foot-and-Mouth Disease Center was established in 1951. Using information gathered from participating countries, the Center developed plans for FMD eradication. By 2000, Chile, Uruguay, Argentina, Paraguay, and parts of Brazil were declared free of FMD. Although many authorities assumed that FMD had been virtually eradicated from Western Europe, a major epidemic in 2001, the first since 1967, costs millions of dollars and resulted in the destruction of more than 1 million animals in the United Kingdom alone. Vaccination is used in countries where the disease is still endemic, but because vaccinated animals test positive for FMD antibodies, countries where vaccination is practiced cannot call their livestock "disease-free" and they cannot export to other nations. British scientists think meat from animals with FMD was illegally brought into England and fed to pigs.

In 1915, Frederick William Twort (1877–1950) discovered that even bacteria could fall victim to diseases caused by invisible viruses. As Jonathan Swift (1667–1745) had suggested in a satirical poem on the microscope, naturalists might use the instrument to prove that fleas were preyed on by smaller fleas that were, in turn, attacked by still smaller fleas. While trying to grow viruses in artificial medium, Twort noted that colonies of certain bacteria growing on agar sometimes became glassy and transparent. If pure colonies of this micrococcus were touched by a tiny portion of material from the glassy colonies, they too became transparent. Like the infectious agent of many mysterious plant and animal diseases, these so-called Twort particles were filterable.

World War I interrupted Twort's work on this problem and his paper had little immediate impact on microbiology. Twort later became obsessed with speculative work on the possibility that bacteria evolved from viruses that had developed from even more primitive forms.

While working on the dysentery bacillus at the Pasteur Institute, Félix d'Hérelle (1873–1949) also discovered the existence of bacterial viruses. In 1917, he published his observations on "An invisible microbe that is antagonistic to the dysentery bacillus." He never acknowledged that Twort, who published two years earlier, had discovered the same phenomenon. Because the invisible microbe could not grow on laboratory media or heat-killed bacilli, but grew well in a suspension of washed bacteria in a simple salt solution, d'Hérelle concluded that the anti-dysentery microbe was an *obligate bacteriophage*, that is, an eater of bacteria. Bacterial viruses were sometimes called Twort–d'Hérelle particles. The invisible microbe was found in stool samples of patients recovering from bacillary dysentery. When an active filtrate was added to a culture of Shiga bacilli, bacterial growth soon ceased and bacterial death and lysis (dissolution) followed. A trace of the lysate produced the same effect on a fresh Shiga culture. More than 50 such transfers gave the same results, indicating that a living agent was responsible for bacterial lysis.

Speculating on the general implications of the phenomenon he had discovered, d'Hérelle predicted that bacteriophages would be found for other pathogenic bacteria. Although the natural parasitism of the invisible microbe seemed species specific, d'Hérelle believed that laboratory manipulations could transform bacteriophages into "microbes of immunity" with activity against human pathogens. d'Hérelle suggested that phages were involved in natural recovery and the end of epidemics. American novelist Sinclair Lewis (1885–1951), in collaboration with medical writer and microbiologist Paul de Kruif (1890–1971), explored this idea in *Arrowsmith* (1925). Although experimental tests of "phage therapy" were generally abandoned when antibiotics appeared as "miracle drugs," the method has been used in the former Soviet Union, and certain traditional Indian cures may employ naturally occurring bacteriophages. In 1896, for example, a Western scientist reported that water from the Ganges River in India, traditionally known for its curative properties, was lethal to the cholera vibrio.

The hope that bacteriophages could be trained in the laboratory to serve as weapons in the war on bacteria was not realized in the twentieth century, but researchers continue to explore the possibility that viruses might be recruited to attack drug-resistant bacteria. An estimated 90,000 Americans died in 2000 of hospital-acquired infections caused by antibiotic-resistant bacteria. Some scientists think that phages that prey on the tubercle bacillus might provide useful insights into the microbe's pathogenicity, as well as new methods of diagnosis and drug screening. Studies of the genomes of phages that attack tubercle bacteria suggest genetic exchanges between phages and their bacterial hosts. Many researchers are skeptical about this approach, primarily because of possible adverse effects caused by introducing a self-replicating virus into a patient's bloodstream. Some drug companies have, however, explored the use of genetic engineering to control potentially useful "therapeutic phages" that could be given orally or as topical treatments.

In order to find a virus that could kill a specific bacterial pathogen, researchers had to use a mixture of viruses. Critics warn that phage preparations might be contaminated with unknown strains. Even if highly purified preparations are used, dangerous strains of viruses might arise through recombination or mutation. Moreover, replicating viruses might also acquire and express genes for toxins or learn how to attack the cells of the patient instead of the bacterial target. Some researchers hope that genetic engineering can be used to produce very specific viruses and, therefore, reduce the risks. Others argue that naturally occurring viruses—already engineered by Mother Nature—are likely to be superior to, as well as less costly to produce, than modified viruses. One approach is to use phages to kill *Salmonella* and *Listeria*, often associated with food poisoning, during food preparation.

In a practical, rather than philosophical sense, many arguments about the nature of viruses faded from the picture as researchers in the 1930s and 1940s examined them with new biochemical techniques. By the 1940s, biochemists were discovering just how complicated biological macromolecules could be. Advances in biochemistry supported the concept of the virus as a complex entity on the borderline between cells, genes, and molecules. Viruses could, therefore, be described as particles composed of a protein overcoat and an inner core of nucleic acid that is capable of entering a host cell and taking over its metabolic apparatus. As to just what viruses are and where they fit into the scheme of things among plants and animals, microbes and macromolecules, living and nonliving, French microbiologist André Lwoff's (1902–1994) paraphrase of a famous line by Gertrude Stein seems the most appropriate answer: "Viruses should be considered viruses because viruses are viruses."

Stories about the Human Genome Project are commonly published in the popular press and newspapers. In contrast, the sequencing of microbial genomes generates little publicity. Microbial genomics may have many practical applications for better vaccines, safer fermented foods and beverages, biodefenses, cleaner environment, and better health. Although the complete genomes of some one hundred microbes were sequenced by 2003, scientists note that we really know very little about the microbial world.

Research on diseases attributed to slow viruses, viroids, and prions suggests that other invisible, mysterious, and perhaps menacing creatures may well exist in the submicroscopic world. Unlike viruses, viroids appear to be pathogens consisting of small, single-stranded RNA molecules without a protein coat. Between 1971, when Theodor O. Diener (1921–) discovered that the infectious agent responsible for potato spindle tuber disease was a novel pathogen consisting of naked RNA, and 2001, about 30 viroid species and hundreds of variants had been studied. Viroid diseases affect many plants, from avocadoes to coconuts, but viroids may also be involved in tumor formation and other diseases of animals. Despite the excitement generated by studies of viroids and other small RNAs, many questions remain about how viroids replicate, move from cell to cell, and cause disease. Viroids have been called evolutionary fossils and relics of pre-cellular evolution, but their discovery has stimulated research into interaction between foreign RNA molecules and human diseases.

Viroids have been called "naked intruders," but because they contain nucleic acid, they still seemed to fit into the fundamental framework, or Central Dogma, of molecular biology, that is, the flow of genetic information from nucleic acids to proteins. Prions, the most bizarre of all the infectious agents discovered in the twentieth century, challenge the Central Dogma, as well as the idea that "viruses are viruses," at least in the case of disorders that were originally attributed to "slow viruses." In 1982, Stanley B. Prusiner (1942–) coined the term prion, which stood for "proteinaceous infectious particle." The diseases attributed to prions are known as transmissible spongiform encephalopathies (TSE), that is, degenerative diseases of the central nervous system. Prion diseases of animals include scrapie in sheep and goats, transmissible mink encephalopathy, chronic wasting disease of mule deer and elk, feline spongiform encephalopathy, and bovine spongiform encephalopathy (BSE, commonly known as mad cow disease). Human diseases attributed to prions include Creutzfeldt–Jakob Disease (CJD) and a new variant (vCJD) that appears to be related to BSE, Fatal Familial Insomnia, Gerstmann–Sräussler–Scheinker syndrome, and kuru.

The idea that some neurological degenerative diseases might be caused by a novel infectious agent was suggested by Carleton Gajdusek's (1923–) studies of kuru, a disease found only among the Fore people of New Guinea. Based on field studies, Gajdusek came to the conclusion that kuru was transmitted by mourning rituals during which women and children handled and ate the brains of deceased relatives. After cannibalism was outlawed, the incidence of the disease decreased. Using brain tissue from victims of kuru, Gajdusek and his associates were able to transmit the disease to chimpanzees. Symptoms did not appear, however, until about two years after inoculation. Laboratory experiments by Gajdusek and others suggested that kuru, scrapie, and CJD might be caused by similar infectious agents. Gajdusek, who was awarded a Nobel

Prize in 1976, thought that the infectious agent must be an unconventional "slow virus."

Many aspects of the history of kuru seem relevant to the still unfolding story of BSE and vCJD. Scrapie, an old Scottish name for a disease of sheep and goats, has been known since the eighteenth century, but until the 1980s when BSE first appeared in England, there was no evidence of transmission to cows or humans. Scientists believe the BSE epidemic began when a nutritional supplement containing the rendered remains of sheep and cows was added to cattle feed. By essentially transforming domesticated herbivores into carnivores, or even cannibals like the Fore victims of kuru, the new dietary regimen presumably created an unprecedented opportunity for scrapie agents to infect cattle. As the mad cow epidemic reached its peak in 1992, millions of cattle were destroyed, but by then contaminated meat products had probably entered the food chain. The World Health Organization warned in 2003 that many countries, particularly in Eastern Europe and Southeast Asia, were at risk for mad cow disease, even though the worst appeared to be over in Britain. Mad cow disease appeared in areas in Europe, Southeast Asia, Canada, North Africa, and the United States that used contaminated feed.

Not all prion infections can be transmitted from one species to another, but the new variant of CJD, designated vCJD, has been attributed to the consumption of beef from animals with BSE. Much about the transmission of prion diseases remains obscure, as demonstrated by the relatively small number of human cases that occurred in Great Britain, compared to the millions of people who must have eaten contaminated meat. The panic caused by mad cow disease has raised awareness of all the prion diseases. Perhaps, the emergence of new diseases, such as BSE and vCJD, might be related to the ways in which human beings have affected the environment, especially through global exchanges of previously isolated plants, animals, and infectious agents.

In 1972, after one of his patients died of CJD, Stanley Prusiner began studying the literature that linked CJD to kuru and scrapie. Creutzfeldt–Jakob Disease appears to strike sporadically, affecting about one in one million people over the age of 60 years throughout the world. When Prusiner isolated the scrapie agent from the brains of diseased hamsters, he was surprised to find that it apparently consisted of a specific protein. All previously known infectious agents, even the smallest viruses, contained genetic material in the form of nucleic acids, either DNA or RNA. Prusiner's "protein only hypothesis" was initially regarded as heresy, but within a few years, genes that encoded prion proteins were found in all animals tested, including humans.

Despite continuing skepticism and controversy, by the early 1990s many scientists had accepted Prusiner's prion hypothesis. In 1997, Prusiner was awarded the Nobel Prize in Physiology or Medicine for discovering prions and establishing a new genre of disease-causing agents. According to Prusiner's theory, prion proteins can exist in two distinct conformations, one of which is quite harmless. Prion proteins can also exist in altered conformations that act as rogue proteins or "evil twins." In the altered conformation, prion proteins are apparently capable of inducing their benign counterparts to undergo the same transformation. As the transformed proteins accumulate and aggregate, they form thread-like structures that ultimately destroy nerve cells and result in fatal brain diseases. Despite many uncertainties about the way in which prions cause brain disease, Prusiner suggests that understanding the three-dimensional structure of prion proteins might lead to useful therapeutic interventions. Moreover, the success of the prion hypothesis in explaining infectious, heredity, and sporadic forms of scrapie-like diseases suggests that similar mechanisms might play a role in other disorders, including Alzheimer's disease, Parkinson's disease, and amyotrophic lateral sclerosis.

In 1972, Sir Frank Macfarlane Burnet, the Australian virologist who shared the Nobel Prize with Peter Medawar in 1960, famously declared that "the most likely forecast about the future of infectious disease is that it will be very dull." Since the 1960s, many physicians and health policy analysts shared the assumption that microbial diseases could be essentially ignored because of the power of antibiotics, vaccines, and other therapeutic agents. By the end of the century, it was clear that predictions about the demise of infectious disease had been grossly exaggerated. Infectious organisms—known and previously unknown—continued to evolve and find ways to exploit new opportunities. By the end of the twentieth century, approximately five hundred million illnesses and six million deaths each year were caused by AIDS, tuberculosis, and malaria. One out of every two deaths in developing countries is due to infectious diseases, but globalization and rapid transportation link all parts of the world.

The "catalog" of human diseases is likely to grow as new diseases appear and old categories, such as "fevers" or "fevers of unknown origin," are re-examined and broken down into specific "new" diseases. The appearance of West Nile virus in New York City in 1999 and its subsequent spread into other states demonstrated how easily pathogens could establish themselves in new regions. Previously unknown diseases, such as AIDS, Legionnaires' disease, Lyme disease, mad cow disease, Ebola fever, Rift Valley fever, SARS, avian influenza, monkey pox, Nipah virus, Lyssavirus, Chandipura virus, and so forth, have appeared and old diseases have spread to new areas while many pathogens have become antibiotic-resistant. For example, antibiotic-resistant strains of *Staphylococcus aureus* have caused fatal pneumonias, heart infections, toxic shock syndrome, and necrotizing fasciitis (flesh-eating bacteria).

Scientists have identified many factors that may affect the distribution and emergence of infectious diseases, including environmental factors, population growth and age distribution, migration, war, international travel and commerce, technological and industrial factors, and national and international commitment to disease control and public health measures. Climate changes produced by global warming might have significant consequences for the global distribution of diseases, especially water-borne diseases and diseases transmitted by mosquitoes. Although the chronic, degenerative diseases of old age have become the major concern of the wealthy, industrialized countries, in much of the world, poverty and the lack of basic sanitary facilities contribute to the continuing burden of infectious diseases. According to the United Nations, at the beginning of the twenty-first century more than one billion people lack clean drinking water and more than two million people die each year from illnesses associated with dirty water and poor sanitation.

## SUGGESTED READINGS

Baldwin, P. (1999). *Contagion and the State in Europe, 1830–1930.* New York: Cambridge University Press.

Barry, J. M. (2004). *The Great Influenza: The Epic Story of the Deadliest Plague in History.* New York: Penguin.

Bashford, A., and Hooker, C, eds. (2001). *Contagion: Historical and Cultural Studies.* New York: Routledge.

Bates, B. (1992). *Bargaining for Life: A Social History of Tuberculosis, 1876–1938.* Philadelphia, PA: University of Pennsylvania Press.

Brock, T. D., ed. (1999). *Milestones in Microbiology.* Washington, DC: ASM Press.

Brock, T. D. (1988). *Robert Koch. A Life in Medicine and Bacteriology.* Madison, WI: Science Tech.

Bullough, B., and Rosen, G. (1992). *Preventive Medicine in the United States, 1900–1990: Trends and Interpretations.* Canton, MA: Science History Publications.

Conrad, L. I., and Wujastyk, D., eds. (2000). *Contagion: Perspectives from Premodern Societies.* Brookfield, VT: Ashgate.

Crosby, A. W. (2003). *America's Forgotten Pandemic: The Influenza of 1918.* New York: Cambridge University Press.

Debré, P. (2000). *Louis Pasteur.* Baltimore, MD: Johns Hopkins University Press.

Dormandy, T. (1999). *The White Death: A History of Tuberculosis.* New York: New York University Press.

Dubos, R., and Dubos, J. (1987). *The White Plague. Tuberculosis, Man, and Society*. New Brunswick, NJ: Rutgers University Press.

Duffy, J. (1990). *The Sanitarians: A History of American Public Health*. Urbana, IL: University of Illinois Press.

Farmer, P. (1999). *Infections and Inequalities. The Modern Plagues*. Berkeley, CA: University of California Press.

Fenner, F., and Gibbs, A., eds. (1988). *A History of Virology*. Basel: Karger.

Garrett, L. (1994). *The Coming Plague; Newly Emerging Diseases in a World Out of Balance*. New York: Farrar, Straus and Giroux.

Garrett, L. (2000). *Betrayal of Trust: The Collapse of Global Public Health*. New York: Hyperion.

Geison, G. L. (1995). *The Private Science of Louis Pasteur*. Princeton, NJ: Princeton University Press.

Grafe, A. (1991). *A History of Experimental Virology*. Berlin: Springer-Verlag.

Guillemin, J. (1999). *Anthrax: The Investigation of a Deadly Outbreak*. Berkeley, CA: University of California Press.

Hammonds, E. M. (1999). *Childhood's Deadly Scourge: The Campaign to Control Diphtheria in New York City, 1880–1930*. Baltimore, MD: Johns Hopkins University Press.

Hays, J. N. (1998). *The Burdens of Disease: Epidemics and Human Response in Western History*. New Brunswick, NJ: Rutgers University Press.

Hughs, S. S. (1977). *The Virus: A History of the Concept*. New York: Science History Publications.

Jarcho, S. (2000). *The Concept of Contagion in Medicine, Literature, and Religion*. Malabar, FL: Krieger.

Kiple, K. F., ed. (1993). *The Cambridge World History of Human Disease*. Cambridge: Cambridge University Press.

Laporte, D. (2002). *History of Shit*. Cambridge, MA: MIT Press.

Latour, B. (1988). *The Pasteurization of France*. Cambridge, MA: Harvard University Press.

Leavitt, J. W. (1996). *Typhoid Mary: Captive to the Public's Health*. Boston, MA: Beacon Press.

Lechevalier, H. A., and Solotorovsky, M. (1974). *Three Centuries of Microbiology*. New York: Dover.

Lederberg, J., Shope, R. E., and Oaks, S. C. Jr., eds. (1992). *Emerging Infections: Microbial Threats to Health in the United States*. Washington, DC: National Academy Press.

Lederberg, J., ed. (1999). *Biological Weapons: Limiting the Threat*. Cambridge, MA: MIT Press.

Parascandola, J., ed. (1980). *The History of Antibiotics: A Symposium*. Madison, WI: American Institute of the History of Pharmacy.

Porter, D. (1999). *Health, Civilization, and the State: A History of Public Health from Ancient to Modern Times*. New York: Routledge.

Prusiner, S. B. (1999). *Prion Biology and Diseases.* Cold Spring Harbor, NY: Cold Spring Harbor Laboratory Press.

Rabenau, H. F., Cinatl, J., and Doerr, H. W., eds. (2001). *Prions: A Challenge for Science, Medicine and the Public Health System.* New York: Karger.

Riley, J. C. (2001). *Rising Life Expectancy: A Global History.* New York: Cambridge University Press.

Rosner, D., ed. (1995). *Hives of Sickness. Public Health and Epidemics in New York City.* New Brunswick, NJ: Rutgers University Press.

Schwartz, M. (2003). *How the Cows Turned Mad.* Berkeley, CA: University of California Press.

Silverstein, A. M. (1981). *Pure Politics and Impure Science: The Swine Flu Affair.* Baltimore, MD: Johns Hopkins University Press.

Summers, W. C. (1999). *Félix d'Hérelle and the Origins of Molecular Biology.* New Haven, CT: Yale University Press.

Tomes, N. (1998). *The Gospel of Germs: Men, Women, and the Microbe in American Life.* Cambridge, MA: Harvard University Press.

Watts, S. (1998). *Epidemics and History: Disease, Power and Imperialism.* New Haven, CT: Yale University Press.

Young, J. H. (1989). *Pure Food: Securing the Federal Food and Drugs Act of 1906.* Princeton, NJ: Princeton University Press.

# 14

# Diagnostics and Therapeutics

For many hundreds of years, medical theory, practice, and even therapies changed so little that Hippocrates and Galen might easily have rejoined the community of learned physicians. But the most knowledgeable physician of the 1880s would be completely mystified by the diagnostic and therapeutic techniques of medicine today, as well as its scientific, institutional, educational, economic, and ethical components. Nevertheless, it could be argued that the conceptual framework within which physicians are educated and within which they practice today belongs to the era of Pasteur and Koch. A century of profound change established the fundamental concept that health and disease can be explained in terms of the biomedical sciences.

Therapeutic theory and practice changed profoundly in the nineteenth century. Since the time of Hippocrates, doctors and patients expected therapy to alter symptoms and visibly remove bad humors or secretions. Although in retrospect, the tendency of orthodox doctors to "bleed, purge, and clyster" seems an undifferentiated approach to therapy, doctors argued that treatment was based on the specific characteristics and the environment peculiar to each patient, such as age, sex, race, occupation, diet, family, climate, seasonal factors, and so forth. Wise and experienced physicians treated the patient, not the disease. Physicians warned their students that they must not prescribe for the name of the disease, but for patient and place. Physicians typically thought of disease in terms of systemic imbalance. Therapy, therefore, was a rational attempt to restore the natural balance of the patient, usually by "depleting" treatments, such as bleeding, cupping, purging, and starvation. Given the system of beliefs, such remedies obviously were "effective"—that is, a feverish, excited patient was likely to become more calm after bleeding and vomiting. By the 1850s, physicians were beginning to believe that most diseases suffered by their patients were debilitating rather than overstimulating. Therefore, restoring a natural balance required therapeutic stimulation instead of depletion. Although the rational for therapeutic interventions has changed throughout history, and varies in different cultures, as William Osler famously declared: "The desire to take medicine is perhaps the greatest feature which distinguishes men from animals." Osler exhibited a healthy skepticism about therapeutics and, rather than succumb to the therapeutic imperative, he was willing to say in his textbook: "No known treatment" or "Medicinal treatment is of little avail."

By the end of the nineteenth century, however, physicians were promoting therapeutic strategies based on experimental science. Physicians were learning to diagnose disease by means of allegedly objective techniques, rather than relying primarily on the patient's account of symptoms. As "scientific practitioners," physicians increasingly focused on specific diseases while minimizing the differences among patients. The new therapeutic rationalization called for treatment to be specific to the disease. "Experimental therapeutics," or "physiological therapeutics" promised that the methods pursued in the laboratory would explain the basic physiological principles of health, disease, and the action of remedies. When therapeutics joined the basic sciences, instead of merely treating symptoms, physicians would prescribe remedies specific to the pathological process. But optimism about a new era of "scientific therapeutics" developed before laboratory science had actually made any substantive contributions to therapeutics. The promise of new scientific therapies did not immediately provide cures, but it probably helped doctors question and abandon older, sometimes dangerous remedies. Truly novel therapeutic strategies, such as serum therapy, did not emerge from the laboratory until the 1890s. One hundred years later, biotechnology and genetic engineering firms were making similar promises of future miracle drugs and breakthroughs.

If we look at the history of medicine from the point of view of the diseased and distressed individual, it seems likely that in terms of dealing with the patient's suffering, hope, despair, expectations, and tendency to disobey medical orders and resort to self-medication, Hippocrates and Galen might well have valuable advice for the modern physician. Indeed, their emphasis on the prevention of disease, the individuality of the patient, the interplay between patients and their environment, the notion of treating the patient as a whole, and the role of the physician in prescribing a life-long, health-promoting regimen would enjoy a powerful resonance with public hopes and expectations today.

By the beginning of the twentieth century, medical microbiology made it possible to identify the cause and means of transmission of many infectious diseases, but it had little impact on therapeutics. As for surgery, if asepsis and antisepsis failed, surgeons were as helpless against infection as their medieval counterparts. The golden age of microbiology was a time of great excitement with respect to the science of medicine, but from the point of view of the sick, naming the causative agent of their disease was not as important as having a remedy. The major public health benefit of germ theory was the guidance it provided in dealing with the threat of waterborne diseases like typhoid fever and cholera through improved sanitation and rational public health measures, such as the purification of drinking water, proper sewer systems, food inspection, and pasteurization. Respiratory diseases, like tuberculosis and diphtheria, however, presented a different set of problems. While public health authorities could rationalize the need for compulsory measures, such as vaccination, isolation of the sick, and the identification of healthy carriers of infectious diseases, such measures conflicted with cherished concepts of individual liberties and the right to privacy.

## THE ART AND SCIENCE OF DIAGNOSIS

The triumphs of medical microbiology tend to overshadow another important aspect of nineteenth-century medicine that grew out of what we might think of as the unhappy intersection between clinical medicine practiced at the patient's bedside and pathological investigations conducted in the autopsy room. Achieving a more precise understanding of the nature and seats of disease within the dead body was eventually coupled with more precise diagnosis of disease in living patients. Symptoms were correlated with internal localized lesions, but, until the development of instruments such as the stethoscope, the lesions could only be detected at the postmortem.

The gradual development and recent enthusiastic reception of the technological aids used in the diagnosis of disease represent remarkable aspects of the evolution of medical practice over the course of the last two hundred years. Beyond their obvious role in transforming the art of diagnosis, medical instruments have profoundly affected the relationship between patient and physician, the education and practical training of physicians, the demarcation between areas of medical specialization, the locus of medical practice, and even the financial structure of medical care and treatment. From the time of Hippocrates until well into the nineteenth century, the average physician relied on essentially subjective information, such as the patient's own account of the course of illness and the physician's observations of notable signs and symptoms. Which signs and symptoms were considered notable was determined by prevailing medical philosophy, tempered by the experience of the individual physician. In general, physical examinations that involving touching the patient were extremely limited, except for some attention to the quality of the pulse. Under these circumstances, the physician could diagnose and prescribe by letter without even seeing the patient. Indeed, the fee for advising the patient by letter was often higher than that for an office visit.

During the nineteenth century, even the average physician was being encouraged to follow the path marked out by the great clinicians and morbid anatomists of the previous century towards a more active role in obtaining objective information concerning signs and symptoms of illness by direct physical examination. In 1761, the year in which Giovanni Battista Morgagni (1682–1771) published his monumental five-volume examination of *The Seats and Causes of Diseases*, Leopold Auenbrugger (1722–1809) of Vienna published another landmark in the history of medicine entitled *Inventum Novum*. In little more than 20 pages, Auenbrugger set forth an account of a new diagnostic method called "chest percussion." Using this method, the physician could gain insight into the internal state of the chest cavity by carefully evaluating the sounds produced by tapping or thumping the patient's chest. Of course a great deal of experience was needed before a doctor learned to distinguish between the sounds of a healthy chest and those which betrayed the earliest signs of tuberculosis or pneumonia produced by a "morbid chest."

Auenbrugger, who was considered a gifted amateur musician and composer, presumably had a better-trained ear than most physicians. Chest percussion, which depends on the differences in sound transmitted through air and fluid, is rather like tapping a wine cask or beer barrel to determine whether it is empty or partially full. Because his father was a tavern keeper, Auenbrugger was probably quite familiar with this phenomenon. Although Auenbrugger considered his method revolutionary, some physicians saw little difference between percussion and other methods of diagnosis by auscultation (listening) dating back to the time of Hippocrates, such as shaking the patient and listening for the sound of fluid sloshing about in the chest, or placing the physician's ear on the patient's chest. Indeed, Auenbrugger's teacher had employed percussion of the abdomen in cases of ascites (fluid accumulation in the peritoneal cavity).

Few physicians expressed any interest in Auenbrugger's work until Jean-Nicolas Corvisart (1755–1821) published a translation and commentary in 1808. By this time, thanks to the work of the so-called Paris school of morbid anatomy, humoralism had been essentially eclipsed by the concept of localized pathological anatomy. Corvisart's disciples, especially René Théophile Hyacinthe Laënnec (1781–1826), established the value of direct (immediate) and indirect (mediate) auscultation and transformed the art and science of physical examination. Working at the Necker Hospital and the Charité, Laënnec adopted the goals and methods of the Paris school of hospital medicine. Eventually, his invention of the stethoscope would make him one of the most famous exemplars of this school, and a symbol of French science, but during his rather brief lifetime, his peers generally treated him with indifference and hostility.

Proponents of early nineteenth-century "hospital medicine" tended to see themselves as disciples of Hippocrates, because of their emphasis on clinical observation, but the context in which they worked, as well as their methods were very different from those of the ancients. Leaders of the French Revolution had imagined a new era in which hospitals, medical schools, and doctors would disappear. Instead, in the aftermath of the Revolution, new hospitals, medical schools, and professional standards emerged. In the major hospitals of Paris, clinicians could see thousands of cases and carry out many hundreds of autopsies. American students flocked to the great hospitals of France to supplement their limited education and gain clinical experience. Becoming disciples of French masters, they translated their writings into English. A note of envy for the extensive opportunities for the observation of disease found only in Europe often crept into their introductory remarks. Somewhat later in the century, schools and hospitals in Germany and Great Britain overtook those of France as centers of clinical studies and laboratory research.

The large scale of nineteenth-century hospital medicine provided the "clinical material" for more active and intrusive methods of physical examination and diagnosis, statistical evaluation of various therapeutic interventions (sometimes known as the numerical method of Pierre Charles Alexandre Louis, 1787–1872), and confirmation of correlations among symptoms, lesions, and remedies by means of investigations conducted in the autopsy room. Although immediate auscultation and chest percussion were becoming valuable aids to diagnosis and research into what Corvisart called "internal medicine," many physicians were reluctant to practice these methods. Given the great abundance of fleas and lice on many patients, and the general neglect of personal hygiene, a certain reluctance to put one's ear on the patient's chest was understandable. The stethoscope not only provided some distance between physicians and patients, it improved the quality of the sounds that could be heard within the chest. The name stethoscope was coined from the Greek for "chest" (*stethos*) and "to view" (*skopein*). It was the first of many "scopes" that gave researchers access to the interior of the body and allowed them to "anatomize" the living before they dissected the deceased.

In *On Mediate Auscultation* (1819), Laënnec described the difficulties he encountered when examining a young woman with signs of heart disease. Discreet percussion with a gloved hand did not reveal anything about the state of the inside of her chest, because of the rather stout state of the outside of her chest. Considerations of propriety precluded immediate auscultation, but in a flash of inspiration, Laënnec took a sheaf of paper and rolled it into a cylinder. When he applied one end of the cylinder to her chest and the other to his ear, he could hear the heartbeat with remarkably clarity. Improvements in the basic cylinder

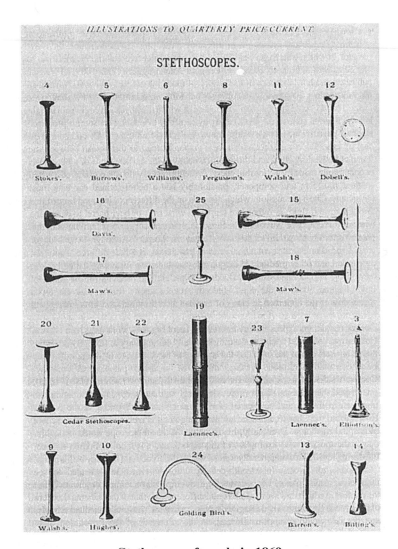

**Stethoscopes for sale in 1869.**

of Laënnec made it possible to listen to many sounds and movements within the chest. Through changes in materials and configuration, and the introduction of stethoscopes that transmitted sound to both ears, doctors tried to improve the stethoscope. The instrument has remained fairly consistent in appearance since the 1920s. The classical stethoscope has been relegated to the status of a "triage tool" to detect obviously suspicious sounds that lead to more sophisticated and expensive tests, such as the echocardiogram.

Laënnec warned physicians not to neglect Auenbrugger's methods when using the stethoscope, because the physician should use as many aids to diagnosis as possible. More important, it was essential to realize that a great deal of practice was required before the instrument could be used effectively. To learn the technique, the young physician should work in a hospital where he had access to many kinds of patients and expert guidance. Moreover, large numbers of postmortems were needed to confirm diagnostic accuracy. Like many of his colleagues, Laënnec succumbed to tuberculosis, the disease that was so often the object of his research. France, which had contributed so much to the study of tuberculosis, had the highest mortality rate from consumption in western Europe well into the twentieth century, perhaps largely due to lingering beliefs that heredity was more significant than contagion and general indifference to public health measures.

Sir John Forbes (1787–1861), who translated excerpts of Laënnec's nine hundred-page treatise on auscultation and diseases of the chest into English in 1821, noted that the stethoscope was extremely valuable, but he doubted that mediate auscultation would ever come into general use among English doctors, because its use required too much time and trouble. His most serious objection was that the instrument was totally foreign in character and incompatible with British traditions. Its use could be imposed on patients in the army and navy and in hospitals, but not on private patients. Like many of his colleagues, Forbes saw something ludicrous about a dignified physician listening to the patient's chest through a long tube. In other words, instruments were associated with surgeons and manual labor, not with the philosophical habits of English physicians. Many physicians believed that the advantages of objective aids to diagnosis were small and uncertain compared to the threat that instruments might disrupt the bond that was supposed to exist between physician and patient.

Obviously, Dr. Forbes proved to be a very poor prophet. The stethoscope soon became the very symbol of medicine and a necessary part of the doctor's wardrobe. Few doctors were able to match Laënnec's extraordinary skill at auscultation, but many learned that it was possible to use the instrument to gain objective information about the nature of a patient's condition and to distinguish between different diseases, such as tuberculosis and pleurisy. The stethoscope made it possible for physicians to "anatomize" the living body, but it was only in the autopsy room that the diagnosis could be confirmed. Even the most selfless patient was unlikely to sympathize with a physician who referred to the postmortem as the best way to diagnose disease because a few autopsies shed more light on pathology than 20 years spent observing symptoms.

It is interesting that the thermometer was not accepted into diagnostics as quickly as the stethoscope, although Santorio Santorio had introduced the clinical thermometer in the seventeenth century. The concept of localized pathology is generally given credit for the acceptance of physical aids to diagnosis, as well as advances in surgery, but the thermometer, which reflected a general condition of bodily heat, did not fit the pattern of a pathology of solids.

The stethoscope was, of course, only the first of the many "scopes" that allowed physicians to view every nook and cranny of the interior of the body. It is obviously a long way from Laënnec's cylinder to computerized axial tomography (CAT scans), nuclear magnetic resonance imaging (MRI), and positron emission tomography (PET scans), but it is a brief interval compared to the many centuries that separated Hippocrates from Laënnec. From the patient's point of view, advances in diagnostics that were not associated with progress in therapeutics were of dubious value. Although increasingly sophisticated and expensive new instruments have contributed to the power and prestige of medicine, and may have saved many patients from the burden of uncertainty, they do not necessarily improve the treatment of disease or the healing of wounds.

One of the persistent complaints issued against the great hospitals of Paris and Vienna was that their physicians were too interested in diagnosis and pathology, but too little interested in therapy. A nineteenth-century cynic assessing the battle between practitioners who favored active interventions and researchers who relied on a passive or expectative approach could conclude that Viennese hospital doctors no longer killed their patients, they just let them die. In the Parisian hospitals, a variety of approaches to therapy competed for attention. Some physicians favored bleeding, others relied on antimony or other chemical remedies, while some remained loyal to complex ancient remedies derived from plants, animals, and minerals. Even the standard definition of therapeutics as the art of curing diseases was called into question by those who claimed that the term referred to the most convenient means of treating disease. Oliver Wendell Holmes suggested that patients might be better off if the entire materia medica, except for quinine and opium, was thrown into the sea. Most doctors, however, agreed that it was better to try something doubtful than do nothing. Moreover, advances in chemistry were providing new drugs—such as morphine, emetine, strychnine, codeine, and iodine—that were unquestionably powerful, even if their safety and efficacy remained in doubt.

An accurate diagnosis at an early stage of a disease like tuberculosis, which was made possible by tuberculin and chest X-rays, could be interpreted as simply increasing the length of time in which the patient brooded on the inevitability of death. Nevertheless, the development of sophisticated diagnostic instruments has become fundamental to the health-care enterprise and is often blamed for the escalating costs of medical care. Although the stethoscope and similar devices introduced the fundamental concept of studying the interior structures and functions of the living body, the trend to ever more sophisticated and expensive diagnostic techniques can be traced to Wilhelm Konrad

Roentgen's (1845–1923) discovery of X-rays in 1895. Roentgen was investigating the properties of cathode rays when he observed a new kind of ray that was able to pass through opaque objects, including clothing, hair, and flesh. Bones, however, stopped the rays, leaving a picture of their shadow on a photographic plate. Roentgen's preliminary report to the Physico-Medical Society of Wurzburg, "On a New Kind of Ray," included several radiographs, including the well-known picture of Frau Roentgen's skeletal hand. When the popular press published stories about X-rays, Roentgen's findings caused worldwide speculation about their potential role in medicine. In 1901, Roentgen, already a universal celebrity, was awarded the first Nobel Prize in Physics.

X-rays gave physicians a new diagnostic tool, as well as a means of investigating the interior of the body. Just as the microscope and telescope made it possible to look at the microcosm and macrocosm in new ways, by making the flesh that clothed the bones essentially transparent X-rays created a new way of looking at the human body. After the initial period of enthusiastic and uncritical use, researchers realized that prolonged exposure to X-rays might cause tissue damage and cancer, in addition to the burns that were more quickly noted.

By the late 1960s, new medical instruments made it possible to visualize interior aspects of the body that had been impossible to see with ordinary X-rays. The methods called the "second wave of imaging technology" included computerized tomography, MRI, ultrasound, mammography, and PET. Sir Godfrey Hounsfield (1919–2004), a British electrical engineer, and Allan Macleod Cormack (1924–1998), a South African physicist, shared the 1979 Nobel Prize in Physiology or Medicine for their independent contributions to the development of computer-assisted tomography. (The brightness of images that appear on the CAT scanner is measured in Hounsfield units.) Neither man had a background in medicine or a doctoral degree, but, according to the Nobel Prize Committee, their revolutionary work "ushered medicine into the space age."

Computed axial tomography allows computers to analyze and produce a series of cross-sectional images from X-rays that are taken from many different angles. Although the original scanner was designed to examine the head, the instrument was adapted to study every organ system in the body. Despite the enormous cost of the device, about seven thousand CAT scanners were in use in American hospitals by 2000. Magnetic resonance imaging (originally called nuclear magnetic resonance or NMR) can create thin-section images of any part of the body from any angle, generating biomedical and anatomical information. MRI has been particularly valuable for diagnosing diseases of the brain and central nervous system. Physicists and chemists used NMR technology in the 1940s, but it became a diagnostic tool, referred to as MRI, in the 1980s.

In less than two hundred years, diagnostic and therapeutic technologies have become central and enormously expensive components of medicine. Technological success has created an avalanche of expectations and questions about the actual risks and benefits associated with this transformation of medical practice. Faith in the diagnostic power of medical instruments led to decreased interest in the procedure that the pioneers in this field thought so fundamental: confirmation at the postmortem.

Autopsies were once routinely performed in a majority of hospital deaths, but since the 1980s, the number of such procedures in the United States and several other countries has dropped sharply. Before 1970, the Joint Commission on Accreditation of Healthcare Organizations mandated autopsies in at least 20 percent of all hospital deaths, but by 1995, the National Center for Health Statistics stopped collecting national autopsy statistics. In most wrongful-death cases against hospitals or physicians, an autopsy is critical to establishing negligence. Doctors and hospital administrators, afraid of being sued over mistaken diagnoses, increasingly avoid autopsies. Attempts to quantify the incidence of medical errors suggest that autopsies uncover missed or incorrect diagnoses in up to 25 percent of hospital deaths. In many cases, the correct diagnoses might have led to changes in therapy or other procedures. Autopsies revealed that many systemic bacterial, viral, and fungal infections had not been diagnosed prior to death. Whatever the cause of death in a particular case, such infections might have been a threat to those who had been in contact with the patient. Similar studies of patients who died in intensive-care units found many instances of incorrect diagnoses, as well as evidence of infections, cancers, and other undiagnosed diseases. Researchers suggested that over-reliance on sophisticated diagnostic imaging techniques sometimes contributed directly to major diagnostic errors.

## SERUM THERAPY

As a new generation of scientists looked back on the golden age of bacteriology, their enthusiasm was tempered by the realization that microbe hunting did not in itself lead to the cure of disease. A re-evaluation of the factors that determined the balance between health and disease involved rejecting too narrow a bacteriological focus and working towards an understanding of human physiological responses to microbial agents. Certainly, the observation that surviving one attack of a particular disease provided protection from subsequent attacks was not new. This was the basis of the immunity earned in exchange for submitting to the risks of smallpox inoculation or vaccination. The Latin term "immunity" originally referred to an "exemption" in the legal sense. Since the introduction of Jennerian vaccination, it was clear that protective vaccines took advantage of the body's own defense mechanisms, but the modern era of immunization began in the 1880s when Louis Pasteur proved that it was possible to attenuate pathogenic microbes and create specific vaccines in the laboratory. Building on the work of Louis Pasteur and Robert Koch, Shibasaburo Kitasato, Emil von Behring, and Paul Ehrlich developed new forms of treatment known as serum therapy and chemotherapy.

Coming from a family with many children and limited resources, Emil Adolf von Behring (1854–1917) attended the Army Medical College in Berlin in exchange for 10 years of service in the Prussian Army. Military medicine provided an important route into the profession for many men of modest means. After working as an assistant to Robert Koch at the Institute for Infectious Diseases, Behring held professorships at Halle and Marburg. Friedrich Althoff (1839–1908), one of the leading officers of the Prussian Ministry of Education and Cultural Affairs, played a major role in advancing Behring's career. When Behring became Director of the Institute of Hygiene at Marburg, he divided the Institute into two departments, a Research Department for Experimental Therapy and a Teaching Department for Hygiene and Bacteriology. Claiming that his health precluded teaching, Behring devoted himself to research and business ventures. In 1914, he founded the Behringwerke for the production of sera and vaccines. His career provides a paradigm for a new era in which studies of basic science could lead to patents and profits.

During the nineteenth century, several particularly virulent outbreaks of a disease variously known as croup, malignant angina, and throat distemper attracted the attention of clinicians and bacteriologists. Pierre Fidèle Bretonneau (1778–1862) suggested the name "diphtheritis" for what he thought of as a specific form of malignant sore throat that killed young children by sudden suffocation. In 1883, *Corynebacterium diphtheriae*, the bacillus that causes the disease was discovered by Theodor Klebs (1834–1913) and Friedrich Loeffler (1852–1915). By the end of the decade, researchers at the Pasteur Institute in Paris had demonstrated that bacteria-free filtrates of diphtheria cultures contained a toxin that produced the symptoms of the disease when injected into experimental animals. Autopsies revealed that the disease caused considerable damage to the internal organs, but the bacteria usually remained localized in the throat. Pasteur's associates Émile Roux (1853–1933) and Alexandre Yersin (1863–1943) proved that diphtheria bacilli release toxins that enter the bloodstream and damage various tissues. Diphtheria is acquired by inhaling bacteria released when a patient or carrier coughs and sneezes. Within a week after infection, the victim experiences generalized illness and the characteristic "false-membrane" at the back of the throat. During virulent outbreaks, the disease had a case fatality rate of 30 to 50 percent, but many people acquired immunity after experiencing fairly mild symptoms. Doctors sometimes performed tracheotomy to prevent death by asphyxiation, but even if this operation produced temporary relief, toxemia might still cause death. Tracheotomy was essentially replaced by intubation in the 1890s.

Shibasaburo Kitasato (1852–1931), a Japanese physician working at Koch's Institute, isolated the tetanus bacillus and proved that, like the diphtheria bacillus, it produced a toxin that caused the symptoms of the disease when injected into experimental animals. Trained as a military doctor in the Listerian era, Behring was intrigued by the possibility of using "internal disinfectants" against infectious diseases. Experiments with iodoform initiated a life-long preoccupation with antitoxic substances and an appreciation for the fact that chemical disinfectants were often more damaging to the tissues of the host than to the invading bacteria. Some preliminary experiments indicated that while iodoform did not kill microbes, it seemed to neutralize bacterial toxins.

Working together on the toxins of diphtheria and tetanus bacilli, Behring and Kitasato demonstrated that when experimental animals were given a series of injections of toxins, they produced *antitoxins*, substances in the blood that neutralized the bacterial toxins. Antitoxins produced by experimental animals could be used to immunize other animals, and could even cure infected animals. Encouraged by these early results, Behring predicted that his toxin–antitoxin preparations would lead to the eradication of diphtheria, which typically killed more than fifty thousand children in Germany each year.

A first step in the transformation of serum therapy from a laboratory curiosity into a therapeutic tool was accomplished by turning sheep and horses into antitoxin factories. Although Behring planned to enter a commercial relationship with Hoechst, the German chemical company producing Koch's tuberculin, his preparations were too variable, unreliable, and weak for routine use or commercial distribution. Fearing that French scientists would make further advances in serum therapy, Behring asked Paul Ehrlich (1854–1915) for help. Having systematically worked out methods of immunization with the plant toxins ricin and abrin, Ehrlich knew how to increase antitoxin strength and measure the activity of antisera with precision. By producing highly active, standardized sera, Ehrlich made serum therapy practical. Behring and Ehrlich established a laboratory in Berlin to obtain serum from sheep and horses.

In 1892, Berhing, Ehrlich, and Hoechst entered into an arrangement to work on diphtheria antitoxin. Production and marketing of the therapeutic serum began two years later. According to their previous agreement, Behring and Ehrlich were to share in the profits from diphtheria antitoxin, but Behring persuaded Ehrlich to give up his share of the profits by promising to help him get his own research institute. For reasons that remain obscure, Behring did not carry out his part of the deal. He did, however, keep his enlarged share of the profits and became a very wealthy man. The immunity provided by Behring's therapeutic serum, which was a result of passive immunity, was short-lived. In 1901, Behring began experiments with attenuated cultures of diphtheria bacilli as a means of establishing active immunization. In 1913, Behring publicly described his diphtheria protective agent, which was called "Toxin–Antitoxin." It contained a mixture of diphtheria toxin and therapeutic serum antitoxin.

Relations between Ehrlich and Behring rapidly deteriorated as Behring became richer and more arrogant. Perhaps Ehrlich could take some comfort in the fact that after their collaboration ended all of Behring's scientific projects were failures. Koch's tuberculin fiasco stimulated Behring's search for an effective therapeutic agent, but he too was unsuccessful. Instead, he attempted to develop a preventive vaccination. Assuming that the tubercle bacillus was primarily transmitted to children through milk, Behring tried to destroy this source of infection by treating milk with formaldehyde. Even if babies or calves could be forced to consume formaldehyde-treated milk, most tuberculosis infections were contracted via the respiratory route. Behring's attempts to establish attenuated tubercle bacteria that could serve as immunizing agents were unsuccessful.

Diphtheria was generally considered a minor disease when compared to tuberculosis, but while tuberculin was causing bitter disappointment, serum therapy was being hailed as a major contribution to medicine. The first Nobel Prize for Physiology of Medicine, awarded in 1901, honored Behring for creating a "victorious weapon against illness and deaths." By making it possible to induce life-saving active and passive immunity, serum therapy seemed to be the ultimate answer to the threat of infectious diseases. Yet within 10 years, the euphoria trigged by the success of the diphtheria antitoxin was replaced by profound disappointment and the dawn of a period that has been called the "Dark Ages of Immunology." Despite the overall success of antitoxin, some patients experienced serious side effects and a few died. Treatment was most successful if given in the early stages of the disease, but doctors were reluctant to use antitoxin until the disease was clearly life threatening. Control programs were complicated by the discovery that many people were asymptomatic carriers.

By the end of the twentieth century, genetic engineers were exploiting the "naturally engineered" properties of various bacterial toxins in order to create hybrid molecules in which toxins are linked to specific antibodies. Diphtheria toxin, for example, was naturally engineered as a protein that could penetrate cell membranes, but it is only one of several bacterial toxins that have found a place in biomedical research and medical practice. The use of botulinum toxin for cosmetic purposes is, perhaps, one of the best-known examples. Previously, *Clostridium botulinum* toxin was universally feared as the cause of paralysis following the ingestion of improperly preserved foods. Just as alchemists once began their quest for powerful elixirs with poisons, genetic engineers have turned to bacterial toxins to find molecules suitable for appropriate modifications. Such novel immunotoxins have been referred to as "poisoned arrows" or "smart bombs," which, at least in theory, can deliver more fire power than the "charmed bullets" first synthesized in the laboratory of Paul Ehrlich, the founder of chemotherapy.

Since the discovery of serum therapy, diphtheria has been the most successfully studied of the once common childhood diseases. Case fatality rates rarely exceeded 10 percent, but, sometimes, exceptional epidemics took a very heavy toll among young victims. Because immunity can be brought about by antibodies directed against the toxin itself, researchers could focus on the toxin rather than the bacillus. In 1928, Gaston Leon Ramon (1886–1963) discovered that diphtheria toxin treated with formaldehyde retained serological specificity and immunogenicity, while losing its toxicity. Modified toxins were called "toxoids." Evidence for the proposition that there is nothing new under the sun can be found in nineteenth-century reports about certain "wizards" in central Africa who told visiting Europeans that they could protect people against snakebites with a potion containing snake heads and ant eggs. Native healers in other parts of the world have employed similar methods. By exploiting the fact that certain ants contain formic acid, so-called primitive healers had accomplished the chemical detoxification of toxins and venoms. Massive immunization campaigns have almost eliminated the threat of diphtheria in the wealthy industrialized nations. Diphtheria remains the only major human infectious disease of bacterial origin that has been so successfully managed by preventive immunizations. Unfortunately, a generation unfamiliar with the threat once posed by diphtheria is unable to understand the dangers posed by the breakdown of "herd immunity."

## ANTIBIOTICS AND IMMUNOLOGY

Throughout his career, Paul Ehrlich (1854–1915) struggled to understand the body's immunological defenses and to develop experimentally based therapeutic systems to augment them. Like Pasteur, his theoretical interests were closely linked to practical problems. This interplay between the theoretical and practical resulted in significant contributions to immunology, toxicology, pharmacology, and therapeutics. Ehrlich's achievements include the development of salvarsan and other drugs, clarification of the distinction between active and passive immunity, recognition of the latent period in the development of active immunity, and an ingenious conceptual model for antibody production and antigen–antibody recognition. Salvarsan, the first chemotherapeutic agent specifically aimed at the microbe that causes syphilis, provided an effective demonstration for Paul Ehrlich's belief that it is possible to fight infectious diseases through a systematic search for drugs that kill invading microorganisms without damaging the host. Such drugs have been called "magic bullets."

Ehrlich's doctoral thesis "A Contribution towards the Theory and Practice of Histological Staining," seems to contain the germ of his life's work: the concept that specific chemicals can interact with particular tissues, cells, subcellular components, or microbial agents. In 1878,

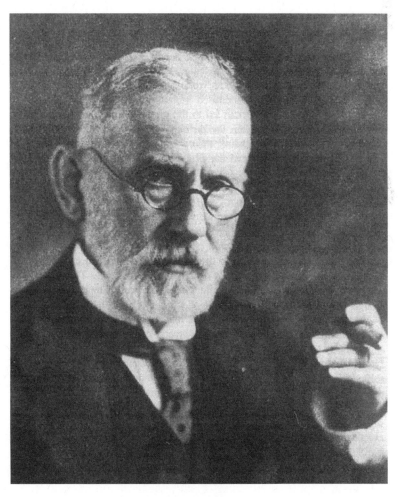

**Paul Ehrlich.**

after studying at the Universities of Breslau, Strasbourg, and Leipzig, Ehrlich graduated and qualified as a doctor of medicine. As assistant to Friedrich Frerichs at the Berlin Medical Clinic, Ehrlich was allowed to continue his research. But Frerichs committed suicide in 1885, and Ehrlich's new supervisor expected his senior physicians to devote more time to the clinic than to research. Depressed and somewhat ill, Ehrlich seized the opportunity provided by a positive tuberculin test to leave the hospital and embark on a consumptive's pilgrimage to Egypt. Returning to Berlin with his health restored, Ehrlich was distressed to find himself almost totally excluded from the academic community. He was not nominated for a professorship or offered a position in a scientific institute for 15 years. During this period, he conducted studies of the nervous system that involved testing the effect of methylene blue on neuralgia and malaria.

Selective staining techniques allowed Ehrlich to distinguish different types of white blood cells and leukemias. Somewhat later, using bacteriological techniques and transplantable tumors, Ehrlich initiated a new approach to cancer research in which cancer cells were treated like microbes and the host organism served as the nutrient medium. Finally, in 1896, Ehrlich was appointed director of a new Institute for Serology and Serum Testing. Facilities at the Institute were rather limited, but Ehrlich told friends he could work in a barn, as long as he had test tubes, a Bunsen burner, and blotting paper. Three years later, the Institute was transferred from Berlin to Frankfurt and renamed the Royal Institute for Experimental Therapy. Next to the Royal Institute, thanks to a large bequest from Franziska Speyer, Ehrlich established the Georg Speyer Institute for Chemotherapy.

In 1908, Ehrlich shared the Nobel Prize in Physiology or Medicine with Élie Metchnikoff (1845–1916) for their work on immunity. Ehrlich's Nobel Prize lecture, entitled "Partial Cell Functions," began with a tribute to the concept of the cell as the unit of life and "the axis around which the whole of the modern science of life revolves." He thought, however, that the problem of cell life had reached a stage of investigation in which it was necessary to "break down the concept of the cell as a unit into that of a great number of individual specific partial functions." Research programs that analyzed the chemical nature of the many processes occurring within the cell would provide a real understanding of vital functions and lead to the "rational use of medicinal substances." Progress in this direction, he explained, had come about as a result of attempts to find the key to the mysterious processes underlying the discovery of the antitoxins. "Key" was the operative word, because as the great organic chemist Emil Fischer (1852–1919) had said of enzymes and their substrates, antibodies and antigens entered into a chemical bond of such strict specificity that they interacted like lock and key.

Ehrlich used the term "immunotherapy" as early as 1906 in a period of great hope that many diseases would be prevented or cured by serum therapy. As the limitations of serum therapy became more apparent, especially in the case of cancer, Ehrlich eventually shifted his focus from immunology to experimental pharmacology and chemotherapy. Further progress, Ehrlich concluded, would have to come from synthetic drugs rather than natural antibodies. In the mid-nineteenth century, many researchers had questioned the value of all remedies, but Ehrlich saw experimental pharmacology as a science with great promise and potential.

In studying the marvelous specificity of the antibodies generated in response to the challenge of poisons, toxins, and other foreign invaders, Ehrlich became convinced that it should be possible to design chemotherapeutic substances by exploiting specific interactions between synthetic chemicals and biological materials. Because the body did not produce effective antibodies for every challenge, Ehrlich considered it the task of medical science to provide chemical agents that would substitute for or augment the body's natural defenses. Antibodies were nature's own magic bullets; chemotherapy was an attempt to imitate nature by creating drugs lethal to pathogenic microbes, but harmless to the patient.

Using the "disinfection" produced by quinine for malaria as a model, Ehrlich planned an extensive series of tests of potential drugs and their derivatives. Despite the ambitious scope of his research program, he encouraged his associates to take time for reflection. Ehrlich believed that the keys to success in research were "Gelt, Geduld, and Gluck" (money, patience, and luck), and that spending too much time in the laboratory meant wasteful use of supplies and experimental animals. Ehrlich closely supervised the work of all his collaborators, to the point that senior associates working in his laboratory complained about the lack of independence. Each day he gave even the most senior researcher little notes (*Blöke*), which might be considered the precursors of "post-it" notes, that told them what they should be doing.

The first targets for Ehrlich's new chemotherapy were the trypanosomes, the causative agents of African sleeping sickness, Gambia fever, and nagana. Following his "chemical intuition" along a path that had begun with his early studies of dye substances, Ehrlich began an investigation of a drug called atoxyl and related arsenic compounds. Atoxyl was quite effective in the test tube, but was not a suitable therapeutic agent because it caused neurological damage and blindness. The distinction between killing microbes in the test tube and killing them in a living being, without causing damage to the patient, is often forgotten. Ehrlich's test tube experiments proved that the accepted chemical formula for atoxyl was incorrect. It was, therefore, possible to create myriads of derivatives, many of which proved to be safer and more effective than atoxyl.

Because spirochetes were thought to be similar to trypanosomes, Ehrlich's group also conducted tests on spirochetal diseases. Fritz Schaudinn (1871–1906) and Erich Hoffmann (1868–1959) had discovered the causative agent for syphilis in 1905. Within a year, scientists succeeded in establishing syphilitic infections in rabbits. Sahachiro Hata (1873–1938), an expert in the use of this model system, conducted systematic tests of Ehrlich's arsenical compounds on the microbes that cause syphilis, chicken spirillosis, and relapsing fever. Some of the atoxyl derivatives were quite toxic, but birds infected with chicken spirillosis were cured by one injection of Preparation 606. This chemical also cured relapsing fever in rats and syphilis in rabbits.

After two physicians offered to be guinea pigs, Ehrlich's collaborators began a series of intramuscular injections of 606 on certain patients with progressive paralysis, an invariably fatal condition thought to be of syphilitic origin. Expecting at most a slight increase in survival, they were surprised at the improvements caused by a single injection of the drug. The possibility that toxic effects might be delayed remained unresolved. Moreover, the remissions, relapses, and complications that were part of the natural history of syphilis made evaluating remedies extremely difficult. Preparation 606, which was given the name salvarsan, underwent testing that was quite extensive compared to the usual practices of the time. After the drug had been tested on almost thirty thousand patients, salvarsan was made available to the medical community at large. When congratulated on this remarkable achievement, Ehrlich often replied that salvarsan accounted for one moment of good luck after seven years of misfortune. With tens of thousands successfully treated for syphilis he could not anticipate the misfortunes still to come.

Alchemists often began the search for their elixirs of life with poisons, because the fact that a substance was a known poison proved that it was powerful. As this ancient approach suggests, it is unreasonable to expect any drug to be both effective and completely harmless. Nevertheless, some of Ehrlich's supporters argued that salvarsan was nontoxic, while his critics accused the drug of causing a wide range of adverse reactions. A dermatologist named Richard Dreuw made one of the first attacks on salvarsan. Although most doctors were complaining that Ehrlich had been too cautious, Dreuw accused Ehrlich of releasing salvarsan without sufficient testing. When medical journals rejected his papers, Dreuw became obsessed with the idea that a "salvarsan syndicate" was controlling the Germany medical community and suppressing all criticism of salvarsan. Joined by some members of the Reichstag and anti-Semitic newspapers, Dreuw attacked Ehrlich personally and demanded that the Imperial Health Office establish a national ban on salvarsan.

Anti-salvarsan crusaders claimed that the drug caused deafness, blindness, nerve damage, and death, but ignored the fact that one million people had been successfully treated. Moreover, deafness, blindness, nerve damage, and death were also caused by syphilis. Compared to the deaths caused by syphilis, and the suffering of its victims, salvarsan was relatively benign, although prolonged treatment involved real dangers of adverse effects in some patients. Another problem was that patients who had been cured often returned to the behaviors that caused them to contract syphilis in the first place; they blamed the "relapse" not on themselves, but on salvarsan.

The most bizarre member of the anti-salvarsan crusade was Karl Wassmann, a writer who habitually dressed as a monk. Hearing prostitutes complain that salvarsan was being forced on them at the Frankfurt Hospital, Wassmann concluded that Prof. Herxheimer, director of the Dermatology Department, was an agent of the "salvarsan syndicate." From 1913 on, Wassmann made the battle between prostitutes and the medical authorities a major theme of his magazine, *The Freethinker*. According to Wassmann, the government was suppressing the truth about the salvarsan syndicate and the appalling effects caused by the drug. Proclaiming himself champion of the abused underclass, Wassmann courted controversy to call attention to himself and his writings. Unwilling to accept these attacks on his professional behavior, Herxheimer sued Wassmann for slander. Salvarsan was so completely vindicated by the evidence brought out at the trial that when the prosecution requested a six-month prison term for Wassmann the court doubled the sentence. Despite this outcome, Ehrlich was extremely distressed by the trial and the futility of trying to present complex scientific and medical issues in the hostile, adversarial environment of the courtroom. Salvarsan, with the addition of mercury and bismuth, remained the standard remedy for syphilis until it was replaced by penicillin after World War II.

Attempts to create an arsenal of magic bullets were largely unsuccessful until the 1930s when Gerhard Domagk (1895–1964) found that a sulfur-containing red dye called prontosil protected mice from streptococcal infections. This led to the synthesis of a series of related drugs called the sulfonamides or "sulfa drugs," which were highly effective against certain bacteria. Domagk was the director of research in experimental pathology and bacteriology at the German chemical firm I. G. Farben. Like Ehrlich, Domagk turned to the study of dyes as a means of understanding pathogenic microorganisms. Preliminary studies of bacterial staining led to a systematic survey of the aniline dyes in hopes of finding chemicals that would kill bacteria.

In a typical experiment, Domagk determined the quantity of bacteria needed to kill inoculated mice (the lethal dose). Then he inoculated mice with 10 times the lethal dose and gave half of the animals a test substance, such as prontosil. By 1932, Domagk had shown that prontosil protected mice against lethal doses of staphylococci and streptococci. As early as 1933, the drug was secretly used in humans with life-threatening staphylococcal and streptococcal infections. However, Domagk's report, "A Contribution to the Chemotherapy of Bacterial Infections," was not published until 1935. Domagk may have delayed publication because of Farben's interest in securing patent protection, but the delay might also have been caused by some difficulties in reproducing the initial results. In 1939, Domagk was awarded the Nobel Prize in Physiology or Medicine "for the discovery of the antibacterial effects of prontosil," but Nazi officials would not allow him to accept it. Germany's leadership in the development of chemotherapeutic agents was essentially lost during the period from 1933 to 1945, because of National Socialistic policies that isolated Germany from the international research community and forced many Jewish scientists to seek refuge in England and America. Domagk finally received the Nobel medal in 1947 and delivered a very emotional lecture on progress in chemotherapy.

As soon as Domagk's results were published, prontosil was tested in laboratories in France, America, and Britain. Researchers at the Pasteur Institute proved that prontosil was inactive until it was split in the animal body. The antibacterial activity was due to the sulfonamide portion of the molecule. Not only was sulfanilamide more active than prontosil, it did not have the disadvantage of being a messy red dye. Prontosil was synthesized and patented by I.G. Farben in 1932, but an account of the synthesis of sulfanilamide had been published in 1908. Thus, Farben could not claim patent protection for derivatives of sulfanilamide. With open season on the sulfa drugs, more than five thousand derivatives were synthesized in the decade after Domagk's report. In the entire series of sulfonamides, so laboriously synthesized and tested, fewer than 20 clinically useful compounds were identified. Chemists began to realize that the odds of synthesizing a safe and effective magic bullet were rather like those of winning the lottery.

Nevertheless, studies of the sulfa drugs flooded the literature. Laboratory tests showed that many of these drugs were effective against various bacteria, at least in the laboratory. Clinical trials in hospitals throughout the world provided promising results in the treatment of pneumonia, scarlet fever, gonococcal infections, and so forth. Unfortunately, drug-resistant strains of bacteria appeared almost as rapidly as new drugs. The sulfa drugs were indiscriminately prescribed for infections of unknown origin, casually given for suspected gonorrheal infections, and liberally sprinkled into wounds.

Hailed as "miracle drugs" in the 1930s, by the end of World War II, the sulfa drugs were considered largely obsolete. Domagk suggested that part of the problem might have been caused by a decrease in natural resistance due to wartime stress and malnutrition, the spread of primary resistant strains enhanced by "the general upheaval during and after the war," and the development of resistant strains during the course of treatment. The same disappointments would follow the use of penicillin, Domagk warned, unless physicians learned to appreciate the factors that led to the development and spread of resistant strains.

The next generation of wonder drugs for infectious disease came from a previously obscure corner of nature's storehouse. By the 1870s, several scientists had called attention to the implications of "antibiosis" (the struggle for existence between different microorganisms), but according to popular mythology, the antibiotic era began in 1928 when Alexander Fleming (1881–1955) discovered penicillin. Of course, the real story is much more complicated. Indeed, in his 1945 Nobel Lecture, Fleming suggested that the discovery of "natural antiseptics" had taken so long because bacteriologists of his generation had taken the fact of microbial antagonisms for granted rather than as a phenomenon to be explored.

Fleming discovered the effect of the mold *Penicillium notatum* on bacteria in 1928. Within a year, he demonstrated that crude preparations of penicillin killed certain bacteria but were apparently harmless to higher animals. Penicillin was not the first antibacterial agent Fleming discovered. In 1922, he found what he called a "powerful antibacterial ferment" in nasal secretions, tears, and saliva. Although this enzyme, which was named "lysozyme," plays a role in the body's natural defense system, it was not a practical magic bullet. As Fleming often said, he was not a chemist. Howard Florey and Ernst Boris Chain, who later tested and purified penicillin, worked out the chemical nature and mode of action of lysozyme.

Alexander Fleming was only seven when his elderly father, a Scottish farmer died. Because his family's resources were limited, Fleming worked as a clerk for several years before a small legacy made it possible for him to attend St. Mary's Medical School in London. More mature than the other students, Fleming excelled at competitive examinations, swimming, and shooting. After graduating in 1908, he became assistant to the eminent and eccentric bacteriologist, Sir Almroth Wright (1861–1947). Fleming's interest in agents that kill bacteria was stimulated by his experience in the Royal Army Medical Corps during the First World War. Attending to the septic wounds that were the common aftermath of battle, Fleming was convinced that chemical antiseptics were generally more lethal to human tissues than to the invading bacteria.

After the war, Fleming returned to St. Mary's to continue his research on antibacterial substances. According to what we might call the penicillin myth, a spore drifted through an open window into Fleming's laboratory and settled in a Petri dish on which he was growing staphylococci. Contamination of bacteriological materials with molds is a common laboratory accident, generally considered a sign of poor sterile technique and general sloppiness. Acknowledging this correlation, Fleming often said that he would have made no discoveries if his laboratory bench had always been neat and tidy. Fortunately, his contaminated plate was left among stacks of dirty Petri dishes when Fleming went off on vacation. On his return, Fleming noticed that staphylococci had been destroyed in the vicinity of a certain mold colony and he decided that this case of antibiosis was worth pursuing.

Scientists who tried to recreate this great moment in medical history suggest an alternative scenario: staphylococci were sown on the famous Petri dish but did not grow because of an unusual cold spell. A spore of the relatively rare *P. notatum* that had previously fallen onto the plate began to grow during this period. Finally, warmer temperatures triggered the growth of the staphylococci and the penicillin that

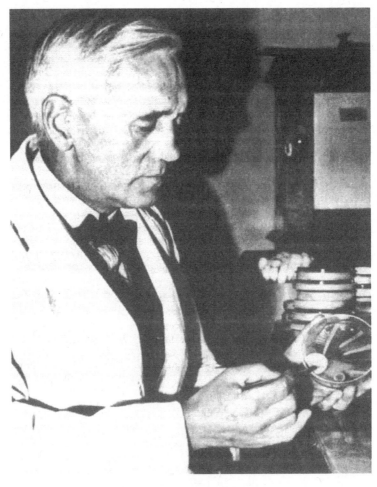

**Alexander Fleming in 1944.**

had been released into the medium around the mold colony killed the growing bacteria. Serendipity had to be working overtime in Fleming's behalf, but it is necessary to propose such a sequence of events in order to explain Fleming's observation, because penicillin cannot dissolve fully grown colonies of staphylococci. Testing the effects of his mold, Fleming discovered that even in crude, dilute preparations, penicillin stopped the growth of bacteria and caused them to die. It was, however, essentially harmless to white blood cells in the test tube. The active agent in his penicillin preparations was apparently unstable and extremely difficult to purify. Not being an active clinician or a chemist, Fleming rarely managed to have a supply of penicillin and a suitable patient available at the same time. Nor did Fleming perform the animal experiments that would have demonstrated penicillin's effectiveness in fighting bacteria in infected animals. In 1930, however, one of Fleming's former students successfully used local applications of crude penicillin in treating eye infections.

In 1928, when Fleming began to work with penicillin, textbooks of therapeutics and pharmacology were still recommending ancient preparations of aromatic substances and heavy metal salts for the treatment of infected wounds, along with relatively new disinfectants such as carbolic acid, hydrogen peroxide, iodoform, and the hypochlorites. Chemists had prepared many modifications of known disinfectants, but physicians generally believed that if any drug were present in the bloodstream in concentrations high enough to kill bacteria, human tissues and organs would be damaged as well. After penicillin had become the new "wonder drug," Fleming complained that neither bacteriologists nor physicians paid any attention to penicillin until the introduction of sulfanilamide changed attitudes towards the treatment of bacterial infections.

Although the story of Fleming's accidental discovery of penicillin is well known, the fact that penicillin remained a laboratory curiosity until World War II is often forgotten. Both aspects of the penicillin story were recognized in 1945 when the Nobel Prize for Physiology or Medicine was awarded to Alexander Fleming, Howard Walter Florey (1898–1968), and Ernst Boris Chain (1906–1979) "for the discovery of penicillin and its curative effect in various infectious diseases." Almroth Wright, however, insisted that all the credit for the discovery should go to Fleming and headlines in some prominent newspapers noted that the Nobel Prize had gone to "Fleming and Two Co-Workers."

In 1938, Florey, Director of the Sir William Dunn School of Pathology at Oxford University, Chain, and Norman Heatley, began a systematic study of naturally occurring antibacterial agents, including lysozyme and substances produced by various microbes. Within two years, partially purified penicillin was tested in mice infected with virulent streptococci. Further experiments proved that penicillin was active against streptococci, staphylococci, and several other pathogens. With penicillin performing as an ideal magic bullet in mice, the Oxford group quickly moved on to human experiments. The first patient was a 43-year-old man who had contracted a mixed infection of staphylococci and streptococci. Although the patient was close to death when treatment began, penicillin produced a remarkable improvement. Unfortunately, even though the drug was recovered from the patient's urine, the supply was soon exhausted and the patient died. An account of the first successful clinical trial was published in the British medical journal, the *Lancet*, but further studies became part of the secret war effort.

With Britain's resources strained by the war, it was obvious that British pharmaceutical companies could not develop a new drug. Florey was forced to seek American support. The path from laboratory curiosity to the industrial production of penicillin was full of obstacles, not all of them technical and scientific. Research on penicillin was closely associated with military needs and goals. Inevitably, the secrecy that surrounded the initial trials attracted reporters and generated wild rumors. Within two years of Florey's visit to the United States, about 16 companies were producing penicillin and major clinical trials were under way. As hundreds of patients were treated with penicillin, researchers became more optimistic about its therapeutic potential. Penicillin was effective in the treatment of syphilis, gonorrhea, and infections caused by pneumococci, staphylococci, and streptococci. Penicillin was hailed as a panacea that would deliver armies from both venereal diseases and battle injuries. Where supplies were limited, military authorities had to decide whether to use it on those wounded in battle, or those "wounded" in the brothels.

In his delayed Nobel Prize Lecture in 1947, Domagk attributed differences in mortality rates for American soldiers in the two world wars to the sulfonamides and penicillin. Of course many other aspects of battlefield conditions, weaponry, military medicine, surgery, and hygiene had changed during the years between the wars, but differences between the nations that had access to penicillin and those that did not reflected, at least in part, the role played by antibiotics. Paradoxically, Florey was more cautious in evaluating the impact of penicillin on battle casualties than Domagk. Direct comparisons of raw mortality figures can be misleading, Florey warned, because in many cases, new therapies and battlefield evacuation techniques extended lives that would have ended abruptly in previous wars. This created increasingly intricate and intractable problems of repair and recovery.

When the war ended, although American and British pharmaceutical firms were selling millions of units of penicillin, there was still a flourishing black market where penicillin bottles were refilled with worthless chemicals and sold for hundreds of dollars. By 1948, pharmaceutical plants all over the world were producing penicillin. When penicillin became readily available, many physicians adopted treatment regimens reminiscent of the era of so-called heroic medicine. Penicillin was combined with bismuth, arsenicals, sulfonamides, and other drugs, and injected at frequent intervals. Further work proved that a single dose of penicillin was effective in treating certain diseases. The promise of a simple cure for the major sexually transmitted diseases drove moralists to denounce penicillin as a stimulus to promiscuity.

During the war, some scientists insisted that chemical synthesis of the penicillin molecule would be more productive than further modifications of fermentation techniques. By the late 1940s, chemists had decided that the synthesis of penicillin was impractical, if not impossible. In commercial terms, this was essentially true, but the total synthesis of penicillin was finally achieved in 1957 by organic chemist John C. Sheehan. Reflecting on the problems that followed his synthesis of penicillin, Sheehan noted that it had taken 23 years to clear up patent disputes.

Inspired by lessons learned and profits earned with penicillin, researchers sifted through samples of dirt from every corner of the world in search of new miracle molds. Quoting Ecclesiastes in his 1952 Nobel Prize Lecture, Selman A. Waksman (1888–1973) reminded his audience: "The Lord hath created medicines out of the earth; and he that is wise will not abhor them." During his search for such medicines, Waksman, a biochemist and pioneer in soil microbiology, discovered streptomycin, neomycin, and many other antibiotics, most of which were too weak or too toxic for human use. Waksman coined the term "antibiotic" to refer to a group of compounds produced by microorganisms that can inhibit the growth of other microorganisms or even destroy them.

According to bacteriological folklore, the normally persistent tubercle bacillus could be destroyed in the soil. Waksman, therefore, turned his systematic studies of soil microbes into a search for agents antagonistic to the tubercle bacillus. More than ten thousand different soil microbes were investigated before Waksman, Elizabeth Bugie, and Albert Schatz isolated streptomycin in 1944. One year later, William H. Feldman and H. Corwin Hinshaw of the Mayo Clinic announced that streptomycin was effective against tuberculosis. A major share of credit for recognizing the value of streptomycin belonged to Feldman and Hinshaw. Evaluating remedies for tuberculosis is very difficult because the disease is unpredictable, develops slowly, and is affected by nonspecific factors, such as diet and rest. The failure of previous miracle cures had left researchers disillusioned and skeptical about the prospects for chemotherapeutic agents. After seeing signs of improvement in patients with life-threatening meningeal and miliary tuberculosis, Feldman and Hinshaw extended their tests to less acute forms of the disease. The early preparations of streptomycin were impure and

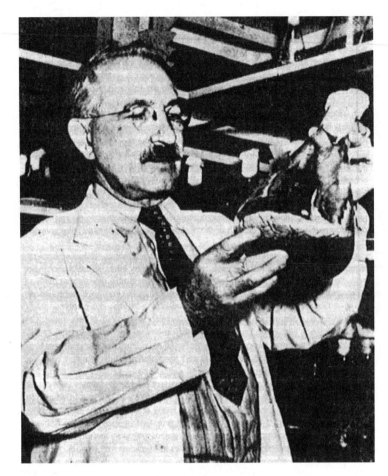

**Selman A. Waksman.**

caused serious side effects, including fever, chills, muscular pains, and deafness. In some tests, only slightly more than half of the streptomycin-treated patients improved after six months. Despite all these problems, in 1948 when eight pharmaceutical companies were producing the drug, demand far exceeded supply. Waksman was awarded the Nobel Prize for the discovery of streptomycin in 1952, two years after the legal settlement of a complex royalty dispute initiated by Schatz. In 1994, Schatz, who insisted that he had not received sufficient credit for the discovery of streptomycin, won the Rutgers University Medal, which is considered a prestigious award, but far short of the Nobel Prize.

Unlike the long barren years between Fleming's discovery of penicillin and the exploitation of its therapeutic potential, streptomycin went from laboratory curiosity to major pharmaceutical product within a few brief years. Indeed, the success of penicillin and streptomycin proved to be a tremendous stimulus to the growth of the pharmaceutical industry and the expansion of research. During the 1940s and 1950s, the golden age of antibiotics, chloramphenicol, neomycin, aureomycin, erythromycin, nystatin, and other valuable antibiotics were discovered. Reflecting the optimism of this period, Waksman predicted that future research would lead to the discovery of more active and less toxic agents and to powerful combinations of antibiotics and synthetic compounds. By the 1960s, however, the golden age of discovery of novel antibiotics was essentially over. Most of the antibiotics introduced since then have been slight modifications of previously known drugs. Moreover, the warnings issued earlier proved to be true. Overuse and misuse of antibiotics revealed adverse side effects and promoted the development of drug-resistant strains of bacteria.

In many countries, antibiotics are readily available, without prescriptions, and people use them until they feel better. So-called underground medical shops help people avoid the expense of consulting a doctor, but antibiotics are ineffective against viruses and usually affect a limited spectrum of bacteria. Some antibiotics are quite dangerous and are only prescribed when no alternatives are available. Moreover, inappropriate use of the drugs contributes to the development of drug-resistant bacteria.

The widespread use of antibiotics to suppress illness and encourage the growth of animals also poses risks. The risk of creating antibiotic-resistant microbes is well known, but another danger is that antibiotics added to animal feed may appear as contaminants in human foods. The sources of contamination may be convoluted and obscure. A European food scare developed in 2002, for example, because of reports that meat was contaminated with chloramphenicol, a powerful antibiotic that can cause a potentially lethal form of anemia. Chloramphenicol is normally restricted to combating life-threatening diseases such as anthrax and typhoid when other antibiotics are ineffective. Chloramphenicol-contaminated meat was linked to contaminated shrimp that had been mixed with other components of animal feed used in Germany, Austria, Denmark, Poland, and Romania. Some shrimp farmers were apparently using the antibiotic, despite laws banning its use.

## NATURAL DEFENSES: HUMORAL OR CELLULAR?

By the 1880s, it was recognized that the virulence of infectious diseases varied with many factors, including the means and duration of exposure, the way in which the germ entered the body, and the physiological status of the host. By the turn of the century, the fundamental question concerning scientists investigating the immune response was: is the mechanism of innate and acquired immunity humoral or cellular?

When Behring was awarded the first Nobel Prize in Medicine for his work on serum therapy, he made a special point of reviewing the history of the dispute between cellular and humoral pathology. He considered antitoxic serum therapy "humoral therapy in the strictest sense of the word." Humoral theory, Behring predicted, would put medicine on the road to a strictly scientific etiological therapy in contrast to traditional, nonspecific, symptomatic remedies. The scientific debate often degenerated into vicious personal attacks, but Joseph Lister, ever the gentleman, delicately referred to this controversial era as the "romantic chapter in pathology."

As serology was transformed into immunology, scientists saw the new discipline rapidly outgrowing its parental disciplines of microbiology and toxicology. Studies of cellular mechanisms of defense seemed to be a relic of a less sophisticated era of biology closely associated with old-fashioned ideas such as those of Élie Metchnikoff (1845–1916). Other immunologists of this period were primarily concerned with serum antibodies and tended to ignore the role played by cells, but Metchnikoff, discoverer of phagocytes (the "eating cells" that devour invading microorganisms) and the process of phagocytosis, was more interested in the defenses of the host than the depredations of the pathogen. While most scientists argued that specific chemical entities in the blood defended the body from bacteria and toxins, Metchnikoff followed his own idiosyncratic hypotheses concerning evolution, inflammation, immunity, senility, and phagocytosis. When he shared the 1908 Nobel Prize for Physiology or Medicine with Paul Ehrlich, Metchnikoff was praised as the first scientist to establish an experimental approach to the fundamental question of immunity, that is, how does the organism overcome disease-causing microbes?

Through personal experience Metchnikoff knew how little physicians could do for victims of infectious diseases. His first wife had been so weakened by consumption that she had to be carried to their wedding. When she died five years later, Metchnikoff tried to end his own life by swallowing a large dose of opium. With his second wife close to death from typhoid fever, Metchnikoff inoculated himself with the spirochetes thought to cause relapsing fever so that his death would be of service to science. Fortunately, the excitement generated by the discovery of phagocytosis rescued Metchnikoff from the depression that had driven him to attempted bacteriological suicide. From 1888 on, the Pasteur Institute provided a refuge in which Metchnikoff could pursue research problems that were creative and original to the point of eccentricity. Primarily a zoologist, influenced as much by Charles Darwin as Pasteur or Koch, Metchnikoff's theories of inflammation and immunity grew out of his evolutionary vision of comparative pathology.

Studies of inflammation that began with starfish larvae led Metchnikoff to the conclusion that phagocytosis was a biological phenomenon of fundamental importance. While observing the interaction between phagocytes and bacteria, Metchnikoff discovered that phagocytosis was greatly enhanced in animals previously exposed to the same kind of bacteria. He, therefore, concluded that mobile phagocytes were the primary agents of inflammation and immunity. In his Nobel Prize lecture, he expressed hope that people would see his work as an example of the "practical value of pure research." Inspired by Metchnikoff's "phagocyte theory," some surgeons attempted to rush white corpuscles to the rescue by introducing various substances into the abdominal cavity or under the skin. Another follower of Metchnikoff's theories systematically applied cupping-glasses and rubber ligatures around the site of abscesses and similar infections. The localized edema produced by these procedures was supposed to attract an army of protective phagocytes.

Confident that science would eventually free human beings from the threat of disease, Metchnikoff applied his theory of the phagocyte to the specter of senility. Reflecting on the principles of comparative pathology, he concluded that phagocytes were primarily responsible for the signs and symptoms of senility. From gray hair and baldness to weakness of bone, muscle, and brain, Metchnikoff saw the telltale footprints of myriads of motile cells "adrift in the tissues of the aged." Noxious influences, such as bacterial toxins and the products of intestinal putrefaction, allegedly triggered the transformation of friendly phagocytes into fearsome foes. Even though Metchnikoff believed that phagocytes caused senility, he warned that destroying these misguided cells would not prolong life, because the body would then be left defenseless in the struggle against pathogenic microbes.

After comparing the life spans of various animals, Metchnikoff concluded that the organs of digestion determined length of life. Specifically, the problem resided in the large intestine where microbial mischief produced "fermentations and putrefactions harmful to the organism." Stopping just short of a call for prophylactic removal of this "useless organ," Metchnikoff suggested that disinfecting the digestive tract might lengthen life. Unfortunately, traditional purges and enemas seemed to harm the intestines more than the microbes. Since acids could preserve animal and vegetable foods, Metchnikoff concluded that lactic fermentation might prevent putrefaction within the intestines. In practical terms, his advice could be summarized by the motto: "Eat yogurt and live longer."

Although scientists generally ignored Metchnikoff's theory of the treacherous phagocytes and the useless large intestine, his ideas about the positive and negative activities of phagocytes and the ambiguity of the inflammatory response were remarkably prescient. When the body responds to noxious stimuli, the site of the injury exhibits what the Roman writer Celsus called the cardinal signs of inflammation and becomes red, swollen, warm, and painful. Although the inflammatory response is most noticeable on the skin, it also occurs internally, in response to viral invaders or spoiled food. Thus, although inflammation is the body's normal protective reaction, in many cases, inflammation can harm the tissues it is meant to heal. This occurs in diseases like rheumatoid arthritis and multiple sclerosis. In the elderly, the destructive effects of inflammation may be involved in other common chronic diseases, such as arteriosclerosis, diabetes, Alzheimer's disease, osteoporosis, asthma, cirrhosis of the liver, some bowel disorders, psoriasis, meningitis, cystic fibrosis, and cancer. Indeed, some researchers suggest that the use of anti-inflammatory drugs like ibuprofen or naproxen may prevent or delay the development of some of the chronic and debilitating diseases of old age, such as Alzheimer's disease.

Of course the body's failure to mount an effective defense against some pathogens was well known, but the discovery by Charles Robert Richet (1850–1935) and Paul Jules Portier (1866–1962) that the immune system could react to certain antigens with life-threatening hypersensitivity was unexpected. Richet, who won the Nobel Prize in 1913, coined the term "anaphylaxis" to describe this dangerous response. Based on the Greek word *phylaxis* meaning protection, anaphylaxis referred to "that state of an organism in which it is rendered hypersensitive, instead of being protected." Violent itching, vomiting, bloody diarrhea, fainting, choking, and convulsions characterized this state of hypersensitivity. In its most severe form, anaphylactic shock could cause death within a few minutes of exposure to the offending antigen. Further investigations proved that just as it was possible to transfer passive immunity, it was also possible to transfer the anaphylactic condition via serum.

Anaphylaxis seemed to be a peculiar exception to the generally beneficial workings of the immune system. Thus, many scientists believed that immunology would provide the key to establishing powerful new approaches to therapeutics. A good example of the optimism characteristic of this early phase of immunology is provided by Sir Almroth Wright (1861–1947), a man who was expected to take the torch from Pasteur and Koch and illuminate new aspects of experimental immunization and medical bacteriology. Wright expected his work in the Inoculation Department at St. Mary's Hospital to bring about a revolution in medicine, but he is generally remembered only as Alexander Fleming's mentor.

A man of broad interests and inflexible opinions, Wright published about 150 books and papers in science, intellectual morality, and ethics. In addition to his scientific articles, Wright often used the British newspapers to vent his opinions on issues ranging from the ignorance of army officials to the campaign for woman suffrage, which he vehemently opposed. While professor of pathology at the Army Medical School in Royal Victoria Hospital, Wright developed sensitive laboratory methods of diagnosing the "army fevers" that killed more soldiers than bullets. Using a diagnostic test based on what he called the agglutination effect (the clumping of microbes in response to serum from patients recovering from a disease), Wright prepared a vaccine that apparently protected monkeys from Malta fever. In the great tradition of scientists who served as their own guinea pigs, Wright injected himself with his vaccine. Unfortunately, Wright was not as lucky as his monkeys.

While recovering from Malta fever, Wright began planning a major study of typhoid fever. During the 1890s, this dreaded disease claimed tens of thousands of lives in the United States and Great Britain. The case fatality rate varied from 10 to 30 percent, but recovery was a slow and unpredictable process. Using himself and his students as guinea pigs, Wright found that heat-killed cultures of typhoid bacilli could be used as vaccines. Sir William Boog Leishman's (1865–1926) study of typhoid cases in the British Army between 1905 and 1909 provided the first significant documentation of the value of antityphoid inoculations. According to Leishman, the death rate of the unvaccinated men was 10 times that of the inoculated group. Nevertheless, at the beginning of World War I, antityphoid inoculations in the British Army were still voluntary.

Openly contemptuous of the "military mentality," Wright was happy to resign from the Army Medical Service when he was offered the position of pathologist at St. Mary's Hospital in 1902. Although he received only a small salary, meager facilities, and was responsible for many tedious and time-consuming duties, he attracted eager disciples and hordes of desperate patients. With the fees charged for vaccine therapy, Wright's Inoculation Department became a flourishing and financially rewarding enterprise. According to Wright, ingestion of microbes by phagocytes required the action of certain substances in the blood that he called "opsonins," from the Greek opsono, meaning, "I prepare victuals for." Wright's vaccines were designed to increase the so-called opsonic index of the blood by making pathogenic microbes more attractive and digestible.

Patients suffering from acne, bronchitis, carbuncles, erysipelas, and even leprosy submitted to Wright's experimental inoculations and blood tests. Doubtless many patients eventually recovered from self-limited infections, despite the therapy rather than because of it. Disdainful of statistical evaluations of medical interventions, Wright exhibited great confidence in his methods and warned reactionary physicians that they would be "degraded to the position of a head nurse" as the art of medicine was transformed into a form of applied bacteriology. By the end of World War II, it was obvious that Wright's opsonically calibrated vaccines were no more successful than Metchnikoff's attempts to neutralize the harmful effects of phagocytes with yogurt. Even Wright's admirers were forced to conclude that the vaccines dispensed by his Inoculation Department were generally "valueless to the point of fraudulence." British playwright and social critic George Bernard Shaw (1856–1950) immortalized Almroth Wright's eccentricities in *The Doctor's Dilemma*, but scientists remembered him as "Sir Almost Wright."

Reviewing what was known about immunology in the 1920s, the eminent physiologist Ernest H. Starling (1866–1927) concluded that the only thing perfectly clear about the immune system was that "immunity, whether innate or acquired, is extremely complex in character." Further studies of the system have added more degrees of complexity and controversies at least as vigorous as those that characterized the conflict between humoral and cellular theory. Immunology is a relatively young field, but its twentieth-century evolution was so dynamic that it ultimately became one of the fundamental disciplines of modern medicine and biology. Discussions of AIDS, cancer, rheumatoid arthritis, metabolic disorders, and other modern plagues are increasingly conducted in the arcane vocabulary of immunobiology.

Modern explanations for the induction of antibodies and their remarkable diversity and specificity can be divided into information, or instructionist theories, and genetic, or selectionist theories. According to the information theory of antibody synthesis, the antigen dictates the specific structure of the antibody by direct or indirect means. Direct instruction implies that the antigen enters a randomly chosen antibody-producing cell and acts as a template for the production of antibodies with a configuration complementary to that antigen. An indirect template theory suggests that when an antigen enters an antibody-producing cell it modifies the transcription of immunoglobulin genes and, therefore, affects the sequence of the amino acids incorporated into the antibodies produced by that cell and its daughter cells.

A genetic or selectionist theory of antibody production assumes that information for the synthesis of all possible configurations of antibodies is contained in the genome and that specific receptors are normally present on immunocompetent cells. Selectionist theories presuppose sufficient natural diversity to provide ample opportunities for accidental affinity between antigen and immunoglobulin-producing cells. In this scenario, the antigen acts as a kind of trigger for antibody synthesis.

One of the first modern theories of antibody formation, Paul Ehrlich's side-chain theory, was an attempt to provide a chemical explanation for the specificity of the antibody response and the nature of toxins, toxoids, and antibodies. According to this theory, antibody-producing cells were studded with "side-chains," that is, groups capable of specifically combining with antigens such as tetanus toxin and diphtheria toxin. When a particular antigen entered the body, it reacted with its special side-chain. In response, the affected cell committed itself to full-scale production of the appropriate side-chain. Excess side-chains became detached and circulated in the body fluids where they neutralized circulating toxins. Like a key in a lock, the fit between antigen and antibody was remarkably specific, although it was presumably due to accident rather than design.

Karl Landsteiner (1868–1943) argued that Ehrlich's theory was untenable primarily because it presupposed an "unlimited number of physiological substances." However, it was Landsteiner's demonstration that the body is capable of making antibodies against "haptens" (small molecules, or synthetic chemical radicals that were linked to proteins) that transformed the supposed number of antibodies from *unlimited*, in the sense of very large, to *unlimited*, in the sense of almost infinite. The implications of this line of research were so startling that Landsteiner, who won the 1930 Nobel Prize in Medicine for his discovery of the human blood groups, considered his development of the concept of haptens and the chemical approach to immunology a much greater scientific contribution.

It had always been difficult to imagine an antibody-producing cell carrying a large enough array of potentially useful side-chains to cope with naturally occurring antigens. Imagining that evolution had equipped cells with side-chains for the synthetic antigens produced by ingenious chemists was essentially impossible. No significant alternative to the genetic theory emerged, however, until 1930 when Friedrich Breinl (1888–1936) and Felix Haurowitz (1896–1988) proposed the first influential instructionist theory, which they called the "template theory." According to this theory, an antigen enters a lymphocyte and acts as a template for the specific folding of an antibody. Many kinds of objections were offered in response to this hypothesis, but proof that antibodies differ in their amino acid sequence made early versions of this theory untenable. A long line of complex clinical puzzles and methodological challenges culminated in the complete determination of the amino acid sequence of an entire immunoglobulin molecule in 1969 by Gerald M. Edelman (1929–) and his associates. Edelman and Rodney R. Porter (1917–1985) were awarded the Nobel Prize in 1972 in recognition of their work on the biochemical structure of antibodies.

The instructionist theory of antibody production was challenged in 1955 by Niels Kaj Jerne's (1911–1994) "natural-selection theory," which has been described as a revised and modernized form of Ehrlich's classical side-chain theory. Jerne worked at the Danish State Serum Institute before earning a medical degree at Copenhagen. He served as the chief medical officer of the World Health Organization from 1956 to 1962 and director of the Institute of Immunology at Basel from 1969 to 1980. According to Jerne's natural-selection theory, an antigen seeks out a globulin with the appropriate configuration, combines with it, and carries it to the antibody-producing apparatus. Although Jerne introduced his theory in the 1950s, it was not until 1984 that he was awarded the Nobel Prize in Medicine or Physiology "for theories concerning the specificity in development and control of the immune system and the discovery of the principle for production of monoclonal antibodies." In his lecture at the Nobel ceremonies Jerne said, "My concern has always been synthetic ideas, trying to read road-signs leading into the future." Jerne's vision of the natural-selection theory of antibody formation and his complex network theory of the immune response provided the framework for a new phase in the development of cellular immunology. Jerne's early publications served as a challenge to the instructionist theories that had become the dominant paradigm of immunology.

The natural-selection theory implied that the body's innate ability to generate a virtually unlimited number of specific antibodies was independent of exposure to foreign antigens. Normal individuals are born with the genetic capacity to produce a large number of different antibodies, each of which has the ability to interact with a specific foreign antigen. When the immune system encounters a novel antigen, the pre-existing antibody molecule that has the best fit interacts with it, thus stimulating the cells that produce the appropriate antibody. In the 1970s, Jerne elaborated his network theory as an explanation for the regulation of the immune response, essentially through an antibody cascade leading to anti-antibodies, anti-anti-antibodies, and so forth, and the ability of the immune system to balance the network by stimulating or suppressing the production of particular antibodies. This theory provided vital insights into the body's response to infectious diseases, cancers, allergies, and autoimmune disease.

Modified versions of antibody-selection theory solved the primary difficulty of Jerne's original concept by substituting randomly diversified cells for his randomly diversified antibody molecules. That is, cells are subject to selection, not antibodies. In particular, the cell, or clonal-selection theory, independently proposed by Sir Frank Macfarlane Burnet (1899–1985) and David Talmage (1919–), revolutionized ideas about the nature of the immune system, the mechanism of the immune response, and the genesis of immunologic tolerance. Burnet's clonal-selection theory encompassed both the defense mechanism aspect of the immune system and the prohibition against reaction to "self." During development, "forbidden clones" (cells that could react against self) were presumably eliminated or destroyed. Macfarlane Burnet and Sir Peter Medawar (1915–1987) were awarded the Nobel Prize in 1960 for their work on immunological tolerance.

When Macfarlane Burnet reviewed the state of immunology in 1967, 10 years after he proposed the clonal-selection theory, he was pleased to report that the field seemed to have "come of age." Unlike Ehrlich and Landsteiner, who had emphasized the importance of a chemical approach to immunology, Burnet's emphasis was on biological concepts: reproduction, mutation, and selection. By the 1980s, the cell-selection theory had gone beyond general acceptance to the status of "immunological dogma." This transformation was stimulated by the explosive development of experimental cellular immunology. Immunology laboratories were awash with T cells and B cells, helper cells, suppressor cells, killer cells, and fused cells producing monoclonal antibodies. Throughout the 1970s and 1980s, immunologists were awarded Nobel Prizes for remarkable theoretical and practical insights into organ transplant rejection, cancer, autoimmune diseases, and the development of new diagnostic and therapeutic tools of great power and precision. A century of research in immunology since the time of Louis Pasteur had created as many questions as it had answered, but it clearly established the fact that much of the future of medical theory and practice would be outgrowths of immunobiology.

With cardiovascular disease and cancer replacing the infectious diseases as the leading causes of morbidity and mortality in the wealthy, industrialized nations, immunology seemed to offer the answer to the riddle of health and disease just as microbiology had provided answers to questions about the infectious disease. In the 1950s, Macfarlane Burnet expressed his belief that immunology was ready for a new phase of activity that would reach far beyond the previous phase inspired by Paul Ehrlich. Microbiology and chemotherapy had provided a powerful arsenal of magic bullets directed against the infectious diseases. By combining molecular biology and immunology, scientists were attempting to create a new generation of genetically engineered drugs, including so-called smart bombs and poisoned arrows. These new weapons would be designed to target not only old microbial enemies, but also modern epidemic conditions and chronic diseases, such as cardiovascular disease, cancer, Alzheimer's disease, autoimmune disorders, allergies, and organ rejection.

When Cesar Milstein (1927–2002) and Georges Köhler (1946–1995) shared the 1984 Nobel Prize with Jerne, they were specifically honored for the discovery of "the principle for production of monoclonal antibodies." In his Nobel Lecture, Milstein stressed the importance of the fact that the hybridoma technology was an unexpected by-product of basic research that had been conducted to understand the immune system. It was, he said, a clear example of the value of supporting research that might not have an obvious immediate practical application. Monoclonal antibody production was one of the principal driving forces in the creation of the biotechnology industry. It opened the way for the commercial development of new types of drugs and diagnostic tests. Monoclonal antibodies could be equipped with markers and used in the diagnosis of a wide variety of illnesses and the detection of viruses, bacteria, toxins, drugs, antibodies, and other substances.

In 1969, Jerne had predicted that all the interesting problems of immunology would soon be solved and that nothing would remain except the tedious details involved in the management of disease. Such drudgery, he suggested, was not of interest to scientists, but would provide plenty of work for physicians. The innovative hybridoma technique developed by Milstein and Köhler in 1975 falsified that prediction and made it possible to explore many unexpected aspects of the workings of the immune system. Contrary to Jerne's prediction, researchers have not run out of questions to ask about the immune system, nor have there been any complaints that the field has become less exciting.

The characteristic of the immune system that is so important in guarding the body against foreign invaders, that is, the ability to produce an almost unlimited number of different antibodies, represents a problem for scientists trying to understand the system. Immunologists who have struggled with the phenomenon of antibody diversity estimate that a mouse can make millions of different antibodies. The technique developed by Milstein and Köhler has transformed the study of antibody diversity and made it possible to order what Milstein called "antibodies à la carte." The new generation of magic bullets that might be derived from hybridomas could be compared to creating derivatives of atoxyl and the aniline dyes. Hybridomas are made by fusing mouse myeloma tumor cells with spleen cells derived from a mouse that was previously immunized with the antigen of interest. The hybrid cells produce large quantities of specific antibodies, which are called monoclonal antibodies (Mabs). By combining the techniques of immunology and molecular biology, scientists expect to design new generations of magic bullets. As Sir Almroth Wright predicted, the healer of the future might well be an immunologist.

By 1980, only five years after Köhler and Milstein first published an account of their technique, monoclonal antibodies were well-established tools in many areas of biological research. By 1990, thousands of monoclonal antibodies had been produced and described in the literature. Researchers predicted that monoclonal antibodies might be used as novel vaccines and in the diagnosis and treatment of cancers. In cancer therapy, monoclonal antibodies might function as smart bombs, targeted against cancer cells to provide site-specific delivery of chemotherapeutic drugs. The concept is simple in theory, but difficult to achieve in practice. In part this is due to the fact that, despite new insights into the etiology of cancer, discussions of "cancer" are rather like nineteenth-century debates about the nature of fevers, plagues, pestilences, and infectious diseases. The complex constellation of disorders subsumed by the category commonly called cancer looks quite different to physicians, patients, pathologists, oncologists, and molecular biologists. There is a great gap between understanding the nature of oncogenes (genes that appear to induce malignant changes in normal cells when they are affected by carcinogenic agents), transforming retroviruses (RNA viruses that can transform normal cells into malignant cells), proto-oncogenes, and so forth, and establishing safe and effective means of preventing and treating cancers.

Studies of viral infections and possible links between cancer and viruses led to hope that some endogenous agent might serve as a universal viral antidote and cancer drug. Interferon, a protein that interferes with virus infections, was discovered in the 1950s by researchers studying the growth of influenza virus in chick embryonic cells. Despite early excitement about interferon, the substance was very difficult to isolate and characterize. By 1983, about 20 distinct human interferons had been identified. The interferons were involved in the regulation of the immune system, nerve function, growth regulation, and embryonic development. Experiments in the late 1960s suggested that, at least in mice, interferon inhibited virus-induced leukemias and the growth of transplantable tumors. Interferon's potential role in cancer treatment attracted the attention of the media, patient advocacy groups, and members of Congress.

Preliminary tests of interferon's clinical efficacy against osteogenic sarcoma (a malignant bone cancer) in the early 1970s interested virologist Mathilde Krim (1926–), who launched a crusade to support research on interferon as an antitumor agent. Krim, who had earned her Ph.D. in 1953 at the University of Geneva, Switzerland, joined the Sloan-Kettering Institute for Cancer Research in 1962. From 1981 to 1985, she served as Director of the Institute's Interferon Laboratory. Interferon was initially promoted as a potential "miracle drug," which would presumably be well tolerated because it was a "natural agent." Clinical trials were, however, quite disappointing in terms of effectiveness and safety. Adverse reactions to interferon included fever, chills, fatigue, loss of appetite, decreased white-blood-cell counts, and hair loss. Through further development, however, interferon gained a role in the treatment of certain cancers and viral diseases. In addition to her interferon work, Krim became well known as a health educator and AIDS activist. She was the founder of the AIDS Medical Foundation (1983), which later became the American Foundation for AIDS Research. In 2000, President Bill Clinton awarded the Presidential Medal of Freedom to Krim for her contributions to AIDS education and research.

Ever since 1971, when President Richard M. Nixon (1913–1994) declared war on cancer, oncologists and cancer patients have been caught in cycles of euphoria and despair. Since the 1970s, the phrase "war on cancer" has been used to stimulate spending on research. Yet the total cancer death rate has not significantly declined since the declaration of war. Critics insisted that the war was profoundly misguided in terms of its overly optimistic predictions and its implementation. Moreover, the rhetoric of the cancer crusade often conveyed false and misleading information to the general public. Premature reports of "breakthroughs" and "miracle cures" convinced many people that cancer is essentially a single disease and that sufficient spending would soon result in the discovery of a magic bullet. Scientists point out that the funds and technologies associated with the war on cancer stimulated revolutionary developments in molecular biology and biotechnology. Congress and the public, however, prefer to support mission-oriented research rather than basic scientific investigations.

## GENETICS, GENOMICS, AND MEDICINE

For diseases that are caused by defective genes rather than microbes or degenerative processes associated with aging, the healer of the future might have to be a genetic engineer rather than an immunologist. On June 26, 2000, leaders of the Human Genome Project announced the completion of working drafts of the complete human genome and their imminent publication in the British journal *Nature* and the American journal *Science*. Francis Collins, director of the National Human Genome Research Institute, predicted that genomics would revolutionize diagnostics, preventive medicine, and therapeutics within decades. Genomics would, in particular, allow physicians to predict the disease patterns and drug reactions of individual patients. With the completion of the Human Genome Project, scientists immediately began to use the partial maps to locate, isolate, and clone specific disease genes. This information can be used to improve diagnostic methods, help prevent disease, design specific agents to treat patients, and, in some cases, might lead to gene therapy that could correct defective genes. Genetic data on hereditary forms of cancer have allowed individuals with particular oncogenes to undergo pre-emptive surgical removal of organs such as the stomach, breast, ovary, uterus, colon, and thyroid gland. Another product of the Human Genome Project is the development of forensic genomics. Originally thought of as a way to establish databases for identifying criminals, forensic DNA analysis can also help identify human remains, even after significant tissue decomposition, by sequencing mitochondrial DNA from hair, teeth, and bones.

Critics of the Human Genome Project warned of potential ethical, social, and legal problems associated with the ability to determine genetic information. To deal with potential problems, the National

Center for Human Genome Research promoted studies of the ethical, legal, and social implications (ELSI) of the genome project. Advocates of patients' rights demanded the passage of laws that would safeguard genetic privacy. Such laws would prevent employers from using genetic information in making employment decisions and would prevent healthcare organizations and medical insurance plans from using genetic information when making enrollment decisions. In 1995, the Equal Employment Opportunity Commission published guidelines that extended the protections specified by the Americans with Disabilities Act to cover discrimination based on genetic information related to illness, disease, or other conditions. Proof that protection against discrimination based on genetic information was necessary was demonstrated in a landmark case in 2001, in which the U.S. Equal Employment Opportunity Commission (EEOC) went to court to stop a company from testing its employees for genetic defects. In this unprecedented legal battle over medical privacy in the workplace, the EEOC argued that basing employment decisions on the results of genetic tests violated the Americans With Disabilities Act. Concerns about the potential abuse of genetic data led many states to ban the use of genetic screening for making employment-related decisions. Because genetic information could lead to new forms of discrimination, many scientists and ethicists have supported the Universal Declaration of the Human Genome and Human Rights, which states that: "No one shall be subjected to discrimination based on genetic characteristics that is intended to infringe or has the effect of infringing human rights, fundamental freedoms and human dignity."

The Human Genome Project stimulated the rapid development of new disciplines, as well as a new vocabulary. With the completion of the first major phase of the Human Genome Project, scientists could directly confront the task of analyzing tens of thousands of human genes and their relationship to the hundreds of thousands of human proteins. In keeping with the new vocabulary spawned by the Human Genome Project, scientists suggested organizing a complete inventory of human proteins, which would be known as the Human Proteome Project (HUPO). The term proteome, which was coined in 1995, refers to the "set of PROTEins encoded by the genOME." Because proteins are involved in disease states, complete descriptions of proteins, could stimulate rational drug design, as well as the discovery of new disease markers and therapeutic targets.

In 1990, the year that the Human Genome Project began in earnest, after many debates about safety and ethical issues, William French Anderson (1936–) and colleagues at the U.S. National Institute of Health won approval from the Recombinant DNA Advisory Committee (RAC) to conduct the first human gene therapy trial in the United States. Researchers were attempting to use genetic engineering to correct a life-threatening inherited disease. The patient in this experiment was a four-year-old girl born with severe combined immunodeficiency disease (SCID), a rare genetic disease of the immune system. Patients with SCID have a defect in the gene for adenosine deaminase (ADA), an enzyme that is necessary for the production of white blood cells in the bone marrow. Unable to fight infections, children with SCID usually die long before reaching adulthood. A retrovirus was used as a vector to introduce copies of the gene for ADA into stem cells taken from the patient's bone marrow. Modified stem cells were then infused into the patient where they developed into white blood cells that produced ADA for several months.

Despite the optimism generated by Anderson's first case, genetic therapy remained very controversial and many critics argued that, given the potential dangers of genetic manipulation and the use of viruses as vectors, human trials were premature. In 1999, the death of 17-year-old Jesse Gelsinger during a gene therapy trial led to new debates about the safety of gene therapy. Gelsinger died of multiple organ failure four days after treatment for ornithine transcarbamylase (OTC) deficiency. (The enzyme OTC is needed to remove ammonia from the blood.) A preparation of modified adenovirus, which was being used as a vector to deliver the gene for OTC, had been infused into Gelsinger's main liver artery. In response to investigations of Gelsinger's death, the Food and Drug Administration stopped several gene therapy studies using adenovirus vectors. All gene therapy fell under intense scrutiny and had to comply with stricter standards. Nevertheless, in 2002, after reports of adverse affects among patients in otherwise promising gene therapy tests for hemophilia B and X-linked SCID, the Food and Drug Administration suspended about 30 gene therapy trials. Subsequent clinical trials were subjected to a higher level of regulatory oversight and stricter requirements that made clinical trials for all forms of gene therapy much more costly and difficult.

## PARADOXICAL PROGRESS

When epidemiologists look at the rise and fall of diseases in a global setting over long periods of time, they provide a perspective quite different from that available to patients and practicing physicians. Such a perspective suggests a cautious response to the hyperbole surrounding the latest "medical miracles." The analysis of specific examples and general trends in mortality and morbidity have led some historians, epidemiologists, demographers, and critics of medicine to question the role of medicine throughout history and, therefore, the probable effect of modern medical technologies on mortality and morbidity in the foreseeable future. Indeed, in looking closely at the leading causes of death in the

United States today, health policy advisors generally suggest that the most important focus of attention is no longer the conquest of disease, but the containment of medical costs. At the beginning of the twenty-first century, the leading causes of death in America were heart disease, cancer, stroke, diabetes, accidents, and Alzheimer's disease. Instead of dying of childhood diseases, or an emergency appendectomy, Americans are more likely to spend decades in a nursing home with Alzheimer's disease or enter an unhappy middle age sprawl and die of liposuction. Whether longer lives represent an increase in quality as well as quantity is open to question, but suicide (which is likely to be underestimated) was number 11 in the listing of the causes of death in the United States.

The United States devotes more of its economy to healthcare than other industrial countries. Americans spent about 14 percent of gross domestic product on healthcare, while other advanced nations spent about 10 percent. In 2000, healthcare accounted for 10.7 percent of the gross domestic product in Switzerland, 10.6 percent in Germany, 9.5 percent in France, and 9.1 percent in Canada. Medicare spending, for the elderly and disabled, rose 7.8 percent in 2001, while spending under Medicaid, the federal-state program for low-income people, increased by 10.8 percent. Prescription drugs were the fastest-growing category of healthcare spending. In 2001, spending on drugs exceeded spending on nursing homes and home healthcare combined. Pharmaceutical companies say prescription drugs consumed only about ten percent of total healthcare spending in 2001. Spending for hospitals and doctors accounted for more than 50 percent.

As measured by life span and infant mortality, however, most developed nations are healthier than the United States. Moreover, Americans do not have more medical services than residents of other nations. In 2001, the United States had 2.7 doctors per thousand people, compared with a median of 3.1 in the countries in the Organization for Economic Cooperation and Development (OECD). The United States has 2.9 hospital beds per thousand people, compared with the OECD median of 3.9. Germany has 6.3. Researchers concluded that Americans are charged more for doctors, hospitals, drugs, and, especially, for administrative expenses.

Although healthcare spending and access to medical care are hotly contested issues, some studies seem to suggest that increased spending on healthcare does not necessarily lead to significant and measurable improvements in health. In contrast to most goods and services, the supply of healthcare (as measured by the numbers of physicians, specialists, diagnostic and therapeutic equipment, and hospitals) seems to drive demand. Many complex economic, political, and cultural factors are involved in patterns of distribution and usage of healthcare resources, but analysts point to major discrepancies in spending that are not reflected in vital statistics. For example, despite major differences between

Medicare spending for senior citizens in Miami and Minneapolis, life expectancy was essentially the same. Studies that analyzed the relation- ship between the availability of neonatal intensive-care facilities and specialists and infant mortality rates reached a similar conclusion. That is, increasing the availability and usage of healthcare resources increases costs, but does not necessarily result in obvious or measurable improve- ments in health and longevity. Nevertheless, the cost of healthcare and the number of Americans without medical insurance are expected to increase rapidly. Some health policy experts argue that debates about how states and individuals should pay for medical care should be informed by a healthy skepticism about the cost-effectiveness of medical treatments and an understanding that newer, more aggressive, more expensive care does not guarantee better care, better health, or longer life expectancy. For example, studies of the mechanism of heart attacks suggested that increasingly popular aggressive treatments, like bypass surgery, angioplasty, and the insertion of stents (wire cages that hold plaque against an artery wall in order to maintain blood flow) might be useless, as well as dangerous. Preventive measures, such as giving up smoking, lowering cholesterol, and controlling blood pressure, seem to be more significant. Many attempts to show that opening a narrowed artery saved lives or prevented heart attacks were unsuccessful, but the call for aggressive intervention was not affected.

One issue raised by the widespread misconception that the infec- tious diseases have been conquered is whether interest in public health and preventive immunizations can be sustained without the threat of epi- demics and direct experience of so-called childhood diseases. In wealthy, industrialized nations few individuals recall the heavy toll once taken by tuberculosis, diphtheria, smallpox, measles, and polio. Moreover, many people mistakenly believe that antibiotics can cure all infectious diseases. Some observers warn that the declining status of state and city public health departments indicates that, in the absence of fear, the essential but generally routine work of such institutions is neither understood nor appreciated. As Rudolf Virchow (1821–1902), the founder of cellular pathology, warned his bacteria-hunting colleagues, simplistically attri- buting contagious diseases to bacteria "hinders further research and lulls the conscience to sleep." At the turn of the century, fear of biological ter- rorism and the threat of newly emerging diseases stimulated concerns about the ability of industrialized nations to respond to particularly viru- lent, contagious, and unfamiliar infectious diseases. According to public health experts, concern did not necessarily lead to funding and planning.

Understanding the tensions that result from changing patterns of health, disease, and demography, and the differences in patterns found in the wealthy nations and impoverished nations requires familiarity with history, geography, ecology, and economics, as well as knowledge of medicine and science. The global spread of AIDS, which has devastated villages and cities in Africa where the disease may have originated, revealed the necessity for a global and historic perspective. AIDS first appeared as a diagnostic entity in 1981 when the Centers for Disease Control began to report that strange clusters of illnesses usually associated with a severely compromised immune system were appearing in previously healthy gay men in New York and Los Angeles. In 1984, the causative agent, a retrovirus referred to as the human immunodeficiency virus (HIV), was identified. Within five years of the first reports, the United States Public Health Service estimated that more than a million Americans were infected with HIV. Further studies of HIV suggested that the virus had not simply appeared in the 1980s, but had been incubating as a silent epidemic in areas of the world where the deaths of children and young adults from fever and diarrheal diseases were not at all uncommon. Presumably, other still unrecognized diseases and pathogens remain submerged among the fevers of unknown origin (FUOs) in the developing world.

Unlike Thomas McKeown (1911–1988), the eminent social philosopher of medicine, who contended that medical intervention had little effect on mortality rates and minor consequences for morbidity, some medical historians believe that public health measures played a very significant role in the control of infectious diseases during the nineteenth century. Some critics of modern medicine have argued that the term "healthcare" is a misnomer. Many wealthy countries actually have created what should more accurately be called an "illness subeconomy" that consumes a substantial and increasing share of gross domestic product in order to deal with chronic illness. Many scholars agree that there is little evidence that therapeutic medicine affected mortality and morbidity rates. McKeown's work, summarized in *The Modern Rise of Population* (1976), challenged then prevailing assumptions about the relationship between medical practice and changing patterns of mortality and morbidity. Between 1800 and 2000, life expectancy at birth rose from about 30 years to a global average of 67 years. In the wealthy, industrialized nations, life expectancy at birth was more than 75 years. Although patterns of morbidity and mortality have undergone remarkable changes in this relatively brief period of human history, major differences in patterns of disease and life expectancy separate the wealthy nations from developing nations. Moreover, the so-called developing world accounts for about 80 percent of global population. In Africa and other parts of the developing world, over 60 percent of deaths are caused by communicable diseases. In Europe only eight percent of deaths are due to communicable diseases.

Perhaps the fears generated by AIDS will reverse the tendency of the wealthy nations to assume that the infectious diseases have been conquered and that the contagious diseases of third world countries are inconsequential. AIDS has made it clear that the most powerful chemotherapeutic agents are ultimately powerless against the onslaught of germs if the natural immunological defenses cannot participate in the battle. Expensive, complex new drug regimens have transformed AIDS from a fatal disease to a chronic disease, at least for those who can afford therapy, but the remedies themselves are not without risks and adverse effects. Of course, in much of the world old enemies, such as tuberculosis, malaria, measles, cholera, and, above all, poverty and malnutrition, have not given up their role as "million-murdering death."

Medical errors have become the subject of extensive studies and of sharp debates since the 1990s. Although the Hippocratic texts reveal an appreciation of the problem of medical errors and the fact that medical interventions frequently led to unintended adverse effects, recent critics of modern medical practice have diagnosed what they called a "terrifying epidemic of medical mistakes." In 1999, the Institute of Medicine of the National Academy of Sciences published a report entitled *To Err is Human*, which estimated that about 100,000 Americans died annually as a result of medical mistakes that occurred in hospitals, including about seven thousand deaths attributed to medication errors and adverse drug reactions. Some experts are sure that these numbers are underestimates.

Adverse drug reactions are compounded by unanticipated interactions between drugs, dietary supplements, and foods, and the probability that toxic reactions to particular drugs will not be detected until large numbers of people have taken a new drug for a significant amount of time. Pharmaceutical companies and researchers have coined a new term, theranostics (diagnostics + therapy) to suggest a strategy for combining diagnostic tests with targeted drug therapy. Diagnostic tests that could identify patients most likely to be helped or damaged by new medications would be combined with drug therapy that targets a specific gene or protein. Since the turn of the century, several such tests have been developed for use in the diagnosis and treatment of leukemia, breast cancer, colorectal cancer, and lung cancer. Skeptics note that, although "personalized medicine" is an admirable goal, drug companies are more likely to pursue drugs that treat many people than drugs that are specific to much smaller groups of patients. Advocates of theranostics argue that increased efficacy and safety would stimulate the development and approval of many more new drugs for chronic diseases and infectious diseases as well as cancers.

Despite sophisticated diagnostic imaging, there is compelling evidence that many errors occur in diagnosis, surgery, and prescriptions. A report published in 2004 found that out of some sixty-four thousand patients who had undergone appendectomies between 1987 and 1998 about 15 percent did not have appendicitis. Among the female patients in this group about 23 percent of the appendectomies were unnecessary. Researchers found that cardiologists missed evidence of significant heart disease about a third of the time. Similar errors were found in reviews of radiologists examining mammograms. Cynics say that the true extent of medical errors is impossible to measure because serious mistakes are buried with the patient, as demonstrated by studies of randomly selected autopsies. Nevertheless, biomedical scientists continue to believe that further advances in technology will provide more sophisticated and accurate diagnostic information. Skeptics insist that techniques that work in the laboratory do not necessarily work under more complex, less structured conditions.

As demonstrated in the controversy that erupted when salvarsan was used to treat syphilis, evaluating the safety and efficacy of any drug or medical innovation entails many difficulties, scientific and political. Indeed, the passage of time and rigorous statistical analyses are likely to demonstrate that various "miracle drugs" are dangerous, ineffective, or no more effective than older remedies. Worse yet, some drugs pose dangers not only to the patients for whom they were prescribed, but also for their future children, as demonstrated by the tragic cases of thalidomide and diethylstilbesterol (DES). DES, a synthetic estrogen, was widely prescribed from the 1940s to the 1970s, in the mistaken belief that it would prevent miscarriages. Not only did DES increase the risk of complications during pregnancy, it caused a rare form of cancer in DES daughters, reproductive disorders in both DES sons and daughters, and increased the risk of various cancers in women who had taken the drug.

During the 1950s, thalidomide entered the German pharmaceutical market as a remedy for insomnia, tension, and morning sickness. The drug was described as more effective and safer than barbiturates. It was so commonly used to sedate children that it was often referred to as the West German baby-sitter. By 1960, when the drug was already available in about fifty countries, members of the German Society for Pediatric Medicine were discussing a suspiciously high number of unusual birth defects. Ultimately, researchers estimated that about ten thousand children were born with abnormalities of the internal organs as well as deformities of the arms, legs, hands, and feet that were grouped together as phocomelia (from the Greek for seal + limb). Widukind Lenz (1919–1995), a pediatrician and professor at the University of Hamburg, became particularly interested in possible links between phocomelia and thalidomide. In 1961, he reported his suspicions about "a frightening increase in deformities" and suggested a link between the birth defects and a new drug.

Eventually, thalidomide was identified as a powerful teratogen (an agent that causes malformations in an embryo or fetus) and the cause of the worldwide epidemic of phocomelia. Because of the work of Frances Kathleen Oldham Kelsey (1914–), a medical officer at the Food and Drug Administration, less than 20 cases occurred in the

United States. The Pure Food and Drug Act of 1906 established the regulatory agency that became the Food and Drug Administration in order to protect consumers from dangerous foods, drugs, and cosmetics. In 1937, for example, the Masengill Company prepared a liquid form of sulfanilamide by dissolving the drug in diethylene glycol, which is a sweet, but highly toxic liquid. About 240 gallons of "sulfanilamide elixir" were distributed, without any tests for safety, and at least 107 people died. This tragedy created demands for federal regulations that would prevent the marketing of unsafe pharmaceutical products. On June 15, 1938, President Franklin D. Roosevelt signed into law the Food, Drug and Cosmetic Act.

Despite claims by the manufacturer, Richardson-Merrell Inc., that no adverse effects occurred when thalidomide was taken for insomnia, nervous tension, asthma, and relief of nausea in early pregnancy, Kelsey delayed approval of thalidomide by repeatedly requesting addition tests and information. Merrell was seeking approval of thalidomide as a sleeping aid, but Kelsey noted that the drug did not make experimental animals sleepy. Despite evidence from England that some patients taking thalidomide experienced serious effects on the nervous system that resulted in tingling, numbness, and burning in their fingers and toes, Kelsey's supervisors and the drug manufacturer exerted considerable pressure on her to expedite approval. According to a 1962 report read into the Congressional Record by Senator Estes Kefauver, Merrell continued to call for routine approval and appealed to Kelsey's superiors. Moreover, even without approval, the law at the time allowed Richardson-Merrell Inc. to enlist hundreds of American doctors to carry out "clinical trials" of thalidomide on their private patients. After the relationship between thalidomide and phocomelia became public knowledge, Merrell revoked its application and eventually withdrew the drug from experimental use. The thalidomide tragedy was one of the factors that stimulated the passage of legislation that gave the FDA additional authority to regulate the introduction of new drugs.

An experienced researcher in pharmacology when she began work at the FDA in 1960, Kelsey had earned a master's degree in pharmacology from McGill University, Montreal (1934), a Ph.D. (1938) in pharmacology, and a medical degree (1950) from the University of Chicago. While teaching at the University, she married fellow faculty member, Dr. Fremont Ellis Kelsey. The Kelseys moved to South Dakota where Frances Kelsey practiced medicine and taught pharmacology. When her husband accepted a position in Washington, DC, Kelsey was hired by the Food and Drug Administration. In 1962, after thalidomide was taken off the market by many European nations, Kelsey was lauded for preventing thalidomide birth defects in thousands of American infants. She received the Distinguished Federal Civilian Service Award from President John Fitzgerald Kennedy (1917–1963). The engraving on her presidential award reads, "Her exceptional judgment in evaluating a new drug for safety for human use has prevented a major tragedy of birth deformities in the United States. Through high ability and steadfast confidence in her professional decision she has made an outstanding contribution to the protection of the health of the American people." The *Washington Post* called Kelsey a "heroine" and praised her for the "skepticism and stubbornness" that prevented a potential American tragedy. The *New York Times* praised Kelsey for leading "a two-year battle with the makers of thalidomide." In 2000, Kelsey, who was still working in the FDA's Center for Drug Evaluation and Research, was inducted into the National Women's Hall of Fame in Seneca Falls, New York.

Germany's federal prosecutor filed a criminal indictment against the manufacturer of thalidomide in 1967. The complex and controversial trial did not end until a negotiated settlement was reached in 1970. Prosecutors agreed to drop charges against the company, and protect the company and individual defendants from future criminal or civil liability, in exchange for an agreement establishing a fund for thalidomide children. The judges explained that it was more important to improve methods of drug development in the future than to punish those associated with marketing thalidomide.

Attempts to balance the need to make drugs available with the need to prevent the adoption of drugs that are potentially dangerous remain problematic. In the 1980s, cancer and AIDS activists demanded more rapid access to new drugs. For patients with deadly diseases, they argued, the benefits of new drugs outweighed any potential risks. The problem of adverse, unexpected interactions between drugs, however, is particularly likely to affect people with severe and chronic diseases. Regulatory agencies typically cite the need for constant vigilance to prevent future thalidomide-like tragedies, while critics of the long, slow, and increasingly expensive process of drug approval insist that new life-saving remedies are held hostage by cold-hearted bureaucrats. Few are likely to remember how Frances Kelsey, serving as a bureaucrat and a "gatekeeper" prevented widespread distribution of thalidomide in the United States. Complicating the argument is the realization that even a drug like thalidomide, with its notorious reputation as a teratogenic agent, may have some value in the treatment of certain diseases, including leprosy, certain AIDS-related conditions such as painful mouth ulcers and severe body wasting, arthritis and other inflammatory disorders, Crohn's disease, multiple sclerosis, Alzheimer's disease, multiple myeloma, myelodysplastic syndrome (also known as preleukemia), and other cancers. Thalidomide seemed to block the normal development of fetal limbs by preventing angiogenesis (the growth of new blood vessels). Obstructing angiogenesis is one of the strategies that might be valuable as a treatment for certain cancers, because like fetal limbs, tumors need new blood vessels in order to grow.

Organizations representing the surviving, adult victims of thalidomide objected to attempts to rehabilitate this highly controversial, teratogenic drug. When thalidomide was licensed for use in the United States in 1998, members of the Thalidomide Victims Association of Canada (TVAC) adopted the unequivocal position that they would "never accept a world with thalidomide in it." Even the remote possibility that a drug might help victims of deadly or debilitating diseases, they warned, could lead to reckless, irresponsible, and unregulated usage, and the possibility of fetal exposure to thalidomide as well as nerve damage in adults. Rather than allowing the possibility of another generation of thalidomide victims, the Association argued for research that would lead to development of thalidomide analogs that would not have its teratogenic effects. However, the potential anticancer effects of thalidomide and its derivatives might involve the same pathways that cause phocomelia. Victims of thalidomide urged the mandatory inclusion of a picture of a thalidomide baby and other educational materials in all packages of thalidomide and the prominent use of that name along with any new trade names.

Both the idea of progress and the role of medicine become problematic when morbidity and mortality are analyzed in terms of a transition from the old epidemic, infectious diseases to diseases of affluence and diseases of medical progress, and when patients find their rising expectations for cure and comfort increasingly frustrated. Many scientists and physicians would agree with what Benjamin Franklin said in 1772: "It appears that the doctrines of life and death in general are yet but little understood." Healthcare controversies have been addressed judiciously in professional journals and the scholarly literature, and passionately in popular books, magazines, and TV talk shows. Another five hundred pages would hardly begin to address these problems, but perhaps even a bare survey of the history of medicine will provide some of the facts and concepts that every person needs to know in order to appreciate the complex relationships among disease, health, medicine, and society. The biomedical sciences are certainly entering a new era in the development of vaccines and therapeutic agents. But as always, there are no remedies without risk. Therefore, the words of the wise doctors of Salerno still provide an appropriate conclusion to any considerations of the history of medicine:

> And here I cease to write, but will not cease
>
> To wish you live in health, and die in peace;
>
> And ye our Physicke rules that friendly read,
>
> God grant that Physicke you may never need.

## SUGGESTED READINGS

Amler, R. W., and Dull, H. B., eds. (1987). *Closing the Gap: The Burden of Unnecessary Illness.* New York: Oxford University Press.

Bäumler, E. (1984). *Paul Ehrlich. Scientist for Life.* New York: Holmes and Meier.

Blaufox, M. D. (2002). *An Ear to the Chest: An Illustrated History of the Evolution of the Stethoscope.* Lancaster, U.K.: Parthenon Publishing.

Brim, O. G., Ryff, C. D., and Kessler, R. C., eds. (2004). *How Healthy Are We? A National Study of Well-Being at Midlife.* Chicago, IL: University of Chicago Press.

Burnet, F. M. (1968). *Changing Patterns: An Atypical Autobiography.* Melbourne, Australia: Heinemann.

Callahan, D. (2003). *What Price Better Health? Hazards of the Research Imperative.* Berkeley, CA: University of California Press.

Christie D. A., and Tansey E. M., eds. (2003). *Genetic Testing.* Wellcome Witnesses to Twentieth Century Medicine. Vol. 17. London: The Wellcome Trust Centre for the History of Medicine.

Clark, R. W. (1985). *The Life of Ernst Chain. Penicillin and Beyond.* New York: St. Martin's Press.

Cooke, R. (2001). *Dr. Folkman's War. Angiogenesis and the Struggle to Defeat Cancer.* New York: Random House.

Cutler, D. M. (2003). *Your Money or Your Life.* New York: Oxford University Press.

Duffin, J. (1998). *To See with a Better Eye: A Life of R. T. H. Laennec.* Princeton, NJ: Princeton University Press.

Dunnill, M. (2000). *The Plato of Praed Street: The Life and Times of Almroth Wright.* London: Royal Society of Medicine Press.

Dutton, D. B. (1988). *Worse than the Disease. Pitfalls of Medical Progress.* New York: Cambridge University Press.

Evans, J. H. (2001). *Playing God? Human Genetic Engineering and the Rationalization of Public Bioethical Debate.* Chicago, IL: University of Chicago Press.

Gordon, C. (2003). *Dead on Arrival: The Politics of Health Care in Twentieth-Century America.* Princeton, NJ: Princeton University Press.

Hilts, P. J. (2003). *Protecting America's Health. The FDA, Business, and One Hundred Years of Regulation.* New York: Alfred A. Knopf.

Hogan, N. C. (2003). *Unhealed Wounds: Medical Malpractice in the Twentieth Century.* New York: LFB Scholarly Publishing LLC.

Illich, I. (1982). *Medical Nemesis: The Expropriation of Health.* New York: Pantheon Books.

Kevles, B. H. (1998). *Naked to the Bone. Medical Imaging in the Twentieth Century.* Reading, MA: Addison-Wesley.

Kohn, L. T., Corrigan, J. M., and Donaldson, M. S., eds. (2000). *To Err is Human: Building a Safer Health System.* Washington, DC: National Academy Press.

Leichter, H. M. (1991). *Free to Be Foolish: Politics and Health Promotion in the United States and Great Britain.* Princeton, NJ: Princeton University Press.

Lerner, B. H. (2001). *The Breast Cancer Wars: Hope, Fear, and the Pursuit of a Cure in Twentieth-Century America.* New York: Oxford University Press.

Marks, H. M. (1997). *The Progress of Experiment: Science and Therapeutic Reform in the United States, 1900–1990.* New York: Cambridge University Press.

Maulitz, R. C., ed. (1988). *Unnatural Causes: The Three Leading Killer Diseases in America.* New Brunswick, NJ: Rutgers University Press.

Mazumdar, P. M. H., ed. (1989). *Immunology, 1930–1980: Essays on the History of Immunology.* Toronto: Wall & Thompson.

McKeown, T. (2003). *The Role of Medicine. Dream, Mirage, or Nemesis?* Princeton, NJ: Princeton University Press.

Medawar, P. B. (1986). *Memoirs of a Thinking Radish: An Autobiography.* Oxford: Oxford University Press.

Panem, S. (1984). *The Interferon Crusade.* Washington, DC: Brookings Institute.

Parascondola, J., ed. (1980). *The History of Antibiotics; A Symposium.* Madison, WI: American Institute of the History of Pharmacy.

Riley, J. C. (2001). *Rising Life Expectancy: A Global History.* New York: Cambridge University Press.

Sharpe, V. A., and Faden, A. I. (1998). *Medical Harm: Historical, Conceptual, and Ethical Dimensions of Iatrogenic Illness.* Cambridge: Cambridge University Press.

Silverstein, A. M. (1989). *A History of Immunology.* New York: Academic Press.

Silverstein, A. M. (2002). *Paul Ehrlich's Receptor Immunology: The Magnificent Obsession.* San Diego, CA: Academic Press.

Stephens, T. D., and Brynner, R. (2001). *Dark Remedy: The Impact of Thalidomide and Its Revival as a Vital Medicine.* Cambridge: Perseus Publishing.

Stevens, R. (1998). *American Medicine and the Public Interest. A History of Specialization.* Berkeley, CA: University of California Press.

Wachter, R. M., and Shojania, K. G. (2004). *Internal Bleeding: The Truth Behind America's Terrifying Epidemic of Medical Mistakes.* RuggedLand.

Zucker, M. B., ed. (1999). *The Right to Die Debate: A Documentary History.* Westport, CT: Greenwood Press.

# Index

591